D0782143

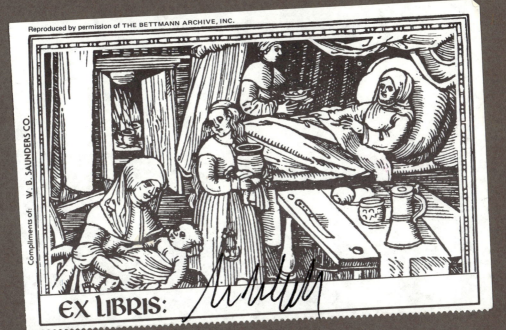

Reproduced by permission of THE BETTMANN ARCHIVE, INC.

Compliments of: W. B. SAUNDERS CO.

EX LIBRIS:

LIBRARY-LRC
TEXAS HEART INSTITUTE

The Pulmonary Circulation

The Pulmonary Circulation: Normal and Abnormal

MECHANISMS, MANAGEMENT, AND THE NATIONAL REGISTRY

ALFRED P. FISHMAN, M.D.

EDITOR

upp UNIVERSITY OF PENNSYLVANIA PRESS
PHILADELPHIA   1990

This publication is supported by a grant from the
National Institutes of Health.

Copyright © 1990 by the University of Pennsylvania Press
All rights reserved
Printed in the United States of America

Library of Congress Cataloging-in-Publication Data
The Pulmonary circulation : normal and abnormal : mechanisms, management, and
    the national registry / Alfred P. Fishman, editor.
        p.   cm.
    Includes bibliographical references.
    ISBN 0-8122-8110-1. — ISBN 0-8122-8110-1
    1. Pulmonary hypertension.   2. Pulmonary circulation.   3. Pulmonary hyper-
tension—United States.   I. Fishman, Alfred P.
    [DNLM: 1. Hypertension, Pulmonary.   2. Pulmonary Circulation.   3. Reg-
istries. WF 600 P9824]
    RC776.P87P844   1989
    616.2'4—dc20
DNLM/DLC
for Library of Congress   89-40403
                                                                               CIP

Designed by Adrianne Onderdonk Dudden

CONTENTS

Acknowledgments   xi
Introduction   xiii
ALFRED P. FISHMAN

PART ONE

THE NORMAL PULMONARY AND BRONCHIAL CIRCULATIONS

1   The Normal Pulmonary Microcirculation   3
JOAN GIL

2   Comparative Biology of the Pulmonary Circulation   17
ANTHONY P. FARRELL

3   Excitation and Contraction in Smooth Muscle   31
ANDREW P. SOMLYO
AVRIL V. SOMLYO

4   Pulmonary Vascular Resistance (P:$\dot{Q}$ Relations)   41
JOHN H. LINEHAN
CHRISTOPHER A. DAWSON

5   Endothelial and Smooth Muscle Cell Interaction   57
JOHN N. EVANS
JANICE T. COFLESKY

6   Endothelial Processing of Biologically Active Materials   69
UNA S. RYAN

7   Endothelin: Mediator of Hypoxic Vasoconstriction?   85
MICHAEL I. KOTLIKOFF
ALFRED P. FISHMAN

8   Mediators in the Pulmonary Circulation   91
KENNETH L. BRIGHAM

9   The Enigma of Hypoxic Pulmonary Vasoconstriction   109
ALFRED P. FISHMAN

10   Central Neural Regulation of the Pulmonary Circulation   131
WALKER A. LONG
D. LESLIE BROWN

11   Bronchial Circulation   151
MICHAEL MAGNO

12   Tone and Responsiveness in the Fetal and Neonatal Pulmonary Circulation   161
SIDNEY CASSIN

PART TWO

VASCULAR INJURY

13   Endothelial Injury Studied in Cell Culture   173
ALICE R. JOHNSON

14   Inhibition of Proliferation of Vascular Smooth Muscle Cells by Heparin   187
WILLIAM E. BENITZ

15   Role of Growth Factors in Pulmonary Hypertension   201
STEVEN M. ALBELDA

16   Oxygen Radicals and Vascular Injury   217
SUSAN L. LINDSAY
BRUCE A. FREEMAN

17   Endothelial Cell Modulation of Coagulation and Fibrinolysis   231
KATHERINE A. HAJJAR
RALPH L. NACHMAN

18   Atherogenesis in the Pulmonary Artery   245
ROBERT W. WISSLER
DRAGOSLAVA VESSELINOVITCH

PART THREE

PULMONARY HYPERTENSION

19 Vascular Remodeling   259
LYNNE M. REID

20 Chronic Hypoxic Pulmonary Hypertension   283
ROBERT F. GROVER

21 Familial Pulmonary Hypertension   301
JOHN H. NEWMAN
JAMES E. LOYD

22 Animal Models of Chronic Pulmonary Hypertension   315
JOHN T. REEVES
ANDREW J. PEACOCK
KURT R. STENMARK

23 The Pathology of Secondary Pulmonary Hypertension   329
WILLIAM D. EDWARDS

24 Pulmonary Veno-Occlusive Disease   343
C.A. WAGENVOORT

25 Pulmonary Hypertension in Collagen Vascular Disease   353
BRUCE H. BRUNDAGE

26 Pulmonary Hypertension Associated with Hepatic Cirrhosis   359
BERTRON M. GROVES   JANET KERNIS
BRUCE H. BRUNDAGE   DAVID R. DANTZKER
C. GREGORY ELLIOTT   ALFRED P. FISHMAN
SPENCER K. KOERNER   KENNETH M. MOSER
JEFFREY D. FISHER   DANIEL A. PIETRO
ROBERT H. PETER   JOHN T. REEVES
STUART RICH   SHARON I.S. ROUNDS

27 Persistent Pulmonary Hypertension of the Newborn   371
MICHAEL A. HEYMANN
SCOTT J. SOIFER

28 Pulmonary Hypertension in the Toxic Oil Syndrome   385
JOSE LÓPEZ-SENDÓN
MIGUEL A. GOMEZ SANCHEZ
MARÍA JOSÉ MESTRE DE JUAN
ISABEL COMA-CANELLA

29   Aminorex Pulmonary Hypertension   397

HANS PETER GURTNER

30   Thromboembolic Pulmonary Hypertension   413

KENNETH M. MOSER

PART FOUR

THE PRIMARY PULMONARY HYPERTENSION REGISTRY

31   Introduction to the National Registry on Primary Pulmonary Hypertension   437

ALFRED P. FISHMAN

32   The Research and Clinical Dilemmas Encountered by the Primary Pulmonary Hypertension Registry   441

EDWARD H. BERGOFSKY
CAROL E. VREIM

33   NIH Registry on Primary Pulmonary Hypertension: Baseline Characteristics of the Patients Enrolled   451

STUART RICH

34   The Histopathology of Primary Pulmonary Hypertension   459

GIUSEPPE G. PIETRA

35   Mortality Follow-Up of Primary Pulmonary Hypertension   473

PAUL S. LEVY
STUART RICH
JANET KERNIS

PART FIVE

TREATMENT OF PULMONARY HYPERTENSION

36   Vasodilator Therapy (General Aspects)   479

LEWIS J. RUBIN

37   Acute Vasodilator Testing and Pharmacological Treatment of Primary Pulmonary Hypertension   485

E. KENNETH WEIR

38 Anticoagulation in the Treatment of Pulmonary Hypertension   501

MARC COHEN
VALENTIN FUSTER
WILLIAM D. EDWARDS

39 The Criteria and Preparation for Heart-Lung Transplantation   511

TIM W. HIGENBOTTAM

Contributors   523
Index   529

ACKNOWLEDGMENTS

Financial support for this book and the international conference that preceded it—at which the results of the National Registry on Primary Pulmonary Hypertension were presented—was provided by the Division of Lung Diseases, Heart, Lung, and Blood Institute of the National Institutes of Health and by an educational grant from the Burroughs Wellcome Co. Dr. Carol Vreim of the National Heart, Lung, and Blood Institute played a key role both in the Registry and in the conference. Dr. Walker Long was instrumental in arranging for the support from the Burroughs Wellcome Co.

INTRODUCTION

Starting in 1981, thirty-five medical centers participated in a nationwide registry designed to collect, collate and analyze data on unexplained ("primary") pulmonary hypertension. The participants saw in this shared experience an opportunity to gain a better understanding of this rare disease and to replace empiricism by science in its management. To accomplish this goal, a steering committee established criteria for inclusion and exclusion and set up specific mechanisms for collecting data in a systematic and standardized way. The advent of pulmonary vasodilator therapy heralded by a rash of case reports further spurred efforts to obtain a firmer grasp of the natural history of the disease and the effects of a variety of touted agents in positively modifying its course.

At the time that the Registry began, it was not clear if primary pulmonary hypertension was more than a clinical syndrome. Suspicion was high that a variety of arcane etiologies could end in pulmonary hypertension for which no cause could be identified at autopsy or by biopsy. Bruited about were putative roles for diet, genetics, thromboembolism, and connective tissue diseases as initiating mechanisms. Confidence in reports of remarkable success using a particular vasodilator agent was shaken by ambiguities in defining a beneficial response and almost invariably rocked by contradictory accounts of either failure or complications using the same agent.

Prompted at least in part by this nationwide effort to get a firmer hold on the clinical entity of primary pulmonary hypertension, interest rekindled in the mechanisms responsible for occlusive pulmonary vascular disease and in the regulation of the pulmonary circulation, normal as well as abnormal. Discoveries in relevant fields, notably in cellular physiology, fueled this renaissance. Fresh insights into cell-cell communication focused attention on the interplay between endothelium and the underlying smooth muscle in effecting a vasomotor response. Heparin proved to exert an inhibitory influence on vascular smooth muscle, suggesting fresh approaches to preventing medial hypertrophy. Improved understanding of local mediators, interplay between blood and endothelium, and mechanisms involved in coagulation led to the replacement of the idea of "multiple pulmonary emboli" by the idea of pulmonary hypertension arising from widespread thrombosis in small pulmonary arteries.

To mark the end of the Registry, a conference was convened in Philadelphia in 1987 under the auspices of the National Heart, Lung, and Blood Institute and of the Burroughs Wellcome Co. The purpose of the Conference was to synthesize current understanding of the pulmonary circulation with particular respect to the development, prevention, and reversal of pulmonary vascular occlusive disease. Investigators from this country and abroad presented results, compared data, and shared experiences. It was evident by the end of the Conference that the past 5 to 6 years had considerably reoriented thinking about the control of the pulmonary circulation and the pathogenesis of primary pulmonary hypertension.

This book was triggered by the Conference but by no means is it a transcript or a recapitulation. Instead, those who seemed to have most to contribute were invited to summarize some aspect of the normal or abnormal pulmonary circulation relating to pulmonary hypertension. Each chapter was edited, drawings were often refashioned, and a serious effort was made to provide a cohesive account. To cap it all off, the book closes with brief summaries of the findings of the National Registry. The end result should be viewed as a perspective of the current understanding of the control of the normal and abnormal pulmonary circulation and a presentation of the leading edges of research that bears on the problem of pulmonary hypertension in general and of primary pulmonary hypertension in particular.

It is fitting to acknowledge those who made possible both the update provided by the meeting and the publication of this book. Dr. Carol Vreim played a critical role in organizing the National Registry; and the National Heart, Lung, and Blood Institute and the Burroughs Wellcome Co., with Dr. Walker Long as intermediary, provided financial support for the meeting and its publication.

At the home front, a considerable part of the editorial responsibility fell to Suzanne Markloff who was involved in shaping the book from beginning to end. Betsy Ann Bozzarello helped to streamline the activities of the Editor to make time available for the processing of the manuscripts. And, last but not least, my wife and daughter, Linda and Hannah, helped to create a setting and a frame of mind that made it possible to bring to fruition this large undertaking.

Alfred P. Fishman
Philadelphia

PART ONE

The Normal Pulmonary and Bronchial Circulations

Joan Gil, M.D.

1

The Normal Pulmonary Microcirculation

STATIC ANATOMY OF THE PULMONARY CIRCULATION

The main purpose of this chapter is to review the structure of the capillary network in the gas exchanging area, i.e., in the alveolar walls. Nevertheless, neither the anatomy nor the function of the pulmonary capillaries can be fully understood without a brief consideration of the conducting arteries and veins and some mention of the interrelations between the pulmonary and the bronchial and pleural circulations.

Several major functional differences between the systemic and pulmonary circulations deserve special mention within the context of this work: (1) the site of flow resistance in the pulmonary vessels resides in the alveolar capillaries; this has been established both by experimental data (1,31) and by computer analysis based on morphometric data (6,41,43); (2) intracapillary pressures are highly variable depending on the location of the capillary probed; the question of whether pressure is also variable inside the same capillary is still wide open; (3) the bronchial and pleural systemic beds drain, in part, into alveolar capillaries after a complex anastomotic pattern (21,35,37); these communications constitute the anatomic basis of a shunt.

With regard to the pathophysiology of the common forms of pulmonary hypertension, it is important to stress that the early structural changes (extension of smooth muscle into peripheral small arteries, medial hypertrophy, intimal fibroelastosis) (28,29,30) are observed in arteries which normally contribute little to the generation of resistance to perfusion. This raises a complex dilemma whenever we attempt to interpret these anatomic changes in conducting vessels as representing the cause or the effect of increased pressure.

Conducting Blood Vessels

It is not within the scope of the present article to describe conducting blood vessels in detail as others have done (21,22,35,38). The progress made in morphometry of both the arterial and venous trees was rendered possible by the introduction of the Strahler ordering system to classify data. In humans, most of our knowledge derives from the painstaking efforts of Horsfield (23,24,32). In cats, the laboratory of Fung (41,43) has reported complete morphometric data of the whole vascular tree. The following characteristics may have functional significance:

1. A comparison of the arterial tree with the bronchial tree reveals that there are many more arteries than airways. This is because of the existence of supernumerary arteries which, unlike the axial arteries, do not follow the bronchus but instead penetrate the lung parenchyma immediately after branching.
2. The literature on pulmonary mechanics stresses the significance of the tethering by alveolar septa around small bronchioles to help in keeping them open. This is equally important for blood vessels. After reaching a certain diameter, arteries loose their muscular media, and their most peripheral branches consist only of an endothelial lining and an internal elastica

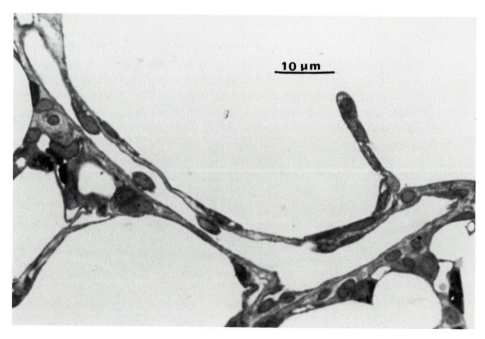

Figure 1: Rabbit lung fixed by vascular perfusion showing small peripheral arteriole without muscle. Note location of the artery and tethering by secondary alveolar speta.

(Figs. 1 and 2). The wall of pulmonary veins is also very thin as compared to systemic veins of the same diameter. They are surrounded by subatmospheric pressure related to the continuity of their adventitial connective tissue sheath with the mediastinum and/or visceral pleura and are subjected to radial pull by alveolar septa which results in increase of their diameter with inflation (3,25). A reduction in the pull of the type that occurs in obstructive airways disease may cause reduction in the diameter of the arteries and veins serving the area of the lesion, thereby contributing to a local reduction in perfusion. In fact, many of the local changes in conducting vessels in human pulmonary pathology are unexplained.

The Hexagonal Network of the Alveolar Wall

OVERALL APPEARANCE

In electron microscopy, a pulmonary capillary does not differ much from a systemic counterpart. It is not fenestrated and its most striking feature may well be the extreme cytoplasmic attenuation visible near the cellular junction, lined by smooth cellular membranes, too thin to host any of the membrane vesicles abundant in other cytoplasmic areas (13). Whether plasmalemmal vesicles can act as transcellular transport shuttles has been the subject of heated controversies (2,8,14); the alternative is that they represent fixed membranous differentiations ("caveolae") and that some of them, by fusing, create permanent or transient racemose transcellular channels (34). Surprisingly, this controversy has not

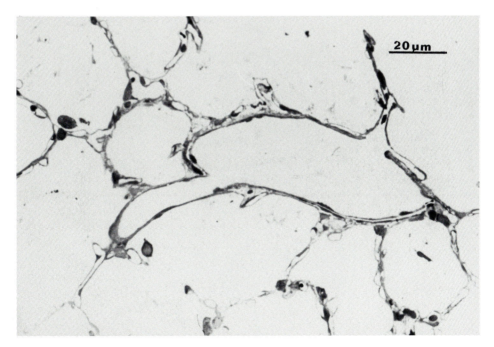

Figure 2: Rabbit lung fixed by vascular perfusion. Conducting vessel shown branching and giving off tiny branches that penetrate alveolar corners.

been extended to the squamous alveolar epithelium which offers striking similarities (13).

The organization of the capillary networks is strikingly different in the systemic and pulmonary circulations. The most common pattern of capillarization in the systemic circulation involves breakdown of the terminal arterioles in a pattern somehow comparable to a spreading brush of evenly spaced capillaries, which later reunite on the venous side to form a venule. Despite the frequency of irregularities and anastomoses, in general, some anatomic connection can be recognized between an individual capillary and an arteriole of origin. This is markedly different in the lung. Our source of knowledge of the unique characteristics of the alveolar network stems from Weibel's seminal book on lung morphometry (38): he viewed the capillaries in the alveolar wall as forming an hexagonal, very dense network, fed and drained in places by the conducting vessels. Attempts to define capillary domains of single pulmonary arteries are controversial and not universally accepted. To overcome the irregularities of biological variability and make biophysical analysis feasible, some modelling is needed. This involves a major intellectual contribution, as a model stresses functionally significant properties and underplays others.

For Weibel, the recognizable pattern was a hexagonal network of short, cylindrical tubes, modified at their bases in the form of wedges to allow for a junction with two adjacent segments. He published data and scattergrams for diameter (6.1–9.6 μm) and length (9–13 μm) of individual capillaries and estimates on their total numbers in terms of what contemporary literature would call a "capillary load," i.e., number of capillaries per unit of alveolar epithelial surface area (118E4–237E4/cm^2). Although these dimensions did not account for recruitment and derecruitment or for functional changes in diameter (which were not known to occur at the time) and although these data were later replaced by more rele-

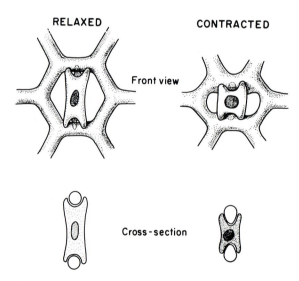

Figure 3: Drawing showing relative positions of the hexagonal capillary network and the contractile myofibroblast in the center of the hexagons. The main effect of cell contraction would be a deformation of the hexagon and possibly of the capillary lumen.

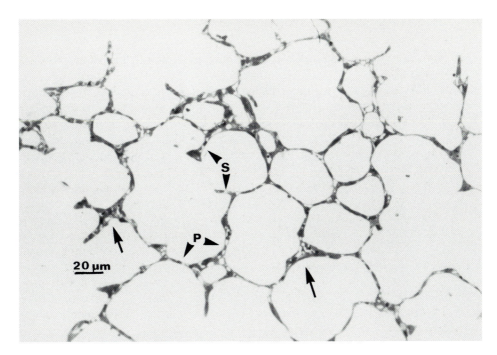

Figure 4: Rabbit lung fixed under zone 2 conditions. Note smoothness of alveolar spaces and corner pleats (arrows). Capillaries of some septal areas are fully open and others are fully closed. Note difference between primary (P) and secondary (S) alveolar walls. Primary septa are between different ducts, secondary between alveoli of the same duct.

vant parameters obtained at the electron microscopy level (such as luminal volume, endothelial volume, or endothelial surface area) (7,42), this quantitative description and the underlying notion of the hexagonal network provided for the first time a basis to approach what had looked like an untreatable problem. More recently, Fung and Sobin (4,5) emphasized a fundamental difference between pulmonary and systemic capillaries: the capillary segments, even if they are tubular as in Weibel's model, are not long enough to allow for the development of Poiseuillian flow; entry and exit conditions prevail throughout the entire network, and flow cannot be calculated using the formulas for tubular flow.

As an alternative, they proposed to regard the alveolar network as a flat sheet bound on both sides by a tissue membrane frequently interrupted by so-called posts (which they compared to the concrete pillars of a parking garage); in Weibel's model, these posts would be the equivalent of the central space of the hexagons (Fig. 3). Much has been made of the difference between the two approaches when, in fact, there is little. These are simply two conceptual simplifications (models) of the same structural reality. The value of the sheet model resides in the formulas that it makes possible to apply. As for the details contrasting the hexagonal and sheet flow models, such as capillary perimeter, it can easily be shown that they vary depending on the set of pressures (zonal conditions) under which they were preserved (10,15).

THE CAPILLARY NETWORK INSIDE THE ALVEOLAR WALL

The capillary network occupies most of the alveolar septum. Evidently, capillary anatomy is closely related to the spatial arrangement of the septa. As we pointed out earlier (10,13), the most evident implication is that since alveolar walls can be subdivided into two types which we call "primary" (at the bottom of the alveoli separating two different ducts) and "secondary" (the lateral walls which separate alveoli open to the same duct) (Fig. 4), and since secondary walls are perpendicular to the primary walls, are relatively short and cannot be erased, sections of the capillary networks can also be subdivided into primary and secondary. The existence of capillary networks perpendicular to each other was noted in Weibel's *Morphometry of the Human Lung* (38) but has not been the object of functional analyses. The differences between primary and secondary walls and their capillaries are obvious: primary walls are constant, secondary walls are irregularly developed; pores of Kohn, to be of any significance, must be located in the primary wall, and arteries and veins feed or drain only capillaries in the primary walls. We interpreted secondary wall capillaries as collaterals (10) outside of the preferential paths located in the primary wall. Based on the observation (see later) that, under zone 2 conditions, secondary walls are the most frequently wholly "derecruited" (i.e., that all their capillaries are simultaneously closed), we speculated that they might be compared to a fountain receiving the blood injection centrally at its insertion basis and draining back peripherally toward the primary walls. Alternatively, if the secondary walls were well developed and of homogeneous height, one could envision a flow of blood inside their capillaries parallel to the primary septum and in the axial direction. This situation would be difficult to analyze because of the confluence of two walls into one which would require merger of two separate capillary networks and probably result in a major turbulence and flow impairment. But, we know of no studies aimed at clarifying this situation.

CONTRACTILE CELLS IN THE ALVEOLAR INTERSTITIUM

The alveolar interstitium that surrounds capillaries differs markedly from the extra-alveolar connective tissue sheaths in several respects (12,13,17): since it is not distensible, it allows the accumulation of only small pockets of fluid which contain few interstitial cells, including fibroblasts and myofibroblasts in the space between neighboring capillaries. It was Kapanci (26) who first pointed out the existence of contractile filaments in these interstitial cells and suggested that they may play a role in flow regulation. While this is an appealing hypothesis, a precise model is needed to understand how this is possible. Figure 3 shows our view of how their contraction might produce a localized deformation of the hexagonal network, conceivably leading to fold formation capable of directing flow or closing capillary domains. We must stress the extraordinary difficulty in setting up experiments to check this theory, which presumes some kind of alignment between the axis of the cell and the septum.

FUNCTIONAL ASPECTS

Recruitment and Derecruitment of Capillaries

With an endothelial surface of about 120 m² on the average, the size of the capillary bed in the human lung is impressive by any standards (7,42). But, since the effectiveness of gas transfer is far below maximal expectations because of ventilation-perfusion irregularities, it is reasonable to question the extent to which the enormous bed is utilized. Moreover, it can be questioned if differences in capillary configuration or condition contribute to the unevenness in perfusion. No major fixed differences in structure are apparent in micrographs of the lung fixed by routine techniques. Therefore, we must consider functional differences.

There is a great methodological difficulty in studying dynamic, unstable alveolar morphology because its configuration changes with the prevailing pressure conditions. However, this can be done in the air-filled lung either by rapid freezing (27,40) or by vascular perfusion (9,15). An analysis of the matter requires fixation following a defined mechanical history and with well-defined air pressure, arterial inflow pressure, and left atrial pressure. Using rapid freezing, West and his colleagues (20,36) showed the variable degrees of filling of the wall capillaries in patches and that, under certain conditions, flow is restricted to capillaries located in alveolar corners. In our laboratory, perfusion-fixation techniques, originally introduced in order to study the morphology of alveolar surfactant (9) and changes in airway configuration related to respiratory movements (15,19), proved to be powerful tools for the study of capillary configurations. We found by proper adjustment of transmural pressures that certain generalizations could be made about capillary configurations: (1) the diameter of the capillaries is variable and can be related to the arterial pressure, an observation also reported by Fung and Sobin (4,5); (2) segments or patches of the capillary bed can be completely closed (derecruited); (3) open capillaries are often confined to alveolar corners, often inside pleats; and (4) when open capillaries are located in the septum away from corners, they tend to be flattened, conceivably due to surface tension forces (see below).

Folds and Pleatings of the Alveolar Wall

The events inside the alveolus during the respiratory movements have always been the object of considerable curiosity, but few authors have discussed the parallelism and interdependence between the alveolar wall and the capillary network that makes up most of it. It has been suggested that intra-alveolar surface tension has the effect of evening out capillaries, causing them to change in profile from round to slitlike (11,33). Studies of lungs fixed by vascular perfusion or rapid freezing have consistently revealed smooth alveolar surfaces, epithelial folds dwelling deeply in the endothelium and capillary lumen, and finally pleats—foldings involving the entire wall at septal junctions which cause the reversible formation of a bundle of capillaries in alveolar corners (15,19). These are contained within a space surrounded by smoothly curved tissue surfaces which protect the capillaries located inside against air pressure (Figs. 5 and 6).

The functional implications of these configurations are considerable. It has

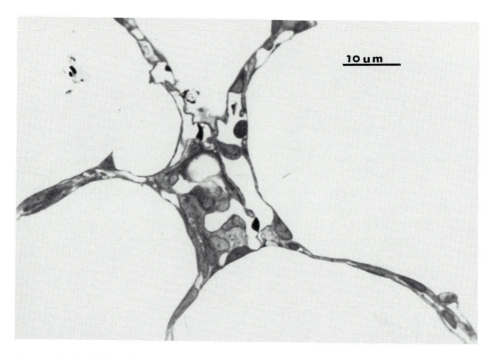

Figure 5: Rabbit lung fixed by vascular perfusion. Septal pleat surrounded by secondary walls. (Two of them show open capillaries, three closed.)

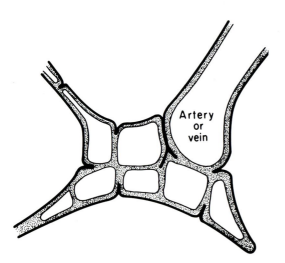

Figure 6: Rendition of reversible septal pleat connected to conducting vessels and containing a bundle of capillaries. These corner capillaries represent a shortcut between arteries and veins and are always protected against high alveolar pressures. From here, the flow may extend into neighboring areas. The non-sectional profile of corner capillaries is circular.

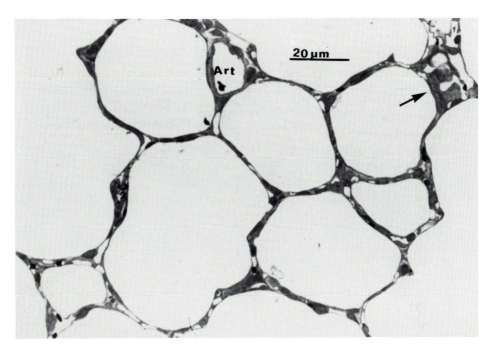

Figure 7: Rabbit lung fixed by vascular perfusion under zone 2 conditions. Note smoothness of walls, slitlike capillary lumen in the septa, completely derecruited areas, and septal pleat with corner capillaries. Art = artery.

been known for years that high intra-alveolar air pressure, e.g., during cough, squeezes blood out of wall capillaries, shifting the blood into extra-alveolar arteries and veins (3,25). To guarantee the continuous flow of blood from the right to the left ventricle, it is important to have capillary areas that cannot be shut off by temporary increases of intra-alveolar air pressures; this seems to be the function accomplished by corner vessels inside septal pleats. Corner vessels might be regarded as protective formations against rising air pressures. This function is important under zone 1 and 2 conditions (see below); to be effective, this function requires that corner vessels constitute a shortcut between the arterial and venous vessels.

ARTERIOVENOUS SHORTCUTS

As mentioned in the previous section, one striking observation is that corner capillaries are always wide open and have round transversal profiles, which is not necessarily true of the rest of the alveolar capillaries in the zone 2 lung (Figs. 4 and 7). We performed serial reconstructions of well-fixed areas which would include a whole septal pleat from the beginning to its end (18). Our observations made in lungs fixed in zone 2 were conclusive: when sectioning deeper toward the bottom of an alveolus, at some point all capillaries surrounding the narrow lumen appear open as the bottom of the structure is approached; the bottom is found to be made up by a septal pleat and the lumen of the airspace disappears blindly inside the pleat.

Sectioning beyond the pleat discloses an opposite arrangement: an air-filled lumen appears within the pleat which continues for a short distance into a widening funnel-like structure surrounded by fully opened capillaries; this funnel eventually blends into the usual parenchymal image. The arrangement is so predictable that a generally reliable way of anticipating a pleat in the nearest serial sections is to follow a narrow airspace completely surrounded by open capillaries.

But another observation was of even greater interest: the pleats are always connected to two conducting blood vessels that approach them through interstitial spaces (Figs. 1 and 2). Sometimes, one single pleat is fed and drained by an artery and a vein; other times, a continuity can be observed between several corner pleats, and the arterial and venous connections may be placed at different pleats. This allows the following interpretation: in the zone 1 and 2 lungs, the pleats develop by folding of alveolar septa at the bottom of air spaces ("alveoli") and bridge a conducting small artery and a vein. The conducting vessels are protected against collapse because of their interstitial location and tethering by alveolar septa; the corner vessels are protected by curvatures surrounding the whole pleat. We do not know how to estimate flow resistance in the capillaries located within the pleat. However, we do know that in the kidney, the glomerular tuft offers very little resistance to flow and we suspect that to be true here too. Therefore, this arrangement is optimal to guarantee patency of the arteriovenous communication regardless of alveolar pressure.

We envision perfusion of the rest of the alveolar area as a form of pressure-related overflow: if transmural pressures permit, blood flow, which is guaranteed to occur only in corners, penetrates into the alveolar wall and penetrates deeply toward alveolar mouths. Although we know of no morphological way of further

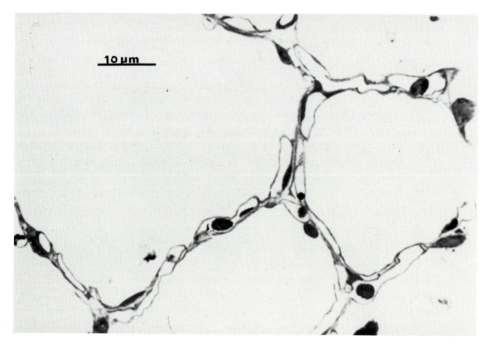

Figure 8: Rabbit lung fixed under zone 3 conditions. Note that all capillaries are open and bulging, no pleats are seen, and the alveolar surface is undulating.

examining the matter, it is evident that this scheme requires flow in two directions. Of great significance, but difficult to interpret, is the fact that under zone 2 entire lateral walls are either completely open or closed, suggesting some kind of dam or functional barrier. (See above section on interstitial contractile cells and Fig. 3). Fung and Yen have offered a hemodynamic analysis of the closure of capillaries (6).

ZONAL PERFUSION MODELS: A SUMMARY

The most important conclusion of our description of the extensive alveolar capillary network is that, in vivo, its configuration, degree of perfusion, and dimensions are highly variable depending on the prevailing arterial, venous, and air pressures. We have performed fixations of rabbit lungs by vascular perfusion under the following conditions:

Zone 1: where air pressure exceeds both the arterial and venous pressures

Zone 2: where air pressure is lower than the arterial pressure but higher than the venous pressure (the situation prevailing in patients on a respirator)

Zone 3: where both arterial and venous pressures exceed the air pressure (the situation prevailing most of the time in the healthy human lung).

Zone 3 resembles the conventionally described static morphology of the alveolar wall (Figs. 2 and 8): all capillaries are open, their cross sections have rounded or oval profiles, the alveolar wall is undulated, and alveolar corner pleats are conspicuously missing. To the extent that alveolar morphology at the septal level results from the interaction between surface tension forces and transmural pressure, it can be concluded that the vascular engorgement confers stiffness to the capillary network and eliminates or prevents pleat formation or total alveolar wall smoothness.

Zone 2 is remarkable for the following (Figs. 1, 4, and 7):

1. Existence of septal pleats containing bundles of circumferential open capillaries and bound by smooth curved surfaces.
2. Existence of alveolar walls with open capillaries and alveolar walls with patches of completely closed capillaries (Fig. 4). Admixture of opened and closed capillaries in the same wall is uncommon.
3. Alveolar walls are flat, possibly due to surface tension effects, and the lumen of capillaries away from corners in perfused walls, due to the above, is slitlike.

Zone 1 (no micrograph shown) represents a variation of zone 2, generally less regular and definable, remarkable mostly for relatively larger corner vessels under the pleats or even in unpleated corners, probably representing dilated capillaries or one-channel shortcuts between arteries and veins and many more completely collapsed wall capillaries than under zone 2.

Figure 9 summarizes the findings of Figures 4, 7, and 8. We envision zones 1 and 2 as a continuum: in the high zone 1, only corners are open (Fig. 9A) and all septal capillaries are closed; in zone 2, corners and many septal capillaries are

PREFERENTIAL PATHS AND
LEVELS OF PERFUSION

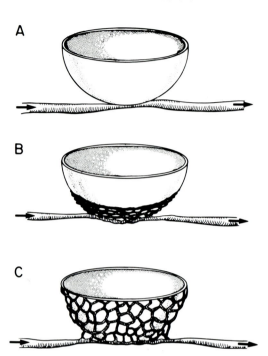

Figure 9: Rendition of the functional situation encountered in zones 1 (A), 2 (B), and 3 (C). The model stresses the observation that circulation through the corners located at the bottom of alveoli is always possible even when alveolar air pressures are high. In A, flow takes place mostly through single, dilated capillaries (conceivably placed in the shortest line between an artery and the nearest vein); in B, more flow takes place inside the pleats with occasional perfusion of portions of the wall emanating out of the corners; in C, the whole parenchyma is being perfused; blood must be flowing in two directions.

open (Fig. 9B); zone 3 differs qualitatively in that there are no corner vessels and the septal wall is no longer flat. Among the issues raised by morphological studies but outside of the experimental possibilities of this methodology is the flow velocity. Since zones 1 and 2 exhibit a markedly reduced cross-sectional capillary luminal area, one would have to assume an increased flow velocity if the right ventricular output stays the same during the existence of high alveolar air pressure.

Lung in a Respirator

Another situation of great practical significance in which corner pleats feature prominently is when the lungs are connected to a positive end-expiratory pressure (PEEP) respirator. The anatomic configuration can be expected to be similar to that existing in rodent lungs fixed by vascular perfusion under zone 2 conditions (described above). The corner vessels present under these conditions are capable of withstanding high air pressures without closing and, by virtue of its location between an artery and a vein, ensure the continuity of blood flow. It must also be noted that capillaries on one side are lined by thin portions of the air blood barrier which have a high capacitance for local gas exchange (Figs. 5 and 6). Flow velocity inside the capillary tufts would be high if substantial parts of the capillary bed are closed. Diffusion capacity in these areas would also be high and limited only by flow velocity. We regard the formation of corner pleats as a true beneficial anatomic factor in facilitating gas exchange.

ACKNOWLEDGMENTS

The author was supported by National Heart, Lung, and Blood Institute Grant No. 34196. The author is indebted to Diana Cira, D.V.M., for her devoted help in the performance of the experiments and in the preparation of the manuscript. Also, the author thanks Mrs. Marva Barbee for her outstanding secretarial assistance.

REFERENCES

1. Bhattacharya J, Staub NC: Direct measurement of microvascular pressures in the isolated perfused dog lung. Science 210:327–328, 1980.

2. Bundgaard M: Vesicular transport in capillary endothelium: Does it occur? Fed Proc 42:2425–2430, 1983.

3. Culver BH, Butler J: Mechanical influences on the pulmonary microcirculation. Annu Rev Physiol 42:187–198, 1980.

4. Fung YC, Sobin SS: Theory of sheet flow in lung alveoli. J Appl Physiol 26:472–488, 1969.

5. Fung YC, Sobin SS: Pulmonary alveolar blood flow, in JB West (ed), *Bioengineering Aspects of the Lung.* New York, Marcel Dekker, 1977, pp 267–359.

6. Fung YC, Yen RT: A new theory of pulmonary blood flow in zone 2 condition. J Appl Physiol 60:1638–1650, 1986.

7. Gehr P, Bachofen M, Weibel ER: The normal lung: Ultrastructure and morphometric estimation of diffusing capacity. Respir Physiol 32:121–140, 1978.

8. Ghitescu L, Fixman A, Simionescu M, Simionescu N: Specific binding sites for albumin restricted to plasmalemmal vesicles of continuous capillary endothelium. Receptor-mediated transcytosis. J Cell Biol 102:1304–1311, 1986.

9. Gil J: Preservation of tissues for electron microscopy under physiological criteria, in D Glick, RM Rosenbaum (eds), *Techniques of Biochemical and Biophysical Morphology*, Vol 3. New York, Wiley Interscience, 1977, pp 19–44.

10. Gil J: Morphologic aspects of alveolar microcirculation. Fed Proc 37:2462–2465, 1978.

11. Gil J: Influence of surface forces on pulmonary circulation, in AP Fishman (ed), *Pulmonary Edema.* Bethesda, American Physiological Society, 1979, pp 53–64.

12. Gil J: Organization of microcirculation in the lung. Annu Rev Physiol 42:177–186, 1980.

13. Gil J: Alveolar wall relations. Ann NY Acad Sci 384:31–43, 1982.

14. Gil J: Number and distribution of plasmalemmal vesicles in the lung. Fed Proc 42:2414–2418, 1983.

15. Gil J, Bachofen H, Gehr P, Weibel ER: Alveolar volume-to-surface area relationship in air- and saline-filled lungs fixed by vascular perfusion. J Appl Physiol 47:990–1001, 1979.

16. Gil J, Martinez-Hernandez A: The connective tissue of the rat lung: electron immunohistochemical studies. J Histochem Cytochem 32:230–238, 1984.

17. Gil J, McNiff JM: Interstitial cells at the boundary between alveolar and extraalveolar connective tissue in the lung. J Ultrastruct Res 76:149–157, 1981.

18. Gil J, Tsai YH: Reconstruction of alveolar capillary networks in lungs perfused with osmium in Zone II. Physiologist 28:371A, 1985.

19. Gil J, Weibel ER: Morphological study of pressure volume hysteresis in rat lungs fixed by vascular perfusion. Respir Physiol 15:190–213, 1972.

20. Glazier JB, Hughes JMB, Maloney JE, West

JB: Measurements of capillary dimensions and blood volume in rapidly frozen lungs. J Appl Physiol 26:65–76, 1969.

21. Harris P, Heath D: *The Human Pulmonary Circulation. Its Form and Function in Health and Disease, 3rd ed.* Edinburgh, Churchill Livingstone, 1986.

22. Hislop A, Reid L: Formation of the pulmonary vasculature, in WA Hodson (ed), *Development of the Lung.* New York, Marcel Dekker, 1977, pp 37–86.

23. Horsfield K: Some mathematical properties of branching trees with application to the respiratory system. Bull Math Biol 38:305–315, 1976.

24. Horsfield K: Morphometry of the small pulmonary arteries in man. Circ Res 42:593–597, 1978.

25. Howell JBL, Permutt J, Proctor DF, Riley RL: Effect of inflation of the lung on different parts of the pulmonary vascular bed. J Appl Physiol 16:71–76, 1961.

26. Kapanci Y, Assimacopoulos A, Irle C, Zwahlen A, Gabbiani G: "Contractile interstitial cells" in pulmonary alveolar septa: A possible regulator of ventilation/perfusion ratio? J Cell Biol 60:375–392, 1974.

27. Mazzone RW, Durand CM, West JB: Electron microscopy of lung rapidly frozen under controlled physiological conditions. J Appl Physiol 45:325–335, 1978.

28. Meyrick B, Clarke SW, Symons C, Woodgate DJ, Reid L: Primary pulmonary hypertension: A case report including electron microscopic study. Br J Dis Chest 68:11–20, 1974.

29. Meyrick B, Reid L: Development of pulmonary arterial changes in rats fed *Crotalaria spectabilis.* Am J Pathol 94:37–51, 1979.

30. Meyrick B, Reid L: Pulmonary hypertension. Anatomic and physiologic correlates. Clin Chest Med 4:199–217, 1983.

31. Nagasaka Y, Bhattacharya J, Nanjo S, Gropper MA, Staub NC: Micropuncture measurement of lung microvascular pressure profile during hypoxia in cats. Circ Res 54:90–95, 1984.

32. Singhal S, Henderson R, Horsfield K, Harding K, Cumming G: Morphometry of the human pulmonary arterial tree. Circ Res 33:190–197, 1973.

33. Staub NC: Effects of alveolar surface tension on the pulmonary vascular bed. Jap Heart J 7:386–399, 1966.

34. Taylor AE, Granger DN: Exchange of macromolecules across the microcirculation, in Renkin EM, Michel CC (eds), *Handbook of Physiology. Sect 2: The Cardiovascular System Circulation, VOL IV: Microcirculation I.* Bethesda, MD, American Physiological Society, 1984, pp 467–520.

35. Von Hayek H: *The Human Lung,* transl by VE Krahl. New York, Hafner, 1960.

36. Warrell DA, Evans JW, Clarke RO, Kingaby GP, West JB: Pattern of filling in the pulmonary capillary bed. J Appl Physiol 32:346–356, 1972.

37. Weibel ER: Die Blutgefassanastomosen in der menschlichen Lunge. Z Zellforsch 50:653–692, 1959.

38. Weibel ER: *Morphometry of the Human Lung.* New York, Academic Press, 1963.

39. Weibel ER, Gil J: Structure-function relationships at the alveolar level, in JB West (ed), *Engineering Aspects of Lung Biology.* New York, Marcel Dekker, 1977, pp 1–81.

40. Weibel ER, Limacher W, Bachofen H: Electron microscopy of rapidly frozen lungs: Evaluation on the basis of standard criteria. J Appl Physiol 53:516–527, 1982.

41. Yen RT, Zhuang FY, Fung YC, Ho HH, Tremer H, Sobin SS: Morphometry of cat pulmonary venous tree. J Appl Physiol 55:236–242, 1983.

42. Zeltner TB, Caduff JH, Gehr P, Pfenninger J, Burri PH: The postnatal development and growth of the human lung. I. Morphometry. Respir Physiol 67:247–267, 1987.

43. Zhuang FY, Fung YC, Yen RT: Analysis of blood flow in cat's lung with detailed anatomical and elasticity data. J Appl Physiol 55:1341–1348, 1983.

Anthony P. Farrell, Ph.D.

2

Comparative Biology of the Pulmonary Circulation

This chapter considers nonavian and nonmammalian vertebrates that are either facultative air breathers (e.g., most air-breathing fish including the Australian lungfish, *Neoceratodus)* or obligate air breathers (e.g., the African lungfish, *Protopterus*, amphibians, and reptiles) and that typically breathe air intermittently. A pulmonary circulation is found in most, but not all, intermittent air breathers. Lungfishes, anuran amphibians, and reptiles possess true lungs. Other air-breathing fishes, which are considered separately from lungfishes in this chapter, lack a true lung but often use an analogous structure, a vascularized swimbladder, as an accessory air-breathing organ (ABO).

These intermittent air breathers characteristically perform a single ventilation or a set of ventilations followed by an apneic period that is highly variable. Apnea typically lasts several minutes, but even in obligate air breathers it can last 20 to 30 min. An extreme example is the turtle that can overwinter underwater for 6 months. Air-breathing fishes, lungfishes, and amphibian larvae also possess gills for water breathing and are, therefore, bimodal breathers.

Intermittent air breathers are an interesting group of animals in terms of pulmonary control. Because they do not continuously ventilate their lungs, large changes in lung perfusion can be expected if ventilation and perfusion are to be matched; as indicated below, ventilation-perfusion matching in intermittent air breathers is achieved differently from matching in birds and mammals. Moreover, shifts in blood flow between lungs and gills can be anticipated in bimodal breathers since both organs are not necessarily used for gas exchange to the same degree at a given period in time.

CIRCULATORY PATTERNS IN INTERMITTENT AIR BREATHERS

Birds and mammals are continuous air breathers that use lungs; fish are generally continuous water breathers that use gills. The respiratory and systemic circulations of fish, birds, and mammals lie in series (Fig. 1). Therefore, in these animals, respiratory blood flow must closely match systemic blood flow over the long term. This is not the case for intermittent air breathers.

During evolution, transition from an aquatic to a terrestrial life-style was accompanied by a transition to air breathing. Among the vertebrates, the transition to air breathing was accompanied by a reduction or loss of the gills, and the development of a lung or an air-breathing organ (ABO) (16). In contrast to birds and mammals, the circulation to the lung or ABO of intermittent air breathers developed in parallel to the systemic circulation (Fig. 1). This circulatory pattern provides the basis for independently varying pulmonary and systemic blood flow so that lung perfusion can match intermittent lung ventilation without compromising systemic perfusion. Moreover, since, with the exception of crocodiles, the two circuits are perfused by a single ventricle, the distribution of the cardiac output is simply a function of the relative resistances of the pulmonary and systemic circuits which are arranged in parallel.

However, a single ventricle does complicate matters in terms of venous return since systemic and pulmonary venous returns may become mixed within the heart. Nonetheless, these animals do have mechanisms to limit intracardiac mixing: laminar flow through the heart makes it possible for right and left atria outputs to remain spatially separated within the ventricle (9,18). Also, evolutionary alterations in cardiac anatomy (Fig. 1) create interconnected chambers within the ventricle: septation creates two atria in lungfishes, amphibians, and reptiles, partial septa in the single ventricle of lungfishes, amphibians and noncrocodilian reptiles and separate pulmonary and systemic outflow tracts from the ventricle. Air-breathing fish have a single aorta and the blood flow to the air-breathing organ (ABO) is situated distal to the gill circulation. The single aorta of lungfishes and truncus arteriosus of amphibians is divided by a septal ridge which separates blood flow to the pulmonary and systemic circuits. Separate pulmonary and systemic outlets are found in reptiles.

Although intracardiac mixing is limited in intermittent air breathers, it is never completely prevented except in crocodiles where there are two ventricles. Intracardiac shunts affect pulmonary flow both quantitatively and qualitatively since they operate to increase systemic venous return to the pulmonary circulation (10).

CARDIOVASCULAR EVENTS ASSOCIATED WITH AIR BREATHING

Blood flow and pressure measurements clearly indicate that heart rate and pulmonary flow decrease progressively during apnea in crocodiles, lizards, snakes, tortoises, turtles, toads, frogs, and the African lungfish, *Protopterus*. Therefore, the cardiovascular events associated with an air breath are more pronounced following longer periods of apnea. For example, in turtles the reflex tachycardia

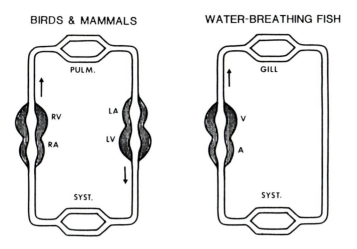

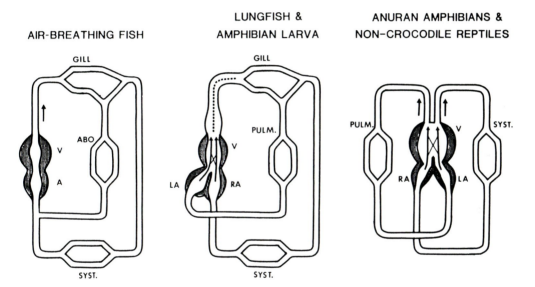

Figure 1: Schematic diagrams of the circulatory patterns in vertebrates. In birds and mammals and water-breathing fish, the respiratory circuit lies in series with the systemic circuit. In contrast, the pulmonary circuit lies in parallel with the sysmetic circuit in intermittent air breathers. In bimodal breathers, the lung circuit is located postbranchially. V = ventricle; A = atrium; LA = left atrium; RA = right atrium; RV = right ventricle; LV = left ventricle; PULM = pulmonary circuit; SYST = systemic circuit; ABO = air-breathing organ.

that accompanies an air breath helps to achieve as much as a 2-fold increase in cardiac output and a 4-fold increase in pulmonary blood flow.

In *Protopterus*, pulmonary flow consistently increases following an air breath (Fig. 2) but not always with an attendant increase in cardiac output or heart rate (12). Pulmonary blood flow has been estimated to vary from less than 20 percent to more than 70 percent of the cardiac output.

In the clawed toad, *Xenopus laevis*, pulmocutaneous blood flow increases 2- to 4-fold above the prebreath level within a few heart beats of the start of ventilation (16,18). The increase in pulmonary flow is often unaccompanied by a change in systemic blood flow or heart rate (Fig. 3); pulmonary flow represents about 50 percent of the total cardiac output. In the bullfrog, *Rana catesbeiana*, 38 percent of cardiac output can go to the lung (20). In the tropical toad, *Bufo marinus*, lung ventilation following short periods of apnea (<1 min) can be accompanied by a 20 to 30 percent increase in pulmonary flow without change in heart rate (21). However, longer apnea (7 min) can double pulmonary flow at the air breath because of reflex tachycardia and increased pulmonary stroke volume.

AFRICAN   LUNGFISH

A

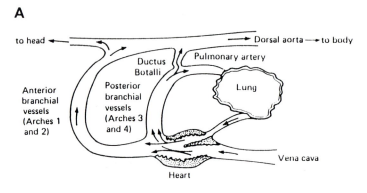

B

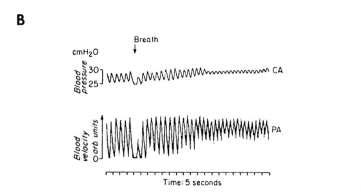

Figure 2:
A. A schematic of the circulatory arrangement in the African lungfish, *Protopterus*.
B. An example of the pronounced cardiovascular changes that accompany an air breath in *Protopterus*. PA = pulmonary artery; CA = conus arteriosus. (Adapted from Johansen et al. [12].)

TURTLE

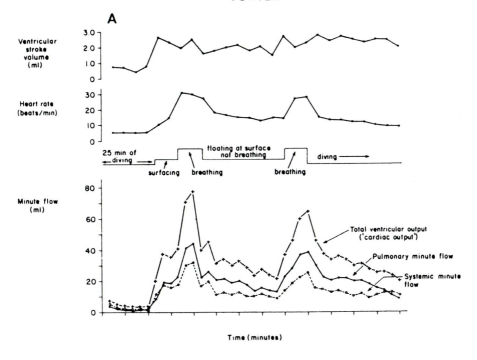

Ventricular stroke volume (ml)

Heart rate (beats/min)

25 min of diving — surfacing — breathing — floating at surface not breathing — breathing — diving —

Minute flow (ml)

Total ventricular output ('cardiac output')

Pulmonary minute flow

Systemic minute flow

Time (minutes)

TOAD

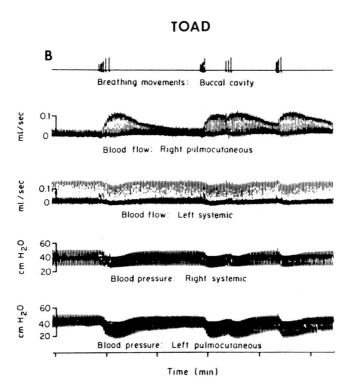

Breathing movements: Buccal cavity

ml/sec — Blood flow: Right pulmocutaneous

ml/sec — Blood flow: Left systemic

cm H₂O — Blood pressure: Right systemic

cm H₂O — Blood pressure: Left pulmocutaneous

Time (min)

Figure 3: Examples of the pronounced cardiovascular changes that accompany intermittent breathing.
A. The turtle, *Chrysemys.* (Adapted from Shelton and Burggren [19].)
B. The toad, *Xenopus.* (Adapted from Shelton: Respir Physiol 9: 183–199, 1970.)

Moreover, pulmonary flow at the end of apnea is linearly related to the length of apnea (1–7 min).

In the turtle, *Chrysemys scripta*, a 10 to 15 min apnea evokes an increase in cardiac output (e.g., from 26.6 to 57.4 ml/min/kg), primarily due to tachycardia (11 to 23 bpm) (Fig. 3). During lung ventilation, about 65 percent of cardiac output can go to the lung and pulmonary flow can increase 3.5-fold while systemic flow increases by only 27 percent. In *Chrysemys picta* (at 15°C), cardiac output was found to increase (e.g., from 18.5 to 71.6 ml/min/kg) after an air breath (10); pulmonary flow, which represented 34 to 43 percent of cardiac output, increased almost 5-fold whereas systemic flow increased 3-fold.

Although changes in heart rate and cardiac output may not occur during short apneic periods, reflex tachycardia contributes significantly to the increase in cardiac output after prolonged apnea. Control of heart rate in these vertebrates is primarily by the vagus nerve, and injections of atropine have shown that bradycardia during apnea is cholinergically mediated.

Interestingly, similar changes in heart rate and perfusion of the ABO also occur in air-breathing fishes, with or without concomitant changes in cardiac output (5,16). Thus, the nature and control of the central cardiac events are apparently independent of whether a lung or an ABO is used for air breathing.

Thus, changes in cardiac output that are synchronized with air breathing can support an increase in pulmonary flow which does not compromise systemic flow. Nevertheless, as indicated in the next section, the distribution of cardiac output ultimately depends on the relative outflow resistances of the systemic and pulmonary circuits.

VASCULAR CONTROL OF PULMONARY FLOW

Since the systemic and pulmonary circuits lie in parallel in intermittent air breathers, it is possible to increase pulmonary flow following an air breath by either increasing systemic resistance or decreasing pulmonary resistance or some combination of the two. As outlined below, the most common strategy is to decrease pulmonary resistance. Moreover, the major change in pulmonary resistance occurs in the pulmonary artery extrinsic to the lung parenchyma and is under vagal control.

Lungfish

Lungfishes are representatives of the first vertebrates to develop a true lung. They are normally found in water where they continuously ventilate their gills and periodically (1 to 30 min) surface to take an air breath. The adult *Protopterus* is an obligate air breather and the lung is the major site for oxygen uptake. During droughts, *Protopterus* can survive out of water for many months by estivating in mud cocoons and breathing air intermittently. They possess four bilateral pairs of gill arches. The two posterior pairs of gill arches have secondary lamellae for gas exchange with the water, whereas the two anterior pairs lack secondary lamellae and they correspond to the carotid and systemic arches of the Amniota. Cardiac output goes directly to the gill arches (Fig. 2). Blood flow to the anterior gill arches bypasses the gas exchange sites and goes directly to the systemic circuit. Blood flow through the posterior arches can perfuse the secondary lamellae for gas exchange with water, and it can also perfuse the postbranchial pulmonary circulation. A further anatomical refinement is a very short muscular vessel, the ductus Botalli, which acts as a postbranchial shunt between the systemic and pulmonary circuits. Clearly, blood leaving the posterior gill arches can enter either the pulmonary artery or the dorsal aorta via the ductus Botalli.

Vascular controls have been studied in *Protopterus* (8). Both the ductus Botalli and the proximal segment of the pulmonary artery are vasoactive. *In vitro* perfusion of the ductus Botalli using hypoxic saline causes it to dilate. Dopamine and prostaglandin E_2 are also potent dilators, whereas the β-agonist, isoproterenol, and acetylcholine are less powerful. Alpha-adrenergic agonists constrict the ductus Botalli. The vascular smooth muscle of the ductus is innervated, probably by cholinergic vagal fibers since adrenergic neurons have not been found in lungfish (15). The pulmonary arterial vasomotor segment (PAVS) is also innervated and is constricted by acetylcholine. Hypoxic saline and α-adrenergic agonists are notably without effect on the pulmonary artery.

Although vascular controls are not completely understood for *Protopterus*, the above information suggests that pulmonary blood flow is regulated by antagonistic vasomotion in the ductus Botalli and the PAVS. The following "extreme case" scenarios can be envisaged. During water breathing, secondary lamellae located on the posterior gill arches are perfused. The ductus is dilated and the PAVS is constricted, so postbranchial blood enters the systemic circulation. Since arterial P_{O_2} is low during apnea (13), the ductus Botalli is probably kept open by local hypoxic vasodilatation, whereas the pulmonary artery is closed by vagal vasoconstriction of the PAVS. During air breathing, blood entering the posterior gill arches bypasses the secondary lamellae by means of shunt vessels located at the base of the lamellae. The control of gill lamellar shunts is not understood, but it may involve passive as well as active components since secondary lamellae tend to collapse in air. In any event, vascular resistance of the posterior gill arches is reduced relative to the anterior gill arches (8), which means that a greater proportion of cardiac output goes to the posterior arches and, thence, to the lung. The ductus Botalli is closed, probably as a result of a high systemic P_{O_2}, and reduced cholinergic tonus to the PAVS keeps the pulmonary artery open. The shunting blood between the pulmonary and systemic circuits afforded by the ductus Botalli is clearly analogous to the role of the ductus arteriosus of the mammalian fetus; so, too, is the apparent mechanism for vasoactivity in the ductus Botalli.

A similar vascular arrangement to that found in the lungfish also exists in fish that utilize a well-vascularized swimbladder for air breathing. The importance of drawing such a comparison is that it is possible to delineate the control mechanisms that are specific to the evolution of a pulmonary circulation. *Hoplerythrinus unitaeniatus* increases heart rate and blood flow to the swimbladder after an air breath without a concomitant increase in cardiac output (7). As in the lungfish, preferentially, perfusion of the posterior branchial arches can increase blood flow to the swimbladder. However, vasomotor control of the swimbladder artery (a branch of the celiac artery) is lacking (16). Thus, control of flow to the ABO is probably achieved by an increase in systemic resistance (α-adrenergic vasoconstriction) rather than a decrease in pulmonary vascular resistance as found in *Protopterus*.

Amphibian Larvae

Amphibian larvae provide an exciting insight into the ontogenic aspect of pulmonary control since, as they develop, larvae demonstrate a clear transition between the controls described above for *Protopterus* and those described below for adult amphibians and reptiles.

Control of the pulmonary circulation has been studied in the salamander larva, *Ambystoma*, which has external gills for water breathing and a lung for air breathing (14). The circulatory pattern is similar to that of the lungfish except that there are two possible routes for blood to flow to the lungs in *Ambystoma* (Fig. 4): a direct, prebranchial route via a pulmonary artery; and an indirect, postbranchial route via the posterior gill arches and ductus arteriosus similar to that in *Protopterus*. Experiments using microspheres have shown that most pulmonary blood flow is derived from the posterior gill arches. The resistance of the pulmonary artery is about three times greater than that in the gill circuit. This probably reflects cholinergic vasoconstriction since the pulmonary artery receives vagal innervation, but adrenergic innervation and vasoactivity are absent. Control of the ductus arteriosus has not been examined. In hypoxic water, *Ambystoma* increases lung ventilation. Lung perfusion increases 3-fold and the relative perfusion of the posterior gill arches also increases. Systemic α-adrenergic vasoconstriction probably redistributes flow between the pulmonary and systemic circuits.

Most (60 to 70 percent) of the blood flowing through the gills passes through lamellar shunt vessels, such as those in *Protopterus*. The control of these shunts is unknown.

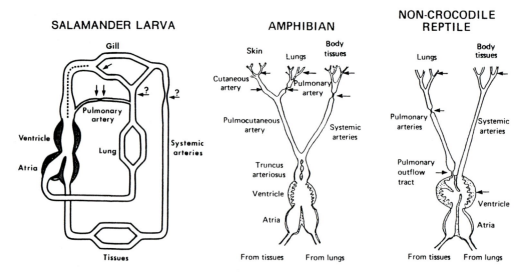

Figure 4: The major vasoactive sites, as indicated by arrows, which influence pulmonary flow in amphibians and noncrocodilian reptiles. (Adapted from Randall et al. [16].)

During metamorphosis, the gills regress, the branchial shunt vessels of the first gill arch develop into the carotid labyrinth, and the shunt vessels of the other gill arches coalesce to form the aortic arches. Although the ductus arteriosus remains the major channel for blood flow to the lung (i.e., of the order of 70 percent), during the metamorphosis, its role gradually diminishes and the pulmonary artery enlarges to dominate pulmonary blood flow in the adult. This ontogenic transition from a control mechanism involving the gill arches and ductus arteriosus to a control mechanism involving the pulmonary artery clearly parallels the evolutionary steps illustrated above for *Protopterus* and below for adult amphibians.

Adult Amphibians and Noncrocodilian Reptiles

Essentially the same principle for vascular control of pulmonary flow obtains in adult anuran amphibians (frogs and toads) and noncrocodilian reptiles (snakes, turtles, tortoises, and lizards) (Fig. 4) (9,16): pulmonary flow is reduced during apnea by a progressive increase in pulmonary vascular resistance with relatively little or no change in systemic resistance. The vasculature associated with the lung parenchyma represents a low resistance circuit, as evidenced by the lower diastolic pressures in the pulmonary versus systemic arteries (2,19). However, the pulmonary artery extrinsic to the lung parenchyma can increase its resistance considerably through reflex cholinergic vasoconstriction. In turtles and snakes, but not in amphibians, an additional resistance site is associated with a band of smooth muscle located in the pulmonary outflow tract immediately proximal to the ventricle (cavum pulmonale). In the snake, this accounts for a major decrease in blood pressure (1). Both the pulmonary artery and the smooth muscle associated with the pulmonary outflow tract receive vagal innervation. Atropine injections produce marked decreases in pulmonary resistance and increases in pulmonary flow. There is also a weak adrenergic dilation of the pulmonary artery in turtles, but not in amphibians.

Amphibians have a pulmocutaneous artery rather than a simple pulmonary artery as in reptiles (Fig. 4). Flow in the pulmocutaneous artery is partitioned between the pulmonary and cutaneous circuits according to the relative resistances of the two circuits. In *Bufo marinus*, only 8 to 14 percent of pulmocutaneous blood flow goes to the skin (21); in *Xenopus*, about 48 percent of pulmocutaneous flow goes to the skin (20). In *Bufo*, α-adrenergic vasoconstriction of the cutaneous artery may enhance pulmonary blood flow since, at the onset of air breathing, cutaneous vascular resistance increases at the same time that pulmonary resistance decreases.

Crocodiles

Crocodiles have two ventricles which normally function in a manner similar to the mammalian heart (right ventricular output goes to the pulmonary circuit and left ventricular output goes to the systemic circuit). Although the left systemic aorta arises from the right ventricle (Fig. 5), a portion of the left ventricular output

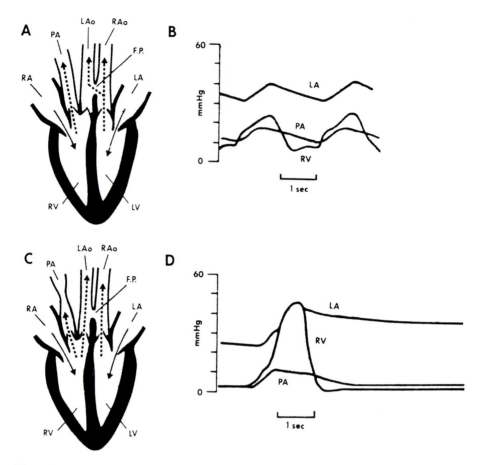

Figure 5: In crocodiles, the systemic and pulmonary outflow from the heart are normally separated (A), as indicated by the pressure differential between the right ventricle and left aorta (B). However, during prolonged submersion, bradycardia is accompanied by some of the right ventricular output going to the systemic circuit (C) because pressure development by the right ventricle increases and matches that in the left ventricle (D). F.P. = foramen Panizzae; LAo = left aorta; RAo = right aorta. (Adapted from White: *Biology of the Reptilia,* Vol 5, 1976, pp 275–334.)

enters the left aorta from the right aorta via the foramen Panizzae. Moreover, because systolic pressure in the left ventricle exceeds that in the right ventricle, the left aortic valve is closed and right ventricular output can only go to the pulmonary circulation. However, during prolonged apnea, crocodiles can vary pulmonary flow without compromising systemic flow because vagal cholinergic constriction of the pulmonary artery increases the outflow resistance of the right ventricle (9). As a result, systolic pressure in the right ventricle increases and matches that in the left ventricle. Thus, the left aortic valve can then open, and the right ventricular output is distributed between the pulmonary artery and left aorta as a function of the relative resistance of the pulmonary and systemic circuits. This right-to-left shunt is clearly a favorable strategy when the lung is not ventilated for long periods and blood oxygen stores need to be diverted to the systemic circuit.

SENSORY INPUT

The cardiovascular changes accompanying intermittent air breathing are largely controlled by reflexes. Although the efferent control of pulmonary flow has been reasonably well defined, much less is known about the afferent arm of the reflex. Nonetheless, vagal afferents convey information about the stage of lung inflation in all lower vertebrates examined to date: in *Protopterus*, amphibians, turtles, snakes, and crocodiles, artificial inflation of the lung with N_2 produces reflex tachycardia and increased pulmonary blood flow that are quantitatively similar to that following a normal air breath (4,10,11). A vago-vagal reflex loop seems to be responsible for coordinating the cardiovascular events associated with intermittent air breathing.

Peripheral and central chemoreceptors, as well as lung stretch receptors, can influence pulmonary flow. When *Bufo marinus* breathe hypercapnic air, they develop bradycardia and reduced pulmonary blood flow; when they breathe a hypercapnic-nitrogen mixture, pulmonary resistance increases 6-fold (21). Chemoreceptors may indirectly influence pulmonary blood flow through their effect on respiratory frequency.

EVOLUTIONARY TRENDS

Definite patterns emerge in terms of the evolution of the control of pulmonary flow at the level of the heart, the arteries, and the arterioles (Table 1). In the lower vertebrates, these patterns can be categorized as follows: (1) Reflex changes in heart rate, which are often central to changes in lung perfusion, are inhibitory, cholinergic, and mediated by the vagus. This mechanism contrasts

TABLE 1 MAJOR CONTROL MECHANISMS INVOLVED IN THE REGULATION OF BLOOD FLOW TO THE LUNG AND AIR-BREATHING ORGAN IN INTERMITTENT AIR BREATHERS

	Fish	Lungfish	Amphibian larva	Adult amphibian	Turtle	Snake	Crocodile
Heart	Chol	Chol	(Chol)	Chol	Chol	Chol	Chol
Pulmonary (or celiac) artery	/	Chol	Chol	Chol ← weak AD →	Chol	Chol	Chol
Systemic circuit	AD	/	AD?	/	/	/	/
Ductus	?	Hypoxia	?	/	/	/	/
Gill arch	+	+	+	/	/	/	/
Gill shunt	/	+	+	/	/	/	/
Inflation reflex	?	+	?	+	+	+	+

AD = adrenergic; Chol = cholinergic; ? = possible or unknown; + = present; / = absent; (Chol) = probable but not tested.

with the usual excitatory adrenergic control of heart rate in birds and mammals. Nevertheless, it should be noted that cholinergic inhibition is the primary mechanism for the bradycardia associated with intermittent breathing in birds and mammals, such as ducks, seals, and whales, that engage in prolonged or forced apneic diving. (2) Large changes in pulmonary flow, independent of systemic flow, are achieved by varying pulmonary rather than systemic resistance. This control is achieved by cholinergic vasoconstriction of the pulmonary artery which is also mediated by the vagus. Adrenergic vasoactivity in the pulmonary circuit of lower vertebrates is either absent or weak and dilatatory. Once again, this situation contrasts with the usual pattern in birds and mammals where systemic and pulmonary flow are closely matched and pulmonary vasoconstriction occurs at the arteriolar level in response to adrenergic and hypoxic stimuli. Diving birds and mammals use the strategy of reducing pulmonary flow in parallel with systemic flow and selectively perfusing vital organs during apnea. (3) Air-breathing fish that lack a true lung apparently vary blood flow to the air-breathing organ (ABO) by means of adrenergic systemic vasoconstriction. (4) In bimodal air breathers, the pulmonary circulation is derived postbranchially. Thus, gill shunts at the arteriolar level and preferential perfusion of the gill arches are important, albeit poorly understood, in controlling pulmonary flow. (5) The afferent arm of the cardiovascular reflexes associated with intermittent air breathing also appears to be vagally mediated.

BLOOD FLOW AT THE CAPILLARY LEVEL

A distinctive feature perhaps of all primary gas exchange sites—lungs, gills, and some ABOs—is their high vascular density. Capillaries usually occupy about 90 percent of the respiratory surface area in the fish gill, the turtle lung, and the mammalian lung. In addition, respiratory capillaries are much more compliant than systemic capillaries. According to sheet blood flow theory, blood flow through respiratory capillaries is directly related to the vascular transmural pressure (VTP). Therefore, VTP is probably an important determinant of the distribution of capillary blood flow in all lungs.

VTP is determined primarily by the difference between intravascular pressure and intrapulmonary pressure. Whether sheet flow theory is applicable to the mammalian lung is debatable. Nonetheless, arterial blood pressure is low (e.g., 25/10 mmHg), and alveolar pressure is fairly uniform throughout the lung. Therefore, hydrostatic pressure, through its effect on VTP, is the primary factor varying blood distribution at the alveolar level. Changes in pulmonary blood pressure and intrapulmonary pressure also affect VTP and alter blood distribution at the alveolar level.

In lower vertebrates, the situation is somewhat different. Arterial blood pressure to the lungs, ABO, or gills is marginally higher than the pulmonary arterial pressure in mammals (9). To compensate, gill capillaries have a much thicker epithelial barrier than lungs, whereas the lung capillaries of intermittent air breathers are protected by the high extrapulmonary resistance of the pulmonary artery. Pressure measurements at the capillary level of intermittent air breathers have not been made. However, it is reasonable to anticipate that (1) capillary pressure will be considerably lower than the pulmonary arterial pressure because of this resistance site, and (2) capillary pressure will oscillate considerably, decreasing during apnea and increasing during each air breath (lung fluid filtration, which is also influenced directly by capillary blood pressure, is low during apnea and increases considerably following an air breath in turtles [3]), and (3) because of the swings in capillary blood pressure, it can be predicted that the alveolar capillary sheet will tend to collapse during apnea as VTP decreases.

Intrapulmonary pressure influences VTP importantly in intermittent air breathers. Normally, the lung is kept inflated during apnea by a fairly constant pressure (2 to 10 mmHg) (16). Such a pressure is significant in counteracting the capillary blood pressure. Although it is recognized that lung perfusion, pulmonary blood pressure, and gas exchange are all reduced during diving in turtles (19), it is possible that the alveolar capillary sheet cannot be perfused during even shallow dives unless pulmonary blood pressure is *increased*. However, despite the reduction in capillary blood flow caused by changes in VTP during apnea, pulmonary flow may still continue in the larger, apparently less compliant vessels associated with alveolar support structures (6). This kind of pulmonary perfusion could explain the anatomical shunts of 10 to 28 percent observed in turtle lungs (17) even though obvious vascular shunts and ventilation in homogeneities have not been detected.

CONCLUDING REMARKS

In this chapter, a number of similarities and evolutionary trends were established for the control of pulmonary flow in lower vertebrates that are intermittent air breathers. Except perhaps for the similarities that exist at the capillary level, most factors affecting pulmonary flow and vasoactivity in intermittent air breathers are clearly different from those in birds and mammals. Why cholinergic inhibitory reflexes dominate in lower vertebrates and adrenergic reflexes dominate in birds and mammals is not entirely clear, but it obviously reflects selection pressures that have acted through the millenia. Intermittent air breathers are clearly 'evolutionary survivors'. A well-developed sympathetic nervous system was not apparently required for their ectothermic, 'wait-and-prey' life-style. In contrast, the evolutionary success of birds and mammals rests on being endotherms with a high cardiovascular scope for activity; the high cardiovascular scope is apparently related to a well-developed sympathetic control of the cardiovascular system.

ACKNOWLEDGMENTS

Financial support was provided by the Natural Science and Engineering Research Council, Canada, and the British Columbia Health Care Research Foundation.

REFERENCES

1. Burggren WW: Circulation during intermittent lung ventilation in the garter snake, *Thamnophis*. Can J Zool 55:1720–1725, 1977.

2. Burggren WW: The pulmonary circulation of the chelonian reptile: morphology, haemodynamics and pharmacology. J Comp Physiol B 166:330–332, 1977.

3. Burggren WW: Pulmonary plasma filtration in the turtle: a wet vertebrate lung? Science 215:77–78, 1982.

4. Delaney RG, Laurent P, Galante R, Pack AI, Fishman AP: Pulmonary mechanoreceptors in the dipnoi lungfish *Protopterus* and *Lepidosiren*. Am J Physiol 244:R418-R428, 1983.

5. Farrell AP: Cardiovascular events associated with air breathing in two teleosts, *Hoplerythrinus unitaeniatus* and *Arapaima gigas*. Can J Zool 56:953–958, 1978.

6. Farrell AP: Relations between capillary dimensions and transmural pressure in the turtle lung. Respir Physiol 45:13–24, 1981.

7. Farrell AP, Sobin SS: Sheet blood flow: Its application in predicting shunts in respiratory systems, in Johansen K, Burggren W (eds), *Cardiovascular Shunts*. Copenhagen, Munksgaard, 1985, pp 269–281.

8. Fishman AP, Delaney RG, Laurent P: Circulation adaptation to bimodal respiration in the dipnoan lungfish. J Appl Physiol 59:285–294, 1985.

9. Johansen K, Burggren WW: Cardiovascular function in the lower vertebrates, in Bourne GH (ed), *Hearts and Heart-like Organs*, vol 1. New York, Academic Press, 1980, pp 61–117.

10. Johansen K, Burggren WW (eds): *Cardiovascular Shunts: Phylogenetic, Ontogenetic and Clinical Aspects*. Copenhagen, Munksgaard, 1985.

11. Johansen K, Burggren WW, Glass M: Pulmonary stretch receptors regulate heart rate and pulmonary flow in the turtle, *Pseudemys scripta*. Comp Biochem Physiol 58:185–192, 1977.

12. Johansen K, Lenfant C, Hanson D: Cardiovascular dynamics in lungfish. Z Vergl Physiol 59:157–186, 1968.

13. Lahiri S, Szidon JP, Fishman AP: Potential respiratory and circulatory adjustments to hypoxia in the African lungfish. Fed Proc 29:1141–1148, 1970.

14. Malvin GM: Cardiovascular shunting during amphibian metamorphosis, in Johansen K, Burggren W (eds), *Cardiovascular Shunts*. Copenhagen, Munksgaard, 1985, pp 163–178.

15. Nilsson S: *Autonomic Nerve Function in the Vertebrates*. Berlin, Springer-Verlag, 1983.

16. Randall DJ, Burggren WW, Farrell AP, Haswell MS: *The evolution of air-breathing in vertebrates*. Cambridge University Press, 1981.

17. Seymour RS: Functional venous admixture in the lungs of the turtle, *Chrysemys scripta*. Respir Physiol 53:99–108, 1983.

18. Shelton G: Functional and evolutionary significance of cardiovascular shunts in the Amphibia, in Johansen K, Burggren W (eds), *Cardiovascular Shunts*. Copenhagen, Munksgaard, 1985, pp 100–115.

19. Shelton G, Burggren WW: Cardiovascular dynamics of the chelonia during apnoea and lung ventilation. J Exp Biol 64:323–343, 1976.

20. Tazawa H, Mochizuki M, Piiper J: Respiratory gas transport by the incompletely separated double circulation in the bullfrog, *Rana catesbeiana*. Respir Physiol 36:77–95, 1979.

21. West NH, Burggren WW: Factors influencing pulmonary and cutaneous arterial blood flow in the toad, *Bufo marinus*. Am J Physiol 247:R884–R894, 1984.

Andrew P. Somlyo, M.D.
Avril V. Somlyo, Ph.D.

3

Excitation and Contraction in Smooth Muscle

Contraction in smooth muscle is generally initiated by excitation of the surface membrane that triggers a rise in cytoplasmic free Ca^{2+}. The latter, through Ca^{2+}-sensitive regulatory protein(s), activates the contractile apparatus. The specific steps are outlined in greater detail in Figure 1. In this chapter, we shall briefly review the evidence demonstrating the mechanisms mediating the above sequence, with an emphasis on their operation in main pulmonary artery smooth muscle.

Smooth muscles have been classified, based on their response to depolarization with high K^+ and their membrane electrical properties, as tonic or phasic (53,65,66). The rabbit main pulmonary artery contains a "prototype" tonic smooth muscle that responds with a maintained contraction to depolarization with high K and is depolarized gradedly, without action potentials, in response to excitatory transmitters (53,65). Tonic smooth muscle is found not only in the main pulmonary artery (53,65,66,68) but in the aorta (54) and trachealis (15) as well. Phasic smooth muscles respond to depolarization with an initial peak ("phasic") in force that declines to a variable plateau; they generate action potentials spontaneously and/or in response to excitatory transmitters or depolarization (33,50). The resting membrane potential of the tonic, main pulmonary artery smooth muscle is generally more negative, approximately $-60mV$ (66), than that of phasic smooth muscles. Tonic smooth muscles in the airways are tracheal rather than bronchiolar (55) and, in the systemic arterial bed (33,38), tend to be in the large vessels and acquire more phasic properties in the smaller arteries.

The major mechanisms of excitation-contraction coupling are electromechani-

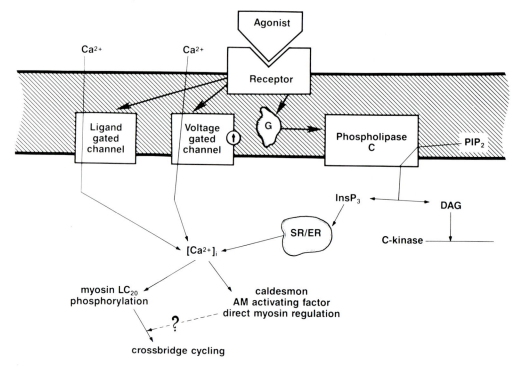

Figure 1: Schematic showing steps involved in the contraction of smooth muscle. The agonist binds to a receptor and activates (1) a ligand-gated channel, (2) a voltage-gated channel, and (3) a specific G protein which activates phospholipase C that ultimately activates diacylgylcerol (DAG). InsP$_3$ affects the SR/ER, releasing calcium and causing an increase in cytosolic CA^{++} [Ca^{2+}]$_i$. The increase in [Ca^{2+}]$_i$ causes phosphorylation of the 20 kDa myosin light chain (LC$_{20}$) through myosin light chain kinase. This is the classic pathway which causes crossbridge cycling. An alternate pathway may involve caldesmon, an actinomyosin (AM) activating factor, or direct myosin regulation. SR = sarcoplasmic reticulum; ER = endoplasmic reticulum.

cal coupling and pharmacomechanical coupling (Table 1). Pharmacomechanical coupling is contractile activation or inhibition through mechanisms that are independent of surface membrane potential. The two mechanisms can operate concurrently. Electromechanical coupling controls tension by regulating cytoplasmic Ca^{2+} through the membrane potential. There is considerable evidence showing that intracellular Ca^{2+} release plays a major role in pharmacomechanical (8,18,19,39) as well as in electromechanical coupling (36,50). The contribution of Ca^{2+} influx through voltage-gated channels is also well established (7,69), although the quantitative contribution of influx to activator Ca^{2+} in different smooth muscles and under different experimental conditions is not known (46). Ligand (ATP)-gated channels have been detected in patch clamp records (3); the existence of norepinephrine- and serotonin-gated Ca^{2+} channels had already been shown by more conventional, electrophysiological methods (56), although recent patch clamp studies (20,44) did not reveal channels operated by α-adrenergic receptors. In addition to regulation by voltage-independent control of cytoplasmic Ca^{2+}, phenomena reflecting pharmacomechanical coupling may be mediated by

TABLE 1 EXCITATION CONTRACTION COUPLING

Electromechanical Coupling: Voltage-Controlled
Release of intracellular, stored Ca^{2+}
Ca^{2+}-influx through voltage-gated channels
Pharmacomechanical Coupling: Voltage-Independent
Ca^{2+}-release by messenger: $InsP_3$
Ca^{2+}-influx through ligand-gated channels
Other (e.g., phosphorylation of myosin light chain
   kinase by kinase A)

Ca^{2+}-independent mechanisms, such as inhibition of myosin light chain kinase (MLCK) by its phosphorylation catalyzed by (cyclic AMP-dependent) kinase A (1,35,45).

The mechanism of electromechanical Ca^{2+} release in either smooth or striated muscle is not understood (51). In contrast, much recent information has been accumulated concerning the role of inositol 1,4,5-trisphosphate ($InsP_3$) in pharmacomechanical Ca^{2+} release (2,5,61,70). The liberation of $InsP_3$ through receptor activated hydrolysis of membrane phosphatidyl-inositol bisphosphate (PIP_2) by phospholipase C has now been well studied in a variety of cell systems (4). $InsP_3$ has also been shown to release intracellular Ca in smooth muscle (5,61,67), and, as shown in rabbit main pulmonary artery, the amount of Ca^{2+} released is sufficient to cause contraction (61). Moreover, the development of force following the release of $InsP_3$ from a photolabile, inactive (caged) precursor of $InsP_3$ is sufficiently rapid (70) for $InsP_3$ to meet the kinetic criteria of a physiological messenger.

Studies on smooth muscles in which the surface membrane was permeabilized to permit the free entry of Ca^{2+} have shown that Ca^{2+} can regulate contraction in smooth muscle (14,21,23,27,33, 48). More recently, the advent of practical and reliable indicators of intracellular free Ca^{2+} (6,25) permitted several laboratories to verify that a rise in cytoplasmic free Ca^{2+} also triggers contraction under physiological conditions in intact smooth muscle (17,22,30). Rhythmic fluctuations in cytoplasmic free Ca^{2+} triggering contractions in a spontaneously active intestinal smooth muscle (Fig. 2) illustrate the physiological relationship between cycling of Ca^{2+} and contraction. Similarly, both the rise in cytoplasmic free Ca^{2+} induced by transmitters (Fig. 3) and Ca^{2+} release detected by electron probe analysis (8), in depolarized smooth muscle in Ca^{2+}-free solution, show that release from an intracellular site (see below) is a major mechanism of pharmacomechanical coupling.

THE SARCOPLASMIC RETICULUM, NOT MITOCHONDRIA, IS THE PHYSIOLOGICAL REGULATOR OF CYTOPLASMIC Ca^{2+}

The structural identity of the organelle that is the sink and source of intracellular Ca^{2+} released by transmitters has been one of the central questions of excitation-contraction coupling in smooth muscle. The existence of a well-developed sarcoplasmic reticulum (SR) in vascular smooth muscle was first demonstrated in main pulmonary artery (19). The volume of the SR is relatively large in this smooth

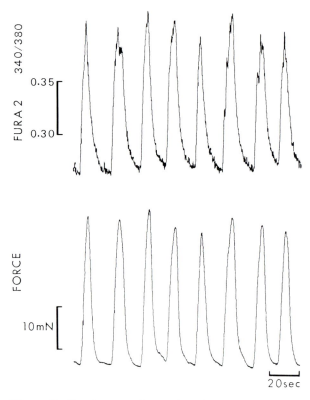

Figure 2: Spontaneous fluctuations in cytoplasmic free Ca^{2+} triggering contractions in guinea pig ileum smooth muscle. The upper trace is the ratio of fluorescence of the Ca^{2+}-indicator FURA 2; the lower trace shows tension. The rhythmic fluctuations of the Ca^{2+} transients occur at rates comparable to the trains of action potentials normally recorded in such intestinal smooth muscle. (Reproduced from Hoar et al. [31].)

muscle (Fig. 4) that can also contract in the absence of extracellular Ca^{2+} (19). These and other observations strongly implicated the SR as the major source of activator Ca^{2+} in smooth muscle. Electron probe microanalytic studies showed directly that the SR can accumulate Ca^{2+} by an ATP-dependent process, and that Ca^{2+} can be released from the SR of pulmonary artery and other smooth muscle (8,37,58). The Ca^{2+} content of the SR is sufficient to trigger maximal contractions even in those smooth muscles that, unlike rabbit main pulmonary artery, contain a rather small volume (less than 2 percent) of SR (8).

Mitochondria, in contrast to the SR, contain relatively low concentrations of Ca^{2+} in normal cells, muscle, or nonmuscle (57), and it is now clear that mitochondria do not play a significant role in the physiological regulation of cytoplasmic-free Ca^{2+}. This, notwithstanding the fact that mitochondria can accumulate massive amounts of Ca^{2+} during pathologically increased Ca^{2+} influx and when cytoplasmic Ca^{2+} reaches abnormally high levels (10,59).

Finally, it must be emphasized that, although the emphasis of this chapter is on the role of organelles in intracellular Ca^{2+} metabolism, the maintenance of steady state total calcium, in the face of Ca^{2+} influx, clearly requires plasma

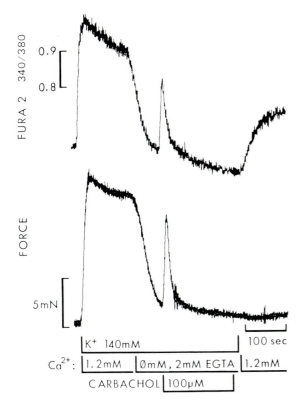

Figure 3: Intracellular calcium release by carbachol in depolarized guinea pig ileal smooth muscle. Following depolarization of the smooth muscle with a high K, 1.2 mM Ca^{2+}-containing solution, the smooth muscle strip was transferred into a Ca^{2+}-free depolarizing solution. The addition of carbachol evoked an increased fura 2 fluorescence, indicative of intracellular Ca^{2+} release and secondary contraction. This result is a demonstration of pharmacomechanical Ca^{2+} release from the intracellular Ca^{2+} store. (Reproduced from Hoar et al. [31].)

membrane transport systems: the most significant of these is probably the Ca^{2+}-ATPase (13,16,71) of the plasma membrane.

CONTRACTILE REGULATION AND THE CONTRACTILE MECHANISM

Initiation of contraction in smooth muscle is generally thought to require the combination of Ca^{2+} with calmodulin, the binding of a Ca^{2+}_4-calmodulin complex to the catalytic subunit of myosin light chain kinase (MLCK), and phosphorylation of serine 19 on the 20 kDa myosin light chain by the Ca^{2+}_4-calmodulin activated MLCK. This phosphorylation enables actin to activate myosin ATPase (27). Relaxation, in this regulatory system, is due to dephosphorylation of myosin by myosin light chain phosphatase (26,27,31,47). Regulation by thin filament-associ-

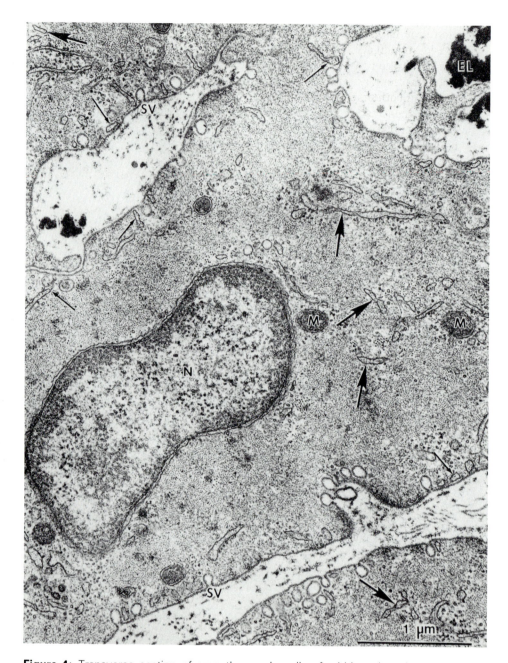

Figure 4: Transverse section of smooth muscle cells of rabbit main pulmonary artery, illustrating the location of SR tubules throughout the cytoplasm (large arrows) as well as at the cell periphery (small arrows). SV = surface vesicle; EL = elastin; M = mitochondrion; N = nucleus. (Reproduced from Kuriyama et al. [38].)

ated proteins, such as caldesmon, or by myosin-regulated mechanisms has been considered (40,49), but evidence for this is still not sufficiently complete to allow the integration into a definite physiological mechanism. An extensive volume, including the majority of significant developments related to contractile regulation in smooth muscle, was recently published (49).

An understanding of the contractile process itself requires knowledge of the structural components of the contractile apparatus and of the relationship between, respectively, the biochemical and structural events underlying contraction. Ultrastructural studies over more than a decade established that the major ultrastructural components of the contractile apparatus are filamentous in smooth, as in striated, muscle (9,52,60,62). These studies revealed that the cytoplasmic and plasma membrane-bound dense bodies are attachment sites for actin, functionally analogous to the Z-lines of striated muscle and that, in addition to actin filaments, myosin is present in filamentous form both in relaxed and in contracted smooth muscle. The demonstration of crossbridges on myosin filaments (52) and, most recently, visualization of crossbridges in a characteristic rigor configuration (63), were clearly consistent with a sliding filament mechanism of contraction mediated through crossbridge cycling. Such a mechanism had already been inferred from the length-active tension (24,29,41) and length-energy consumption (28) relationships.

The sliding filament mechanism of contraction of striated muscle is considered to be mediated by a cyclic attachment/detachment process between myosin crossbridges and actin filaments, accompanied and energized by the biochemical reactions of the actomyosin ATPase cycle. Major features of this mechanism are that, in the absence of ATP (rigor), crossbridges are attached to actin filaments in a rigorlike configuration and that reattachment into a force-generating state is preceded by ATP-induced detachment of rigor bridges. The presence of both rigor bridges and rigor stiffness in smooth muscle (63) is consistent with a crossbridge mediated mechanism of contraction. Detachment of crossbridges, from rigor, also precedes reattachment and force generation when ATP is released from caged ATP, by a laser pulse, onto smooth muscle (63). These studies and the temporal relation between myosin light chain phosphorylation and force development (27,34) also established that, under physiological conditions, the rate limiting process of force development in smooth muscle is the activity of the myosin light chain kinase/phosphatase system, rather than the intrinsic rate of actomyosin reactions.

A potentially important finding of the laser flash photolysis studies (63) was the demonstration of cooperativity in smooth muscle. Cooperativity, originally observed in striated muscle (43), is a process through which a few attached crossbridges permit the attachment of other crossbridges, without the physiologically necessary Ca^{2+} activation. A major feature of smooth muscle is its ability to maintain force at low levels of energy expenditure and myosin light chain phosphorylation (11,12,42); this latch or "catchlike" state may be mediated by cooperativity between phosphorylated and nonphosphorylated crossbridges (63).

ACKNOWLEDGMENTS

Supported by HL15835 to the Pennsylvania Muscle Institute. We thank Ms. M. Tokito for preparation of illustrations and Mrs. B. Tyrcha for typing of the manuscript.

REFERENCES

1. Adelstein RS, Hathaway DR: Role of calcium and cyclic adenosine 3',5'-monophosphate in regulating smooth muscle contraction. Am J Cardiol 44: 783–787, 1979.

2. Baron CB, Cunningham N, Strauss JF, Coburn RF: Pharmacomechanical coupling in smooth muscle may involve phosphatidyl inositol metabolism. Proc Natl Acad Sci USA 81: 6899-6903, 1984.

3. Benham CD, Tsien RW: A novel receptor-operated Ca^{2+}-permeable channel activated by ATP in smooth muscle. Nature 328: 275–278, 1987.

4. Berridge MJ, Irvine RF: Inositol trisphosphate, a novel second messenger in cellular signal transduction. Nature 312: 315–321, 1984.

5. Bitar KN, Bradford PG, Putney JW, Makhlouf GM: Stoichiometry of contraction and Ca^{2+} mobilization by inositol 1,4,5-trisphosphate in isolated gastric smooth muscle cells. J Biol Chem 261: 16591–16596, 1986.

6. Blinks JR: Intracellular $[Ca^{2+}]$ measurements, in Fozzard HA, Haber E, Jennings RB, Katz AM, Morgan HE (eds), *The Heart and Cardiovascular System*. New York, Raven Press, 1986, pp 671–701.

7. Bolton TB: Mechanisms of action of transmitters and other substances on smooth muscle. Physiol Rev 59: 606–718, 1979.

8. Bond M, Kitazawa T, Somlyo AP, Somlyo AV: Release and recycling of calcium by the sarcoplasmic reticulum in guinea pig portal vein smooth muscle. J Physiol 355: 677–695, 1984.

9. Bond M, Somlyo AV: Dense bodies and actin polarity in vertebrate smooth muscle. J Cell Biol 95: 403–413, 1982.

10. Broderick R, Somlyo AP: Calcium and magnesium transport *in situ* mitochondria: Electron probe analysis of vascular smooth muscle. Circ Res 61: 523–530, 1987.

11. Butler TM, Siegman MJ: Chemical energetics of contraction in mammalian smooth muscle. Fed Proc 41: 204–208, 1982.

12. Butler TM, Siegman MJ, Mooers SU: Slowing of crossbridge cycling rate in mammalian smooth muscle occurs without evidence of an increase in internal load, in Siegman MJ, Somlyo AP, Stephens NL (eds), *Regulation and Contraction of Smooth Muscle*. New York, Alan R. Liss, 1987, pp 289–303.

13. Carafoli E: Molecular, mechanistic, and functional aspects of the plasma membrane calcium pump, in *Epithelial Calcium and Phosphate Transport: Molecular and Cellular Aspects*. New York, Alan R. Liss, 1984, pp 13–17.

14. Cassidy PS, Kerrick WGL, Hoar PE, Malencik DA: Exogenous calmodulin increases Ca^{2+} sensitivity of isometric tension activation and myosin phosphorylation in skinned smooth muscle. Pflügers Arch 392: 115–120, 1981.

15. Coburn RF, Yamaguchi T: Membrane potential-dependent and -independent tension in the canine tracheal muscle. J Pharmacol Exp Ther 201: 276–284, 1977.

16. Daniel EE: The use of subcellular membrane fractions in analysis of control of smooth muscle function. Experientia 41: 905–913, 1985.

17. DeFeo TT, Morgan KG: Calcium-force relationships as detected with *aequorin* in two different vascular smooth muscles of the ferret. J Physiol 369: 269–282, 1985.

18. Deth R, Casteels R: A study of releasable Ca fractions in smooth muscle cells of the rabbit aorta. J Gen Physiol 69: 401–416, 1977.

19. Devine CE, Somlyo AV, Somlyo AP: Sarcoplasmic reticulum and excitation-contraction coupling in mammalian smooth muscle. J Cell Biol 52: 690–718, 1972.

20. Droogmans G, Declerck I, Casteels R: Effect of adrenergic agonists on Ca^{2+}-channel currents in single vascular smooth muscle cells. Pflügers Arch 409: 7–12, 1987.

21. Endo M, Kitazawa T, Yagi S, Iino M, Kakuta Y: Some properties of chemically skinned smooth muscle fibers, in Casteels R, Godfraind T, Ruegg JC (eds), *Excitation-Contraction Coupling in Smooth Muscle*. Amsterdam, Elsevier/North-Holland, 1977, pp 199–209.

22. Fay FS, Shlevin HH, Granger WC, Taylor SR: Aequorin luminescence during activation of single isolated smooth muscle cells. Nature 280: 506–508, 1979.

23. Filo RS, Bohr DF, Ruegg JC: Glycerinated skeletal and smooth muscle: Calcium and magnesium dependence. Science 147: 1581–1583, 1963.

24. Gordon AR, Siegman MJ: Mechanical properties of smooth muscle. I. Length tension and force-velocity relations. Am J Physiol 221:1243–1249, 1971.

25. Grynkiewicz G, Poenie M, Tsien TY: A new generation of Ca^{2+} indicators with greatly improved fluorescence properties. J Biol Chem 260:3440–3450, 1985.

26. Haeberle JR, Hathaway DR, DePaoli-Roach AA: Dephosphorylation of myosin in catalytic subunit of a type-2 phosphate produces relaxation of chemically skinned uterine smooth muscle. J Biol Chem 250:9965–9968, 1985.

27. Hartshorne DJ: Biochemistry of the contractile process in smooth muscle, in Johnson LR (ed), *Physiology of the Gastrointestinal Tract*. New York, Raven Press, 1987, pp 423–482.

28. Hellstrand P, Paul RJ: Vascular smooth muscle: Relations between energy metabolism and mechanics, in Barnes CD (ed) *Metabolic, Tonic and Contractile Mechanisms*. New York, Academic Press, 1985, pp 1–35.

29. Herlihy JT, Murphy RA: Length-tension relationship of smooth muscle of the hog carotid artery. Circ Res 33:275–283, 1973.

30. Himpens B, Somlyo AP: Free calcium and force transients during depolarization and pharmacomechanical coupling in guinea pig smooth muscle. J Physiol (Lond) 395:507–530, 1988.

31. Hoar PE, Pato MD, Kerrick GL: Myosin light chain phosphatase: Effect on the activation and relaxation of gizzard smooth muscle skinned fibers. J Biol Chem 260:8760–8764, 1982.

32. Iino M: Tension responses of chemically skinned fibre bundles of the guinea-pig taenia caeci under varied ionic environments. J Physiol (Lond) 320:449–467, 1981.

33. Johansson B, Somlyo AP: Electrophysiology and excitation-contraction coupling, in Bohr DF, Somlyo AP, Sparks HV (eds), *The Handbook of Physiology: The Cardiovascular System. Vol II: Vascular Smooth Muscle*. Bethesda, American Physiological Society, 1980, pp 301–324.

34. Kamm KE, Stull JT: The function of myosin and myosin light chain kinase phosphorylation in smooth muscle. Annu Rev Pharmacol Toxicol 25:593–620, 1985.

35. Kerrick WGL, Hoar PE: Inhibition of smooth muscle tension by cyclic AMP-dependent protein kinase. Nature 292:253–255, 1981.

36. Kobayashi S, Kanaide H, Nakamura M: K⁺-depolarization induces a direct release of Ca^{2+} from intracellular storage sites in cultured vascular smooth muscle cells from rat aorta. Biochem Biophys Res Commun 129:877–884, 1985.

37. Kowarski D, Shuman H, Somlyo AP, Somlyo AV: Calcium release by noradrenaline from central sarcoplasmic reticulum in rabbit main pulmonary artery smooth muscle. J Physiol (Lond) 366:153–175, 1985.

38. Kuriyama H, Ito Y, Suzuki H, Kitamura K, Itoh T: Factors modifying contraction-relaxation cycle in vascular smooth muscles. Am J Physiol 243:H641–H662, 1982.

39. Leijten PA, van Breemen C: The effects of caffeine on the noradrenaline-sensitive calcium store in rabbit aorta. J Physiol (Lond) 357:327–339, 1984.

40. Marston SB, Smith CW: The thin filaments of smooth muscles. J Muscle Res Cell Motil 6:669–708, 1985.

41. Mulvany MJ, Warshaw DM: The active tension-length curve of vascular smooth muscle related to its cellular components. J Gen Physiol 74:85–104, 1979.

42. Murphy RA, Ratz PH, Hai CM: Determinants of the latch state in vascular smooth muscle, in Siegman MJ, Somlyo AP, Stephens NL (eds), *Regulation and Contraction of Smooth Muscle*. New York, Alan R. Liss, 1987, pp 411–415.

43. Murray JM, Weber A: Cooperativity of the calcium switch of the regulated rabbit actomyosin system. Mol Cell Biochem 35:11–15, 1980.

44. Nelson MT, Laher I, Worley J: Membrane potential regulates dihydropyridine inhibition of single calcium channels and contraction of rabbit mesenteric artery. Ann NY Acad Sci, 1987. In press.

45. Pfitzer G, Ruegg JC, Zimmer M, Hofmann F: Relaxation of skinned coronary arteries depends on the relative concentrations of Ca^{2+}, calmodulin and active cAMP-dependent protein kinase. Pflügers Arch 405:70–76, 1985.

46. Ratz PH, Murphy RA: Contributions of intracellular and extracellular Ca^{2+} pools to activation of myosin phosphorylation and stress in swine carotid media. Circ Res 60:410–421, 1987.

47. Ruegg JC: *Calcium in Muscle Activation: A Comparative Approach*. New York, Springer-Verlag, 1986.

48. Ruegg JC, Pfitzer G: Modulation of calcium sensitivity in guinea pig taenia coli: Skinned fiber studies. Experientia 41:997–1001, 1985.

49. Siegman M, Somlyo AP, Stephens NL (eds): *Regulation and Contraction of Smooth Muscle: Progress in Clinical and Biological Research*. New York, Alan R. Liss, 1987.

50. Somlyo AP: Excitation contraction coupling and the ultrastructure of smooth muscle. Circ Res 57:497–507, 1985.

51. Somlyo AP: Excitation-contraction coupling. The messenger across the gap. Nature 316:298–299, 1985.

52. Somlyo AP, Devine CE, Somlyo AV, Rice RV: Filament organization in vertebrate smooth muscle. Philos Trans R Soc Lond [Biol] 265:223–296, 1973.

53. Somlyo AP, Somlyo AV: Vascular smooth muscle: I. Normal structure, pathology, biochemistry and biophysics. Pharmacol Rev 20:197–272, 1968.

54. Somlyo AP, Somlyo AV: Pharmacology of excitation-contraction coupling in vascular smooth muscle and in avian slow muscle. Fed Proc 28 : 1634–1642, 1969.

55. Somlyo AP, Somlyo AV: Biophysics of smooth muscle excitation and contraction, in Bouhuys A (ed), *Airway Dynamics*. Springfield, IL, Charles C. Thomas, 1970, pp 209–229.

56. Somlyo AP, Somlyo AV: Electrophysiological correlates of the inequality of maximal vascular smooth muscle contraction elicited by drugs, in Bevan JA, Furchgott RF, Maxwell RA, Somlyo AP (eds), *Vascular Neuroeffector Systems*. Basel, S. Karger AG, 1971, pp 216–228.

57. Somlyo AP, Somlyo AV, Bond M, Broderick R, Goldman YE, Shuman H, Walker JW, Trentham DR: Calcium and magnesium movements in cells and the role of inositol trisphosphate in muscle, in Eaton DC, Mandel LJ (eds), *Cell Calcium and the Control of Membrane Transport*. New York, Rockefeller University Press, 1987, pp 77–92.

58. Somlyo AP, Somlyo AV, Shuman H: Electron probe analysis of vascular smooth muscle: Composition of mitochondria, nuclei and cytoplasm. J Cell Biol 81 : 316–335, 1979.

59. Somlyo AP, Somlyo AV, Shuman H, Endo M: Calcium and monovalent ions in smooth muscle. Fed Proc 41 : 2883–2890, 1982.

60. Somlyo AV: Ultrastructure of vascular smooth muscle, in Bohr DF, Somlyo AP, Sparks HV (eds), *The Handbook of Physiology. The Cardiovascular System. Vol II: Vascular Smooth Muscle*. Bethesda, American Physiological Society, 1981, pp 33–67.

61. Somlyo AV, Bond M, Somlyo AP, Scarpa A: Inositol-trisphosphate (InsP$_3$) induced calcium release and contraction in vascular smooth muscle. Proc Natl Acad Sci USA 82 : 5231–5235, 1985.

62. Somlyo AV, Butler TM, Bond M, Somlyo AP: Myosin filaments have nonphosphorylated light chains in relaxed smooth muscle. Nature 294 : 567–570, 1981.

63. Somlyo AV, Goldman YE, Fujimori T, Bond M, Trentham DR, Somlyo AP: Crossbridge transients initiated by photolysis of caged nucleotides and crossbridge structure, in smooth muscle, in Siegman M, Somlyo AP, Stephens NL (eds), *Regulation and Contraction of Smooth Muscle, Progress in Clinical and Biological Research*. New York, Alan R. Liss, 1987, pp 27–41.

64. Somlyo AV, Somlyo AP: Vasomotor function of smooth muscle in main pulmonary artery. Am J Physiol 206 : 1196–1199, 1964.

65. Somlyo AV, Somlyo AP: Electromechanical and pharmacomechanical coupling in vascular smooth muscle. J Pharmacol Exp Therap 159 : 129–145, 1968.

66. Somlyo AV, Vinall P, Somlyo AP: Excitation-contraction coupling and electrical events in two types of vascular smooth muscle. Microvasc Res 1 : 354–373, 1969.

67. Suematsu E, Hirata M, Hashimoto T, Kuriyama H: Inositol 1,4,5-trisphosphate releases Ca^{2+} from intracellular store sites in skinned single cells of porcine coronary artery. Biochem Biophys Res Commun 120 : 481–485, 1984.

68. Suzuki H, Twarog BM: Membrane properties of smooth muscle cells in pulmonary arteries of the rat. Am J Physiol 242 : H900–H906, 1982.

69. van Breemen C, Cauvin C, Johns A, Leijten P, Yamamoto H: Ca^{2+} regulation of vascular smooth muscle. Fed Proc 45 : 2746–2751, 1986.

70. Walker JW, Somlyo AV, Goldman YE, Somlyo AP, Trentham DR: Kinetics of smooth and skeletal muscle activation by laser pulse photolysis of caged inositol 1,4,5-trisphosphate. Nature 327 : 249–251, 1987.

71. Wuytack F, De Schutter G, Casteels R: Partial purification of (Ca^{2+} + Mg^{2+})-dependent ATPase from pig smooth muscle and reconstitution of an ATP-dependent Ca^{2+}-transport system. Biochem J 198 : 265–271, 1981.

John H. Linehan, Ph.D.

Christopher A. Dawson, Ph.D.

4

Pulmonary Vascular Resistance (P:Q̇ Relations)

Measurements of both the flow and the inlet and outlet pressures of the pulmonary vascular bed provide access to important and useful information about pulmonary vascular and right heart function. In terms of pulmonary vascular function, two aspects are of particular interest. One is the separation of active (e.g., changes in vasomotor tone, chronic changes in vessel wall properties, etc.) from passive (e.g., changes in vessel transmural pressures due to changes in left atrial pressure, cardiac output, transpulmonary pressures, etc.) pulmonary hemodynamic responses. A second is the identification of the longitudinal (arterial, venous, or capillary) location within the vascular bed where such responses occur. The separation of active and passive responses can be accomplished with the help of the mean pressure and flow data while the longitudinal location of pulmonary vascular changes is more readily decipherable from steady-state oscillatory pressure-flow data or from transient perturbations in the mean pressure-flow relations than from the mean pressure-flow relations alone.

PULMONARY VASCULAR RESISTANCE

The pulmonary vascular resistance is probably the least invasive and least technically difficult hemodynamic parameter to obtain from measurements of pressure and flow in vivo. The pulmonary vascular resistance (R) in the normal postnatal circulation is defined as the ratio of the mean pulmonary arterial-left atrial pressure difference and the cardiac output ($\dot{Q}$).

$$R = (Ppa - Pla)/\dot{Q} \tag{1}$$

where Ppa is the mean pulmonary artery pressure, and Pla is the mean left atrial pressure. The units of pulmonary vascular resistance are also defined by Eq. (1); namely, the units of pressure per unit of flow often expressed as dyn·sec/cm^5 or mmHg·min/L (7,15,16).

Wedge Pressure

In practice, Pla is generally replaced in Eq. (1) by the pulmonary arterial wedge pressure (Pw). The Pw is obtained by measuring the pressure at the tip of a catheter passed into a pulmonary branch artery. The catheter is then used to occlude the artery in which the catheter tip resides. The occlusion is accomplished by inflating a balloon located just upstream from the catheter tip, or by advancing the catheter tip until it is "wedged" in an artery whose diameter is the same as the catheter tip diameter. Thus, the flow in the smaller arteries, the capillaries, and the veins subtended by the occluded artery ceases. The tip of the wedged catheter is then open downstream through the resulting stagnant column of blood extending from the catheter tip through the microvascular bed to a vein of about the same diameter as the occluded artery. As long as this stagnant fluid column is continuous, the catheter tip pressure will be equal to the venous pressure at the confluence of this vein with the next larger vein carrying flowing blood. If the occluded artery is fairly large (on the order of 3 mm or larger), as is usually the case when a balloon-tipped catheter is used, the confluence will also be in a large vein, and the wedge pressure will normally be very close to left atrial pressure. The mean pulmonary artery pressure and the thermal dilution cardiac output can be measured using the same catheter. Thus, the mean pressures and flow in Eq. (1) can be obtained using a single percutaneous venous catheter (18).

One problem in obtaining the left atrial pressure from the wedge pressure is that the alveolar capillaries are collapsible (7,18,19,20). Thus, if the hydrostatic pressure at the relevant venous confluence is less than alveolar pressure, a condition referred to as the zone 2 condition, the catheter tip can be facing a blind termination in capillaries collapsed by the alveolar pressure. Under these conditions, Pw will no longer be a useful estimate of left atrial pressure. This problem is normally avoided by wedging the catheter in arteries which are below the level of the left atrium (zone 3). However, during positive pressure ventilation, even this precaution does not guarantee equivalence of Pw and Pla. Another potential problem is that of large vein obstruction in which a significant wedge pressure-left atrial pressure gradient could develop and go undetected without a measure of the pressure in the left atrium. Although the pulmonary arterial wedge pressure has also been referred to by alternative names, the term pulmonary capillary wedge pressure should probably be avoided since, in zone 3, Pw is generally a pressure downstream from the capillaries and closer to Pla.

In addition to the mean wedge pressure, the transient wedge pressure decay obtained immediately following balloon inflation contains potentially useful information. This information concerns the longitudinal location of pulmonary vascular responses and it has been used to estimate pulmonary capillary pressure (3,4,11). This approach is related to the vascular occlusion methods used in experimental

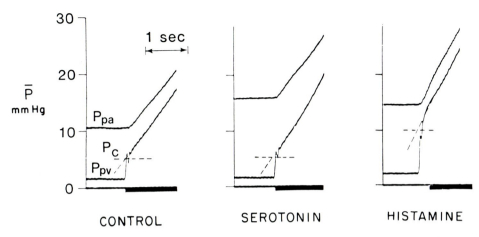

Figure 1: Pulmonary venous occlusion. Data obtained from a dog lung lobe perfused by a pump at a constant inflow rate. Before the venous occlusion (thin portion of abscissa line), the pulmonary arterial pressure, Ppa, and pulmonary venous pressure, Ppv, were constant. At the instant of occlusion, Ppv rapidly increased and then rose more slowly in a nearly linear fashion. After the rapid jump in Ppv, Ppa followed a time course nearly parallel to Ppv. A simple model consisting of series arterial and venous resistances separated by a microvascular compliance in parallel with the venous resistance can be used to interpret these data (see text). According to the model, the dashed horizontal line graphically separates the preocclusion arterial-venous pressure difference into the pressure drops upstream and downstream from the pressure of the microvascular compliance, Pc. Serotonin infusion increased the upstream pressure drop and histamine increased the downstream pressure drop. (Data from Dawson et al. [5].)

animal preparations (5,9,14). The information contained in the arterial and/or venous pressure curves when the inflow or outflow to a lung lobe is suddenly occluded can be appreciated by reference to Figure 1 which shows the transient pulmonary arterial and venous pressures which result when the venous outflow from a pump perfused dog lung lobe was suddenly occluded. The tracing of venous pressure (Pv) increases rapidly just after the occlusion and then follows a time course which is nearly linear in time. After the rapid jump in venous pressure, the arterial pressure (Pa) follows a time course roughly parallel to that of the venous pressure curve. The curves labeled serotonin and histamine were obtained during infusion of these vasoconstrictor agents. During serotonin infusion, the rapid rise in venous pressure is roughly equal to that under control conditions. In contrast, the rapid rise in venous pressure during histamine infusion is significantly larger than during control conditions. These features of the data can be explained by a simple model in which the vascular bed is represented by an arterial and venous vascular resistance separated by a microvascular compliance in parallel with the venous resistance (5). Prior to venous occlusion, there is a steady flow through the two series resistances, and the pulmonary arterial-venous pressure difference is the sum of the pressure drops across the resistances. When the venous outflow is occluded, the flow through the venous resistance stops and venous pressure rapidly rises to equal the microvascular or capillary pressure. Since flow continues through the arterial resistance and the continuously increasing volume is stored in the microvascular compliance, the pressure drop across the arterial resistance remains unchanged after occlusion. Hence, the pressure difference between the linear portions of the arterial and venous pressure curves is the arterial pressure drop. The data in Figure 1 are thus interpreted as indicating that the arterial pressure drop increased during serotonin infusion, while during histamine infusion the venous pressure drop increased.

Although this simple model understates the complexity of the actual distribution of vascular resistance and compliance (2,14), it is a useful conceptualization for interpreting the pressure decay at the tip of the balloon catheter when the balloon is inflated. Holloway et al. (11) and others (3,4) observed that after balloon inflation there was an initial rapid fall in pressure that was followed by a slower decay, reminiscent of the response predicted by the simple resistance compliance model used to explain Figure 1; that is, when the arterial inflow to the portion of the lung lobe subtended by the catheterized artery is stopped, the pressure at the catheter tip falls rapidly to the capillary pressure. This pressure then decays more slowly as the volume stored within the microvascular compliance discharges through the venous resistance.

This approach has the promise of being useful for deducing the sites of elevated pulmonary vascular resistance in vivo. While it can be difficult to identify a clear break in the pressure decay curve for specifying capillary pressure per se, and the extrapolation of the exponential decay curve backward in time can be equivocal, pulmonary vasoconstriction with arterial or venous constrictors does show clear differences in the exponential decay of the catheter tip pressure to the steady wedge pressure. Figure 2 is an example of the time course for the fall in pressure at the tip of a Swan Ganz catheter placed in a pulmonary artery of an anesthetized dog. The preocclusion pressure was increased by both serotonin and histamine infusion reflecting the vasoconstriction induced by these agents. Although the mean pressures were increased in both cases, the patterns of the changes in pulsatile pressure were different. When the balloon was inflated, the

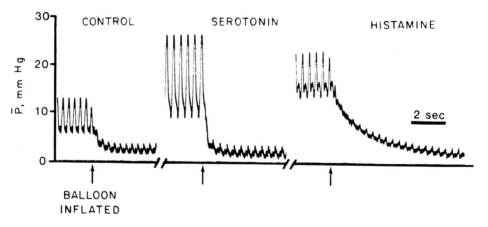

Figure 2: Serotonin or histamine infusion into a sublobar artery in an anesthetized dog. Pressures were recorded at the tip of a Swan Ganz catheter under control conditions and during the infusion of serotonin or histamine. The rate of fall in the pressure after balloon inflation (arrows) contains information about the site of vasoconstriction induced by serotonin or histamine.

time courses for the pressure decay down to the steady wedge pressure were also different. The large pulse pressure and rapid fall to the wedge pressure during serotonin infusion are consistent with arterial constriction while the relatively small change in pulse pressure and slow fall to the wedge pressure during histamine infusion are consistent with venous constriction. According to the simple model, consisting of resistances upstream and downstream from a microvascular compliance, the rapid fall (e.g., during serotonin infusion) occurs because a major fraction of the vascular volume is able to empty quickly through the low venous resistance; the slow fall (e.g., during histamine infusion) reflects slow emptying through a high venous resistance. Thus, when the pulmonary diastolic pressure is elevated, a rapid fall in the catheter tip pressure to the steady wedge pressure suggests that capillary pressure is close to left atrial pressure. On the other hand, a slow fall in pressure suggests that capillary pressure is closer to arterial pressure. Therefore, methods for objectively evaluating these pressure curves should prove useful for evaluating the site of elevated resistance.

Resistance and Mechanical Energy Balance

Equation (1) is only a definition of pulmonary vascular resistance. Its physical meaning is derived from consideration of the physical principles that relate pressure and flow, i.e., the fluid mechanical energy balance (8,15). As applied to the lung, this energy balance is

$$Ppa - Pla = \Delta KE + \Delta PE + LE \tag{2}$$

ΔKE represents the difference in kinetic energy of the flowing blood at the outlet and inlet of the pulmonary circulation. $\Delta KE = \rho v_v^2/2 - \rho v_a^2/2$, where ρ is the blood density and v_v and v_a are the mean pulmonary venous and arterial velocities, respectively. Since the mean pulmonary arterial and venous flow rates are virtually identical and $\dot{Q} = Av$, only the difference in cross-sectional area, A, between inlet and outlet would contribute to the measured $Ppa - Pla$ difference; the effect of this difference is generally assumed to be small enough to be ignored. ΔPE is the difference in potential energy or, equivalently, the hydrostatic pressure difference. This term is equal to ρgh where g is the acceleration due to gravity and h is the vertical elevation difference between the outlet and inlet. In practice, this term is eliminated from consideration by referencing both inlet and outlet pressures to a common vertical level rather than to the site of measurement. The last term in Eq. (2), LE, represents the loss of mechanical energy that results from the effects of friction (viscosity) as the blood flows through the vessels. Ignoring the changes in potential and kinetic energy between inlet and outlet, the pressure difference between inlet and outlet is the sum of the frictional losses from the inlet to the outlet. Thus, the definition of pulmonary vascular resistance in Eq. (1) is an explicit statement that the pressure difference due to the frictional losses is related to the mean blood flow rate by the proportionality factor, R, which is the mechanical energy dissipated into heat per unit of blood flow under the conditions of the measurements.

The analogy between Eq. (1) and Ohm's law for the steady flow of electrical current is often used to put Eq. (1) in perspective. This can be useful if the analogy is not carried too far. One utility of this analogy is in determining the contribution of serial and parallel resistances to this total vascular resistance of the organ. In accordance with this analogy, series resistances are additive while it is the reciprocals of the parallel resistances that are additive. Thus, the pulmonary vascular resistance can change as a result of changes in local serial resistances or by changing the number of perfused parallel vessels. The reciprocal rule for addition of parallel resistances helps to put the appropriate normalization of resistance with respect to body size into perspective. Since resistance falls with an increase in the number of parallel vessels, normalization with respect to body size (e.g., surface area or weight) should be done by forming the product of the resistance defined according to Eq. (1) and the body size or, equivalently, the normalized resistance is (Ppa − Pw)/cardiac index.

The local hemodynamic resistance is dependent on how the local geometric properties of the vasculature and the blood viscosity play their respective roles in the dissipation of mechanical energy. To this end, another useful concept is Poiseuille's law. For the steady, laminar (low Reynolds number) flow of a homogeneous Newtonian fluid in a long, cylindrical tube, the Poiseuille resistance is $8\eta l/\pi r^4$ (where l is vessel length) which is independent of the flow and the transmural pressure. The interrelationships defined by Poiseuille's law are very important, particularly as they provide insight concerning the role of blood viscosity (η) and the strong relationship which exists between vessel radius (r) and hemodynamic resistance. On the other hand, literal application to the vascular bed coupled with the implication that R is a constant in analogy with Ohm's law can be misleading. In the vascular bed, the existence of bifurcations, flow pulsations, the nonhomogeneous particulate nature of the blood and, particularly, the change in the geometry of the vascular bed with changes in transmural pressure, result in a situation in which R is not a constant independent of transmural pressure and flow. For instance, in the large vessels where there is a large pulsatile flow component and velocities can be high, the average velocity profiles over the flow cross section are blunted, resulting in mechanical energy losses due to viscosity that are larger than predicted by Poiseuille's law. The branching of the vessels and the small length to diameter ratios for the vessels also distort the mean velocity profile from the parabolic profile associated with the minimum resistance predicted by Poiseuille's law. In the small vessels (less than about 300μ), hematocrit, which is an important determinant of blood viscosity, is less than in the large vessels (the Fahraeus effect). This reduction in hematocrit causes the resistance in the small vessels to be smaller than that predicted using the large vessel blood viscosity.

The strong dependence of the vascular resistance on the luminal dimensions in distensible, collapsible vessels results in the resistances of the pulmonary vessels being dependent on transmural pressure. The pulmonary vessels can be classified according to the factors determining their perivascular pressure. The vessels, whose perivascular pressure is essentially alveolar pressure, are referred to as "alveolar vessels." Vessels whose perivascular pressure is determined by pleural pressure are called "extra-alveolar vessels." The extra-alveolar vessels can be further subdivided into two classes: those which are outside the lung parenchyma (the main pulmonary artery and lobar arteries and veins) and whose effective perivascular pressure is pleural or intrathoracic pressure, and those which are imbedded in the parenchyma and whose effective perivascular pressure is determined by both the pleural pressure and the interdependence between the vessels and surrounding parenchyma (7). When the transmural pressure is positive, the vessel diameters are directly proportional to the transmural pressure. The importance of this effort on vascular resistance can be put into perspective by observing that, according to the Poiseuille resistance, a 10 percent increase in vessel diameter will decrease the vascular resistance in that vessel by about 46 percent. Thus, when flow increases and intravascular pressures increase, the change in the arterial-left atrial pressure difference would be less than is expected if the vessels were rigid. When the transmural pressure becomes negative, vessel collapsibility, particularly for alveolar vessels, results in a situation in which the effective driving pressure controlling the flow rate is no longer the arterial-venous pressure difference which represents the total mechanical energy loss due to the flow.

This apparent dichotomy complicates the interpretation of how pressure depends on flow. To put this into perspective, consider that, when alveolar pressure exceeds the intravascular pressure at the venous end of the collapsible alveolar vessels, the alveolar vessels are compressed and the arterial-alveolar pressure difference becomes the driving pressure for the flow. Under these conditions, referred to as zone 2 conditions (20), the flow through the alveolar vessels has been likened to the flow over a waterfall or sluice gate, in which case the height of the waterfall, analogous with the difference between alveolar and left atrial pressures, does not influence the flow (19). Although changes in the alveolar-left atrial pressure difference (occurring under zone 2 conditions as the geometry of the alveolar vessels varies) are not necessarily accompanied by an alteration in flow, these changes always reflect changes in total vascular resistance and, hence, changes in the mechanical energy dissipated. The increased resistance associated with the narrowing of the alveolar vessels is commonly referred to as the "Starling resistance." The influence of this behavior of the alveolar vessels on pressure-flow relations in the lungs is used to help explain the normal gravity-dependent vertical gradient in pulmonary blood flow (20). The mechanical phenomenon involved in the low Reynolds number flow in the alveolar vessels has been discussed in detail by Fung (8). Additionally, the concept that active wall tension can have an effect on pulmonary artery pressure-flow relations in a manner similar to alveolar pressure by producing a Starling resistor-like phenomenon in pulmonary vessels even when vascular pressures exceed alveolar pressure has also been used to interpret pulmonary vascular pressure-flow relations as discussed below.

The Pulmonary Vascular Pressure-Flow Curve

In an attempt to understand better the meaning of pulmonary vascular resistance, particularly as it relates to detection of active pulmonary vascular responses, the pulmonary arterial-venous pressure difference has been measured over a range of flow rates (with other variables such as transpulmonary pressure and left atrial pressure held constant) (14,17). In Figure 3, the mean pressure versus flow data is shown from experiments on isolated perfused cat lungs (14). The pressure versus flow curve has a hyperbolic appearance, concave to the flow axis. The slope of the chord connecting the origin at zero flow with any point on the curve is the pulmonary vascular resistance (R) at that flow rate as defined by

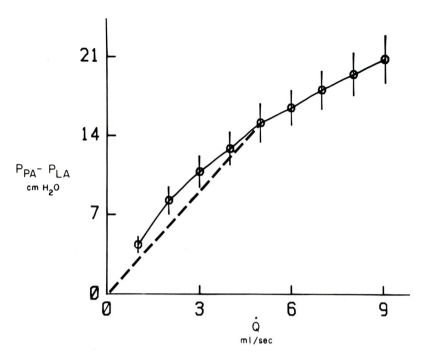

Figure 3: Pressure-flow data from isolated perfused cat lungs. Flow was varied over the indicated range while the downstream pressure, Pla, was held constant. The slope of the chord (dashed line) connecting any point on the curve with the zero flow origin is the pulmonary vascular resistance, Eq. (1). As flow increases, the slope of the chord decreases, indicating a decrease in pulmonary vascular resistance. (Data from Kristnan et al. [14].)

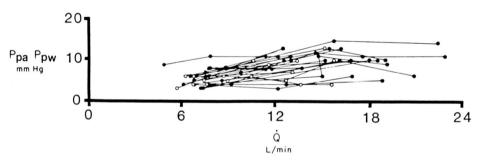

Figure 4: Pressure-flow curves from exercising humans. The mean pulmonary artery pressure, $\bar{P}pa$, minus the mean pulmonary artery wedge pressure, $\bar{P}pw$, is plotted against cardiac output ($\dot{Q}$). Cardiac output was increased by exercise. For normal subjects, the pressure-flow curve is quite flat. (Data from Ekelund and Holmgren [6].)

Eq. (1). Since the slope of the chord decreases with increasing flow, it is clear that the pulmonary vascular resistance decreases with increasing flow. Over the higher range of physiological flow rates, the curve appears to approach a linear asymptote which has a slope smaller than the vascular resistance. The advantage of the pressure versus flow curve over a single measurement of the pressures and flow can be appreciated by noting that changes in vasomotor tone are commonly associated with changes in cardiac output. If both the cardiac output and the arterial-venous pressure difference were to change in the same direction, a concomitant change in vasomotor tone would be difficult to recognize if only the pulmonary vascular resistance were calculated. On the other hand, a change in vasomotor tone could be observed as a shift in the whole pressure versus flow curve if the arterial-venous pressure differences were measured over a range of flows.

In man, the pressure-flow curve has been studied by making measurements of pressures and cardiac output at varying intensity of exercise (6,13,18). This usually results in an increase in wedge pressure as well as pulmonary artery pressure with an increasing cardiac output. This is in contrast to experiments such as that shown in Figure 3 in which left atrial pressure is generally held constant. When the Ppa − Pw difference is plotted versus flow in exercising man, the resulting pressure-flow curve can be even flatter than curves obtained with constant left atrial pressure in animal experiments. This is presumably due, at least in part, to the additional vascular distension that results from the increase in left atrial pressure. Figure 4 shows pressure-flow curves from normal exercising human subjects (2). The flat curves reflect, in some cases, rather marked decreases in pulmonary vascular resistance with increasing flow.

To obtain additional insights from changes in the shape of the pressure-flow curve, attempts have been made to explain the curve in terms of the vessel mechanics which might be responsible for its shape. One popular view is to assume that the pulmonary vascular bed consists of parallel vascular pathways of essentially nondistensible vessels, with the flow through each pathway controlled by the pulmonary artery pressure and a range of critical closing pressures among the parallel pathways (16).

According to this view, the resistance in each pathway can be conceptually divided into two series components; one a constant resistance which is the resistance of the open rigid pathway, and the other a Starling resistance. The constant resistance has sometimes been referred to as the Ohmic resistance of the pathway (to distinguish it from the variable Starling resistance). According to this model, this closing pressure that controls the Starling resistance can be the alveolar pressure surrounding the alveolar vessels or an effective pressure such as that generated by smooth muscle tone. The latter could result, even under zone 3 conditions, in narrowing within some flow limiting segment of the vasculature (e.g., in muscular arteries or veins). According to this concept, the closing pressure is a force that controls the Starling resistance when downstream pressures within a given parallel pathway are low relative to this closing pressure. Flow is then determined by the arterial pressure-closing pressure difference existing across the Ohmic resistance. When arterial pressure is below the closing pressure, the pathway is closed.

With the parallel pathways presenting a range of closing pressures, the shape of the pressure-flow curve can be explained. Near the origin, the pressure rises rapidly with increasing flow, but resistance falls as flow is distributed among increasing numbers of parallel vessels as their respective closing pressures are exceeded. Eventually, when the arterial pressure has become high enough such that all of the parallel pathways are open, the slope of the pressure-flow curve becomes constant. The intercept of the linear portion of the curve extrapolated back to zero flow is interpreted to be a pressure equal to a weighted average of the closing pressures for the entire pulmonary vascular bed. In this model then, the arterial pressure-mean closing pressure difference is considered to control the flow, and the slope of the linear portion of the pressure-flow curve is the harmonic mean of the parallel Ohmic resistances upstream from the locus of the closing pressures (16). This model is appealing because it provides a conceptual basis for a two-parameter (slope and intercept) description of the pressure-flow curve as fitted with a straight line. Specifically, the slope of the line is the upstream Ohmic resistance and the intercept is the mean closing pressure.

One problem with interpreting this model, particularly for its application to the zone 3 lung, is that the shape of the pressure-flow curve alone is not sufficient evidence to demonstrate the uniqueness of this model. In particular, the model ignores the potential influence of the distensibility of the small resistance vessels. Recently, Fung and his co-workers (8) have demonstrated that a pressure-flow curve, with a shape that appears to be experimentally indistinguishable from that typically observed for lungs, can be obtained using a model in which the vessels are distensible but without closing pressures. Thus, the description of the pressure-flow curve strictly in terms of closing pressures and nondistensible vessels probably overstates the importance of the Ohmic and Starling resistor dichotomy. This dichotomy also has the consequence that, as long as the slope of the pressure-flow curve continues to be constant with increasing flow, all pressures downstream from the locus of the critical closing pressure must remain less than the critical closing pressure. If at some point along the pressure-flow curve the downstream pressure exceeded the critical closing pressure, the controlling pressure difference would then become the arterial-left atrial pressure difference and the slope of the pressure-flow curve would increase. Since this has not been generally observed, the implication would be that the pressure drop downstream from the critical closing pressure is a very small fraction of the total arterial-venous pressure difference. If one assumes that the capillaries (1) and/or veins (8,12) contribute substantially to the total resistance in the zone 3 lung, the anatomical location for the closing pressure must be close to the venous outflow from the vascular bed, and it is not clear how the closing pressure would be generated in these vessels.

The Ohmic-Starling resistor model for explaining the pulmonary pressure-flow curve has been used to interpret the influence of pulmonary vasoconstriction in terms of its apparent effects on the mean closing pressure and vessel diameters. According to this model, a parallel shift in the pressure-flow curve to higher pressures indicates an increase in closing pressures with the result that the Starling resistance is increased. On the other hand, an increase in slope indicates a decreasing diameter of the Ohmic resistance vessels, thereby resulting in an increase in the Ohmic resistance. A parallel shift, such as has been observed with hypoxic vasoconstriction (16,17), has been used as evidence in favor of this dichotomy of effects.

Recently, however, Mitzner and Huang (17) have shown that a parallel shift of the pressure-flow curve can be theoretically produced in a distensible vessel model when vasoconstriction increases both the resistance and compliance of the constricted vessels. Thus, a distensible vessel model of vascular resistance appears to account for the response to vasoconstriction equally as well as the Ohmic-Starling resistor model.

On closer examination, the two concepts may not need to be considered as mutually exclusive as they seem. Consider the fact that the compliance of a vessel under Starling resistor conditions is very large when compared to the compliance that is obtained when the transmural pressure is positive over the entire length of the vessel (8). Thus, increasing closing pressures would cause a large increase in vessel compliance when fully open vessels develop a Starling resistance. Moreover, the model of Mitzner and Huang (17) may be a demonstration that, although the all-or-none Starling resistor model is a conceptual oversimplification, it does incorporate certain aspects of the relevant physics. In light of the above discussion, however, the previous interpretations of the slope and intercept are now obscured in that, while these parameters may be useful empirical descriptors of the pressure-flow curve, their physical meaning is not so clear. Their utility then comes from the fact that a shift in the pressure-flow curve in the absence of substantial changes in other relevant variables, such as pleural or left atrial pressure, is convincing evidence for an active pulmonary vascular response.

Knowledge of the shape of the normal pulmonary vascular pressure-flow curve is necessary to put the concept of pulmonary vascular resistance into practical perspective. A change in the calculated resistance from one time, or condition, to another is indicative of some change in pulmonary vascular geometry. However, given the normal pulmonary vascular pressure versus flow curve, it is difficult to see any particular advantage of calculating the vascular resistance for an individual set of Ppa, Pla, and $\dot{Q}$ measurements since it is the values of Pa, Pw or Pla, and $\dot{Q}$ themselves that are needed to interpret the resistance value. A comparison of measured Ppa with normal values indicates whether there is pulmonary hypertension. A comparison of Pw with normal values indicates whether the pulmonary hypertension is the result of high left atrial pressure or high pulmonary vascular resistance. Due to the relative flatness of the pulmonary artery pressure versus flow curve, cardiac output would have to be rather high to produce a substantially elevated Pa pressure. A low cardiac output along with an elevated Pa pressure and normal Pw could be indicative of rather severe obstruction whereas a low cardiac output and a high resistance with a normal pulmonary artery pressure might not indicate any pulmonary vascular involvement.

While the full pressure-flow curve is not readily available in clinical practice, the use of an exercise test to evaluate the pulmonary circulation derives its utility from the same principle. In other words, a reduced distensibility of the pulmonary vascular bed is clearly demonstrated by an inordinate increase in Ppa − Pw with increased cardiac output. The use of a vasodilator to detect an active vasomotor component in pulmonary hypertension also has to be evaluated with an appreciation for the shape of the pressure-flow curve. For example, a decrease in pulmonary vascular resistance accompanied by an increase in cardiac output does not necessarily imply pulmonary vasodilation.

OSCILLATORY PRESSURE FLOW RELATIONS, INPUT IMPEDANCE

The pulmonary arterial input impedance can be calculated from measurements of pulsatile pressure and flow near the entrance of the pulmonary artery (7,10,15). An advantage of pulsatile pressure flow data over the mean pressures and flow is that they contain information about the elastic properties as well as the geometry of the pulmonary arterial tree. The input impedance, defined as the ratio of the amplitudes of oscillatory pressure to oscillatory flow at a given frequency, can be determined from the measured phasic pressure and flow curves when they are mathematically resolved into their sinusoidal components.

To calculate the input impedance, the measured pulsatile pressure ($P[t]$) and flow ($\dot{Q}(t)$) are expressed as the sum of sinusoidal waves of various amplitudes, frequencies, and phase angles as follows:

$$P(t) = \bar{P} + \sum_{k=1}^{k_{max}} P_k \cos(k\omega t - \beta_k) \tag{3}$$

and

$$\dot{Q}(t) = \bar{\dot{Q}} + \sum_{k=1}^{k_{max}} \dot{Q}_k \cos(k\omega t - \alpha_k) \tag{4}$$

where k represents successive positive integer multiples (harmonics) of the fundamental angular frequency, ω, in radians ($\omega = 2\pi f$ where f is the heart rate) up to an arbitrary maximum value, k_{max}; $\bar{P}$ and $\bar{\dot{Q}}$ are respectively the mean pulmonary artery pressure and flow; P_k and $\dot{Q}_k$ are the amplitudes of the pressure and flow waves for the kth harmonic, respectively; and β_k and α_k are their respective phase angles. To calculate the input impedance, each harmonic of the above series can be written in terms of a complex number according to

$$p_k = P_k \{\exp[j(k\omega t - \beta_k)]\} \tag{5}$$

and

$$q_k = \dot{Q}_k \{\exp[j(k\omega t - \alpha_k)]\} \tag{6}$$

where $j = \sqrt{-1}$. The input impedance is then a complex number defined as:

$$Z(k\omega) = p_k/q_k = (P_k/\dot{Q}_k)\exp[j(\alpha_k - \beta_k)] \tag{7}$$

which is characterized by a modulus, $Z_k = P_k/\dot{Q}_k$, and a phase angle, $\phi_k = (\alpha_k - \beta_k)$, for each frequency, $k\omega$.

An assumption underlying the concept of the input impedance is that the pulmonary arterial tree behaves as a linear system, i.e., the pressure and flow of a given frequency are independent of the magnitude of the pressure, and the pressure and flow waves of each frequency are independent of those of other frequencies. The assumption of linearity can be only an approximation in real blood vessels, but it appears to be adequate such that nonlinearities do not appear to confuse the interpretation of the calculated impedance (15).

The impedance spectrum, in terms of modulus and phase angle, is dependent on both the geometry and compliance of the pulmonary arterial tree. In the normal lung, the modulus of the pulmonary arterial input impedance first decreases from the zero frequency value and then fluctuates between relative maxima and minima with increasing frequency. The phase angle is negative (flow leads pressure) for low infrequencies and then becomes positive near the first minimum in the modulus. The modulus at zero frequency represents the input resistance, i.e., the mean arterial pressure divided by mean flow, although sometimes the pulmonary vascular resistance defined by Eq. (1) is used. The fluctuations in the impedance modulus with frequency are due to reflections from regions within the vascular bed in which there is a change in the characteristic impedance. Although such changes are essentially continuous through the vascular bed, relatively sharp changes occur in the distal arterial tree. This results in fairly consistent fluctuations in the normal impedance spectrum. The frequencies of these fluctuations are dependent on the distance between the measuring site and the sites of major reflections as well as the compliance and the wave speed in the arteries; thus, they are dependent on body size. The negative phase angle at low frequencies indicates the dominance of the arterial compliance while the positive phase angle at higher frequencies reveals the dominance of inertial effects including reflections. The characteristic impedance of the pulmonary artery is the value of the input impedance had there been no reflections. Thus, the characteristic impedance cannot be measured directly in vivo. An estimate of the characteristic impedance of the pulmonary artery is generally obtained by averaging the impedance moduli for frequencies equal to or greater than the frequency of the first minimum.

The characteristic impedance, the frequency of the first minimum and maximum, and other specific features of the input impedance spectrum then provide objective means of characterizing changes in the input impedance spectrum. Narrowing or dilation of the small arteries changes the input resistance and wave reflections and, thus, the magnitudes of the maxima and minima and the frequencies at which they occur. A decrease in compliance of the large arteries shifts the maxima and minima to higher frequencies. The characteristic impedance is increased by stiffening and/or narrowing of the arteries. As in the case of the vascular resistance, interpretation of the measured input impedance in terms of active responses of the pulmonary arterial tree is complicated by the fact that the vessel elastic properties and geometry are influenced by both active and passive factors. Thus, evaluation of the contribution of active and passive phenomena can be problematic. In general, an increase in the characteristic impedance is evidence for a decrease in compliance of the large arteries whereas an increase in the input resistance is consistent with increased resistance in small vessels or elevated left atrial pressure. The stiffening of the larger pulmonary arteries reflected by an increase in characteristic impedance results in an increase in the pulsatile component of right ventricular work for a given mean flow and, thus, a less efficient ventricle. Figure 5 shows examples of how the pulmonary input impedance spectrum can vary in patients with pulmonary vascular disease.

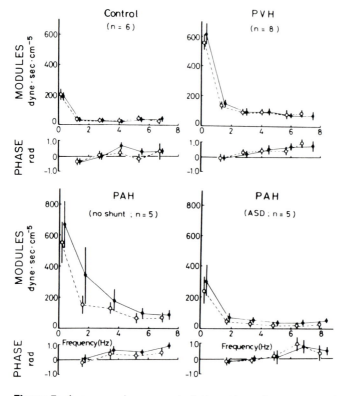

Figure 5: Average pulmonary arterial input impedance spectra in a control group of human subjects and in patients with pulmonary venous hypertension (PVH group), in patients with pulmonary arterial hypertension (PAH group), and in patients with pulmonary arterial hypertension and atrial septal defect (ASD). The continuous lines and solid circles were obtained while the subjects breathed room air; the dashed lines and open circles while the subjects breathed oxygen. Pulmonary artery pressure and flow velocity were measured using catheter tip transducers. (Reproduced from Haneda et al. [10].)

In conclusion, changes in the pulmonary vascular pressure flow relationship can provide considerable insight into the hemodynamic function of the lung vasculature. However, interpretation of changes in vascular resistance and impedance also requires some insight into the factors that influence the normal pulmonary hemodynamics. Some of these factors can be conceptualized by the use of simple analogies and models which can be quite useful if kept in proper perspective.

REFERENCES

1. Bhattacharya J, Staub NC: Direct measurement of microvascular pressures in isolated perfused dog lung. Science 210 : 327–328, 1980.

2. Bronikowski TA, Dawson CA, Linehan JH: Limits on continuous distribution of pulmonary vascular resistance versus compliance from outflow occlusion. Microvasc Res 30 : 306–313, 1985.

3. Collee GG, Lynch KE, Hill RD, Zapol WM: Bedside measurement of pulmonary capillary pressure in patients with acute respiratory failure. Anesthesiology 66 : 614–620, 1987.

4. Cope DK, Allison RC, Parmentier JL, Miller JN, Taylor AE: Measurement of effective pulmonary capillary pressure using the pressure profile after pulmonary artery occlusion. Crit Care Med 14 : 16–22, 1986.

5. Dawson CA, Linehan JH, Rickaby DA: Pulmonary microcirculatory hemodynamics. Ann NY Acad Sci 394 : 90–106, 1982.

6. Ekelund LG, Holmgren A: Central hemodynamics during exercise. Circ Res 20:I-33; I-43 (Suppl I), 1967.

7. Fishman AP: Pulmonary circulation, in Fishman AP, Fisher AB (eds), *Handbook of Physiology. Sect 3: The Respiratory System, Vol I: Circulation and Nonrespiratory Functions.* Baltimore, American Physiological Society, 1985, pp 93–165.

8. Fung YC: *Biodynamics: Circulation.* New York, Springer-Verlag, 1984.

9. Hakim TS, Michel RP, Chang HK: Partitioning of pulmonary vascular resistance in dogs by arterial and venous occlusion. J Appl Physiol 52 : 710–715, 1982.

10. Haneda T, Nakajima T, Shirato K, Onodera S, Takishima T: Effects of oxygen breathing on pulmonary vascular input impedance in patients with pulmonary hypertension. Chest 83 : 520–533, 1983.

11. Holloway H, Perry M, Downey J, Parker J, Taylor A: Estimation of effective pulmonary capillary pressure in intact lungs. J Appl Physiol 54 : 846–851, 1983.

12. Hyman AL: Effects of large increases in pulmonary blood flow on pulmonary venous pressure. J Appl Physiol 27 : 179–185, 1969.

13. Janicki JS, Weber KT, Likoff MJ, Fishman AP: The pressure-flow response of the pulmonary circulation in patients with heart failure and pulmonary vascular disease. Circulation 72 : 1270–1278, 1985.

14. Krishnan A, Linehan JH, Rickaby DA, Dawson CA: Cat lung hemodynamics: Comparison of experimental results and model predictions. J Appl Physiol 61 : 2023–2034, 1986.

15. Milnor WR: *Hemodynamics.* Baltimore, Williams and Wilkins, 1982.

16. Mitzner W: Resistance of the pulmonary circulation. Clin Chest Med 4 : 127–137, 1983.

17. Mitzner W, Huang I: Interpretation of pressure-flow curves in the pulmonary vascular bed, in Will JA, Dawson CA, Weir EK, Buckner CA (eds), *The Pulmonary Circulation in Health and Disease.* Orlando, FL, Academic Press, 1987, pp 215–230.

18. O'Quin R, Marini JJ: Pulmonary artery occlusion pressure: Clinical physiology, measurement, and interpretation. Am Rev Respir Dis 128 : 319–326, 1983.

19. Permutt S, Bromberger-Barnea B, Bane HN: Alveolar pressure, pulmonary venous pressure, and the vascular water fall. Med Thorac 19 : 239–260, 1962.

20. West JB, Dollery CT: Distribution of blood flow and the pressure-flow relations of the whole lung. J Appl Physiol 20 : 175–183, 1965.

John N. Evans, Ph.D.
Janice T. Coflesky, Ph.D.

5

Endothelial and Smooth Muscle Cell Interaction

The pulmonary circulation normally functions as a low pressure system despite the fact that it continually receives the entire cardiac output. This unique property is generally ascribed to its being a highly compliant system in which the contribution of active smooth muscle tone is low. A high level of compliance may result from reduced amounts of smooth muscle in the pulmonary arterial wall when compared to systemic vessels of comparable size and/or a lower level of activation of these muscle cells. Pulmonary vessel wall tension is dependent upon both the active tone of medial smooth muscle cells and passive mechanical properties. The latter of these components is largely determined by structural elements, particularly the connective tissue matrix. Pulmonary vascular resistance can be significantly increased in disorders of the lung resulting in pressures approaching those of the systemic circulation. Increases in pulmonary arterial pressure arise from a reduction in total vascular cross-sectional area through some combination of vessel obliteration and lumen narrowing due to increased wall tension.

It has become evident that endothelial cells play a vital role in the biology of the vascular wall. They provide a barrier function, actively metabolize vasoactive compounds, regulate cell proliferation, and modulate the contractile responses of smooth muscle cells to a variety of mediators. This chapter concentrates on specific interactions between the endothelial cell and underlying smooth muscle within the pulmonary blood vessel wall. We discuss three topic areas: pharmacological responses, vessel wall metabolism, and cellular proliferation. In order to relate these topics to the development of pulmonary hypertension, we describe the results of experiments which utilized a model of pulmonary hypertension induced by exposure of rats to elevated fractions of oxygen.

ENDOTHELIAL RELATED SMOOTH MUSCLE RELAXATION

Since Furchgott and Zawadzki first reported that endothelial cells are required for the relaxation of isolated blood vessels by acetylcholine, a number of laboratories have demonstrated the importance of a functional endothelium in the maintenance of vascular tone within both the systemic and pulmonary circulations (3,11). Endothelial cells produce an inhibitory factor termed endothelium-derived relaxing factor (EDRF) which is a highly labile substance with a very short half-life. This factor has been implicated in the relaxations of precontracted blood vessels to a variety of pharmacological agents. Palmer et al. have recently published data which indicate that EDRF may be nitric oxide (15). Whether there are multiple EDRFs is unclear at the present time.

Whatever the factor, one mechanism of action appears to be the stimulation of soluble guanylate cyclase and a resultant increase in levels of cyclic guanosine $3'5'$-monophosphate (cGMP) which are then responsible for the dilatory effect. Recently, Ignarro et al. have shown that bovine intrapulmonary vessels contain cGMP and that these levels of cGMP are significantly reduced when the endothelium is removed (12). Interestingly, they also reported that smaller vessels had a higher concentration of cGMP than those which were larger and more central. This finding may have important implications for the control of vascular responsiveness at various levels of the pulmonary circulation.

Given the demonstrated importance of the endothelium in the control of vascular tone, we chose to investigate endothelium-dependent pharmacological responses in an animal model of pulmonary hypertension (7). Male Sprague-Dawley rats were exposed to 85% O_2 for 7 days and the response of isolated vessel segments was assessed. Segments of immediately intrapulmonary vessels were isolated and mounted on two small parallel wires in a myograph which permitted the measurement of circumferential tension development at controlled muscle lengths in response to selected agents. This system was chosen based upon the knowledge that chronic exposure of rats to elevated fractions of inspired oxygen for 21 days results in endothelial cell injury and the development of pulmonary hypertension (8). This hypertension is associated with significant vascular remodelling and changes in the contractile properties of isolated pulmonary arteries. Following 7 days of in vivo exposure to 85% O_2, examination of the vessel luminal surfaces by scanning electron microscopy revealed marked swelling and sloughing of the endothelium with focal areas of necrosis. There was also evidence of inflammatory cell influx and adherence of platelets to the injured wall. Concentration response curves to prostaglandin $F_{2\alpha}$ in vessels from the oxygen-exposed rats demonstrated increased sensitivity. The experimental dose to produce 50 percent of the maximum response was reduced while the maximal response itself was unchanged. The functional state of the endothelium was assessed in vessels precontracted with $PGF_{2\alpha}$ by determining the degree of relaxation to the cumulative addition of acetylcholine (Fig. 1). Control vessels were fully relaxed by acetylcholine while arteries isolated from the oxygen exposed rats relaxed by only 30 per-

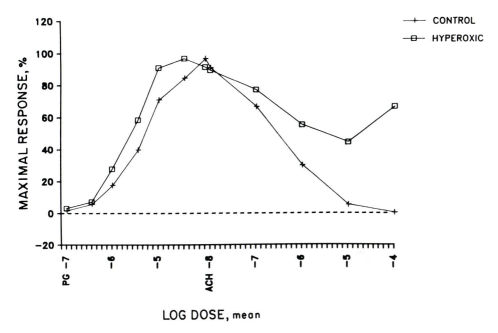

Figure 1: Concentration-response curves: adult proximal intrapulmonary arteries. Concentration-response curves to prostaglandin $F_{2\alpha}$ (PG) were generated for each isolated control (+) and hyperoxic (□) vessel. Increasing concentrations of acetylcholine (ACh) were added to the precontracted vessels to assess relaxant effects. Each point represents the mean + SEM of six experiments.

cent. The response to acetylcholine was abolished in both groups by the addition of atropine (10^{-6}M).

To verify that the smooth muscle cells were indeed capable of complete relaxation, we tested responses to the addition of sodium nitroprusside, a non-endothelium-dependent dilator. In both the control and treated tissues, sodium nitroprusside caused full relaxation of the contraction induced by $PGF_{2\alpha}$. Methylene blue, a specific blocker of soluble guanylate cyclase, reversed the relaxation induced by acetylcholine, thus indicating a role for cGMP and supporting the concept that acetylcholine was working through an endothelial cell-mediated mechanism.

These results have important implications for our understanding of the mechanisms underlying the control of pulmonary vascular resistance. They demonstrate that altered pharmacological responses of the vasculature can be induced by physiological injury to the endothelium which do not extend to complete cell denudation as has been performed in most in vitro experiments. Taken from this perspective, the endothelial cell damage occurring during hyperoxic injury to the lung represents an in vivo model of cellular derangement in which specific alterations in vascular response may be assessed as they contribute to the development of pulmonary hypertension. These results bear further on the fact that it is clearly not sufficient to assume that the histological presence of an endothelium implies its functional integrity in the vessel wall.

Recent research has supported evidence of an in situ endothelial-dependent system in the lung. Several investigators have studied perfused lung preparations to evaluate the role of the endothelium in determining pharmacological responsiveness in both normal and injured lungs. Rounds et al. demonstrated increased pulmonary vascular reactivity to hypoxia and angiotensin II in rats with acute lung injury induced by administration of α-naphthylthiourea (ANTU) (18). This treatment causes injury of the endothelial cell and supports the contention that the endothelium is important in maintaining low tone in the lung. Cherry and Gillis have further demonstrated that acetylcholine reduces pulmonary arterial pressure in a bed whose pressure had previously been elevated by cyclooxygenase blockade (4). The dilatory response is blocked by quinacrine and hemoglobin which are known to antagonize endothelium-dependent relaxation of vascular smooth muscle. This finding suggests that endothelium-dependent factors may be released within the pulmonary circulation and contribute to the regulation of blood flow in the lung.

VESSEL WALL METABOLISM

The pulmonary vasculature plays a vital role in metabolic processes by generating, activating, and inactivating biologically potent compounds (1). Metabolism of these substances by the lung can produce local effects on vascular tone, airway reactivity, and microvascular permeability, while also regulating the composition of blood passing through the pulmonary circuit. The homeostatic functions of the endothelium are altered during acute injury to the lung. These alterations contribute to inflammatory responses, initiate metabolic changes in the vessel wall, and ultimately result in local variations in vascular tone during the development of pulmonary hypertension.

Following damage to the endothelium, excessive formation and reduced degradation of compounds such as prostaglandins, thromboxanes, leukotrienes, platelet-activating factor, activated complement, and proteolytic enzymes have been reported (19). Considerable evidence has linked these substances to various pulmonary manifestations of hyperoxic lung injury. Although the pathophysiology of pulmonary oxygen toxicity has been studied extensively, much remains unknown about the factors which trigger metabolic changes, the mechanism of their activation or release, the interactions among them, and their relative importance in eliciting structural and functional changes within the pulmonary circulation. Recent attention has focused on the role of potent metabolites of arachidonic acid (i.e., prostaglandins, thromboxanes, and leukotrienes) in mediating inflammatory processes and pulmonary edema formation during acute lung injury. In particular, the ability of these substances to increase vascular permeability and elicit prominent vasomotor responses has been emphasized.

We hypothesized that changes in the relative production of dilatory and constrictor substances by the vessel wall during hyperoxic injury may alter vascular reactivity and contribute to the development of pulmonary hypertension. To address this question, we examined the accumulation of arachidonic acid metabolites by pulmonary arteries isolated from rats exposed in vivo to 85% O_2 (5). The accumulation of these products was measured in vessel organ cultures under basal and stimulated experimental conditions. Individual arterial samples were placed in Waymouth's culture medium and incubated for 24 hr at 37°C with

95% air–5% CO_2. At the end of the 24-hr period, media was removed from the samples and immediately frozen at $-70°C$ for later assay of basal accumulation levels of metabolites. Following transfer of tissues to new culture plates, fresh medium was added and product accumulation was stimulated by the addition of acetylcholine (ACh) $(10^{-5}M)$. Accumulation of prostacyclin (PGI_2), thromboxane A_2 (TXA_2), prostaglandin E_2 (PGE_2), and peptidyl leukotrienes (LT) (C_4,D_4,E_4) was measured by radioimmunoassay. Measured levels of arachidonic acid metabolites in the media were normalized to milligrams of explant tissue protein and expressed as ng/mg protein.

Prostacyclin was the predominant vessel wall product measured among isolated arteries and was present in amounts 3-fold greater than thromboxane A_2, the next most abundant metabolite (Fig. 2). The basal levels of prostaglandin E_2 and peptidyl leukotriene were relatively minimal. Significantly greater amounts of PGI_2 were measured among adult control proximal pulmonary arteries com-

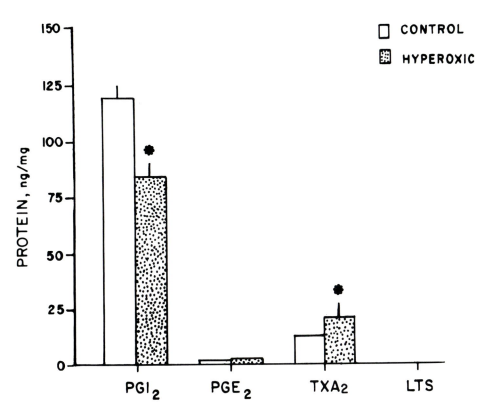

Figure 2: Proximal pulmonary artery: products of vessel wall metabolism. The results reflect the basal accumulation of stable metabolites of prostacyclin (PGI_2), prostaglandin E_2 (PGE_2), thromboxane A_2 (TXA_2), and peptidyl leukotrienes C_4, D_4, and E_4 (LTS) by organ cultures during a 24-hr incubation period following vessel isolation. Individual vessel samples were cultured in Waymouth's culture media at 37°C with 95% air/5% CO_2. At the end of the incubation period, media were removed and frozen at $-70°C$ for subsequent assay. For each product, control and hyperoxic tissues are compared (n = 10). (* indicates a significant difference between hyperoxic and control at $p < .05$.)

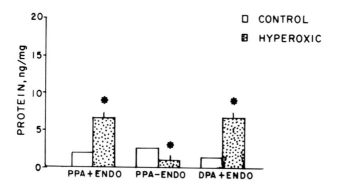

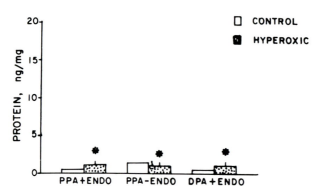

Figure 3: Stimulated accumulation of prostacyclin (PGI$_2$) (upper panel) and thromboxane (TXA$_2$) (lower panel). The figures show the accumulation of the stable metabolites of PGI$_2$ and TXA$_2$ during a 1-hr incubation of explant cultures of hilar intrapulmonary arteries in the presence of 10^{-5} M ACh. The three groups of arteries include: adult proximal pulmonary artery with intact endothelium (PPA + ENDO); adult proximal pulmonary artery with endothelium removed (PPA − ENDO); and adult distal pulmonary artery with intact endothelium (DPA + ENDO). Comparisons are made between hyperoxic and control within arteries within each group (n = 10). Not shown are the results indicating that, in the presence of media alone, accumulation of product during 1 hr was not detectable. Data are expressed as ng product/mg protein. (* indicates a significant difference between hyperoxic and control at p < .05.)

pared to hyperoxic tissues under conditions of basal accumulation. This difference between control and hyperoxic arteries was also observed among proximal pulmonary arteries stripped of endothelium. It was possible to stimulate accumulation of prostacyclin with 10^{-5}M ACh in proximal and distal pulmonary arteries (Fig. 3, upper panel). Stimulation of hyperoxic arteries produced significantly greater amounts of PGI$_2$ than control vessels. When hyperoxic pulmonary arteries were mechanically stripped of endothelium, accumulation of PGI$_2$ in response to ACh was reduced. This result suggests that the endothelium of hyperoxic pul-

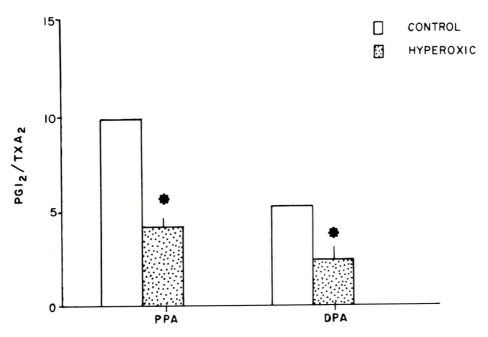

Figure 4: Ratio of prostacyclin (PGI$_2$) to thromboxane A$_2$ (TXA$_2$) production. The data represent the ratios of stable metabolites of PGI$_2$ and TXA$_2$ in explant cultures of proximal and distal intrapulmonary arteries following a 24-hr incubation period after vessel isolation. For each ratio, separate comparisons between control and hyperoxic tissues are shown (n = 10). PPA = proximal pulmonary artery; DPA = distal pulmonary artery. (* indicates a significant difference between hyperoxic and control at p < .05.)

monary arteries contributes to the enhanced accumulation of PGI$_2$ upon stimulation with Ach, since its removal reduced the amount of product measured.

Hyperoxic arterial explants accumulated greater amounts of the stable metabolite TXA$_2$ than control tissues during 24-hr basal incubation (Fig. 2). Significant increases in this product were noted in both adult proximal and distal artery sites. Additionally, hyperoxic arteries accumulated greater amounts of TXB$_2$ upon stimulation with acetylcholine (Fig. 3, lower panel). This response was reversed upon mechanical stripping of the endothelium, implying a role for the hyperoxic endothelium in enhancing thromboxane levels measured in response to exogenous stimuli.

In order to depict changes in the relative amounts of potent vasodilators and vasoconstrictors in the pulmonary arterial wall, we compared the ratio of prostacyclin to thromboxane A$_2$ accumulation under basal conditions (Fig. 4). This ratio was significantly decreased in both adult hyperoxic proximal and distal arteries when compared to control vessels. Although these ratios do not necessarily reflect the relative potency of the products in the intact tissues, the apparent balance between vasodilating and vasoconstricting thrombogenic substances is shifted in favor of vasoconstriction following hyperoxic damage to the lung.

Organ culture methodologies provide an effective and sensitive means of assaying the products of vessel wall metabolism in intact samples of isolated control and injured pulmonary arteries. Significant differences exist in the amounts of specific metabolites accumulated by control, oxygen-exposed, and mechanically denuded pulmonary arteries. Of further importance is the demonstration that hyperoxic injury and mechanical removal of the endothelium disrupt normal vessel wall metabolism to alter the accumulation of potent vasoactive substances over short periods of time. This point needs to be considered in extrapolating responses from mechanically denuded tissues to the behavior of arteries remodelled following in vivo physiologic disturbances in the endothelium resulting from pulmonary injury or disease.

The alterations in arachidonic acid metabolism which we report have further implications for the interpretation of responses routinely recorded in tissue-bath bioassay systems. The release of endothelium-derived relaxing factor in response to acetylcholine, calcium ionophore, and several other agents has been much publicized (11). Our demonstration that acetylcholine can simultaneously elicit effects on the production of arachidonic acid metabolites by arterial explants suggests a more generalized vessel wall response to this type of stimulus. The overall sum of vasoconstricting and vasodilating substances released into the circulation by these mechanisms may confound a simple interpretation of specific EDRF effects. Ultimately, it is the local composition of the circulating milieu that determines vascular tone within the intact lung and that becomes altered under various conditions of pulmonary injury.

RESTRUCTURING OF THE ARTERIAL WALL IN INJURY

Cellular Proliferation

The role of endothelial cell mediated control of smooth muscle proliferation has been most extensively studied in systemic blood vessels with particular regard to atherogenesis. Endothelial cells have been shown to secrete several smooth muscle cell growth factors including a PDGF-like peptide, an endothelium-derived growth factor, a somatomedin C-like growth factor, a fibroblast growth factor, and a growth inhibitory factor (17). Enhanced production of these factors has been particularly increased in models of vessel wall injury and repair (16). Under these conditions, endothelial cell denudation results in the removal of factors that are normally being secreted to inhibit smooth muscle proliferation in the intact vessel wall. Injury to the endothelium impairs this regulatory function and permits blood-borne cells such as neutrophils, macrophages, and platelets to interact with the medial layer and release metabolites which can have modifying effects on the smooth muscle.

Specifically, smooth muscle cells can undergo phenotypic changes and proliferate in response to local mitogens such as platelet-derived growth factor (PDGF) (20). Frank endothelial cell loss may not be an essential requirement for increases in growth factor production. Instead, these changes may be triggered by shifts in the amounts of growth stimulatory versus inhibitory factors produced in response to altered gas tension, shear stress, or wall tension.

Vender et al. have recently demonstrated that bovine pulmonary arterial endothelial cells respond to hypoxia in situ by producing a factor which stimulates proliferation of isolated smooth muscle cell cultures in vitro (22). In rats exposed to hypoxia in vivo, formation of new muscle cells has been shown to take place in the small nonmuscular and partially muscular arteries of the lung, whereas medial thickening in the large pulmonary arteries involves hypertrophy of preexisting smooth muscle cells and an increase in the amount of connective tissue. The pulmonary hypertension that develops during chronic oxygen injury to the lung is similarly associated with hypertrophy of the pulmonary arterial wall. Remodelling of the pulmonary vasculature includes increased muscularity of vessels, neomuscularization of previously nonmuscular vessels, and obliteration of capillaries (13).

The precise contribution of cellular hypertrophy and hyperplasia to the changes occurring in the pulmonary arterial wall has not been described for vessels remodelled in hyperoxia. However, the recovery of endothelial cell surface area following 85% O_2 exposure proceeds following vessel wall damage as an adaptive response to injury (9). Whether these responses are specific to the continual presence of toxic oxygen radical species or the presence of blood-borne growth factors has not been addressed in this model of pulmonary hypertension. In a series of experiments aimed at depicting the time course of vessel wall remodelling, we examined the proliferative changes in large intrapulmonary arteries isolated from rats exposed to hyperoxia.

Exposure of rats to 85% O_2 over a period of 10 days produced a significant increase in the number of cells undergoing DNA synthesis as evidenced by a greater percentage of cells labelled with thymidine (6). Although the level of thymidine incorporation in the pulmonary endothelium was significantly increased by day 3 in hyperoxia, cells of the endothelium, media, and adventitia all showed the greatest elevation in DNA synthesis at the end of 7 days in 85% O_2. These increases in DNA synthesis were further translated into an increased total number of cells within the hyperoxic vessel wall by the end of the week. Adventitial fibroblasts and endothelial cells demonstrated the most marked proliferative responses to hyperoxia at this time point. While structural changes which occur within the pulmonary circulation remodelled in hyperoxia have generally been described for the alveolar-capillary unit, our results establish that cellular hyperplasia also occurs in proximal portions of the pulmonary arterial bed during early injury to the lung.

Changes in Actin Phenotypes

The relative production of contractile and noncontractile proteins in the blood vessel wall changes during development as well as in response to elevated strain during the progression of systemic hypertension (2,10). Apart from their contractile role, vascular smooth muscle cells are capable of synthesizing extracellular proteins such as elastin and collagen. Recently, specific increases in smooth muscle elastogenic factors have been identified in a hypoxic model of pulmonary hypertension (14). The involvement of the smooth muscle cell in the production of extracellular connective tissue proteins, as well as in the production of the intracellular contractile proteins actin and myosin, implies that a shift in the relative synthesis of these two types of proteins could result in changes in force development by the vessel wall. Previous studies of mechanical changes in hypertensive pulmonary arteries demonstrate that the active contractile capabilities of arterial segments remodelled in chronic hyperoxia are reduced (8). An increase in wall strain during the development of hypertension may be a stimulus for changes in protein synthesis and cellular proliferation within the vessel wall, although the mechanisms by which these processes are initiated are unclear.

Developing an understanding of the concentration, distribution, and function of contractile and cytoskeletal proteins in remodelling vascular smooth muscle is essential to understanding vessel wall response in injury. A number of important changes occur in the actin and intermediate filament composition and distribution in remodelling vascular smooth muscle (21). This has become especially obvious in studies of endothelial damage and atherosclerosis. Fifteen days after endothelial cell injury, cells that have migrated into the intima contain lesser amounts of actin and desmin and higher amounts of vimentin than is characteristic of the smooth muscle cell population as a whole. The normal predominance of alpha smooth muscle actin is replaced by increases in both beta nonmuscle and gamma smooth muscle actins. These changes are similar to those observed when aortic smooth muscle cells are put in culture in the presence of 10 percent serum. Smooth muscle cells grown in plasma-derived serum or very low concentrations of serum retain a pattern of actin isoforms more like that observed in vivo (21). This effect on prolonging the differentiated function and phenotype of isolated smooth muscle cells may be similarly achieved by culturing these cells in the presence of feeder layers of endothelial cells (2). In the absence of these feeder layers, muscle cells gradually dedifferentiate to resemble fibroblasts and undergo rapid proliferation to confluency.

In order to examine whether alterations in vessel contractility following remodelling were associated with additional changes in vascular smooth muscle proteins, we quantitated the relative changes in actin isoforms by two-dimensional gel electrophoresis (6). We were particularly interested in associating changes in actin phenotypes with the smooth muscle proliferation observed following hyperoxic injury to the vessel wall. Our findings revealed a 10 percent increase in the relative amounts of beta and gamma actin as a percentage of total actin in pulmonary arteries isolated from rats at the end of 7 days' exposure to high oxygen concentrations. Control vessels retained a normal predominance of alpha actin as the greatest percentage of their total actin content.

These results reflect the initial findings of a time course study which identified changes in muscle proteins during restructuring of the pulmonary vasculature in hyperoxia. Whether these shifts are a general response of the remodelling medial compartment or are specific to subpopulations of smooth muscle cells in the vessel wall is unknown. The precise contribution of these shifts in muscle protein phenotypes to measures of responsiveness that rely upon circumferential tension development must be further considered in light of the spatial reorientation of cells within the smooth muscle layers of the remodelled media.

SUMMARY

This brief review highlights several areas which are relevant to an understanding of the interactions between endothelial and smooth muscle cells in the normal and injured lung. These interactions are important in regulating vascular reactivity as well as the metabolic and structural state of the vessel wall. Marked endothelial cell damage in hyperoxia is associated with changes in vascular reactivity and tissue remodelling during the development of pulmonary hypertension. The responses of vasodilators known to be dependent upon the presence of an intact endothelium are impaired during injury to the vessel wall. This may be indicative of a diminished release of EDRF in response to normally circulating and neuronally released mediators or reflect a general reduction in arterial sensitivity.

The vessel culture experiments address an additional factor in the control of tone, i.e., change in the relative production of constrictor versus dilator metabolites of arachidonic acid by the vessel wall. The low level of tone in the normal pulmonary circulation may reflect enhanced release of vasodilating substances such as EDRF and prostacyclin relative to vasoconstricting substances such as thromboxane. Changes in the production of these potent vasoactive products may increase resting smooth muscle tone and thereby enhance pulmonary vascular resistance during vessel wall injury.

Pulmonary vascular resistance is not only a function of smooth muscle tone but is also highly dependent on wall structure. Endothelial cell denudation exposes the smooth muscle cell to circulating monocytes, particularly platelets, which can then release PDGF to initiate proliferation. If the wall is thickened by cellular hypertrophy/hyperplasia and/or its mechanical characteristics are altered by changes in the connective tissue matrix, the lumen of the vessel can be reduced. These types of changes involve the interaction of not only endothelial and smooth muscle cells but also fibroblasts. Endothelial cells can generate growth factors for smooth muscle cells and fibroblasts. Conversely, disruptions in endothelial integrity during vessel wall injury can result in the removal of normally occurring growth inhibitory factors. The precise interaction of these cell types in the control of growth and protein synthesis in the pulmonary circulation is not well described.

In summary, we demonstrate that in the hyperoxic model of pulmonary hypertension, vascular damage disrupts the normal communications between endothelial and smooth muscle cells. Vessel wall injury is associated with pronounced changes in vascular tone, arachidonic acid metabolism, and cellular proliferation. The particular signals which initiate these events remain to be identified. Further insight into the interactions of endothelial and smooth muscle cells in the pulmonary vasculature is critical to increasing our understanding of structure and function within the normal lung and of the mechanism(s) by which it is altered during the pathogenesis of pulmonary hypertension.

REFERENCES

1. Bakhle YS, Ferreira SH: Lung metabolism of eicosanoids: Prostaglandins, prostacyclin, thromboxane, and leukotrienes, in Fishman AP, Fisher AB (eds), *Handbook of Physiology. Sect 3: The Respiratory System, Vol I: Circulation and Nonrespiratory Functions.* Baltimore, American Physiological Society, 1985, pp 365–386.

2. Chamley-Campbell J, Campbell GR, Ross R: The smooth muscle in culture. Physiol Rev 59: 1–61, 1979.

3. Chand N, Altura B: Acetylcholine and bradykinin relax intrapulmonary arteries by acting on endothelial cells: Role in lung vascular diseases. Science 213: 1376–1379, 1981.

4. Cherry PD, Gillis NC: Evidence for the role of endothelium-derived relaxing factor in acetylcholine-induced vasodilation in the intact lung. J Pharmacol Exp Ther 241 : 516–520, 1987.

5. Coflesky JT, Adler KB, Evans JN: Alterations in pulmonary vascular responsiveness following hyperoxic injury to the lung. Chest 93 : 147S–148S, 1988.

6. Coflesky JT, Adler KB, Woodcock-Mitchell J, Mitchell J, Evans JN: Proliferative changes in the pulmonary arterial wall during short-term hyperoxic injury to the lung. Am J Pathol 132 : 563–573, 1988.

7. Coflesky JT, Evans JN: Pharmacologic properties of isolated proximal pulmonary arteries after seven-day exposure to in vivo hyperoxia. Am Rev Respir Dis 138 : 945–951, 1988.

8. Coflesky JT, Jones RC, Reid LM, Evans JN: Mechanical properties and structure of isolated pulmonary arteries remodeled by chronic hyperoxia. Am Rev Respir Dis 136 : 388–394, 1987.

9. Crapo JD, Barry BE, Foscue HA, Shelburne J: Structural and biochemical changes in rat lung occurring during exposure to lethal and adaptive doses of oxygen. Am Rev Respir Dis 122 : 123–143, 1980.

10. Dilley RJ, McGeachie JK, Prendergast FJ: A review of the proliferative behaviour, morphology and phenotypes of vascular smooth muscle. Atherosclerosis 63 : 99–107, 1987.

11. Furchgott RF, Zawadzki JV: The obligatory role of endothelial cells in the relaxation of arterial smooth muscle by acetylcholine. Nature 288 : 373–376, 1980.

12. Ignarro LJ, Harbison RG, Wood KS, Kadowitz PJ: Activation of purified soluble guanylate cyclase by endothelium-derived relaxing factor from intrapulmonary artery and vein: Stimulation by acetylcholine, bradykinin and arachidonic acid. J Pharmacol Exp Ther 237 : 893–900, 1987.

13. Jones R, Zapol WM, Reid L: Pulmonary artery remodelling and pulmonary hypertension after exposure to hyperoxia for 7 days: A morphometric and hemodynamic study. Am J Pathol 117 : 273–285, 1984.

14. Mecham RP, Whitehouse LA, Wrenn DS, Parks WC, Griffin GL, Senior RM, Crouch EC, Stenmark KR, Voelkel NF: Smooth muscle-mediated connective tissue remodeling in pulmonary hypertension. Science 237 : 423–426, 1987.

15. Palmer RMJ, Ferrige AG, Moncada S: Nitric oxide release accounts for the biological activity of endothelium-derived relaxing factor. Nature 327 : 524–526, 1987.

16. Reidy MA: A reassessment of endothelial injury and arterial lesion formation. Lab Invest 53 : 513–520, 1985.

17. Ross R, Raines EW, Bowden-Pope DF: The biology of platelet-derived growth factor. Cell 46 : 155–169, 1986.

18. Rounds S, Farber HW, Hill NS, O'Brien RF: Effects of endothelial cell injury on pulmonary vascular reactivity. Chest 88 : 213S–216S, 1985.

19. Said SI: Prostaglandins and the lung. Bull Eur Physiopathol Respir 17 : 487–488, 1981.

20. Schwartz SM, Campbell GR, Campbell JH: Replication of smooth muscle in vascular disease. Circ Res 58 : 427–444, 1986.

21. Skalli O, Bloom WS, Ropraz P, Azzarone B, Gabbiani G: Cytoskeletal remodeling of rat aortic smooth muscle cells in vitro: Relationship to culture conditions and analogies to in vivo situations. J Submicrosc Cytol 18 : 481–493, 1986.

22. Vender RL, Clemmons DR, Kwock L, Friedman M: Reduced oxygen tension induces pulmonary endothelium to release a pulmonary smooth muscle cell mitogen. Am Rev Respir Dis 135 : 622–627, 1987.

Una S. Ryan, Ph.D.

6

Endothelial Processing of Biologically Active Materials

When the pulmonary endothelium made its debut into the world of nonventilatory functions of the lungs (16), its metabolic activities deserved less than a page; now they are the subject of numerous recent books (30,32). Much of the ever-burgeoning literature can be attributed to reports of new properties, new factors, or new interactions with other cells and molecules. The first group of endothelial activities to be documented was the processing of endogenous biologically active molecules. These metabolic activities most frequently represent a degradation of an active substance, hormone, or prohormone to one with less or different activity, but can result in liberation of a more active compound. It has been a constantly reiterated idea, first put forward by Vane (47), that the lung, by nature of its position and large vascular surface area, can exert a very powerful influence on the quality of the blood entering the systemic circulation. Many of the recently described properties of endothelial cells in culture have yet to be shown to be relevant in vivo, but it is clear that the selective processing properties of pulmonary endothelial cells constitute a very real and important physiological function. Moreover, it is now possible to consider endothelial functions in a much more sophisticated light. The pulmonary endothelium can be regarded as representing not only a barrier, transport and processing surface but also a regulatory surface capable of transducing blood-borne signals and of providing a potent surface for rapid amplification of local inflammatory and other reactions.

ENDOTHELIUM AS A REGULATORY SURFACE

Metabolism of Circulating Endogenous Substrates by the Pulmonary Endothelium

Pulmonary endothelial metabolism of endogenous biologically active substances, ranging from simple amines through fatty acids to more complex polypeptides, has been studied extensively over the past two decades (9,29). Many of these metabolic processing reactions affect vascular tone, blood fluidity, and/or the functions of target organs downstream.

For many years, the adenine nucleotides were known to disappear during passage through the lungs (1). The role of endothelium in this process was shown by cytochemical localization of the requisite enzymes (44) on pulmonary endothelial caveolae (Fig. 1a and b). The fate of adenine nucleotides, including the potent platelet aggregatory substance adenosine diphosphate (ADP), upon contact with pulmonary endothelium has been (17) shown to be due to sequential processing by discrete endothelial ectonucleotidases which degrade adenosine triphosphate (ATP) and the potentially harmful ADP to much less active nucleotides like adenosine monophosphate (AMP) and, from the point of view of vascular patency, the positively beneficial purine, adenosine. Thus, the failure of adenine nucleotides to accumulate in the circulation during shock, platelet aggregation, or ischemia can largely be attributed to the efficiency of endothelial processing. In parallel, studies have been carried out on the pulmonary endothelial uptake and metabolism of adenosine itself (3). Endothelial purine receptors, which can stimulate a range of cellular responses, are classified into P_1 (adenosine) and P_2 (ATP and ADP). Endothelial cells transport adenosine through sites that are blocked by dipyridamole and most of the adenosine transported undergoes intracellular phosphorylation to form ATP, ADP, and AMP. Adenosine also interacts with a separate site on the endothelial surface to stimulate the intracellular formation of cyclic AMP and its export from the cells. The P_2 purinoceptor on endothelial cells is of the P_2Y subtype and induces the production of prostacyclin (PGI_2) and endothelium-derived relaxing factor (EDRF) (14). When stimulated, endothelial cells can selectively release purines in sufficient amounts to exert local biological effects. Thus, an integrated system exists on the endothelial surface involving specific release of purines, release of endothelial secretory products via stimulation of purinoceptors, regulated metabolism by ectonucleotidases, and uptake of adenosine, the final product of metabolic reactions. This very complex system controls plasma concentrations of purines and mediates vascular responses to them.

It is also widely known that vasoactive amines such as norepinephrine and 5-hydroxytryptamine (5-HT) undergo pulmonary endothelial uptake and intracellular metabolism by monoamine oxidase and other enzymes (13). On the other hand, several amines that are similar in structure are neither taken up nor metabolized within the pulmonary circulation; thus, both epinephrine and dopamine escape degradation during intrapulmonary transit (13), indicating a fine selectivity by endothelial cells for circulating molecules.

The metabolism of the vasoactive polypeptides, angiotensin I and bradykinin, has been shown to be the result of interaction of the blood-borne substrates with the peptidyldipeptide hydrolase, angiotensin converting enzyme (ACE), kininase

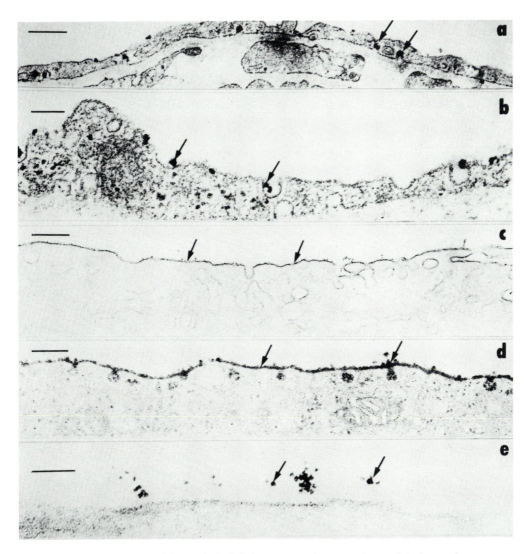

Figure 1: Enzymes of the endothelial plasma membrane and associated caveolae.

a. Cytochemical localization indicating sites of ATPase activity (arrows). Bar = 0.2 μm.

b. Cytochemical localization showing sites of 5'-nucleotidase activity (arrows). Bar = 0.1 μm.

c. Immunocytochemical localization of angiotensin converting enzyme (ACE) (arrows). Bar = 0.2 μm.

d. Immunocytochemical localization of carboxypeptidase N (CPN) (arrows). Bar = 0.2 μm.

e. Immunocytochemical localization of carbonic anhydrase (arrows). Bar = 0.05 μm.

(From Ryan US, Ryan JW: Cell biology of pulmonary endothelium. Circulation 70: III-46–III-62, 1984. Reprinted by permission.)

II (EC 3.4.15.1), situated on the surface of pulmonary endothelial cells (28,38) (Fig. 1c). In the few seconds required for the blood to transit the pulmonary vascular bed, a hypotensive substance (bradykinin) is inactivated and a potent hypertensive substance (angiotensin II) is released into the systemic circulation. Thus, it is the pulmonary endothelium that is responsible for the major role played by the lungs in the control of blood pressure.

Carboxypeptidase N (kininase I, arginine carboxypeptidase, serum carboxypeptidase B or anaphylatoxin inactivator A: EC 3.4.17.3) cleaves the C-terminal basic amino acid of kinins, anaphylatoxins, fibrinopeptides, and enkephalins. The enzyme is present in plasma and has been localized on pulmonary endothelial cells (37) (Fig. 1d). Anaphylatoxin metabolism by carboxypeptidase N indicates an endothelial potential for limiting inflammatory reactions localized within the lung, e.g., in ARDS, disseminated intravascular coagulation, O_2 toxicity or in any situations where complement activation may occur. Enkephalin metabolism by the pulmonary endothelium may be an important function in cases of stress or injury where endogenous enkephalin levels are elevated. Another enzyme, a neutral endopeptidase (NEP) or "enkephalinase," also hydrolyzes biologically active substrates of ACE and cleaves them at the amino side of certain hydrophobic amino acids. Both ACE and NEP are capable of hydrolysis of substance P and neurotensin (43), but the two enzymes differ in susceptibility to inhibitors and substrate preferences. ACE cleaves short peptides while NEP cleaves longer peptides such as the B chain of insulin (12). A newly described, membrane-bound enzyme, carboxypeptidase M, with optimal activity at neutral pH, could inactivate or modulate the activity of peptide hormones before or after their interaction with plasma membrane receptors (42).

Another powerful function of the lung is the selective degradation of some fatty acid derivatives such as prostaglandins of the D, E, and F series. Yet to date, despite the assumption that this process occurs in the pulmonary endothelium, no direct demonstration has been provided by either in vitro or in vivo studies. It may be that the prostaglandins are taken up by endothelium but transported to extravascular sites for processing. On the other hand, pulmonary endothelial cells not only degrade but also generate vasoactive prostaglandins like PGI_2 and PGE_1 from membrane-bound arachidonic acid (6). The stimulus-induced release of endothelial products such as PGI_2 is considered further in a subsequent section.

The ability of the pulmonary endothelium to mobilize arachidonic acid reserves and produce the cyclooxygenase derivative, PGI_2, when appropriately stimulated, would tend toward maintaining blood flow and counteracting the release of mediators of vasoconstriction or platelet aggregation. Arachidonic acid can also be metabolized by the lipoxygenase pathway which generates hydroxyeicosatetraenoic acids (HETEs) and leukotrienes (LTs). Endothelial production of the powerful vasoconstrictor peptide leukotrienes and chemoattractant LTB_4 would seem to work counter to the role of endothelium in guarding against inflammatory vasospastic episodes. In fact, several authors (4,8,45) failed to show any leukotriene production by human umbilical or porcine aortic endothelial cells incubated with ^{14}C-arachidonic acid or ^{35}S-cysteine and stimulated with A23187. However, endothelial cells appear to produce 11, 12 and 15 hydroxyeicosatetraenoic acid (HETEs) (20). The HETEs have been shown to exert an inhibitory influence upon platelet and leukocyte lipoxygenase (46) and, thereby, may modulate the production of leukotrienes by the very cells which tend to interact with, and adhere to, the endothelium in situations of vascular damage. It has also been shown that treatment with LTB_4, LTC_4, and LTD_4 can enhance the production of PGI_2 by endothelial cells (20).

Endothelial cells have also been found to metabolize LT_3 in culture, e.g., LTC_4 is converted to LTD_4 and LTE_4 (20). Even more interesting is conversion of LTA_4 from leukocytes to other LTs by endothelial cells when the two cell types are in communication (4,8). The foregoing has implications for endothelial modulation of the properties of adherent neutrophils in conditions such as pulmonary edema, ARDS, and sepsis. The mechanism of conversion may represent attempted detoxification of LTA_4 via endothelial glutathione.

Endothelial cells are capable of metabolism of other highly active substances such as platelet-activating factor (PAF) (2,7) which could have an important influence on interactions between endothelial cells and circulating platelets and leukocytes in situations where PAF is released as a mediator of lung damage and an activator of leukocytes. However, PAF also exerts marked effects on endothelial cells causing morphological changes, activation of protein kinase C, downregulation of β-adrenergic receptors, and alterations in levels of PGI_2 and thromboxane release (15). Furthermore, it is synthesized by endothelial cells (24).

Although the pulmonary endothelium is remarkably selective in its metabolic properties, there are many opportunities for interaction between specific metabolic activities. For example, xanthine oxidase (XO) activity has been demonstrated in microvascular endothelial cells of certain species (26), and the ability of pulmonary endothelial cells to generate superoxide anion in response to phagocytosis of bacteria has been demonstrated (31). Thus, mechanisms exist for production of O_2 radicals with the potential for damaging the vasculature and other endothelial cells. In cases of ischemia and existing lung damage, released adenine nucleotides would be metabolized to hypoxanthine which could serve as a substrate for endothelial XO, thereby fueling further lung vascular damage.

The regulation of procoagulant and fibrinolytic activity by the endothelial cell, involving splitting of plasma protein precursors to form active molecules by endothelial enzymes, may be considered a form of metabolism and has important implications for vascular patency but is beyond the scope of this chapter (5).

There are a number of other endothelial surface enzymes that process bloodborne substrates not normally considered vasoactive substances. For example, carbonic anhydrase of pulmonary endothelial cells (Fig. 1e) facilitates the release of CO_2 and helps to maintain blood pH (41).

Metabolism of Xenobiotic Substances by Pulmonary Endothelial Cells

A number of drugs with diverse pharmacological properties are sequestered upon passage through the pulmonary circulation and are subsequently metabolized or gradually released unchanged (35).

As is true for endogenous substances, the major site where xenobiotic compounds first encounter living tissue occurs at the lung/blood interface. Thus, pulmonary endothelial cells are among the first type of cell to have intimate contact with intravenously administered drugs and are in a position to influence profoundly the concentrations of xenobiotic compounds reaching the systemic side of

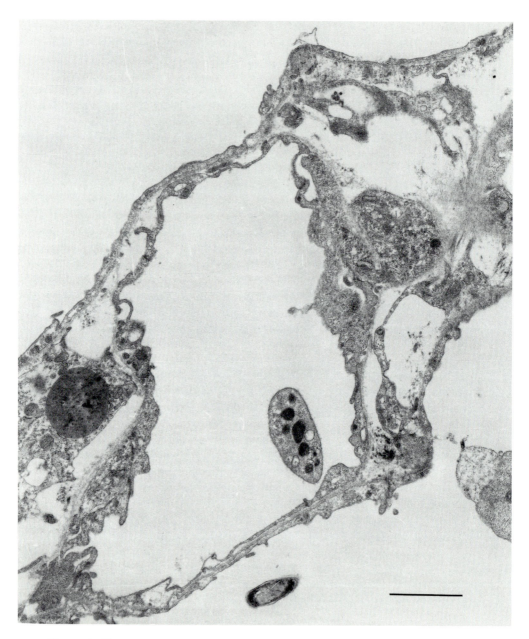

Figure 2: Electron micrograph of thin section from a rat lung 4 hr after ANTU treatment. Endothelial cell damage, e.g., blebbing and vacuolization of the endothelium, has occurred in the thing gas exchanging region and 'scalloping' occurs adjacent to the interstitial regions. The interstitial regions are grossly distended, containing several large spaces. Bar = 0.5 μm. (From Ryan and Grantham [36].)

the circulation. Of the drugs concentrated in the lungs, many pharmacological classes are represented, such as sympathomimetics, antihistamines, antimalarials, morphinelike analgesics, anorectics, tricyclic antidepressants, and anesthetics (35). The rapidity with which drug binding occurs in the lungs suggests a predominantly endothelial locus for interaction between such xenobiotics and pulmonary tissue. Although in many cases the definitive studies using cultured endothelial cells have not been carried out, there is accumulating evidence to suggest that pulmonary endothelium has the potential for being a powerful processor of blood-borne xenobiotic compounds. If a xenobiotic molecule bears structural similarities in terms of chemical groups and charge distribution to an endogenous substrate for pulmonary endothelial uptake, it may itself be a likely candidate for uptake. The subsequent intracellular fate of a xenobiotic upon entering the endothelial cell depends on whether it can interact successfully with the numerous enzyme systems located within the cell, either organelle-associated or cytosolic. Cellular uptake without further processing can represent a form of inactivation, provided that uptake results in retention of the xenobiotic substance, thereby, lowering its concentration in the systemic circulation. Even if the chemical is released again unchanged, a common mechanism among drugs taken up by the lungs, its slow leakage back into the circulation may never reach a biologically active level provided that the rate of metabolism at other sites such as liver and kidney keeps pace with pulmonary release. Alternatively, the pulmonary endothelial cell bears an array of ectoenzymes (described above) which offer the possibility of extracellular xenobiotic metabolism (35).

A number of drugs and chemicals, unrelated to those substances already discussed, are known to cause injury to pulmonary endothelial cells. For example, Figure 2 shows the damage to rat lung microvascular endothelium by α-naphthylthiourea (ANTU). Other examples are bleomycin, nitrofurantoin, mitomycin C, and paraquat. In many cases, the evidence indicates that the injury is related to the generation of oxygen radicals probably resulting from metabolism of these chemicals by some oxidative enzyme system of the endothelial cell. Thus, in some instances, endothelial cell attempts at processing come at the cost of cell integrity.

ENDOTHELIUM AS A TRANSDUCING SURFACE

Responses to Agonists

When pulmonary endothelial cells became available in routine culture (34,38), they were found to be capable not only of processing vasoactive substances but also of responding to them, in some cases to yield an endothelial product. For example, bradykinin is degraded as a consequence of interaction with endothelial cell ACE (28,38) but also binds to receptors on the endothelial surface. One consequence of bradykinin action is to yield an amplification in the release of PGI_2 from endothelial cells (6). Thrombin, ATP, and the calcium ionophore A23187 also cause an increase in endothelial cell PGI_2 production (50).

In 1980 Furchgott and Zawadzki (10) showed that a dilator response to acetylcholine could be obtained in isolated arterial strips only if the endothelium was preserved during preparation, whereas acetylcholine applied directly to smooth muscle led to a constrictor response. Experiments excluding a role for prostacyclin led to the recognition of another vasodilator agent known as endothelium-derived relaxing factor (EDRF) (11). Nitric oxide can account for many of the biological activities of EDRF (25) but, since nitric oxide is a highly reactive molecule, how it is controlled and exported by endothelial cells remains to be elucidated. Agents reported to cause release of EDRF include adenosine diphosphate, adenosine triphosphate, 5-hydroxytryptamine, thrombin, acetylcholine, vasoactive intestinal polypeptide, bradykinin, substance P, cholecystokinin, calcium gene-related peptide, neurotensin, bombesin, noradrenaline, histamine, A23187, clonidine, ergometrine, electrical stimulation, potassium, fatty acids, and shear stress (see Johns et al. [18] for review). Thus, many of the same substances that stimulate release of PGI_2 also stimulate release of EDRF and several of these (e.g., bradykinin, thrombin, ATP, and A23187) also cause the release of another endothelial product, PAF (24).

It is now clear that endothelial cells bear receptors for a host of substances (Fig. 3), occupation of which leads to release of a variety of active substances from the endothelium. Many endothelial functions require the presence of receptors on the surface of the plasma membrane, and there is considerable overlap between substances that are degraded or otherwise processed by endothelial cells and substances that elicit endothelial responses. At present, there is evidence for the existence on endothelial cells of muscarinic, alpha- and beta-adrenergic, purine (adenosine, ATP), insulin, histamine, bradykinin, lipoprotein, thrombin, receptors for the Fc portion of IgG, for complement components C3b and C1q, as well as receptors for PAF, fibrinogen, extracellular matrix proteins, interleukins,

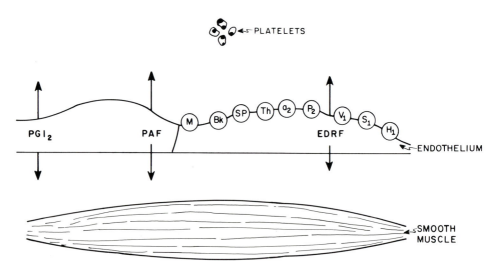

Figure 3: A pictorial representation of receptors on the endothelial surface known to cause release of endothelium-derived products such as EDRF, PGI_2, and PAF. Each of these substances exerts its effects both on platelets and smooth muscle cells (SMC). M = muscarinic receptor; Bk = bradykinin receptor; SP = substance P receptor; Th = thrombin receptor; V_1 = V_1-vasopressaminergic receptor; S_1 = serotonergic receptor; H_1 = histaminergic receptor. (From Ryan US: Endothelial cell receptors. Adv Drug Delivery Revs, 1988, in press.)

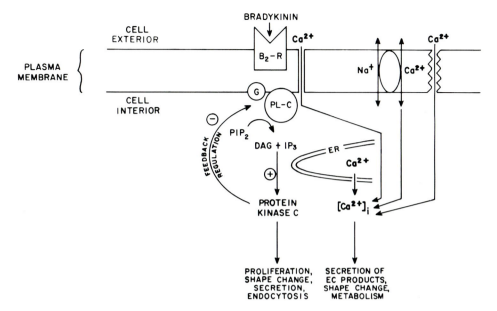

Figure 4: Schematic diagram of signal transduction mechanisms involved in endothelial cell responses to occupation of membrane receptors such as the bradykinin (B_2) receptor. Elevation of intracellular calcium $[CA^{2+}]_i$ can be achieved via liberation from intracellular stores such as the endoplasmic reticulum (ER) or by entry from extracellular sites via receptor operated channels, membrane pumps, or via a leak mechanism. PIP_2 = phosphatidyl inositol bisphosphate; DAG = diacylglycerol; IP_3 = inositol trisphosphate; G = guanine nucleotide binding protein; EC = endothelial cell.

certain growth factors, albumin and other plasma macromolecules, to name only a few. For some of these substances, only the existence of binding sites on endothelial cells is known for sure. Traditionally, agonist binding must elicit a response for the binding site to be considered a receptor; in some cases, the nature of the response resulting from the interaction of a substance with the endothelium remains unclear. There is little argument that proper understanding of the role of the endothelium in homeostasis in general, depends heavily on a sound knowledge of endothelial receptors: their structure, ligand selectivity, association with other plasmalemmal and intracellular molecules, mechanisms of signal propagation, and resistance or adaptation to pathophysiologic changes in the internal environment.

The mechanisms of signal transduction leading to release of the specific product are not yet fully elucidated but are summarized in Figure 4. So far, the cascade of intracellular processes initiated by agonist-receptor interaction and culminating in the secretion of PGI_2 and EDRF remains obscure. Circumstantial evidence supports the suggestion that their release is triggered by an increase in free cytoplasmic calcium concentration ($[Ca^{2+}]_i$); prostacyclin and EDRF are secreted in response to calcium ionophore (19); and agonists that stimulate release of PGI_2 and EDRF induce elevation of $[Ca^{2+}]_i$ in endothelial cells (33). Thus, the mechanisms of agonist-stimulated increase in $[Ca^{2+}]_i$ have been investigated in some detail. Using the fluorescent probes (FURA-2 and INDO-1) in surface-attached endothelial monolayers, the peak elevation of $[Ca^{2+}]_i$ can be partly attributed to mobilization of Ca^{2+} from intracellular stores (33). At the same time, there is evidence that entry of extracellular Ca^{2+} also plays an important role in receptor-mediated elevation of $[Ca^{2+}]_i$ increase in endothelial cells. The stimulation of ^{45}Ca influx in response to thrombin has been shown in bovine pulmonary artery endothelial cells grown on glass cover slips (19,21). The exact mechanism of agonist-induced Ca^{2+} entry is not fully understood. It is unlikely that agonists activate voltage operated calcium channels since they have not been found in endothelial cells (19). In bovine pulmonary artery endothelial cells, thrombin and bradykinin activate ionic currents that may be due to nonspecific influx of divalent cations (19). The current was linearly dependent on membrane potential, and the extrapolated reversal potential was $+4$ mV. Based on these results, it was suggested that extracellular Ca^{2+} enters endothelial cells via receptor-operated channels (19).

We examined the contributions of intracellular Ca^{2+} mobilization, and Ca^{2+} entry via the putative receptor-operated channels, to the total agonist-induced $[Ca^{2+}]_i$ in endothelial cells and have begun to elucidate the mechanisms of receptor coupling to second messenger systems (33).

Thus, studies of GTPγs and GDPβs regulation of PI turnover in cultured endothelial cells show that coupling of the bradykinin receptor (B_2-type) to PI turnover requires guanine nucleotides and involves a G protein which is not a substrate for pertussis toxin. Consequences of activation of PI turnover by bradykinin causing inositol phosphate production would include mobilization of Ca^{2+}, diacylglycerol formation, and stimulation of protein kinase C, and could thus regulate coupling of G protein(s) to phospholipase C. Thus, the mechanisms of stimulus-secretion coupling on endothelial cells include an increase in cytosolic free calcium derived from both intracellular and extracellular sources, activation of phosphoinositol turnover and may involve a feedback mechanism resulting from activation of protein kinase C (33).

As suggested in Figure 4, the same transduction mechanisms may also be involved in endothelial cell changes of shape and behavior (31). Overall, it is clear that endothelium has a great capacity for handling vasoactive signals with a wide spectrum of responses.

Responses to Particulates

Pulmonary endothelial cells respond to blood-borne particulate materials as well as to molecules in solution. Although one does not normally think of endothelium as phagocytic, we have shown that pulmonary endothelial cells in culture can phagocytize polystyrene beads (5 to 20 μm), cholesterol crystals, fixed swelled red cells (10 μm), and a variety of living and killed bacteria (31). Both confluent and dividing cultures ingest particles in a time-dependent manner. Within minutes, S. aureus are bound, entrapped by pseudopodia, and internalized. After several hours, the cells are engorged with bacteria (greater than nine per cell profile). Recognition and entrapment of a bacterium appears to elicit further pseudopod activity, and bacteria frequently are taken up consecutively and internalized as clusters. We have developed a system for time-lapse video recording of endothelial cells that measures parameters of activation, such as division and migration behavior. The data are analyzed by a computer program written in this laboratory. The program can (1) print several statistical reports relating the data from various perspectives of analysis, (2) print genealogy charts for each cell with its relation to its clone members, (3) print a trace of the cell's migration pattern, and (4) create data files that can be interfaced with spreadsheet and graphical software packages such as Lotus 1-2-3.

Through the use of this system, we can define the parameters of endothelial activation in terms of migratory and replicative ability. Phagocytosis appears to stimulate both endothelial cell migration, division, and further phagocytic activity (31). At division, particles are apportioned between the daughter cells. Normally, endothelial cells do not express Fc receptors, but after phagocytosis they show a positive rosette assay with IgG-coated erythrocytes (EA 7S) indicating that Fc receptors have become unmasked (29,31,40). Thus, phagocytosis appears to activate this aspect of endothelial cells as well.

Like professional phagocytes, endothelial cells are capable of discriminating on the basis of surface molecules. For example, endothelial cells derived from bovine pulmonary artery phagocytize the Re mutant of *S. minnesota* in much greater numbers than the wild type (31). Since the Re mutant is distinguished from wild type *S. minnesota* by its ability to bind C1q, and since endothelial cells possess receptors for C1q (51), we examined the role of C1q in the phagocytosis of *S. minnesota* Re mutant (Re) (39). When endothelial cells were preincubated with C1q-enriched medium, subsequent ingestion of Re increased. When Re were preincubated with C1q-enriched medium, the numbers of ingested bacteria were greatly increased. Preincubation of both endothelial cells and bacteria with C1q-enriched media resulted in increased phagocytosis above control levels but less than when either cells or bacteria were preincubated separately in C1q-enriched media. If serum depleted of C1q was used for preincubation of endothelial cells or bacteria, phagocytosis was considerably reduced below control levels. These data indicate that C1q plays an important role in the initial steps (recognition, binding, and ingestion) of phagocytosis. Endothelial cells are able to generate and secrete O_2^-. The signal transduction mechanism of O_2^- release by endothelial cells appears to involve synergistic effects of protein kinase C and Ca^{2+} mobilization (23,31).

It may well be that both Ca^{2+} influx and activation of C-kinase are required for eliciting full physiologic responses from pulmonary endothelial cells. C1q also appears to play a role in the respiratory burst response of endothelial cells to phagocytosis of Re. The level of superoxide anion released from endothelial cells 15 min after phagocytosis of Re (100 bacteria per endothelial cell) was increased (35 nmoles $O_2^-/3 \times 10^6$ endothelial cells). These data point to a role of C1q both in the ingestion and the response of endothelial cells to the Re mutant of *S. minnesota*.

Thus, it is clear that endothelium is capable of the same fine discrimination to surface bound molecules as it displays to circulating solutes. In addition to its known sieving function, the pulmonary vascular bed can ingest particles and respond with a respiratory burst causing release of oxygen radicals and activation of other macrophage-like properties including increased migration, division, and propensity for further phagocytosis (31).

ENDOTHELIUM AS AN AMPLIFICATION SURFACE

Inflammatory reactions and immunity involve close interactions between immunocompetent cells and the vessel wall. Leukocyte localization and extravasation at inflammatory sites involve adhesion to, and passage through, endothelium. Inflammatory lymphokines released by lymphocytes and macrophages are potent regulators of endothelial cell functions such as proliferation, migration, production of colony stimulating factors, and expression of Class II (Ia) histocompatibility antigens. Interferon-gamma regulates the expression of Ia antigens in vascular endothelium (27). IL-1 and TNF affect endothelial cell production of PGI_2, procoagulant activity, plasminogen activator inhibitor, PAF, release of von Willebrand factor, and leukocyte adherence. IL-1 and TNF induce an early, transient expression of mRNA of the c-fos protooncogene, and this may be an important step in the reprogramming of endothelium (22). In addition to responding to lymphokines, endothelial cells can produce them. They can be stimulated to release IL-1 and colony stimulating factor and to augment release of IL-6. Thus, endothelial receptors for cytokines provide opportunities for amplification of local events involving cell-mediated immune reactions, leukocyte recruitment, hemostasis, and proliferative and migratory responses of vessel wall cells. It is clear from this and the previous sections that endothelial cells can act as both a target and source of a number of bioactive molecules. The circulating signals can arrive in fluid or solid phase, and the endothelial response can involve release of a different active molecule (transduction) or release of the same molecule (amplification). In many instances, transduction of blood-borne signals can involve a change in shape or behavior of the endothelial cells and frequently results in a change in behavior of blood cells or neighboring cells of the vascular wall. The "source and target" concept is well exemplified in the case of oxygen radicals and endothelial cells. The vascular lining is a primary target of damage from oxygen radicals produced, for example, by neutrophils. However, as described above, endothelial cells themselves can generate oxygen radicals and release them extracellularly. Therefore, in conditions such as ischemia-reperfusion injury or the sepsis associated with ARDS, the endothelial cell is capable of contributing to the oxidant burden on the vasculature.

CONCLUDING COMMENTS AND FUTURE DIRECTIONS

Endothelial cells provide a dynamic interface for interaction with substrates and formed elements arriving via the blood and for interaction with the underlying layers of the vascular wall (29). However, it is the same anatomic location that makes endothelial cells an immediate target of vascular injury in a wide range of conditions. Endothelial cells, especially those of the pulmonary circulation, are now known from in vivo and in vitro studies to be highly active and capable of selectively metabolizing blood-borne substrates, including peptides, biogenic amines, prostaglandins, and adenine nucleotides, and of degrading a variety of drugs and anesthetics to spare the systemic circulation (35). In addition, endothelial cells possess receptors for a spectrum of agonists and hemostatic factors. The receptor mediated responses of endothelial cells include release of substances that affect vascular tone and blood fluidity. Thus, the presence or absence of endothelium determines (via endothelium-dependent substances) whether the outcome of interaction with platelet products, for example, results in vasospastic or vasodilatory responses of the vascular wall (48). In addition, endothelial cells engage in complex interactions with neutrophils and complement components that have important bearing on inflammatory processes (49). The activities of pulmonary endothelium are not limited to constitutive properties that depend on an intact monolayer. Endothelial cells are also capable of inducible functions, many of them receptor-mediated. Thus, they can respond to stimuli in ways that alter their hemostatic and immunologic potential and that alter their shape and behavior (29).

For all the complex functions of endothelial cells, there are equally complex structural and ultrastructural correlates. Overall, a comprehensive understanding of endothelial processing must include the concept of transduction of circulating signals to yield products affecting interactions with neighboring endothelial cells and other cell types and will require a thorough knowledge of the cellular and molecular biology of the endothelial cell.

ACKNOWLEDGMENTS

It is a pleasure to thank Linda Mayfield for typing the manuscript. The work was supported by NIH grants HL-21568 and HL-33064.

REFERENCES

1. Binet L, Burstein M: Poumon et action vasculaire de l'adenosinetriphosphate (A.T.P.). Presse Med 58 : 1201–1203, 1950.

2. Blank ML, Spector AA, Kaduce TL, Lee T, Snyder F: Metabolism of platelet activating factor (1-alkyl-2-acetyl-sn-glycero-3-phosphocholine and 1-alkyl-2-acetyl-sn-glycerol) by human endothelial cells. Biochim Biophys Acta 876 : 373–378, 1986.

3. Catravas JD, Bassingthwaighte JB, Sparks HV: Adenosine transport and uptake by cardiac and pulmonary endothelial cells, in Ryan US (ed), *Endothelial Cells*, Vol III. Boca Raton, CRC Press, 1988, pp 65–84.

4. Claesson HE, Haeggstrom J: Metabolism of leukotriene A4 by human endothelial cells: evidence for leukotriene C4 and D4 formation by leukocyte-endothelial cell interaction, in Samuelsson B, Paoletti R, Ramwell PW (eds), *Advances in Prostaglandin, Thromboxane, and Leukotriene Research*, vol 17. New York, Raven Press, 1987, pp 115–119.

5. Crutchley DJ: Hemostatic potential of the pulmonary endothelium, in Ryan US (eds), *Pulmonary Endothelium in Health and Disease*. New York, Marcel Dekker, 1987, pp 237–273.

6. Crutchley DJ, Ryan JW, Ryan US, Fisher GH: Bradykinin-induced release of prostacyclin and thromboxanes from bovine pulmonary artery endothelial cells. Studies with lower homologs and calcium antagonists. Biochim Biophys Acta 751 : 99–107, 1983.

7. d'Humieres S, Russo-Marie F, Vargaftig BB: Platelet activating factor acether is involved in thrombin-induced synthesis of prostacyclin by human endothelial cells, in Samuelsson B, Paoletti R, Ramwell PW (eds), *Advances in Prostaglandin, Thromboxane, and Leukotriene Research*, vol 17. New York, Raven Press, 1987, pp 212–215.

8. Feinmark SJ, Cannon PJ: Endothelial cell neutrophil interactions lead to endothelial cell leukotriene C4 synthesis, in Samuelsson B, Paoletti R, Ramwell PW (eds), *Advances in Prostaglandin, Thromboxane, and Leukotriene Research*, vol 17. New York, Raven Press, 1987, pp 120–125.

9. Fishman AP, Pietra GG: Handling of bioactive

materials by the lung. N Engl J Med 291 : 884–890; 953–959, 1974.

10. Furchgott RF, Zawadzki JV: The obligatory role of endothelial cells in the relaxation of arterial smooth muscle by acetylcholine. Nature 288:373–376, 1980.

11. Furchgott RF: Studies on relaxation of rabbit aorta by sodium: the basis for the proposal that the acid-activatable inhibitory factor from bovine retractor penis is inorganic nitrite and the endothelium-derived relaxing factor is nitric oxide, in Vanhoutte PM (ed), *Mechanisms of Vasodilation*, Vol IV. New York, Raven Press, 1988, in press.

12. Gee NS, Matsas R, Kenny AJ: A monoclonal antibody to kidney endopeptidase-24.11. Biochem J 214 : 377–386, 1983.

13. Gillis CN, Pitt BR: The fate of circulating amines within the pulmonary circulation. Annu Rev Physiol 44 : 269–281, 1982.

14. Gordon JL, Martin W: Stimulation of endothelial prostacyclin production plays no role in endothelial-dependent relaxation of the pig aorta. Br J Pharmacol 80 : 179–186, 1983.

15. Grigorian GY, Ryan US: Platelet activating factor effects on bovine pulmonary artery endothelial cells. Circ Res 61 : 389–395, 1987.

16. Heinemann HO, Fishman AP: Nonrespiratory functions of mammalian lung. Physiol Rev 49 : 1–47, 1969.

17. Hellewell PG, Pearson JD: Adenine nucleotides and pulmonary endothelium, in Ryan US (ed), *Pulmonary Endothelium in Health and Disease*. New York, Marcel Dekker, 1987, pp 327–343.

18. Johns A, Khalil RA, Ryan US, van Breemen C: Endothelium-derived relaxing factor, in Ryan US (ed), *Endothelial Cells*, Vol III. Boca Raton, CRC Press, 1988, pp 51–60.

19. Johns A, Lategan TW, Lodge NJ, Ryan US, van Breemen C, Adams DJ: Calcium entry through receptor-operated channels in bovine pulmonary artery endothelial cells. Tissue Cell 19 : 733–745, 1987.

20. Johnson AR, Revtyak GE, Ibe BO, Campbell WB: Endothelial cells metabolize but do not synthesize leukotrienes. Prog Clin Biol Res 199 : 185–196, 1985.

21. Lambert TL, Kent RS, Whorton AR: Bradykinin stimulation of inositol polyphosphate production in porcine aortic endothelial cells. J Biol Chem 261 : 15288–15293, 1986.

22. Mantovani A, Dejana E: Modulation of endothelial function by IL-1. A novel target for pharmacological intervention? Biochem Pharmacol 36 : 301–305, 1987.

23. Matsubara T, Ziff M: Superoxide anion release by human endothelial cells: Synergism between a phorbol ester and a calcium ionophore. J Cell Physiol 127 : 207–210, 1986.

24. McIntyre TM, Zimmerman GA, Satoh K, Prescott SM: Cultured endothelial cells synthesize both platelet-activating factor and prostacyclin in response to histamine, bradykinin and adenosine triphosphate. J Clin Invest 76 : 271–280, 1985.

25. Palmer RM, Ferrige AG, Moncada S: Nitric oxide release accounts for the biological activity of endothelium-derived relaxing factor. Nature 327 : 524–526, 1987.

26. Phan SH, Gannon DE, Varani J, Ryan US: Xanthine oxidase activity in rat pulmonary artery endothelial cells and its alteration by activated neutrophils. J Clin Invest, 1988, in press.

27. Pober JS: Lymphokine modulation of endothelial cell morphology and surface antigens, in Ryan US (ed), *Endothelial Cells*, Vol II. Boca Raton, CRC Press, 1988, pp 259–272.

28. Ryan US: Processing of angiotensin and other peptides by the lungs, in Fishman AP, Fisher AB (eds), *Handbook of Physiology. Sect 3: The Respiratory System, Vol I: Circulation and Nonrespiratory Functions*. Bethesda, American Physiological Society, 1985, pp 351–364.

29. Ryan US: Metabolic activity of pulmonary endothelium: Modulation of structure and function. Annu Rev Physiol 48 : 263–277, 1986.

30. Ryan US (ed): *Pulmonary Endothelium in Health and Disease*. New York, Marcel Dekker, 1987.

31. Ryan US: Phagocytic properties of endothelial cells, in Ryan US (ed), *Endothelial Cells*, Vol III. Boca Raton, CRC Press, 1988, pp 33–49.

32. Ryan US (ed): *Endothelial Cells*, Vol I–III. Boca Raton, CRC Press, 1988.

33. Ryan US: Structural basis for endothelial cell function: Role of calcium, polyphosphoinositide turnover and G-proteins, in Catravas JD, Gillis CN, Ryan US (eds), *Vascular Endothelium: Receptors and Transduction Mechanisms*. New York, Plenum Publishing Corporation, 1988, in press.

34. Ryan US, Clements E, Habliston D, Ryan JW: Isolation and culture of pulmonary artery endothelial cells. Tissue Cell 10 : 535–554, 1978.

35. Ryan US, Grantham CJ: Metabolism of endogenous and xenobiotic substances by pulmonary vascular endothelial cells. Pharmacol Ther, 1988, in press.

36. Ryan US, Johns A, van Breemen C: Role of calcium in receptor mediated endothelial cell responses. Chest 93 : 105S–109S, 1988.

37. Ryan US, Ryan JW: Endothelial cells and inflammation, in Ward PA (ed), *Clinics in Laboratory Medicine*, Vol 3. Philadelphia, W.B. Saunders, 1983, pp 577–599.

38. Ryan US, Ryan JW, Whitaker C, Chiu A: Localization of angiotensin converting enzyme (kininase II). II. Immunocytochemistry and immunofluorescence. Tissue Cell 8 : 125–146, 1976.

39. Ryan US, Schultz DR, Goodwin JD, Vann JM, Selvaraj MP, Hart MA: Role of C1q in phagocytosis of *S. minnesota* by pulmonary endothelial cells. Infect Immun, 1988, submitted.

40. Ryan US, Schultz DR, Ryan JW: Fc and C3b receptors on pulmonary endothelial cells. Induction by injury. Science 214:557–559, 1981.

41. Ryan US, Whitney PL, Ryan JW: Localization of carbonic anhydrase on pulmonary artery endothelial cells in culture. J Appl Physiol 53:914–919, 1982.

42. Skidgel RA, Davis RM, Tan F: Human carboxypeptidase M: Purification and characterization of a membrane-bound carboxypeptidase that cleaves peptide hormones. J Biol Chem 264:2236–2241, 1989.

43. Skidgel RA, Engelbrecht S, Johnson AR, Erdös Eg: Hydrolysis of substance P and neurotensin by converting enzyme and neutral endopeptidase. Peptides 5:769–776, 1984.

44. Smith U, Ryan JW: Pinocytotic vesicles of the pulmonary endothelial cell. Chest 59:12S–15S, 1971.

45. Thomson AR, Revtyak GE, Ibe BO, Campbell WB: Endothelial cells metabolize but do not synthesize leukotrienes. Prog Clin Biol Res 199:185–196, 1985.

46. Vanderhoeck JY, Bryant RW, Bailey JM: Regulation of leukocyte and platelet lipoxygenase by hydroxyeicosanoids. Biochem Pharmacol 31:3463–3467, 1982.

47. Vane JR: The release and fate of vasoactive hormones in the circulation. Br J Pharmacol 35:209–242, 1969.

48. Vanhoutte PM, Houston DS: Platelets, endothelium and vasospasm. Circulation 72:728–734, 1985.

49. Warren JS, Ward PA, Johnson KJ Mechanisms of damage to pulmonary endothelium, in Ryan US (ed), *Pulmonary Endothelium in Health and Disease.* New York, Marcel Dekker, 1987, pp 107–120.

50. Weksler BB, Ley CW, Jaffe EA: Stimulation of endothelial cell prostacyclin production by thrombin, trypsin, and the ionophore A23187. J Clin Invest 62:923–930, 1978.

51. Zhang SC, Schultz DR, Ryan US: Receptor-mediated binding of C1q on pulmonary endothelial cells. Tissue Cell 18:13–18, 1986.

Michael I. Kotlikoff, V.M.D., Ph.D.
Alfred P. Fishman, M.D.

7

Endothelin: Mediator of Hypoxic Vasoconstriction?

A vigorous search is currently underway for the cellular and molecular mechanisms underlying hypoxic pulmonary vasoconstriction. A series of recent reviews have traced the various ways and byways that culminated in the present effort (2,14,19). This chapter focuses on one double-pronged promising lead: the evidence implicating the pulmonary endothelial cell as the cellular O_2 transducer and the discovery of endothelin, a novel peptide constricting factor that is secreted by pulmonary endothelium and has been proposed as a potential mediator of hypoxic pulmonary vasoconstriction (HPV).

In attempting to assess the role of this compound in HPV, criteria presented over a decade ago for the establishment of a chemical mediator of HPV will be used as a benchmark. These criteria are as follows: (1) the mediator or its precursors must exist in the lungs, (2) the source of mediator must be proximate to the resistance vessels, (3) application of the mediator substance to pulmonary blood vessels must cause vasoconstriction, (4) a mechanism for secretion or activation of the mediator by hypoxia must exist, (5) agents which block the pressor response to the substance should similarly block the effects of exogenously applied mediator, and (6) inhibition or depletion of the mediator should depress the hypoxic response (2).

SITE OF O₂ SENSING

Although it is clear that the final effector mechanism of hypoxic pulmonary vasoconstriction involves contraction of smooth muscle cells in the pulmonary vasculature, considerable uncertainty exists about the cell type that senses hypoxia and begins the cascade of O_2-transduction. The two major categories of possibilities, i.e., direct and indirect, are described in the previous chapter. In a word, sensing could occur within vascular smooth muscle cells, per se, to generate intracellular signals that activate myofilaments or sensing could occur in nonmuscle cells to effect a cascade of reactions including the release of intercellular signals that couple oxygen-sensing to smooth muscle contraction. With respect to the latter "indirect" model, pulmonary vascular endothelial cells are the most likely sensing cells on two accounts: (1) their interposition between the blood and smooth muscle puts them in a unique position, and (2) they have proved to be capable of synthesizing and releasing substances with potent vasoactive effects (3,18,21).

In some nonpulmonary tissues, under some experimental conditions, hypoxia and/or anoxia elicit vasoconstriction that is endothelium-dependent and in which endothelial cells are the O_2 sensors (1,4,17). For example, in the coronary artery of the dog, hypoxic vasoconstriction fails to occur if there is no endothelium. Moreover, hypoxia contracts the denuded coronary artery if endothelium is layered on the preparation, implying that a soluble factor is released by endothelial cells during hypoxia (17). Subsequently, an endothelium-derived constricting factor was shown to be produced by cultured aortic (7) and pulmonary (16) endothelial cells: the factor, which proved to be a small molecular weight peptide, evoked sustained contractions of slow onset in pulmonary and coronary vascular strips (7,16). As in the experiments demonstrating endothelium-dependent hypoxic contraction of isolated coronary arteries, contractile activity of the pressor substance was not blocked by receptor antagonists to serotonin, histamine, norepinephrine, leukotrienes, angiotensin II, or substance P receptors; it was also insensitive to cyclooxygenase or lipoxygenase inhibitors (16). Although these observations offer no proof that this factor is involved in eliciting hypoxic vasoconstriction in the pulmonary circulation, they do argue strongly for a physiological role of endothelial cells in regulating vascular smooth muscle contraction in systemic beds.

With respect to adducing evidence concerning the pulmonary vasculature, a major experimental hurdle has been the inability to obtain preparations of pulmonary microvasculature that demonstrate hypoxic vasoconstriction in vitro. Recently, some success was obtained in this regard using small vessels (6). However, the small size of the vessels used and the attendant difficulties in measuring tension made evaluation of the role of the endothelium impossible. In another series of experiments using small isolated pulmonary vessels, acute hypoxia caused depolarization and contraction that was dependent on external calcium and associated with an increase in membrane conductance (5,6,12). Removal of the endothelium abolished not only the pressor responses to hypoxia, but also to all agonists, so that interpretation of the results became equivocal (D. Harder, personal communication).

As one resort to circumvent problems inherent in the use of small pulmonary vessels, investigators have turned to large pulmonary arteries (9). These vessels demonstrated hypoxia-induced contractions that were attenuated approximately 6-fold upon removal of the endothelium, even though the normal contractile responses to norepinephrine were retained. However, unlike experiments with the carotid artery, preparations layered with endothelium did not regain their hypoxic responsiveness.

The vasoconstrictor peptide is found in conditioned media from pulmonary as well as aortic endothelial cells (16). However, the peptide failed to elicit vasoconstriction in the rat lung even though it did elicit sustained pressor responses in the rabbit heart and rat kidney.

In essence, dependence of hypoxic pulmonary vasoconstriction on pulmonary vascular endothelium has not been proved. Indeed, data concerning this point are conflicting. In a recent study, individual cells in pure cultures of smooth muscle cells from the pulmonary artery contracted upon exposure to hypoxia (15). In these cells, measurements of myosin light chain phosphorylation showed a marked increase in ^{32}P uptake under hypoxic conditions. Although these reports are preliminary, they do urge caution in accepting the endothelium-derived constricting factor as the long sought mediator of hypoxic pulmonary hypertension.

ENDOTHELIN

The demonstration that endothelium can produce a vasoconstrictor substance was followed by the isolation, cloning, and sequencing of a novel vasoconstrictor peptide, "endothelin" (8,10,20,21). This substance, first isolated from conditioned media bathing confluent porcine aortic endothelial cells, is a peptide with potent vasoconstricting properties; it is effective on systemic and pulmonary vascular smooth muscle at subnanomolar concentrations. The size of the compound (21 residues, 2492 MW) proved to be quite similar to that proposed for the vasoconstrictor substance previously reported (16), and the physiologic effects of endothelin and the vasoconstrictor factor were quite similar. Also, as in the studies using conditioned endothelial cell culture media, the purified peptide had contractile effects that were sustained and demonstrated a dependence on extracellular calcium; contractions were completely abolished in calcium-free solutions and inhibited by low concentrations of nicardipine, a dihydropyridine calcium channel blocker, indicating that the contractile mechanism probably involves calcium influx through dihydropyridine-sensitive calcium channels. Also in line with the earlier studies using partially purified media, the action of endothelin is resistant to receptor antagonists and inhibitors of cyclooxygenase and lipoxygenase. Finally, in smooth muscle cells grown in culture, endothelin seems to stimulate an increase in the intracellular concentration of calcium that is blocked by removal of extracellular calcium and is not associated with increased phosphatidylinositol metabolism (8).

Determination of the amino acid sequence of purified porcine endothelin yields some insight into the molecular structure of the compound. The short peptide contains two intrachain disulphide bonds, and synthetic endothelin cross-linked in this way is biologically active (21). This structure, i.e., multiple disulphide bonds within a short peptide, is uncommon in biological peptides but is characteristic of a group of peptide toxins that interact functionally with membrane ion channels. The similarity in structure, as well as the dependence of endothelin on extracellular calcium for vasoactivity and the antagonism by dihydropyridines, has led to the hypothesis that endothelin acts functionally as a voltage-dependent calcium channel agonist (8,21).

All in all, it seems likely that endothelin is one or more of the soluble vasoconstrictive factors identified in earlier physiological studies (7,16,17): the production of this substance by cultured endothelial cells, the dependence of its physiological effects on extracellular calcium, and the inability of specific receptor antagonists or cyclooxygenase/lipoxygenase inhibitors to block these effects suggest that endothelin and the endothelium-derived constricting factor of systemic vessels (4,7,16) are the same substance. Less convincing is the evidence that endothelin is responsible for hypoxic pulmonary vasoconstriction even though it does satisfy some of the criteria for a unique mediator of this pressor response (17) and it does seem to act like a suitable voltage-dependent calcium channel agonist (6,11,12,13). Indeed, one telling argument against a major vasoconstrictive role for endothelin on the pulmonary circulation is that preproendothelin mRNA could not be found in the porcine lung (21). Although it is possible that the substance could be transported to the lungs from systemic vessels, the potent effects of endothelin on systemic and pulmonary vascular smooth muscle makes this prospect unlikely. Instead, endothelin may well prove to be only the first in a series of vasoconstrictor peptides that endothelium can produce and that either it, or a counterpart, will be shown to originate in pulmonary vascular endothelium. Even if this prophecy should come true, past experience also predicts that it will still be a great experimental challenge to prove that a soluble vasoconstrictor released in the lungs is the unique mediator of hypoxic pulmonary vasoconstriction.

SUMMARY

A definitive answer to speculation about the role of endothelin in eliciting hypoxic pulmonary vasoconstriction is not possible at this time. Certain critical links in the chain of evidence favoring endothelin as the mediator of the hypoxic pressor response are still missing. For example, pulmonary endothelial cells have not been shown to secrete endothelin in vivo. Nor has endothelin been shown to elicit vasoconstriction of the resistance vessels of the lungs. Whether hypoxia triggers endothelin secretion by pulmonary endothelium is unknown and the presence of the peptide in the lung during hypoxic vasoconstriction remains to be demonstrated. Finally, it is unknown if agents that suppress the release of endothelin or block its effects will inhibit hypoxic pulmonary vasoconstriction. The availability of synthetic endothelin, cDNA probes for preproendothelin, and the production of antibodies to endothelin make it likely that the answers to questions such as these will soon be provided.

REFERENCES

1. DeMey JG, Vanhoutte PM: Anoxia and endothelium-dependent reactivity of the canine femoral artery. J Physiol 335:65–74, 1983.

2. Fishman AP: Hypoxia in the pulmonary circulation: How and where it acts. Circ Res 38:221–231, 1976.

3. Furchgott RF, Zawadzki JV: The obligatory role of endothelial cells in the relaxation of arterial smooth muscle by acetylcholine. Nature 288:370–373, 1980.

4. Gillespie MN, Owasoyo JO, McMurtry IF, O'Brien RF: Sustained coronary vasoconstriction

provoked by a peptidergic substance released from endothelial cells in culture. J Pharmacol Exp Therap 236:339–343, 1986.

5. Harder DR, Madden JA, Dawson CA: A membrane electrical mechanism for hypoxic vasoconstriction in small pulmonary arteries from cat. Chest 88:233S, 1985.

6. Harder DR, Madden JA, Dawson C: Hypoxic induction of Ca^{2+}-dependent action potentials in small pulmonary arteries of the cat. J Appl Physiol 59:1389–1393, 1985.

7. Hickey KA, Rubanyi G, Paul JR, Highsmith RF: Characterization of a coronary vasoconstrictor produced by cultured endothelial cells. Am J Physiol 248:C550-C556, 1985.

8. Hirata Y, Yoshimi H, Takata S, Watanabe TX, Kumagai S, Nakajima K, Kakakibara S: Cellular mechanism of action by a novel vasoconstrictor endothelin in cultured rat vascular smooth muscle cells. Biochem Biophys Res Commun 154:868–875, 1988.

9. Holden WE, McCall E: Hypoxia-induced contractions of porcine pulmonary artery strips depend on intact endothelium. Exp Lung Res 7:101–112, 1984.

10. Itoh Y, Yanagisawa M, Ohkubo S, Kimura C, Kosaka T, Inoue A, Ishida N, Mitsui Y, Onda H, Fujino M, Masaki T: Cloning and sequence analysis of cDNA encoding the precursor of a human endothelium-derived vasoconstrictor peptide, endothelin: identity of human and porcine endothelin. FEBS Lett 231:440–444, 1988.

11. Kennedy T, Summer W: Inhibition of hypoxic pulmonary vasoconstriction by nifedipine. Am J Cardiol 50:864–868, 1982.

12. Madden JA, Dawson CA, Harder DR: Hypoxia-induced activation in small isolated pulmonary arteries from the cat. J Appl Physiol 59:113–118, 1985.

13. McMurtry IF, Davidson AB, Reeves JT, Grover RF: Inhibition of hypoxic pulmonary vasoconstriction by calcium antagonists in isolated rat lungs. Circ Res 38:99–104, 1976.

14. McMurtry IF, Stanbrook HS, Rounds S: The mechanism of hypoxic vasoconstriction: a working hypothesis, in Loeppky JA, Riedesel ML (eds), *Oxygen Transport to Human Tissues.* New York, Elsevier-North Holland, 1982, pp 77–88.

15. Murray TR, Macarak EJ, Marshall BE: Hypoxic pulmonary vasoconstriction in cell culture. Anesthesiology, in press.

16. O'Brien RF, Robbins RJ, McMurtry IF: Endothelial cells in culture produce a vasoconstrictor substance. J Cell Physiol 132:263–270, 1987.

17. Rubanyi GM, Vanhoutte PM: Hypoxia releases a vasoconstrictor substance from the canine vascular endothelium. J Physiol 364:45–56, 1985.

18. Vanhoutte PM, Rubanyi GM, Miller VM, Houston DS: Modulation of vascular smooth muscle contractions by the endothelium. Annu Rev Physiol 48:307–320, 1986.

19. Voelkel NF: Mechanisms of hypoxic pulmonary vasoconstriction. Am Rev Respir Dis 133:1186–1195, 1986.

20. Yanagisawa M, Inoue A, Ishikawa T, Kasuya Y, Kimura S, Kumagaye S, Nakajima K, Watanabe TX, Sakakibara S, Goto K et al: Primary structure, synthesis, and biological activity of rat endothelin, an endothelium-derived vasoconstrictor peptide. Proc Natl Acad Sci USA 85:6964–6967, 1988.

21. Yanagisawa M, Kurihara H, Kimura S, Tomobe Y, Kobayashi M, Mitsui Y, Yazaki Y, Goto K, Masaki T: A novel potent vasoconstrictor peptide produced by vascular endothelial cells. Nature 332:411–415, 1988.

Kenneth L. Brigham, M.D.

8

Mediators in the Pulmonary Circulation

Historically, most studies of functions of the pulmonary circulation have focused on pulmonary vascular resistance, i.e., global vasoconstriction and vasodilation. A disconcertingly immense catalogue of mediators which cause one or the other effect on pulmonary vascular resistance could be compounded, with some value—the global control of pulmonary vascular resistance is important, particularly to the right ventricle which must accommodate to an afterload imposed by the lungs.

But interactions of vasoactive humoral mediators with the pulmonary circulation are much broader and more subtle than implied by investigations in which mediators are given and pulmonary vascular resistance measured. Control of the parallel distribution of vascular resistances in the lungs affects matching of perfusion to ventilation and, thus, gas exchange. Changes in the series distribution of resistance may profoundly influence pressure in exchange vessels. Vasoreactivity, the magnitude of vasoconstrictor responses to a variety of stimuli, may be altered without necessarily altering baseline resistance. The pulmonary microcirculation serves as the principal barrier to fluid and solute movement from the intravascular space, produces and processes mediators which may affect the systemic vascular bed and provides a large, more or less amiable, surface over which the blood flows. All of these functions may involve interactions of humoral mediators with the lungs, the consequences of which determine not only pulmonary function, but functions of other organs as well.

This chapter will try to elucidate some of the subtleties without giving too short shrift to the global control of resistance. In doing so, it is not possible to provide an exhaustive list of mediators which can be produced by or affect pulmonary circulatory function. Rather, selected examples will illustrate interactions between the pulmonary circulation and some potentially important mediators, highlighting what is and what is not known (or currently thought) about pulmonary pathophysiology.

PULMONARY VASCULAR RESISTANCE

In spite of its enormous blood flow, the pulmonary circulation is normally under low pressure because pulmonary vascular resistance is normally low. Sustained increases in pulmonary vascular resistance are deleterious to both the right ventricle and the gas exchange function of the lungs. Is the normally low pulmonary vascular resistance a simple function of the anatomy, or are there vasodilator mediators constantly produced which are necessary to maintain the vascular bed in a dilated state?

The anatomy of the lung vascular bed favors low resistance. The arterial vessels are thin-walled compared to systemic vessels, and there is a large cross-sectional area, both features which minimize resistance to blood flow. However, in the baseline state, it is difficult to decrease pulmonary vascular resistance consistently by infusing even potent vasodilator drugs, implying that, unlike systemic vessels, pulmonary vessels are maximally (or nearly) dilated under baseline conditions. In fact, in order to demonstrate that a mediator dilates the pulmonary circulation, it is commonly necessary to preconstrict the vascular bed (37). Since the pulmonary vasculature is capable of constricting but is, under normal conditions, virtually flaccid, it has been inferred that the pulmonary circulation is under the chronic influence of vasodilator substances, the production of which is essential for maintaining low pulmonary vascular pressure (88).

The search for such substances has not been very fruitful. Several endogenous mediators are potent pulmonary vasodilators, and some of these are produced in the lungs under abnormal conditions. For example, prostacyclin, the principal product of arachidonic acid metabolism in endothelial cells (61), dilates the pulmonary circulation, and the large vascular surface area in the lungs provides an abundant potential source of this substance. The ether lipid, platelet-activating factor (PAF), produced by many cell types, including endothelium (73), is also a pulmonary vasodilator, at least in low doses (51). Pulmonary endothelium may also be capable of producing endothelium-derived relaxing factor (EDRF) (21,86). Increased production of these mediators can be demonstrated with pathological interventions, but demonstration that their chronic production serves a physiological role is more difficult.

With the advent of nonsteroidal, anti-inflammatory agents which appear to act principally by inhibiting prostanoid synthesis, several investigators studied the effects of preventing endogenous generation of prostanoids on pulmonary circulatory function. Because these drugs inhibit generation of other prostanoids than prostacyclin, including some potent vasoconstrictor substances, these studies do not address the role of prostacyclin specifically, but they do provide some insight into the question of whether vasodilator prostanoids are important to the physiology.

Administration of the cyclooxygenase inhibitor, indomethacin, to unanesthe-

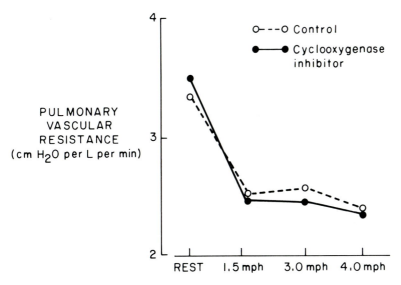

Figure 1: Effects of exercise on pulmonary vascular resistance in unanesthetized sheep. Cyclooxygenase inhibition did not alter baseline resistance and did not prevent the fall in resistance with exercise. (Redrawn from Newman et al. [62].)

tized dogs causes pulmonary vascular resistance to increase acutely (88). However, studies in other species are not consistent with the obvious interpretation that chronic production of vasodilator prostanoids is essential to maintenance of low pulmonary vascular resistance. For example, administration of indomethacin to lambs (47) or administration of another cyclooxygenase inhibitor, meclofenamate, to sheep does not increase baseline pulmonary vascular resistance. Further, as illustrated in Figure 1, the normal fall in pulmonary vascular resistance which occurs with exercise in chronically instrumented sheep is unaffected by cyclooxygenase inhibition (62). The response to exercise ought to be a severe test of the hypothesis since it tests the capacity of the pulmonary circulation to accommodate large increases in cardiac output. These studies indicate that production of vasodilator prostanoids is not essential for maintaining low pulmonary vascular tone at least in unanesthetized sheep. There may well be species differences, but at least the prostacyclin theory is not a generally applicable one.

However, even in sheep, chronic inhibition of cyclooxygenase does increase pulmonary vasoreactivity and cause sustained pulmonary hypertension, including structural remodelling of the pulmonary circulation (57). Figure 2 shows pulmonary vascular resistance in sheep treated chronically with daily subcutaneous indomethacin. Resistance began to increase by 1 week of indomethacin treatment and was sustained; the same animals showed morphological changes of chronic pulmonary hypertension.

Is it possible that vasodilator prostanoids are chronically produced in small quantities and that, although they are not important for short-term control of resistance, they do act in some way to prevent evolution of chronic pulmonary hypertension? A "one mediator, one response" interpretation of these data is

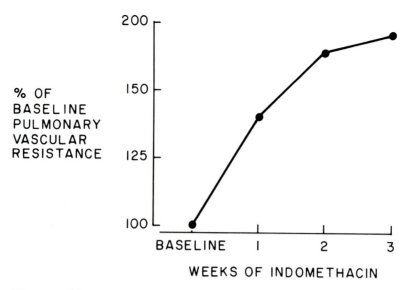

Figure 2: Effects of repeated administration of indomethacin on pulmonary vascular resistance in chronically instrumented sheep. Pulmonary vascular resistance began to rise by 1 week of indomethacin treatment and reached twice the baseline value by 3 weeks. (Redrawn from Meyrick et al. [57].)

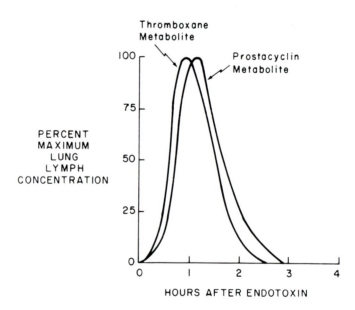

Figure 3: Time course of appearance of thromboxane and prostacyclin metabolites in lung lymph of chronically instrumented sheep following infusion of endotoxin. (Redrawn from Brigham and Snapper [17].)

likely overly simplistic. For example, sheep given indomethacin chronically also accumulate neutrophils in the lung periphery (57), and several interventions which cause chronic pulmonary inflammation also cause sustained pulmonary hypertension (55). The paradox of inflammation caused by an anti-inflammatory agent may illustrate interdependence of mediator effects (cyclooxygenase inhibition might result in generation of proinflammatory leukotrienes) and certainly illustrates some of the complexities involved in determining in vivo roles of specific mediators.

The pulmonary vascular bed constricts in response to a number of stimuli; the most common physiological stimulus is alveolar hypoxia. Since the teleology suggests that hypoxic pulmonary vasoconstriction is a device for matching perfusion to ventilation, that response will be discussed in the next section.

The pulmonary vascular bed also constricts in response to many interventions which cause diffuse lung injury, and much of the information related to mediators of pulmonary vasoconstriction has been obtained in such models. The most common approach has been to determine what mediators are produced with the insult, to describe effects of exogenous administration of the mediator(s), and to determine effects of inhibitors of mediator production or action on the pulmonary vascular response to the insult.

Based on these kinds of studies, several interventions appear to cause pulmonary vasoconstriction by causing endogenous generation of vasoconstrictor prostanoids, probably thromboxane A_2. When infused into a variety of animal preparations, a thromboxane A_2 mimic (a stable analog of prostaglandin H_2) is a potent pulmonary vasoconstrictor. Authentic thromboxane A_2, although difficult to study because of its lability, is also a potent pulmonary vasoconstrictor (4). Either intravascular complement activation (71) or infusion of bacterial endotoxin (65) into experimental animals causes increased concentrations of the stable metabolite of thromboxane A_2 (thromboxane B_2) to appear in blood and lung lymph, and the 2,3 dinor metabolite to appear in urine (45). Cyclooxygenase inhibition (80), more specific inhibition of thromboxane synthesis (33), or administration of a specific thromboxane receptor antagonist (45) all inhibit the immediate pulmonary hypertension. Thromboxane A_2 appears to be an important endogenous mediator of pulmonary hypertension in at least some situations.

There are a host of other mediators, produced in the body, which alter pulmonary vascular resistance. Angiotensin II, produced by enzymatic cleavage of angiotensin I on the surface of endothelial cells (77), is a pulmonary vasoconstrictor. Other vasoconstrictors include serotonin (6), histamine (2), prostaglandins $F_{2\alpha}$ and E_2 (41,42) (and several other prostanoids), leukotrienes C_4 and D_4 (87), and the peptide cytokines, interleukin-2 (44) and tumor necrosis factor (39).

Histamine and PGE_2 responses are interesting because they illustrate qualitative differences between responses in the pulmonary and systemic circulations. Histamine, a classic mediator of inflammation, causes vasodilation in the systemic vascular bed, but vasoconstriction in the lung (2). Interestingly, if histamine is administered to a preconstricted pulmonary vascular bed, it may cause vasodilation (83). Similarly, PGE_2 dilates systemic vessels (91) and constricts pulmonary vessels (42).

There are also examples in which one mediator serves as a sort of second messenger for a physiological effect of another. For example, in sheep, infusion of leukotriene D_4 causes vasoconstriction. LTD_4 also causes release of thromboxane, and cyclooxygenase inhibition prevents the pulmonary vasoconstrictor response to LTD_4 infusion in some preparations (1,66).

Many interventions which cause pulmonary vasoconstriction also cause endogenous production of increased quantities of the vasodilator prostanoid, prostacyclin. Although it is tempting to postulate that this is a homeostatic response, that is difficult to prove. Endothelial cells in culture produce prostacyclin in response to a bewildering number of interventions, and this may be a nonspecific response to endothelial perturbation (9). However, in some preparations, there does appear to be a temporal relationship between release of mediators and the physiological response which is consistent with the notion that there is a homeostatic interaction between mediators having opposite effects. For example, Figure 3 shows the time course of appearance of thromboxane and prostacyclin metabolites in lung lymph from sheep after infusing endotoxin (17). Thromboxane concentrations rise slightly faster than do prostacyclin concentrations. Pulmonary artery pressure increases as thromboxane concentrations rise and begins to decrease as peak concentrations of prostacyclin are reached. These kinds of relationships have led some investigators to suggest that the magnitude of constriction is determined by the relative concentrations of constrictor and dilator substances.

DISTRIBUTION OF BLOOD FLOW IN THE LUNGS

The distribution of perfusion to the large pulmonary microcirculation must have the potential for controlled inhomogeneity in order to preserve the lungs' essential function of gas exchange in the face of inhomogeneous ventilation. This necessity is met by the hypoxic pulmonary vasoconstrictor response, a response which is opposite to systemic vascular responses to hypoxia and is highly localized (75).

The stimulus for hypoxic pulmonary vasoconstriction appears to be mainly alveolar hypoxia. If animals (including humans) are made to ventilate hypoxic gas, pulmonary artery pressure and pulmonary vascular resistance increase. Localization of the hypoxic response is demonstrated by experiments in which portions of the lung are ventilated with hypoxic gas and diversion of blood flow away from the hypoxic area occurs (29). These kinds of data impel teleologic explanations of ventilation-perfusion matching in which the hypoxic vascular response is the principal factor.

In most species in which it has been studied, chronic ventilation of animals with hypoxic gas causes not only acute pulmonary hypertension, but sustained elevations in pulmonary vascular resistance which, with time, result in structural remodelling of the pulmonary vascular bed (74). This chronic effect results in chronic pulmonary hypertension which does not reverse (or does so only very slowly) even when the hypoxic stimulus is removed.

Is there a mediator of hypoxic pulmonary vasoconstriction? Attempts to answer this question have a long and somewhat disappointing history (see chapter by Fishman). Almost every substance which can cause pulmonary vasoconstriction has been proposed, at one time or another, as the mediator of the hypoxic response, including histamine, serotonin, angiotensin, prostanoids, and recently leukotrienes (52,85). To date, there is no conclusive evidence for a humoral mediator of the response.

Recent studies implicating lipoxygenase products of arachidonic acid in the hypoxic response are interesting. In some preparations, hypoxia can stimulate production of such substances in the lungs, and lipoxygenase inhibitors can moderate the response (59,60). This has led to the theory that hypoxia may result in increased production of free radicals in lung cells which can trigger generation of lipoxygenase products (86). Such a sequence appears theoretically possible, although there remain questions about whether a hypoxic challenge which will cause pulmonary vasoconstriction is severe enough to cause the postulated biochemical changes (8).

Endogenous humoral mediators may modulate hypoxic vasoconstriction. Particularly, the vasodilator prostanoid, prostacyclin, has been suggested as having this effect. Prostacyclin is a potent pulmonary vasodilator (37). When prostacyclin is infused intravenously, it can reverse hypoxic pulmonary vasoconstriction, even with continuing hypoxia (27). In some preparations, cyclooxygenase inhibition can augment hypoxic pulmonary vasoconstriction (27). In experimental models of acute lung injury, including oxygen toxicity (63) and endotoxin induced lung injury (36), the hypoxic vasoconstrictor response disappears. Weir and colleagues found that dogs treated with cyclooxygenase inhibitors and then given endotoxin preserved the hypoxic response (90). However, the vasodilator activity of prostacyclin is short-lived in vivo so that continued production of the substance would be necessary to explain prolonged loss of the constrictor response. In this case, it should be possible to cause the hypoxic response to return after it is lost by administering cyclooxygenase inhibitors.

Figure 4 shows data from unanesthetized sheep experiments in which the pulmonary vascular hypoxic response was measured before, and 4 hr after, infusing

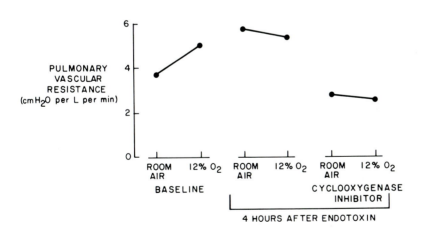

Figure 4: Effects of ventilation of hypoxic gas on pulmonary vascular resistance in unanesthetized sheep before and 4 hr after infusion of endotoxin. The normal hypoxic pulmonary vasoconstrictor response is lost after endotoxin infusion. Although administration of a cyclooxygenase inhibitor (meclofenamate) reduced pulmonary vascular resistance, the drug did not restore the hypoxic vasoconstrictor response. (Redrawn from Hutchison et al. [36].)

endotoxin (36). The response was lost following endotoxemia. However, as shown in the same figure, treatment with the cyclooxygenase inhibitor, ibuprofen, did not cause the response to return. These data are not consistent with endogenous generation of prostacyclin (or other vasodilator prostanoids) as the explanation for loss of the hypoxic response.

It is clear that the lungs have the capacity to adjust resistances to flow in parallel and, thus, to alter the distribution of pulmonary blood flow. It is also clear that alveolar hypoxia causes pulmonary vasoconstriction and that this is a localized phenomenon. Paralysis of the hypoxic response in situations where ventilation is inhomogeneous results in perfusion of poorly ventilated areas and increased shunting of hypoxic blood to the left side of the circulation. It is not yet clear whether there is a mediator or mediators of hypoxic pulmonary vasoconstriction or how the response is modulated by endogenous production of vasodilator substances.

PULMONARY VASOREACTIVITY

Here I present a hypothesis which is largely speculative, although not without some experimental basis. The hypothesis is that the pulmonary circulation may become hypersensitive to vasoconstrictor stimuli and that this hyperreactive state may both adversely affect pulmonary function acutely and, over time, result in structural remodelling of the pulmonary circulation and irreversible pulmonary hypertension. The hyperreactive state could be thought of as a sort of asthma of the pulmonary circulation.

Some experimental manipulations can exaggerate the hypoxic pulmonary pressor response. For example, treatment of animals with cyclooxygenase inhibitors can result in a greater hypoxic pulmonary vasoconstriction than when prostanoid synthesis is intact (29,75). This observation has fostered the notion that vasodilator prostanoids modulate hypoxic vasoconstriction.

The ether lipid, platelet-activating factor (PAF), is a pulmonary vasodilator when given to a preconstricted pulmonary vascular bed (51,75) and, when lungs are treated with a PAF antagonist and then exposed to constrictor stimuli, the constrictor response is exaggerated (32). PAF also increases airway reactivity, an effect which persists for long periods of time following a single exposure to PAF (19).

Some animal models of chronic pulmonary hypertension in which the evolution of the physiological alterations has been studied, demonstrate increased pulmonary vasoconstriction to hypoxia and pharmacological agents during the evolution of structural remodelling of the pulmonary arterial circulation. This is illustrated in Figure 5 where the time course of vasoconstrictor responses in chronically instrumented sheep following bilateral thoracic irradiation is compared to the evolution of pulmonary hypertension (70). At least theoretically, increased reactivity of the pulmonary vascular bed could result from production of a sensitizing mediator or loss of production of a vasodilator necessary for modulating constrictor responses. PAF has been shown to be released in the lungs in some situations (84). Damaged endothelial cells could also lose their ability to produce prostacyclin and endothelial relaxant factor.

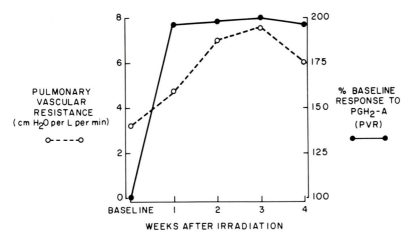

Figure 5: Pulmonary vasoreactivity and pulmonary vascular resistance in chronically instrumented sheep following bilateral thoracic irradiation. The pulmonary vasoconstrictor response to bolus injections of a thromboxane mimic (PGH$_2$-A) was doubled by 1 week after irradiation when pulmonary vascular resistance had just started to increase. Three to 4 weeks after irradiation, pulmonary vascular resistance was almost twice baseline and vasoreactivity remained high. (Redrawn from Perkett et al. [70])

THE PULMONARY MICROCIRCULATION

In addition to their function as conduits for blood and sites of gas exchange, pulmonary capillaries are the principal exchange vessels and their walls are the main barrier which controls the quantity and compositon of fluid reaching the pulmonary interstitium (7). Transcapillary movement of fluid and solutes is determined by relationships defined by Starling (81) and by Kedem and Katchalsky (43), in which hydrostatic pressure is a major force. Longitudinal distribution of resistance to blood flow through the lungs determines pressure in the pulmonary capillaries.

Under normal conditions, about half of the overall pulmonary vascular resistance is located upstream to the exchange vessels (25). A number of interventions have been shown to alter this distribution of resistances. For example, serotonin or histamine increases the fraction of resistance downstream to the capillaries so that for a given pulmonary artery pressure, capillary pressure is higher than in baseline conditions (20). Alveolar hypoxia may also increase downstream resistance and, thus, increase capillary pressure out of proportion to the rise in pulmonary artery pressure at least in young animals (31).

The relevance of alterations in longitudinal distribution of pulmonary vascular resistances is well illustrated by responses to endotoxemia. When endotoxin is infused into sheep, it causes both pulmonary hypertension and, if sufficient quantities of endotoxin are given, pulmonary edema (23). Several different lines of evidence, including ultrastructural studies, indicate that there is capillary injury and increased lung vascular permeability (13). However, other studies show that if pulmonary vascular pressures are not permitted to increase, endotoxin causes

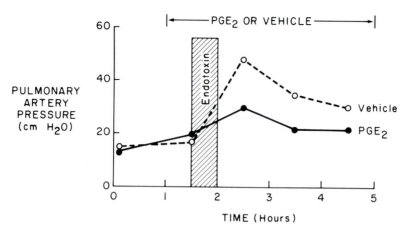

Figure 6: Effects of endotoxin infusion on pulmonary vascular pressures in unanesthetized sheep. Endotoxin infusion caused a rapid increase in pulmonary artery pressure which remained above baseline for several hours. Although left atrial pressure fell, peripheral pulmonary artery wedge pressure increased, suggesting venoconstriction. (Redrawn from Parker and Brigham [68].)

less edema (26). Is the edema caused by increased permeability or increased capillary pressure?

The answer is probably both. Figure 6 illustrates data from unanesthetized sheep in which pressures were measured in the pulmonary artery, in the left atrium, and in a small catheter wedged very peripherally in the arterial side of the circulation (68). Following endotoxin infusion, left atrial pressure fell, but both pulmonary artery pressure and peripheral wedge pressure increased, implying that there was small vein constriction, i.e., increased pressure downstream to the exchange vessels. The resulting increase in capillary pressure would increase transcapillary filtration, an effect which would be greatly exaggerated when permeability of the capillaries was also increased.

It seems very likely that the alteration in pulmonary vascular resistance following endotoxemia is a result of release of endogenous vasoactive mediators. There is evidence implicating histamine (15), serotonin (67), prostanoids and lipoxygenase products of arachidonic acid (65), all of which have the potential for constricting both the arterial and the venous sides of the pulmonary circulation. However, it is not yet clear how these mediators interact to result in the overall response in intact animals.

Under some circumstances, the pulmonary microcirculation may lose its ability to function as an effective barrier to fluid and solute filtration. This increase in pulmonary vascular permeability results in pulmonary edema without requisite increases in pulmonary vascular pressures; this is thought to be the primary abnormality in the human condition called the adult respiratory distress syndrome (ARDS). Much investigative work over the past 15 years has focused on identification of a mediator of increased pulmonary vascular permeability.

Histamine increases permeability in systemic vessels (18) and remains one of the most popular mediators of the inflammatory response. Infusion of histamine into experimental animals can cause pulmonary edema, but histamine is a pulmonary vasoconstrictor and separating hemodynamic effects from effects on capillary permeability has not been easy. Based on observations of the leakage of carbon particles from the microcirculation, histamine has been said to increase permeability of bronchial but not pulmonary vessels in the lungs (72). Infusion of histamine into sheep causes sustained increases in flow of protein-rich lung lymph, changes which are typical of increased permeability in the pulmonary vascular bed (11). However, when left atrial pressure is elevated to maximally recruit lung exchange vessels, and then histamine is infused, it appears that there are two separable effects (3). There is an early increase in flow of protein-rich lung lymph (increased permeability), but this is a transient response followed by a fall in lymph protein concentrations typical of the response to increased pressure (69). This transient effect on permeability can be demonstrated in pulmonary vascular endothelium studied in vitro (54) and also occurs in systemic vascular beds (18). Thus, it appears that effects of histamine are not an adequate explanation for the prolonged increases in pulmonary vascular permeability which occur in animal models of ARDS.

PRODUCTION AND PROCESSING OF MEDIATORS IN THE LUNGS

A number of vasoactive mediators can be produced in the lungs by either constituent lung cells or leukocytes. These mediators could affect either the pulmonary circulation or the systemic circulation or both.

The lungs are rich in mediator producing leukocytes, including mast cells, macrophages, and neutrophils. Mast cells located in the pulmonary interstitium around airways and blood vessels have long been implicated as a source of substances which may cause the bronchoconstriction typical of asthma. Histamine has received most of the attention but, more recently, prostaglandin D_2 and its bioactive metabolite, $9\alpha,11\beta$-PGF_1, have been implicated in bronchoconstrictor reactions (78). Histamine is a pulmonary vasoconstrictor in the relaxed pulmonary vascular bed but may dilate a preconstricted bed (83). PGD_2 is a pulmonary vasoconstrictor (14). Mast cells remain a potential source of mediators which cause or modulate pulmonary hypertension, although it has been difficult to assign them a unique role.

There is a large marginated pool of neutrophils in the pulmonary circulation normally (82), which may be a result of the physics of particle flow in small vessels (49) and humoral conversation between neutrophils and microvascular endothelial cells (5). Many interventions which cause alterations in functions of the pulmonary circulation also cause increased sequestration of neutrophils in the lungs. It is widely believed that sequestration of activated neutrophils in the pulmonary microcirculation is a critical part of the pathogenesis of diffuse lung injury (12,76).

Activated neutrophils produce leukotriene B_4, a lipoxygenase product of arachidonic acid which is a potent activator of neutrophils (24). Not only does LTB_4 stimulate neutrophils, providing a mechanism for self-perpetuation of the activation response, but it also affects endothelial cells so as to make them more adherent to neutrophils (34). On the other hand, prostaglandin E_2, a product of endothelial cells, especially in the microcirculation (28), inhibits LTB_4 release from activated neutrophils (30). Some of the same stimuli which cause sequestra-

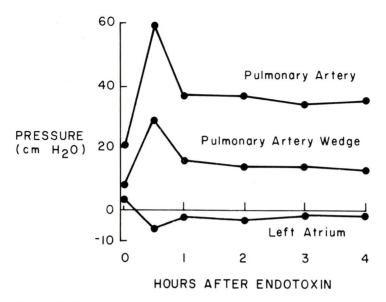

Figure 7: Effects of prostaglandin E_2 (PGE$_2$) on the pulmonary vasoconstrictor response to endotoxin infusion in unanesthetized sheep. Although PGE$_2$ is a pulmonary vasoconstrictor, the drug diminished endotoxin-induced pulmonary hypertension. (Redrawn from Brigham et al. [16])

tion of neutrophils in the lungs also stimulate endothelial cells to produce PGE$_2$. It may be that the magnitude and consequences of leukocyte sequestration in the lungs are dictated by humoral dialogue between neutrophils and endothelial cells, a dialogue in which LTB$_4$ and PGE$_2$ are the vocabulary (10).

This kind of humoral interaction may result in paradoxical effects of exogenously administered mediators. For example, PGE$_2$ is, under normal conditions, a pulmonary vasoconstrictor (42). Endotoxemia causes marked pulmonary neutrophil sequestration in unanesthetized sheep (and all other species in which it has been studied), and one of the principal physiological consequences is pulmonary hypertension. However, as illustrated in Figure 7, if endotoxin is given in the presence of PGE$_2$, the pulmonary hypertension is attenuated (16).

A large population of macrophages is normally present in the pulmonary airspaces. These "alveolar macrophages" serve important defense functions, but they are also a source of mediators which may affect trafficking of other inflammatory cells and may directly affect pulmonary function as well. Alveolar macrophages can produce and release thromboxane (a pulmonary vasoconstrictor), PGE$_2$, and substances (including LTB$_4$) (48) which are chemotactic for neutrophils (35). In some models of pulmonary inflammation, alveolar macrophages can be shown to generate neutrophil chemotaxins (22) which may be important in the pathogenesis of the inflammatory response.

Recently, another population of pulmonary macrophages has been described in some species. These cells, variously called intravascular monocytes (53) or pulmonary intravascular macrophages (PIMs) (89), are located in the lumen of small blood vessels but appear closely adherent to the vascular endothelium. Ultrastructural studies indicate that these cells may become activated, e.g., following endotoxemia (53). Figure 8 is a transmission electron micrograph of an activated intravascular monocyte in the lungs following endotoxemia in a sheep.

The importance of intravascular monocytes as a source of mediators which might affect pulmonary function is not yet clear. It seems possible, even likely, that the generation of thromboxane, responsible for the early pulmonary hypertension following endotoxemia (64), may be principally from these cells since platelets (the usual source of thromboxane) are not the source in the endotoxin model in sheep (79).

Endothelial cells can release a host of mediators which could affect function of the pulmonary circulation either directly or indirectly. The principal eicosanoid produced by pulmonary artery endothelial cells in culture is prostacyclin, and it seems likely that endothelium is the main source of this vasodilator in the several experimental models which stimulate prostacyclin release from the lungs. Endothelial cells also produce PGE_2, and microvascular endothelium cultured from several organs (28), including the lungs (56), can produce large amounts of this prostanoid. Although cultured endothelial cells have been reported to produce

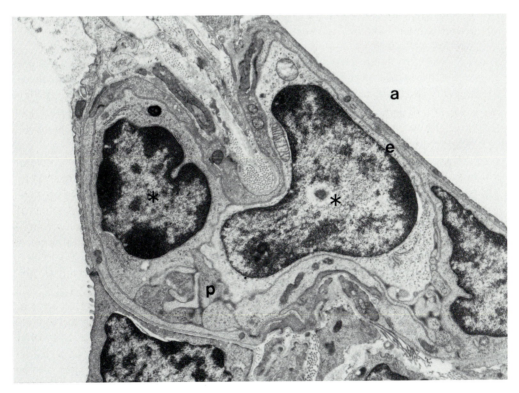

Figure 8: Electron micrograph of an alveolar capillary from a sheep given repeated infusions of endotoxin (three per week) over an 8-week period. The capillary is completely occluded by two pulmonary intravascular macrophages or activated monocytes (*) and their processes (p). e = endothelium; a = alveolus. ×12,300. (Courtesy of Dr. Barbara Meyrick.)

lipoxygenase products of arachidonic acid as well (40), these do not appear to be major products. Endothelial cells from some organs can produce the lipid mediator, platelet-activating factor (PAF) (50), which could be yet another important modulator of pulmonary vascular function as discussed above.

Some endothelial cells in culture can produce peptide cytokines, especially interleukin-1. Endothelial cells stimulated by exposure to either tumor necrosis factor or endotoxin produce increased amounts of interleukin-1, apparently by increasing transcription of the genetic message (46). Interleukin-1 might affect pulmonary vascular responses indirectly by affecting communication among inflammatory cells.

There are anatomic features of the pulmonary circulation which provide the potential for a unique role in regulating the vasculature of systemic organs. All of the cardiac output must pass through the lungs before entering the systemic circulation, and the immense microvascular surface area in the lungs affords the opportunity for altering composition of the blood.

Several vasoactive substances are either removed from or processed by the pulmonary vascular endothelium. Serotonin is extracted from blood by pulmonary capillary endothelium (58). Angiotensin converting enzyme, located on the luminal surface of lung microvascular endothelium, converts angiotensin I to the potent pressor, angiotensin II (77); the same enzyme metabolizes bradykinin, a systemic vasodilator released under some pathologic conditions. The pulmonary circulation may be an important regulator of systemic blood pressure.

There are even more subtle possibilities. Adenosine infused into the kidney attenuates systemic hypertension by inhibiting renin release. Perfusion of the lungs with angiotensin II causes release of adenosine into the vascular effluent (38). These observations provide the elements of a feedback mechanism between the kidneys and the lungs in which the lungs both produce the pressor (angiotensin II) and control production of the precursor (angiotensin I).

REFERENCES

1. Ahmed T, Marchette B, Wanner A, Yerger L: Direct and indirect effects of leukotriene D$_4$ on the pulmonary and systemic circulations. Am Rev Respir Dis 131:554–558, 1985.

2. Aviado DM: *The Lung Circulation*, Vol 1. London, Pergamon Press, 1965.

3. Bernard GR, Snapper JR, Hutchison AA, Brigham KL: Effects of left atrial pressure elevation and histamine infusion on lung lymph in awake sheep. J Appl Physiol 56:1083–1089, 1984.

4. Bowers R, Ellis E, Brigham KL, Oates J: Effects of prostaglandin cyclic endoperoxides on the lung circulation of sheep. J Clin Invest 63:131–137, 1979.

5. Boxer LA, Allen JM, Baehner RL: Diminished polymorphonuclear leukocyte adherence: Function dependent on release of cyclic AMP by endothelial cells after stimulation of β-receptors by epinephrine. J Clin Invest 66:268–274, 1980.

6. Braun K, Stern S: Pulmonary and systemic blood pressure response to serotonin: Role of chemoreceptors. Am J Physiol 201:369–373, 1961.

7. Brigham KL: Lung lymph composition and flow in normal and abnormal states, in Fishman AP (ed), *Update: Pulmonary Diseases and Disorders.* New York, McGraw-Hill, 1982, pp 101–111.

8. Brigham KL: Lipid mediators in the pulmonary circulation: Conference summary. Am Rev Respir Dis 136:785–788, 1987.

9. Brigham KL: Mechanisms of endothelial injury, in Ryan US (ed), *Pulmonary Endothelium in Health and Disease.* New York, Marcel Dekker, 1987, pp 207–236.

10. Brigham KL: Mediators of the inflammatory process: Prostanoids, in Henson P, Murphy R (eds), *Handbook of Inflammation, vol 6: Mediators of the Inflammatory Process.* Amsterdam, Elsevier Science Publishers, 1987, in press.

11. Brigham K, Bowers R, Owen P: Effects of antihistamines on the lung vascular response to histamine in unanesthetized sheep: Diphenhydramine prevention of pulmonary edema and increased permeability. J Clin Invest 58:391–398, 1976.

12. Brigham KL, Meyrick B: Interactions of granulocytes with the lungs. Circ Res 54:623–635, 1984.

13. Brigham KL, Meyrick BO: Endotoxin and lung injury: State of the art review. Am Rev Respir Dis 133:913–927, 1986.

14. Brigham KL, Ogletree ML: Effects of prostaglandins and related compounds on lung vascular permeability. Bull Eur Physiopathol Respir 17:703–722, 1981.

15. Brigham KL, Padove SJ, Bryant DM, McKeen CR, Bowers RE: Diphenhydramine reduces endotoxin effects on lung vascular permeability in sheep. J Appl Physiol 49:516–520, 1980.

16. Brigham KL, Serafin W, Zadoff A, Blair I, Meyrick B, Oates JA: Prostaglandin E_2 attenuation of sheep lung responses to endotoxin. J Appl Physiol 64:2568–2574, 1988.

17. Brigham KL, Snapper JR: Lung lymph composition and flow in normal and abnormal states, in Fishman AP (ed), *Pulmonary Disease and Disorders*, 2nd ed. New York, McGraw-Hill, 1988, pp 909–918.

18. Carter R, Joyner W, Renkin E: Effects of histamine and some other substances on molecular selectivity of the capillary wall to plasma protein and dextran. Microvasc Res 7:31–48, 1974.

19. Cuss FM, Dixon CM, Barnes PJ: Effects of inhaled platelet activating factor on pulmonary function and bronchial responsiveness in man. Lancet 2:189–192, 1986.

20. Dawson CA, Linehan JH, Bronikowski TA, Rickaby DA: Pulmonary microvascular hemodynamics: Occlusion methods, in Will J, Dawson C, Weir K, Buckner C (eds), *The Pulmonary Circulation in Health and Disease*. New York, Academic Press, 1987, pp 175–197.

21. DeMey JG, Claeys M, Vanhoutte PM: Endothelium-dependent inhibitory effects of acetylcholine, adenosine triphosphate, thrombin and arachidonic acid in the canine femoral artery. J Pharmacol Exp Ther 222:166–173, 1982.

22. Duke SS, Bolds JM, Loyd JE, Brigham KL: Endotoxin-induced neutrophilic alveolitis and macrophage chemotaxin production in sheep. Am J Med Sci 296:381–386, 1988.

23. Esbenshade AM, Newman JH, Lams PM, Jolles H, Brigham KL: Respiratory failure after endotoxin infusion in sheep: Lung mechanics and lung fluid balance. J Appl Physiol 53:967–976, 1982.

24. Ford-Hutchison AW, Bray MA, Doig MV, Shipley ME, Smith MJ: Leukotriene B, a potent chemokinetic and aggregating substance released from polymorphonuclear leukocytes. Nature 286:264–265, 1980.

25. Gaar KA, Taylor AE, Owens LJ, Guyton AE: Pulmonary capillary pressure and filtration coefficient in the isolated perfused lung. Am J Physiol 213:910–914, 1967.

26. Gabel JC, Hansen TN, Drake RE: Effect of endotoxin on lung fluid balance in unanesthetized sheep. J Appl Physiol 56:489–494, 1984.

27. Gerber JG, Voelkel NF, Nies AS, McMurtry IF, Reeves JT: Moderation of hypoxic vasoconstriction by infused arachidonic acid: Role of PGI_2. J Appl Physiol 49:107–112, 1980.

28. Gerritsen ME, Cheli CD: Arachidonic acid and prostaglandin endoperoxide metabolism in isolated rabbit and coronary microvessels and isolated cultivated coronary microvessel endothelial cells. J Clin Invest 72:1658–1671, 1983.

29. Hales CA, Rouse ET, Slate JL: Influence of aspirin and indomethacin on variability of alveolar hypoxic vasoconstriction. J Appl Physiol 45:33–39, 1978.

30. Ham EA, Soderman DD, Zanetti ME Dougherty HW, McCauley E, Kuehl FA Jr: Inhibition by prostaglandins of leukotriene B_4 release from activated neutrophils. Proc Natl Acad Sci USA 80:4349–4353, 1983.

31. Hansen TN, Haberkern CM, Hazinski TA, Bland RD: Lung fluid balance in hypoxic lambs. Pediatr Res 18:434–440, 1984.

32. Haynes J, Chang S, Voelkel N: Platelet activating factor decreases vascular reactivity in rat lungs. Fed Proc 46:11–12, 1987.

33. Henry CL, Ogletree ML, Brigham KL, Hammon JW Jr: Thromboxane A_2 mediates the pulmonary vascular response to endotoxin. Surgical Forum 35:134–136, 1985.

34. Hoover RL, Karnovsky MJ, Austen KF, Corey EJ, Lewis RA: Leukotriene B_4 action on endothelium mediates augmented neutrophil-endothelial interactions. Proc Natl Acad Sci USA 81:2191–2193, 1984.

35. Hunninghake GW, Gadek JE, Fales HM, Crystal RG: Human alveolar macrophage-derived chemotactic factor for neutrophils: Stimuli and partial characterization. J Clin Invest 66:473–483, 1980.

36. Hutchison AA, Ogletree ML, Snapper JR, Brigham KL: Effect of endotoxemia on hypoxic pulmonary vasoconstriction in unanesthetized sheep. J Appl Physiol 58:1463–1468, 1985.

37. Hyman AL, Kadowitz PJ: Pulmonary vasodilator activity of prostacyclin (PGI_2) in the cat. Circ Res 45:404–409, 1979.

38. Jackson E et al: Angiotensin II induced release of adenosine from perfused rat lungs (Abstract). Clin Res. In Press.

39. Johnson J, Meyrick B, Jesmok G, Wickersham N, Brigham KL: Infusion of recombinant human tumor necrosis factor alpha (rTNF) into sheep causes changes in pulmonary hemodynamics, pulmonary vascular permeability and leukocyte trafficking similar to those induced by endotoxin (Abstract). Am Rev Respir Dis. In Press.

40. Johnson AR, Revtyak G, Campbell WB: Arachidonic acid metabolites and endothelial injury. Studies with cultures of human endothelial cells. Fed Proc 44:19–24, 1985.

41. Joiner PD, Kadowitz PJ, Hughes JP, Hyman AL: Actions of prostaglandins E$_1$ and E$_{2\alpha}$ on isolated intrapulmonary vascular smooth muscle. Proc Soc Exp Biol Med 150:414–421, 1975.

42. Kadowitz PJ, Joiner PD, Hyman AL: Effect of prostglandin E$_2$ on pulmonary vascular resistance in intact dog, swine and lamb. Eur J Pharmacol 31:72–80, 1975.

43. Kedem O, Katchalsky A: A physical interpretation of the phenomenological coefficients of membrane permeability. J Gen Physiol 45:143–179, 1961.

44. King LS, Kubo K, Duke S, Brigham KL, Newman JH: Human recombinant interleukin 2(IL2) infusion causes acute changes in lung vascular function in awake sheep (Abstract). Physiologist. In press.

45. Kuhl PG, Bolds JM, Loyd JE, Snapper JR, FitzGerald GA: Thromboxane receptor-mediated bronchial and hemodynamic responses in ovine endotoxemia. Am J Physiol 254:R310–R319, 1988.

46. Libby P, Ordovas JM, Auger KR, Robbins AH, Birinyi LK, Dinarello CA: Endotoxin and TNF induce IL-1 gene expression in adult human vascular endothelial cells. Am J Pathol 124:179–185, 1986.

47. Lock JE, Olley PM, Soldin S, Coceani F: Indomethacin-induced pulmonary vasoconstriction in the conscious newborn lambs. Am J Physiol H639–H651, 1980.

48. MacDermot J, Kelsey CR, Waddell KA, Richmond R, Knight RK, Cole PJ, Dollery CT, Landon DN, Blair IA: Synthesis of leukotriene B$_4$ and prostanoids by human alveolar macrophages: Analysis by gas chromatography/mass spectrometry. Prostaglandins 27:163–179, 1984.

49. Martin B, Wright J, Thommasen H, Hogg J: The effect of pulmonary blood flow on the exchange between the circulation and marginating pool of polymorphonuclear leukocytes (PMN) in dog lungs. J Clin Invest 69:1277–1285, 1982.

50. McIntyre TM, Zimmerman GA, Satoh K, Prescott SM: Cultured endothelial cells synthesize both platelet activating factor and prostacyclin in response to histamine, bradykinin and adenosine triphosphate. J Clin Invest 76:271–280, 1985.

51. McMurtry IF, Morris KG: Platelet-activating factor causes pulmonary vasodilation in the rat. Am Rev Respir Dis 134:757–762, 1986.

52. McMurtry IF, Raffenstin B: Potential mechanisms of hypoxic pulmonary vasoconstriction, in Will J, Dawson C, Weir K, Buckner C (eds), *The Pulmonary Circulation in Health and Disease.* New York, Academic Press, 1987, pp 455–468.

53. Meyrick B, Brigham KL: Acute effects of *Escherichia coli* endotoxin on the pulmonary microcirculation of anesthetized sheep: Structure:function relationships. Lab Invest 48:458–470, 1983.

54. Meyrick BO, Brigham KL: Increased permeability associated with dilatation of endothelial cell junctions caused by histamine in intimal explants from bovine pulmonary artery. Exp Lung Res 6:11–25, 1984.

55. Meyrick B, Brigham KL: Repeated *E. coli* endotoxin induced pulmonary inflammation causes chronic pulmonary hypertension in sheep: Structural and functional changes. Lab Invest 55:164–176, 1986.

56. Meyrick B, Hoover R, Jones M, Berry LC, Brigham KL: In vitro effects of endotoxin on bovine and sheep lung microvascular and pulmonary artery endothelial cells. J Cell Physiol 138:165–174, 1989.

57. Meyrick B, Niedermeyer ME, Ogletree ML, Brigham KL: Pulmonary hypertension and increased vasoreactivity caused by repeated indomethacin treatment in sheep. J Appl Physiol 59:443–452, 1985.

58. Morel DR, Dargent F, Bachmann M, Suter PM, Junod AF: Pulmonary extraction of serotonin and propranolol in patients with adult respiratory distress syndrome. Am Rev Respir Dis 132:479–484, 1985.

59. Morganroth ML, Reeves JT, Murphy RC, Voelkel NF: Leukotriene synthesis and/or receptor blockers block hypoxic pulmonary vasoconstriction. J Appl Physiol 56:1340–1346, 1984.

60. Morganroth ML, Stenmark KR, Zirrolli JA, Mauldin R, Mathias M, Reeves JT, Murphy RC, Voelkel NF: Leukotriene C$_4$ production during hypoxic pulmonary vasoconstriction in isolated rat lungs. Prostaglandins 28:867–875, 1984.

61. Nawroth PP, Stern DM, Kaplan KL, Nossel HL: Prostacyclin production by perturbed bovine aortic endothelial cells in culture. Blood 64:801–806, 1984.

62. Newman JH, Butka BJ, Brigham KL: Thromboxane A$_2$ and prostacyclin do not modulate pulmonary hemodynamics during exercise in sheep. J Appl Physiol 61:1706–1711, 1986.

63. Newman JH, Loyd JE, English DK, Ogletree ML, Fulkerson WJ, Brigham KL: Effects of 100% oxygen on lung vascular function in awake sheep. J Appl Physiol 54:1379–1386, 1983.

64. Nichols FC, Schenkein HA, Rutherford RB: Prostaglandin E$_2$, prostaglandin E$_1$ and thromboxane B$_2$ release from human monocytes treated with C3b or bacterial lipopolysaccharide. Biochem Biophys Acta 927:149–157, 1987.

65. Ogletree ML, Begley CJ, King GA, Brigham KL: Influence of steroidal and non-steroidal anti-inflammatory agents on accumulation of arachidonic acid metabolites in plasma and lung lymph after endotoxemia in awake sheep: Measurements of prostacyclin and thromboxane metabolites and 12-HETE. Am Rev Respir Dis 133:55–61, 1986.

66. Ogletree ML, Snapper JL, Brigham KL: Direct

and indirect effects of leukotriene D_4 on the lungs of unanesthetized sheep. Respiration 51:256–265, 1987.

67. Olson NC: Role of 5-hydroxytryptamine in endotoxin-induced respiratory failure in pigs. Am Rev Respir Dis 135:93–99, 1987.

68. Parker RE, Brigham KL: Effects of endotoxemia on pulmonary vascular resistances in unanesthetized sheep. J Appl Physiol 63:1058–1062, 1987.

69. Parker RE, Roselli RJ, Harris TR, Brigham KL: Effects of graded increases in pulmonary vascular pressures on lung fluid balance in unanesthetized sheep. Circ Res 49:1164–1172, 1981.

70. Perkett EA, Brigham KL, Meyrick B: Increased vasoreactivity and chronic pulmonary hypertension following thoracic irradiation in sheep. J Appl Physiol 61:1875–1881, 1986.

71. Perkowski SZ, Havill AM, Flynn JT, Gee MH: Role of intrapulmonary release of eicosanoids and superoxide anion as mediators of pulmonary dysfunction and endothelial injury in sheep with intermittent complement activation. Circ Res 53:574–583, 1983.

72. Pietra GG, Szidon JP, Leventhal MM, Fishman AP: Histamine and interstitial pulmonary edema in the dog. Circ Res 29:323–337, 1971.

73. Prescott SM, Zimmerman GA, McIntyre TM: Human endothelial cells in culture produce platelet-activating factor when stimulated with thrombin. Proc Natl Acad Sci USA 81:3534–3538, 1984.

74. Rabinovitch M, Gamble W, Nadas AS, Meittinen OS, Reid L: Rat pulmonary circulation after chronic hypoxia: hemodynamic and structural changes. Am J Physiol 236:H818-H827, 1979.

75. Reeves JT, McMurtry IF, Voelkel NF: Possible role of membrane lipids in the function of the normal and abnormal pulmonary circulation. Am Rev Respir Dis 136:196–199, 1987.

76. Repine JE, Bowman CM, Tate RM: Neutrophils and lung edema. State of the art. Am Rev Respir Dis 81S:47S–50S, 1982.

77. Ryan US: Processing of angiotensin and other peptides by the lungs, in Fishman AP, Fisher AB (eds), *Handbook of Physiology. Sect 3: The Respiratory System, Vol I: Circulation and Nonrespiratory Functions*. Bethesda, American Physiological Society, 1985, pp 351–364.

78. Seibert K, Sheller JR, Roberts LJ: 9 alpha,11 beta-prostaglandin F_2: Formation and metabolism by human lung and contractile effects on human bronchial smooth muscle. Proc Natl Acad Sci USA 84:254–260, 1987.

79. Snapper JR, Hinson JM Jr, Hutchison AA, Lefferts PL, Ogletree ML, Brigham KL: Effects of platelet depletion on the unanesthetized sheep's pulmonary response to endotoxemia. J Clin Invest 74:1782–1791, 1984.

80. Snapper JR, Hutchison AA, Ogletree ML, Brigham KL: Effects of cyclooxygenase inhibitors on the alterations in lung mechanics caused by endotoxemia in the unanesthetized sheep. J Clin Invest 72:63–76, 1983.

81. Starling EH: On the absorption of fluid from connective tissue spaces. J Physiol 19:312–326, 1986.

82. Staub NC, Schultz EL, Albertine KH: Leukocytes and pulmonary vascular injury. Ann NY Acad Sci 384:332–342, 1982.

83. Stecenko AA, Lefferts P, Mitchell J, Snapper JR, Brigham KL: Vasodilatory effect of aerosol histamine during pulmonary vasoconstriction in the unanesthetized sheep. Pediatr Pulmonol 3:94–100, 1987.

84. Stenmark KR, Eyzaguirre M, Westcott JY, Henson PM, Murphy RC: Potential role of eicosanoids and PAF in the pathophysiology of bronchopulmonary dysplasia. Am Rev Respir Dis 136:770–772, 1987.

85. Voelkel NF: Mechanisms of hypoxic pulmonary vasoconstriction. Am Rev Respir Dis 133:1186–1195, 1986.

86. Voelkel NF, Chang SW, McDonnell TJ, Westcott JY, Haynes J: Role of membrane lipids in the control of normal vascular tone. Am Rev Respir Dis 136:214–217, 1987.

87. Voelkel NF, Stenmark KR, Reeves JT, Mathias MM, Murphy RC: Actions of lipoxygenase metabolites in isolated rat lungs. J Appl Physiol 57:860–867, 1984.

88. Walker BR, Voelkel NF, Reeves JT: Pulmonary pressor response following prostaglandin synthesis inhibition in conscious dogs. J Appl Physiol 52:705–709, 1982.

89. Warner AE, Barry BE, Brain JD: Pulmonary intravascular macrophages in sheep. Lab Invest 55:276–288, 1986.

90. Weir K, Mlczoch J, Reeves J, Grover R: Endotoxemia and the prevention of hypoxic pulmonary vasoconstriction. J Lab Clin Med 88:975–983, 1976.

91. Wennmalm A: Participation of prostaglandins in the regulation of peripheral vascular resistance. Adv Prostaglandin Thromboxane Leukotriene Res 10:303–331, 1982.

Alfred P. Fishman, M.D.

9

The Enigma of Hypoxic Pulmonary Vasoconstriction

Before the 1940s, when the pulmonary circulation of intact animals and humans was still relatively inaccessible for blood sampling or for measuring blood pressures, interest in how it was regulated centered primarily on extrapulmonary influences, notably autonomic nerves and hormones (see Chapter 10), and on distinguishing between active and passive influences responsible for changes in pulmonary vascular resistance.

Things changed in the 1940s and 1950s: (1) the determination that acute hypoxia is a powerful pulmonary vasoconstrictor (106) directed attention from nerves to the chemical control of the pulmonary circulation; (2) the hypothesis that the vasopressor response to acute hypoxia is an automatic device by which local pulmonary blood flow is matched to alveolar ventilation was quickly put to the test in several laboratories using a variety of techniques and different experimental preparations; (3) the automatic adjustment was shown to be largely a local phenomenon and to operate without benefit of nerves; and (4) the advent and standardization of right heart catheterization in humans not only provided ready access to the previously remote pulmonary circulation but also paved the way to exploring how the pulmonary circulation responded to acute hypoxia and was regulated under natural, or near-natural, conditions, in health and disease (23).

Since the 1940s, the hypoxic pressor response has been tested in humans, in a wide variety of animals and animal preparations, and in models. Comparisons have also been made of the effects of age and sex. Although the pressor response has been elicited in virtually all mammals tested, in the fetus and neonate as well as in the adult, and in lower vertebrates, the hypoxic pressor response has proved not to be equally strong in all spaces or at all ages or in both sexes (95). Moreover,

TABLE 1 FACTORS INFLUENCING THE HYPOXIC PRESSOR RESPONSE

Genetics
Species
Age
Sex
Temperature
Experimental manipulation
Anesthesia
Composition of perfusate
Wall structure
Wall tension

in some experimental circumstances, e.g., the isolated perfused lung subjected to severe hypoxia, the pressor response can give way to a dilator response (13,95). Finally, the hypoxic pressor response can be strongly influenced by the setting in which it is tested (Table 1): anesthesia, body cooling, surgical manipulation and blood loss, atelectasis, abnormal perfusates, and artificial internal and external environments can blunt the pressor response (21,67,80,94).

Nonetheless, the experience to date does make it possible to generalize about certain aspects of the hypoxic pulmonary pressor response in intact unanesthetized humans as well as conventional laboratory animals, e.g., dog, cat, and cow: (1) the major component of the hypoxic pressor response begins and ends within the lungs; (2) extrapulmonary influences, such as reflexes from the peripheral chemoreceptors, which ordinarily play only a modest role in the hypoxic pressor responses, can be greatly exaggerated during severe stress; and (3) physiological consequences of hypoxia depend on how much of the lungs is rendered hypoxic: (a) hypoxia of *both lungs* elicits a characteristic constellation that features pulmonary vasoconstriction, a modest increase in cardiac output, a decrease in pulmonary blood volume, and diversion of pulmonary blood flow towards the periphery of the lungs, i.e., toward the apices and subpleural regions (16); the resultant increase in pulmonary arterial pressure improves the uniformity of blood flow throughout the lungs, but only improves slightly the ventilation-perfusion relationships throughout the lungs; (b) hypoxia confined to *one lung* diverts pulmonary blood flow contralaterally, i.e., to the better oxygenated lung with less of an increase in pulmonary arterial pressure (4,78); and (c) hypoxia applied to small segments of a lung evokes intense vasoconstriction, i.e., exerts an important effect in adjusting local alveolar ventilation to blood flow (91); taken together, the experiments involving bilateral hypoxia, unilateral hypoxia, and segmental hypoxia indicate that the smaller the area of the lung rendered hypoxic, the greater the degree of hypoxic vasoconstriction (45,48,61).

PULMONARY VASCULAR RESPONSIVENESS

It has been noted above that even though acute hypoxia has elicited pulmonary vasoconstriction in virtually every species tested, the magnitude of the response has varied with species, age and sex, and the experimental preparation. The response also depends on the antecedent ambient P_{O_2} (95). In part, the vigor of the response can be attributed to the muscle mass in the pulmonary small arteries and arterioles: the thicker vessel walls of calves and pigs (99) can generate more of a hypoxic pulmonary pressor response than can the sparser muscles of the hamster (108). However, anatomy and architecture are not the whole story: the influence of age (84,99), genetic background, gender (113), and experimental circumstance (95) imply a functional component that is difficult to quantify.

Initial Tone

The responsiveness of the pulmonary vasculature is determined not only by the inherent properties of the vascular wall but also by its initial tone, i.e., the level of preexisting sustained partial contraction. In sea dwellers, initial tone is quite low. The reason for this low tone is speculative but is increasingly attributed to vasodilators released locally, particularly prostacyclin and endothelium-derived relaxing factor (EDRF). Other substances, such as bradykinin, vasoactive intestinal peptide, histamine, substance P, and acetylcholine, seem to act as modulators or co-mediators (66).

Because of the low initial tone, attempts to vasodilate the normal pulmonary circulation are destined to be fruitless unless initial tone is artificially heightened, e.g., by administration of a vasopressor agent before challenging the pulmonary circulation with acetylcholine. At the opposite extreme from the relaxed normal pulmonary circulation is the artificially fully constricted pulmonary circulation, as in the case of "gnarly" lungs produced in the rabbit by massive doses of a powerful vasoconstrictor agent, e.g., norepinephrine. Gnarly lungs can be considered a measure of the maximum potential of the pulmonary vascular bed to constrict. Between these extremes of vasodilation and vasoconstriction are intermediate degrees of initial tone that are apt to occur under natural conditions. For example, in native residents at high altitude, initial tone is higher than in sea level dwellers. Also, during intense autonomic activity, as during "fight-or-flight" reactions, the pulmonary circulation, along with vascular beds elsewhere, tenses everywhere and undergoes a massive increase in resistance.

As a general rule, the further removed the preparation and experimental circumstances from natural conditions, the less the initial tone and the more blunted the hypoxic pressor response. Perfusion of the isolated lung with physiologic saline instead of plasma renders it poorly reactive to hypoxia, a situation that can be improved by certain additives, e.g., angiotensin II (64); red blood cells in the perfusate enhance reactivity (67). Acidity (60,79), temperature, electrolyte composition, the extent of autonomic innervation, the electrolyte and protein composition of the bath or perfusate, and access to local and remote hormones influence the threshold, pattern, and magnitude of the vasomotor response. Indeed, it has become commonplace for investigators using certain preparations to introduce biologically active substances into the environs of test circulations, vessels, or vessel strips in order to restore some degree of responsiveness. The use of pharmacologic agents as enhancers automatically poses problems in distinguishing between physiologic and pharmacologic effects on the one hand and on specificity and side actions on the other, especially in the lungs where resistance vessels are inextricably buried within pulmonary parenchyma made up of multiple cell types.

An important element in setting initial tone and in shaping pulmonary vascular responsiveness is the presence and interplay of intrinsic biologically active modulators. Depending on the circumstance, some biologically active substances can reach the lungs from afar: among these are beta agonists, angiotensin (64), and "growth factors"; others are generated locally: prostacyclin (29,105), endothelium-derived relaxing factor, histamine, vasoactive intestinal polypeptide (VIP), substance P, and acetylcholine. Even this bevy is suspected of being incomplete. For example, interest is currently high in "endothelin," a powerful vasoconstrictor polypeptide that is a naturally occurring component of mammalian endothelium that presumably acts as a modulator of voltage-dependent ion channels (115) and is homologous with the sarafotoxins, lethal components of snake venom (47,53). Clearly, the natural interplay that sets initial tone and determines responsiveness is complex and vulnerable to distortion by experimental conditions.

ALVEOLAR HYPOXIA OR MIXED VENOUS HYPOXIA

For the sake of convenience, acute hypoxia has traditionally been induced by decreasing the oxygen tension of inspired gas, thereby lowering the alveolar oxygen tension (P_{O_2}). As a result, the research for the mechanism by which acute hypoxia evokes a pulmonary pressor response has focussed on *alveolar* hypoxia. Unfortunately, this practice runs the risk of beclouding the mechanism since it raises the prospect of a unique sensing mechanism either within the airways or somehow related to alveolar structures. However, specialized structures that could trigger the hypoxic pressor response have not been identified in the alveoli. Nor have neuroepithelial cells in the airways been proven to have functional significance as hypoxic sensors. Instead, the alveoli seem designed only to serve as biological tonometers.

As a corollary, overemphasis on "alveolar hypoxia" has distracted attention from any contributions that might be made by the mixed venous P_{O_2}, or reflexly by systemic arterial P_{O_2}, to the hypoxic pulmonary pressor response. A more realistic view seems to be that hypoxia acts as a stimulus to pulmonary vasoconstriction, either directly or indirectly, by stimulating strategically located sensors in muscular pulmonary vessels, that the intensity of the stimulus is a function of the amount of oxygen that reaches the site (be it via air or blood or by a combination of the two), and that the rigor of the response is a function of the mass of the media. Ordinarily, the influence of alveolar hypoxia predominates over mixed venous hypoxia, due to the shape of the oxyhemoglobin dissociation curve (Fig. 1), the thicker media of precapillary vessels, the influence of pulmonary parenchymal and vascular geometry on limiting oxygen diffusion to the sensors, and possibly the adaptation of pulmonary precapillary blood to lifelong exposure to hypoxemic mixed venous blood (5,62,97).

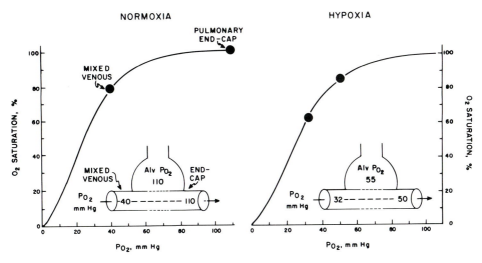

Figure 1: Oxygen dissociation curves during normoxia (left) and hypoxia (right). Shown on each curve are the respective points for mixed venous blood and pulmonary end-capillary blood. The corresponding blood gas tensions are shown schematically beneath each oxygen dissociation curve for a pulmonary microvessel (arteriole, capillary, and vein) traversing the alveolar portion of the lungs. While breathing a hypoxic inspired mixture that decreases alveolar P_{O_2} by about 50 mmHg, the mixed venous P_{O_2} undergoes a relatively small decrease of about 8 mmHg whereas end-capillary P_{O_2} decreases much more, i.e., by about 18 mmHg.

SITES OF HYPOXIC PULMONARY VASOCONSTRICTION

Although by the 1970s the bulk of the evidence favored the small muscular arteries and arterioles as the predominant site of hypoxic pulmonary vasoconstriction, there was still room for debate (22). Since then, the issue seems to have been settled by micropuncture studies in open-chest cats which showed that the increase in resistance during hypoxia is due primarily to constriction of precapillary vessels even though alveolar and venous resistance also increase to a much lesser extent (76). In keeping with these hemodynamic studies, the small pulmonary arteries and arterioles (30–200 μ) of the bullfrog have been seen to constrict in response to local hypoxia (48). All in all, there seems little reason to doubt that acute hypoxia causes vascular smooth muscle throughout the lungs to undergo vasoconstriction but that the predominant effect is on the small muscular arteries and arterioles.

THE STRENGTH OF THE HYPOXIC PRESSOR RESPONSE

Certain cattle are genetically predisposed to develop pulmonary hypertension at altitude; these cattle are endowed with hypertrophied muscle in the media of the pulmonary resistance vessels (112). Dogs raised above sea level (1600 m) have greater pressor responses than their counterparts at sea level (111). Acidosis and products of the lipoxygenase pathway do augment hypoxic pulmonary hypertension (73,76,87).

However, it is much easier to blunt the hypoxic pressor response experimentally than to augment it. Almost all experimental manipulations involving anesthesia (8) and abnormal perfusates can do so (104); so can pregnancy (72) and certain diseases, e.g., liver cirrhosis (17,75), pneumonia (52), and oxygen toxicity (77). Moreover, in some of the less conventional animal species, the pressor response may be difficult to elicit (95).

Different mechanisms have been invoked to account for the dampening of the hypoxic vasoconstrictor response in different conditions: (1) mechanical, such as an increase in cardiac output (88) or left atrial pressure, (2) release of vasodilator substances, e.g., prostaglandins (28), or the presence of estrogens (32), (3) concomitant biochemical abnormalities, e.g., respiratory alkalosis (4), and (4) the presence of inflammatory products and mediators in adjacent pulmonary parenchyma, e.g., hyperoxic lung injury (77).

In many respects, the loss or blunting of the hypoxic pulmonary pressor response in pathological states underscores the vulnerability of the response in animal preparations and isolated vessels to influences that upset homeostatic balances and expose the pulmonary circulation and the enveloping lungs to abnormal internal environments. Finally, therapeutic agents, given for other purposes, can either enhance (e.g., almitrine [85]), depress (e.g., nifedipine [9]), or leave unchanged (e.g., terbutaline [104]) the hypoxic pressor response.

HYPOXIA, ACIDOSIS, AND ALKALOSIS

In the same paper that described the pulmonary pressor response to acute hypoxia, von Euler and Liljestrand showed that hypercapnia also had a pressor effect: addition of 6% CO_2 to the inspired air raised pulmonary arterial pressure. No comment was made about the decrease in the hypercapnic pressor response when a higher concentration (18.7%) CO_2 was breathed. Nor was it possible for them to sort out the effects of hypercapnia from those of acidosis since determinations of blood pH were not yet practical. In 1962, Bergofsky et al. showed that acute acidosis induced by the infusion of hydrochloric acid elicited pulmonary vasoconstriction (7).

Since then, it has become widely accepted that under near-natural conditions, acidosis, per se, elicits pulmonary vasoconstriction and that the hypoxic pressor response is enhanced by extracellular acidosis and diminished by extracellular alkalosis (54,87). However, there is still no consensus (60). One reason for the lack of unanimity is the different ways used to induce acidosis, e.g., metabolic or respiratory on the one hand and a variety of anions on the other. Another major cause, as in the case of testing the effects of hypoxia on the pulmonary circulation, is artifacts introduced by experimental manipulations, differences in the experimental preparations, dissimilar levels of disturbance in acid-base balance, and side effects arising from the impact of different levels of acidosis or alkalosis on either the endothelium or on the blood constituents, resulting in the release of vasoactive substances (1,32).

Respiratory acidosis is often a deliberate or inadvertent complication of experiments involving anesthesia. An increase in P_{CO_2} as well as a decrease in pH can heighten the pulmonary pressor response to hypoxia. However, the relative roles of molecular CO_2 and of [H$^+$] in modifying the hypoxic pressor response are not entirely clear: in unanesthetized humans, the hypercapnic pressor response seems to depend not on molecular CO_2 but on the concentration of hydrogen ions; the opposite seems to be true in anesthetized dogs (22,59,95). This distinction may be important with respect to how, why, and where acidosis, hypercapnia, and hypoxia exert their pulmonary pressor effects.

Another important distinction is between the opposite effects of *extracellular* and *intracellular* alkalosis on the hypoxic pulmonary pressor response (82). For example, *extracellular* alkalosis depresses the hypoxic pulmonary pressor response whereas *intracellular* alkalosis enhances it (69). Whether a single factor, such as the release of prostacyclin or the inhibition of leukotriene synthesis (74), can account for blunting of the hypoxic pressor response during extracellular alkalosis is problematic since so many other undetected elements may be involved, e.g., an opposite change in intracellular pH, a decrease in the intracellular concentration of ionized calcium, or the local release of mediators other than products of arachidonic acid metabolism.

It may bear repeating that although much is uncertain about the relationships between disturbances in acid-base balance and hypoxic pulmonary vasoconstriction, it does seem clear that under near-natural conditions, extracellular acidosis, per se, elicits pulmonary vasoconstriction and that the hypoxic pressor response is enhanced by extracellular acidosis and diminished by extracellular alkalosis. Inevitably, more experiments are in the offing. Therefore, it seems worth emphasizing the need for a continuing alert to possible side effects of stressful or intolerable levels of derangements in acid-base balance and to the introduction of pathophysiological "viruses" as experimental conditions and preparations become further and further removed from natural conditions. In these abnormal circumstances, a positive, or a heightened, response is more apt to be meaningful in physiological terms than is a blunted response that often represents an artifact of the preparation, the manipulation, or the perfusate.

RELATION BETWEEN THE EFFECTS OF HYPOXIA ON SYSTEMIC VESSELS AND STRUCTURES AND THE HYPOXIC PULMONARY PRESSOR RESPONSE

Acute hypoxia stimulates the ventilation via the carotid bodies, dilates systemic resistance vessels, and constricts the ductus arteriosus. It seems reasonable to ask if similar mechanisms are involved in the afferent limb of the hypoxic pulmonary pressor response.

Hypoxic Stimulation of Ventilation via the Carotid Bodies

Hypoxia reflexly stimulates ventilation and heart rate as well as eliciting pulmonary vasoconstriction. Peripheral chemoreceptors in the carotid bodies are responsible for the bulk of the increase in ventilation. But, if there are structure-function similarities between the carotid bodies and the initiators of the hypoxic pulmonary pressor drive, they have to date eluded detection. Each carotid body is a highly vascularized structure made up primarily of glomus and sustenacular cells. The glomus cell appears to be the site of transduction of the hypoxic signal and of the release of neurochemical mediators (catecholamines and peptides) that stimulate electrical activity in the glossopharyngeal nerves. No such complicated counterparts exist in pulmonary vascular walls. Nonetheless, even though strikingly different in appearance, the possibility of shared molecular mechanisms is still very much alive. One prime example of viable prospects are the O_2 sensors: cytochromes of the respiratory chain, O_2-binding proteins, P_{O_2}-sensitive enzymes, depolarization and ionic pumps, redox systems, and an oxygen-sensing, membrane-bound protein receptor. Unfortunately, none of these proposed mechanisms have as yet withstood experimental testing. In contrast to the lack of an identifiable common denominator that would initiate the hypoxic pressor response and the hypoxic increase in ventilation, it seems settled that an increase in cytoplasmic $[Ca^{2+}]$ is involved in the effector pathway.

Hypoxia on Extrapulmonary Resistance Vessels

As a rule, systemic arteries, such as those of the coronary and cerebral circulations, respond to hypoxemia by vasodilating (39). Teleologically, this vasodilation increases oxygen delivery to hypoxic tissues. Although metabolic intermediaries such as ATP depletion or the formation of adenosine have been suggested as likely mechanisms, how systemic vasodilation is effected remains obscure.

The demonstration that the bronchial circulation in the sheep is admirably suited for hemodynamic studies (58) has prompted reexamination of the response of the bronchial (systemic) circulation to acute hypoxia. Recent evidence supports the view that while the pulmonary circulation is constricting during acute hypoxia, the systemic vessels to the lungs (and elsewhere) are dilating (107). The basis for this tantalizing discrepancy is unknown. Quite tantalizing are the observations that administration of endothelium-derived vasoconstrictor polypeptide, endothelin, to intact-chest cats, constricts pulmonary vessels and dilates systemic vessels (53). The role played by endothelium-derived mediator(s) in the opposite effects of hypoxia on the pulmonary and systemic circulation awaits clarification.

Hypoxia on the Ductus Arteriosus

In fetal life, the ductus arteriosus (a remnant of the 6th left bronchial arch) links the pulmonary artery and aorta, i.e., it links two circulations that respond oppositely to acute hypoxia (Fig. 2): in humans and in conventional laboratory animals, the ductus is dilated by hypoxia and constricts in response to oxygen, i.e., it behaves like a systemic artery in response to changes in the oxygen tension in its environment. Moreover, its vasomotor responses rely heavily on vasodilator prostaglandins, in particular those generated via the cyclooxygenase pathway of the arachidonic acid cascade. The heavy dependence of the tone of the ductus on at least one biologically active substance, not only in contemporary animals but also in the first terrestrial animals (24), has encouraged those seeking a unique mediator as the basis for hypoxic pulmonary vasoconstriction.

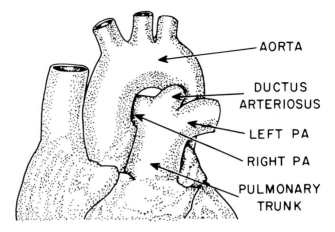

Figure 2: Relationship of the ductus arteriosus to the aorta and pulmonary artery. In contrast to the pulmonary vessels but like the aorta, the ductus dilates during hypoxia.

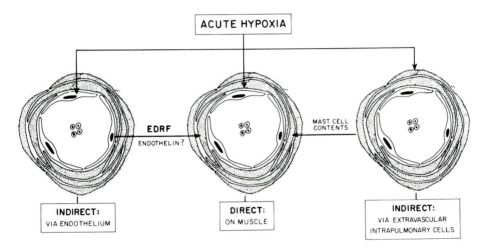

Figure 3: Schematic representation of a small pulmonary artery indicating that a change in tone can be effected in one of three ways: indirectly via the endothelium (left), indirectly via extravascular cells in the lungs (right), or directly via a sensing mechanism in vascular smooth muscle (middle).

MECHANISMS OF HYPOXIC PULMONARY VASOCONSTRICTION

The fact that hypoxia elicits pulmonary vasoconstriction in the isolated perfused lung has directed attention to the substance of the lung as the source, as well as effector, of the hypoxic pressor response. In the 1940s, the search was on for either an intrapulmonary reflex or a direct depressant effect on the contractile machinery. However, neither depressed contractility nor an intrapulmonary reflex proved to be durable explanations. Since then, as the pace of muscle physiology and cell physiology quickened and understanding of biological transduction deepened, a large number of possible candidates have surfaced. Some of these could act *directly* on pulmonary vascular smooth muscle, via an oxygen-sensing mechanism contained with it, to elicit pulmonary vasoconstriction. Others could accomplish the same effect *indirectly*, e.g., via a biological mediator that originates in pulmonary parenchyma in the vicinity of pulmonary vascular smooth muscle (Fig. 3).

Although proponents of either position differ with respect to the sensing (and transduction) mechanisms, both groups agree that an increase in calcium ion concentration within the vascular smooth muscle cells underlies the effector mechanism responsible for the hypoxic pulmonary pressor response.

Although the issue of direct versus indirect is not yet settled, it is instructive to consider certain mechanisms that have been proposed to account for the hypoxic pulmonary pressor response.

Direct

The traditional explanation, still popular in many laboratories, is that the hypoxic pulmonary pressor response represents a *direct* effect of hypoxia on pulmonary vascular smooth muscle (11). Hypoxia could exert a direct effect in a variety of ways, including electromechanical coupling (which could also be effected by a mediator), an intracellular oxygen sensor, cellular metabolism and energetics, oxygen radicals, or an increase in the intracellular concentration of calcium ions from extra- or intracellular sources (Fig. 4). Of the wide array of mechanisms that have been invoked to account for a direct effect—either at the cell surface or within the plasma membrane or cytosol—only a few are still viable.

ELECTROMECHANICAL COUPLING

No matter how hypoxia is sensed, i.e., directly or indirectly via mediators, it seems likely that membrane depolarization is involved in the transduction process and that an increase in calcium ion within the smooth muscle cell is part of the effector process (36,69,92,98).

In the isolated, suffused small pulmonary artery of the cat, a decrease in P_{O_2} causes membrane depolarization, generation of action potentials, and an increase in permeability to Ca^{2+} (and possibly to Na^+), presumably due to voltage-dependent mechanisms (37,98). Both the depolarization and contraction can be blocked by agents that prevent entry of calcium ions into the muscle. Although consistent with the idea of a sensing mechanism in the vessel wall that causes opening of calcium channels in the cell membrane (direct effect), these observations do not exclude the possibility of signals from hypoxic endothelium or the release of a biologically active mediator, e.g., endothelin (indirect effect) (57). It is also unclear if the electrochemical events and ion fluxes at the cell surface relate to a decrease in oxidative metabolism and in mitochondrial ATP generation that acute hypoxia can cause.

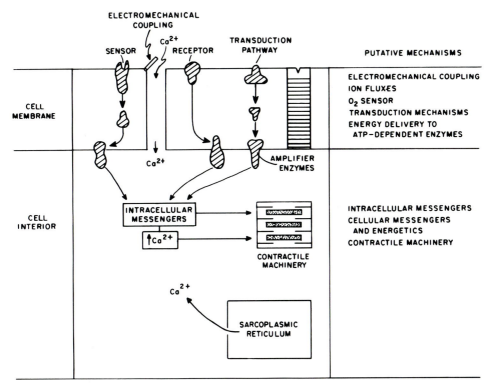

Figure 4: Schematic representation of a cell illustrating hypothetical mechanisms by which a direct effect of hypoxia may operate to increase the intracellular concentration of calcium ions and, thereby, increase vascular tone. (Modified after Berridge MJ, Scient. Amer. Oct 1985, p. 146.)

OXYGEN SENSOR

Over the years, the idea of an O_2 sensor has been transfigured from microscopically visible structures, such as nerve endings and neuroepithelial bodies (21,23,51), to submicroscopic substances, such as an O_2-binding protein (95). Currently, the designation "O_2 sensor" is used to signify either an oxygen-sensitive structure or an oxygen-dependent reaction. Although an oxygen sensor, operating by way of a specific ligand-dependent conformational change in a heme protein, has been shown to be responsible for hypoxic stimulation of the production of erythropoietin (30), the relevance of this observation to hypoxic stimulation of pulmonary vascular smooth muscle is unknown. Oxygen-dependent enzymes, oxygenases, and oxidases have also had their turn (69). However, none of these has lived up to expectations. Cytochrome P_{450}, a recent prospect, was recently discounted by showing that it could only elicit the hypoxic pulmonary pressor response at intolerable levels of P_{O_2} (96). Nonetheless, the possibility remains that some enzyme—as yet unidentified—could cause vasoconstriction when its heme-binding site is not occupied by oxygen.

For those favoring a direct action, the leading candidate for sensor of the hypoxic pressor response seems to be related to a hypoxic decrease in mitochondrial cytochrome oxidase and oxidative phosphorylation (62,69). Unfortunately, much of the evidence in favor of this hypothesis rests on the use of metabolic inhibitors (about which reservations were expressed above). Nonetheless, despite the prevalent enthusiasm for mediators and the inconclusiveness of the observations based on the use of inhibitors, it is difficult to discount the idea that somehow a sensor is triggered to elicit hypoxic pulmonary hypertension by depressing mitochondrial oxidative phosphorylation and decreasing the energy state. This type of explanation could also account for the divergent systemic and pulmonary responses to hypoxia and the loss of the pulmonary pressor response during severe hypoxia. Whether a mitochondrial cytochrome oxidase operates as the sensor is uncertain.

CELLULAR METABOLISM AND ENERGETICS

It is intuitively attractive to look to hypoxic depression of oxidative phosphorylation within vascular smooth muscle for the mechanism that evokes hypoxic pulmonary hypertension (and the opposite effects on the systemic circulation). Among the likely mechanisms are impaired O_2 delivery to vascular smooth muscle (114), reduction in ATP production (86), a decrease in energy level as reflected in the phosphate potential: [ATP]/[ADP][Pi], or delivery of ATP to a sensing mechanism within the cell or cell membrane (90). However, ATP production, per se, has been discounted as the critical factor (35), while the role of other mechanisms involved in oxidative phosphorylation remains uncertain at best (49). Nor has the increase in lactate production accompanying hypoxia proved to be the responsible mechanism (55). Unfortunately, the traditional reliance on metabolic inhibitors has not lived up to expectations, in part because they are generally administered in pharmacological doses in abnormal settings and because they almost invariably lack specificity. These have supported the view that oxidative phosphorylation can be involved; they do not prove that they do.

OXYGEN RADICALS

The possibility has been raised that oxygen radicals could be involved in the hypoxic pressor response. One of several processes could be responsible (112). Among these is a proposed interplay between cGMP and H_2O_2 that would enable the duo to function as an intracellular sensor "within the (pulmonary) arterial wall" (14). However, proposals such as these relating oxygen radicals and H_2O_2

TABLE 2 CRITERIA FOR A UNIQUE CHEMICAL MEDIATOR IN THE HYPOXIC PRESSOR RESPONSE*

1. The mediator or its precursors must exist in the lungs.
2. The source of the mediator must be strategically disposed with respect to the resistance vessels so as to gain ready access to their media during acute hypoxia.
3. The effect of the mediator must be mimicked by the application of the proposed mediator to the pulmonary blood vessels.
4. The mechanism must be present to turn on, and to inactivate, the mediator.
5. Agents which modify the pressor response elicited by the mediator should have similar effects on responses to the exogenously administered mediator.
6. Inhibition or depletion of the mediator, as by pharmacological agents, should depress the hypoxic response.

* From Fishman 1976 (22).

cannot settle the issue of "direct" versus "indirect" on pulmonary resistance vessels since the experiments are done on full-thickness walls of large arteries. Nor have they established as yet that the hypoxic challenge is severe enough to liberate the oxygen radicals required to start the cascade that ends in vasoconstriction.

Indirect Mediators

A long trail of biologically active substances that failed to make the grade marks the search for the unique mediator of the hypoxic pulmonary pressor response (Table 1). Along the way are products of mast cells, e.g., histamine (6), and serotonin (64,99), and neurotransmitters released by intrapulmonary nerve endings, e.g., α-adrenergic agents and angiotensin II (64). Virtually all of these now qualify as substances that can *modify* the hypoxic pressor response, i.e., they can act as *modulators*. Currently, two categories, i.e., products of the arachidonic acid metabolites (15) and endothelium-derived products (26,101), are still in the running as the unique mediator (Table 2). But two of these products of arachidonic acid are fading fast whereas endothelium-derived products—still running strong—are too new for accurate appraisal of their role in the hypoxic pulmonary pressor response (15,31,40).

ARACHIDONIC ACID METABOLITES

Both the cyclooxygenase and lipoxygenase pathways have taken a turn at being implicated as mediators of hypoxic pulmonary vasoconstriction (12). But each has proved to behave more like a modulator than a unique mediator. Several instructive reasons can be preferred for ambiguities in defining the role of individual products of arachidonic acid metabolism in the hypoxic pulmonary pressor response: (1) the complexity of the arachidonic acid cascade that produces an array of evanescent, as well as enduring, biologically active substances; (2) the continuing interplay between the biologically active substances of the cyclooxygenase and lipoxygenase pathways; and (3) overreliance on the specificity of inhibitors used experimentally.

The case for a component of the cyclooxygenase pathway to be involved as the mediator of the hypoxic pressor response rested heavily on augmentation of the hypoxic pulmonary pressor response by inhibitors of the cyclooxygenase pathway (indomethacin and meclofenamate) (110). However, in principle, the cyclooxygenase inhibitors seem more likely to provide insight into the inhibition of the production of prostacyclin, a powerful pulmonary vasodilator, rather than into the liberation of a mediator of the hypoxic pulmonary pressor response (33).

As the case for a component of the cyclooxygenase pathway waned, interest shifted to the lipoxygenase pathway and the leukotrienes that is produces (2,73,104). Circumstantial evidence in favor of the lipoxygenase pathway is that hypoxia causes mast cells in the sheep to degranulate, presumably releasing leukotrienes that could elicit pulmonary vasoconstriction—a return to the old days of the mast cell but substituting slow-reacting substance of anaphylaxis for histamine (2). Also, leukotrienes C_4 appear in bronchoalveolar washings of the isolated lung during acute hypoxia (reviewed in 56). However, interpretation is even more complicated than for products of the cyclooxygenase pathway: leukotrienes are produced by a variety of cells of the lungs in response to diverse stimuli; the appearance in bronchoalveolar fluid of leukotrienes does not mean that they are mediators; the specificity of the inhibitors is not entirely certain. The case against the leukotrienes as mediators of the hypoxic pulmonary pressor response has become convincing (28,56,89).

ENDOTHELIAL VASOMOTOR MEDIATORS: YIN YANG

By now, no one seriously regards endothelium as a passive membrane interposed between the blood and tissue. More reasonable is the view of endothelium as a "distributed organ," one that is dispersed throughout the body as a continuous vascular lining rather than as a conventional solid organ. It is involved in blood coagulation, fibrinolysis, processing biologically active neurohumoral substances, platelet interactions, the extravascular passage of neutrophils, macrophages and lymphocytes, antigen presentation, and smooth muscle proliferation.

Several lines of evidence indicate that endothelium is involved in local vaso-regulation: (1) its ability to generate and release powerful vasodilators, notably prostacyclin and endothelium-derived relaxing factors (26,27,34,40,102); (2) its ability to generate and liberate strong vasoconstricting substances (18), including the polypeptide endothelin (115); and (3) the presence in endothelium of mechano-receptors for monitoring local hemodynamic forces (50).

How these endothelium-derived factors relate to the hypoxic pulmonary pressor response is not yet clear (see Chapter 7). Hypoxia does release vasoconstrictor substance(s) from endothelial cells (18,41). Less credible is that hypoxia exerts its pressor effect by inhibiting endothelium-derived relaxing factors, one of which has been identified as nitric oxide. The understanding of EDRF and endothelin is still in its infancy. Clearly, it is an oversimplification to picture EDRF and endothelin as the sole mediators, neatly poised to counterbalance each other's effects (19). For example, EDRF is short-lived and binds to albumin and hemoglobin whereas endothelin is more prolonged in its effects (31).

One recent insight is that systemic vasodilation is accompanied by an increase in the concentration of cGMP in vascular smooth muscle and that methylene blue inhibits both the vasodilator response and the increase in cGMP levels (63,109). Methylene blue also blocks reversibly the hypoxic pulmonary pressor response in the cat, thereby suggesting that the hypoxic pulmonary pressor response may entail a decrease in the level of cGMP in the pulmonary resistance vessels, presumably by inhibiting soluble guanylate cyclase (42,43). Although these intriguing observations do underscore the vasomotor potential of endothelium, they do not distinguish between a *direct* effect on vascular smooth muscle and an *indirect* effect involving the release of an intermediate factor from endothelium. They also seem to have large and unexplored implications for the vasomotor regulation of abnormal blood vessels in which the structure and function of endothelium may be abnormal (as seen in atherosclerosis, hypertension, and thrombosis).

Platelet-activating factor (acetyl glyceryl ether phosphorylcholine) is released from vascular endothelial cells in response to a variety of stimuli. It is a membrane-derived phospholipid of diverse biological properties including platelet aggregation, activation of leukocytes, and increased capillary permeability. In the isolated rat lung, low doses have been reported to inhibit hypoxic pulmonary vasoconstriction (68) whereas in other preparations and species, higher doses have elicited vasoconstriction (38). High levels of platelet-activating factor have also been found in bronchoalveolar lavage fluid from chronically hypoxic (pulmonary hypertensive) calves (104). Despite mounting circumstantial evidence relating platelet-activating factor to pulmonary vasomotor activity and hypoxia, it is still unclear if endothelial cells release platelet-activating factor during acute hypoxia and if this factor is involved, in any way, in the hypoxic pressor response (69).

INTRACELLULAR CALCIUM ION CONCENTRATION [Ca^{2+}]

Hypotheses about direct or indirect mechanisms for hypoxic pulmonary vasoconstriction generally converge on the idea that the major effector pathway is an increase in the intracellular concentration of calcium ions. The concentration of calcium ions in the vicinity of the contractile machinery represents a balance between the inflow and outflow across the cell membrane on the one hand and the intracellular release and uptake on the other. Within the cell, calcium can be mobilized from the sarcoplasmic reticulum, mitochondrial membranes, or the inner aspect of the cell membrane. Although the bulk of the evidence favors an influx of calcium from extracellular fluid (65,67), the relative contribution of differential mobilization from intracellular stores is unsettled. Also unclear is the mechanism responsible for intracellular mobilization of calcium. One proposed mechanism involves the operation of intracellular phosphate ratios via the regulation of the redox status of certain intermediaries within the cell, e.g., pyridine nucleotides and sulfhydryl groups (70). Parenthetically, confidence in the role of the calcium ion as the effector mechanism stands in marked uncertainty concerning the sensing and transduction mechanisms involved in the hypoxic pulmonary pressor response.

Conclusion: Direct or Indirect?

The question remains unsettled. How acute hypoxia evokes pulmonary vasoconstriction is still enigmatic. Every time that a newly discovered biological mediator fails to withstand experimental scrutiny, confidence is restored in the likelihood of hypoxia exerting a direct effect. Currently, endothelium is being intensively explored as a possible source of a mediator. Meanwhile, proponents of a direct effect have taken heart and have returned either to cellular metabolism or to molecular transduction mechanisms in the plasma membrane or to a combination of the two. However, although sensing and transduction mechanisms remain befogged, it does seem clear that as in vascular smooth muscle elsewhere, an increase in tone is effected by an increase in the free-calcium concentration in the myoplasm and that the increment can derive from two major sources: *the extracellular fluid* (via receptor operated channels, potential-sensitive channels, and calcium leak); and *within the cell* (from the sarcoplasmic reticulum and inner plasmalemmal surface) (100).

CHRONIC HYPOXIA

Life at high altitude where hypoxia prevails is associated with chronic pulmonary arterial hypertension (see Chapter 20). This generalization applies to newcomers, to sojourners, and to native residents. The degree of pulmonary hypertension depends on the altitude, ordinarily modest at tolerable altitudes but approaching systemic levels if alveolar hypoventilation and systemic arterial hypoxemia become severe, as in chronic mountain sickness. As hypoxia is prolonged, anatomical changes in the pulmonary resistance vessels add to the pressor effect of vasoconstriction. The anatomical changes affect endothelium and adventitia as well as the media. "Remodeling" of the media entails both hypertrophy and peripheral extension of pulmonary vascular smooth muscle and right ventricular hypertrophy (44,83). Pulmonary hypertension and vascular hypertrophy can be prevented in chronically hypoxic rats by administering angiotensin II, which presumably prompts the release of dilator prostaglandins, e.g., prostacyclin (81). Prophylaxis can also be accomplished in rats by administering polyunsaturated fats (fish oil) which tilt the balance of constrictor-dilator prostaglandins in favor of the dilators, e.g., from thromboxane A_2 to prostaglandin I_3 (3). However, generalizations about pulmonary reactivity and anatomical vascular changes at altitude are precluded by striking species differences in responsiveness and uncertainties about the extent to which genetic influences shape the responsiveness of individual species.

Vascular smooth muscle not only hypertrophies but releases (in culture) a factor that stimulates the production of elastin by adventitial cells (71). In addition, chronic hypoxia causes structural and functional changes in the vicinity of vascular smooth muscle: endothelium undergoes morphological change (10), and mitogen (PDGF) is released (103). Chronic hypoxia also affects collagen production: inhibition of collagen production in chronically hypoxic rats ameliorates chronic hypoxic pulmonary hypertension (46) (see also Chapter 22).

It has been tacitly assumed that the vasomotor mechanisms underlying the sustained increase in pulmonary vascular tone during chronic hypoxia are directly related to, if not the same as, those that operate during acute hypoxia (81). This may not be so (93). For example, a decrease in the vascular reactivity of hypertensive vessels is presumably a concomitant of the structural changes in the vascular walls (20). The process of remodelling the vascular wall under the influence of sustained high pressures and of growth factors released by both platelets and endothelium automatically ensures changes in spatial arrangements and physical contacts among the various constituents of the vascular wall, between individual cell types, and between matrix and cells. Also, under the influence of chronic hypoxia, metabolic pathways may be inclined to pursue alternate pathways, and altered energetics may modify both pulmonary vascular tone and reactivity. This kind of reasoning has prompted a trial of fish oil diets to prevent pulmonary vascular remodelling: fish oil could act by a direct effect on pulmonary vascular smooth muscle, by decreasing endothelial formation of PDGF (25) and by decreasing platelet activity (3).

All in all, it is much easier to imagine a direct, rather than an indirect, basis for the sustained pulmonary hypertension elicited by chronic hypoxia, e.g., at high altitude. However, even for a direct mechanism it would be necessary to sort out events at the cell surface and in the cell membrane from those within the cytosol. Unfortunately, much more is now known about structural changes in the pulmonary arterial tree resulting from chronic hypoxia than about the biochemical and molecular processes that lead to the pulmonary vascular change and sustain them.

CONCLUDING COMMENTS

This review was undertaken on the assumption that hypoxic pulmonary hypertension is a distinct and reproducible biological entity, elicitable, albeit with some degree of variability, in virtually all conventional species. No reason has surfaced to challenge this assumption. Indeed, over the last 30 years hypoxia has emerged as the most effective, uncomplicated, and consistent stimulus to pulmonary hypertension that has yet been discovered.

The intrapulmonary component of the hypoxic pressor response has been characterized in many ways, ranging from time course to gender and genetic variability. Considerable attention has been paid to interplay with biologically active substances, such as hydrogen and calcium ions, in the internal environment. However, in addition to the dominant intrapulmonary regulation of the hypoxic pulmonary pressor response, an important extrapulmonary element of control resides in the adrenergic innervation of the pulmonary vasculature. The importance of the adrenergic innervation varies from fetus to adult, from species to species, and from state to state. One important contribution of this adrenergic mechanism may be in setting the level of initial tone that is required for hypoxia to act. But the extrapulmonary adrenergic contribution appears to be only one of many factors that interplay to set both the threshold for, and sensitivity of, the hypoxic pressor response.

Most of the experiments considered have required technical ingenuity and often elegant preparations to gain insight into the regulation of the pulmonary circulation. Inevitably, the artificial conditions have resulted in depressed responsiveness of the pulmonary vascular smooth muscle. Taken together, observations made on all sorts of preparations have led to two alternatives about how acute hypoxia exerts its pulmonary pressor effects; directly on pulmonary vascular smooth muscle, or indirectly via a mediator within the lung. Failure to uncover a unique chemical mediator lends conviction to the predominant view that mediators are more apt to set initial tone than to constitute a unique messenger. But the issue is far from closed and the search for a unique mediator presses on.

Chronic hypoxia is widely viewed as entailing the same basic mechanisms for the hypoxic pulmonary pressor response as acute hypoxia. The sustained contraction is easier to rationalize in terms of a direct than an indirect effect. However, hypertrophy and peripheral extension of the media implies growth factors that can evoke diverse effects, including vasoconstriction.

Finally, the pressor response in the pulmonary circulation elicited by hypoxia has to be reconciled conceptually with hypoxic vasoconstriction of the ductus arteriosus and with hypoxic dilation of systemic arteries, including the bronchial arteries: the ductus arteriosus, a link between the two circulations during fetal life and in air-breathing fish, constricts via a direct effect of hypoxia on its media, i.e., without a unique chemical intermediate; the mechanism underlying systemic vasodilation in response to acute hypoxia remains to be uncovered.

REFERENCES

1. Adnot S, Chabrier PE, Brun-Buisson C, Viossat I, Braquet PL: Atrial natriuretic factor (ANF) attenuates the pulmonary pressor response to hypoxia. J Appl Physiol 65 : 1975–1983, 1988.

2. Ahmed T, Oliver W Jr: Does slow-reacting substance of anaphylaxis mediate hypoxic pulmonary vasoconstriction? Am Rev Respir Dis 127 : 566–571, 1983.

3. Archer SL, Johnson GJ, Gebhard RL, Castleman WL, Levine AS, Westcott JY, Voelkel NF, Nelson DP, Weir EK: Dietary fish oil alters lung lipid profile and reduces chronic hypoxic pulmonary hypertension. J Appl Physiol (In Press).

4. Benumof JL, Wahrenbrock EA: Blunted hypoxic pulmonary vasoconstriction by increased lung vascular pressures. J Appl Physiol 38 : 846–850, 1975.

5. Bergofsky EH: Mechanisms underlying vasomotor regulation of regional pulmonary blood flow in normal and disease states. Am J Med 57 : 378–394, 1974.

6. Bergofsky EH: Active control of the normal pulmonary circulation, in Moser KM (ed), *Pulmonary Vascular Diseases. Vol 14: Lung Biology in Health and Disease*. New York, Marcel Dekker, 1979, pp 233–277.

7. Bergofsky EH, Lehr DE, Fishman AP: The effect of changes in hydrogen ion concentration on the pulmonary circulation. J Clin Invest 41 : 1492–1502, 1962.

8. Bindslev L, Jolin A, Hedenstierna G, Baehrendtz S, Santesson J: Hypoxic pulmonary vasoconstriction in the human lung: Effect of repeated hypoxic challenges during anesthesia. Anesthesiology 62 : 621–625, 1985.

9. Bishop MJ, Cheney RW: Comparison of the effects of minoxidil and nifedipine on hypoxic pulmonary vasoconstriction in dogs. J Cardiovasc Pharmacol 5 : 184–189, 1983.

10. Bisio JM, Breen RE, Connell RS, Harrison MW: Pulmonary capillary endothelial dysfunction in hypoxia and endotoxemia: a biochemical and electron microscope study. J Trauma 23 : 730–739, 1983.

11. Bohr DF: The pulmonary hypoxic response: State of the field. Chest 71 : 244–246, 1977.

12. Brigham KL: Conference summary. Lipid mediators in the pulmonary circulation. Am Rev Respir Dis 136 : 785–788, 1987.

13. Brower RG, Gottlieb J, Wise RA, Permutt S, Sylvester JT: Locus of hypoxic vasoconstriction in isolated ferret lungs. J Appl Physiol 63 : 58–65, 1987.

14. Burke-Wolin T, Wolin MS: H_2O_2 and cGMP may function as an O_2 sensor in the pulmonary artery. J Appl Physiol 66 : 167–170, 1989.

15. Busse R, Bassenge E: Endothelium and hypoxic responses. Bibl Cardiol 38 : 21–34, 1984.

16. Capen RL, Wagner WW Jr: Intrapulmonary blood flow redistribution during hypoxia increases gas exchange surface area. J Appl Physiol 52 : 1575–1580, 1982.

17. Daoud FS, Reeves JT, Schaefer JW: Failure of hypoxic pulmonary vasoconstriction in patients with liver cirrhosis. J Clin Invest 51 : 1076–1080, 1971.

18. De Mey JG, Vanhoutte PM: Anoxia and endothelium-dependent reactivity of the canine femoral artery. J Physiol (Lond) 335 : 65–74, 1983.

19. De Nucci G, Gryglewski RJ, Warner TD, Vane JR: Receptor-mediated release of endothelium-derived relaxing factor and prostacyclin from bovine aortic endothelial cells is coupled. Proc Natl Acad Sci USA 85 : 2334–2338, 1988.

20. Fishman AP: Respiratory gases in the regulation of the pulmonary circulation. Physiol Rev 41 : 214–280, 1961.

21. Fishman AP: Dynamics of the pulmonary circulation, in Hamilton WF, Dow P (eds), *Handbook of Physiology. Circulation: II*. Washington, DC, American Physiological Society, 1963, pp 1667–1743.

22. Fishman AP: Hypoxia on the pulmonary circulation: How and where it acts. Circ Res 38 : 221–231, 1976.

23. Fishman AP: Pulmonary circulation, in Fishman AP, Fisher AB (eds), *Handbook of Physiology. Sect 3: The Respiratory System, Vol I: Circulation and Nonrespiratory Functions*. Bethesda, MD, American Physiological Society, 1985, pp 93–166.

24. Fishman AP, Delaney RG, Laurent P, Szidon PJ: Blood shunting in lungfish and humans, in Krogsgaard-Larsen P, Brogger Christensen S, Kofod H (eds), *Cardiovascular Shunts* (Proceedings of the Alfred Benzon Symposium 21). Copenhagen, Munksgaard, 1984, pp 1–8.

25. Fox PL, DiCorleto PE: Lipids containing omega-3 fatty acids specifically inhibit production of a platelet-derived growth factor-like protein by endothelial cells (Abstract). J Cell Biol 105 : 22A, 1987.

26. Furchgott RF: Role of endothelium in response of vascular smooth muscle. Circ Res 53 : 557–573, 1983.

27. Furchgott RF, Zawadzki JV: The obligatory role of endothelial cells in the relaxation of arterial smooth muscle by acetylcholine. Nature 288 : 373–376, 1980.

28. Garrett RC, Foster S, Thomas HM III: Lipoxygenase and cyclooxygenase blockade by BW 755C enhances pulmonary hypoxic vasoconstriction. J Appl Physiol 62 : 129–133, 1987.

29. Gerber JG, Voelkel N, Nies AS, McMurtry IF, Reeves JT: Moderation of hypoxic vasoconstriction by infused arachidonic acid: Role of PGI_2. J Appl Physiol 49 : 107–112, 1980.

30. Goldberg MA, Dunning SP, Bunn HF: Regulation of the erythropoietin gene: Evidence that the oxygen sensor is a Heme Protein. Science 242: 1412–1415, 1988.

31. Gordon J: Vascular biology. Put out to contract. Nature 332: 395–396, 1988.

32. Gordon JB, Wetzel RC, McGeady ML, Adkinson NF Jr, Sylvester JT: Effects of indomethacin on estradiol-induced attenuation of hypoxic vasoconstriction in lamb lungs. J Appl Physiol 61: 2116–2121, 1986.

33. Gottlieb JE, McGeady M, Adkinson NF Jr, Sylvester JT: Effects of cyclo- and lipoxygenase inhibitors on hypoxic vasoconstriction in isolated ferret lungs. J Appl Physiol 64: 936–943, 1988.

34. Griffith TM, Edwards DH, Davies RL, Harrison TJ, Evans KT: EDRF coordinates the behaviour of vascular resistance vessels. Nature 329: 442–445, 1987.

35. Harabin AL, Peake MD, Sylvester JT: Effect of severe hypoxia on the pulmonary vascular response to vasoconstrictor agents. J Appl Physiol 50: 561–565, 1981.

36. Harder DR, Madden JA, Dawson C: A membrane electrical mechanism for hypoxic vasoconstriction of small pulmonary arteries from cat. Chest 88: 233S–235S, 1985.

37. Harder DR, Madden JA, Dawson C: Hypoxic induction of Ca^{2+}-dependent action potentials in small pulmonary arteries of the cat. J Appl Physiol 59: 1389–1393, 1985.

38. Heffner JE, Shoemaker SA, Canham EM, Patel M, McMurtry IF, Morris HG, Repine JE: Acetyl glyceryl ether phosphorylcholine-stimulated human platelets cause pulmonary hypertension and edema in isolated rabbit lungs. J Clin Invest 71: 351–357, 1983.

39. Heisted DD, Abboud FM: Circulatory adjustments to hypoxia. Circulation 61: 463–470, 1980.

40. Hickey KA, Rubanyi G, Paul RJ, Highsmith RF: Characterization of a coronary vasoconstrictor produced by cultured endothelial cells. Am J Physiol 248: C550–C556, 1985.

41. Holden WE, McCall E: Hypoxia-induced contractions of porcine pulmonary artery strips depend on intact endothelium. Exp Lung Res 7: 101–112, 1984.

42. Hyman AL, Kadowitz PJ: Methylene blue selectively and reversibly blocks hypoxic pulmonary vasoconstriction in the cat. J Appl Physiol (In Press).

43. Hyman AL, Kadowitz PJ: Methylene blue selectively inhibits pulmonary vasodilator responses in cats. J Appl Physiol 66: 1513–1517, 1989.

44. Jones R, Langleben D, Reid LM: Patterns of remodeling of the pulmonary circulation in acute and subacute lung injury, in Said SI (ed), *The Pulmonary Circulation and Acute Lung Injury.* New York, Futura Publishing Co., 1985, pp 137–188.

45. Kato M, Staub NC: Response of small pulmonary arteries to unilobar hypoxia and hypercapnia. Circ Res 19: 426–440, 1966.

46. Kerr JS, Riley DJ, Frank MM, Trelstad RL, Frankel HM: Reduction of chronic hypoxic pulmonary hypertension in the rat by β-aminopropionitrile. J Appl Physiol 57: 1760–1766, 1984.

47. Kloog Y, Ambar I, Sokolovsky M, Kochva E, Wollberg Z, Bdolah A: Sarafotoxin, a novel vasoconstrictor peptide: Phosphoinositide hydrolysis in rat heart and brain. Science 242: 268–270, 1988.

48. Koyama T, Horimoto M: Blood flow reduction in local pulmonary microvessels during acute hypoxia imposed on a small fraction of the lung. Respir Physiol 52: 181–189, 1983.

49. Kramer RS, Pearlstein RD: Reversible uncoupling of oxidative phosphorylation at low oxygen tension. Proc Natl Acad Sci USA 80: 5807–5811, 1983.

50. Lansman JB: Endothelial mechanosensors. Going with the flow. Nature 331: 481–482, 1988.

51. Lauweryns JM, de Bock V, Decramer M: Effects of unilateral vagal stimulation on intrapulmonary neuroepithelial bodies. J Appl Physiol 63: 1781–1787, 1987.

52. Light RB, Mink SN, Wood LDH: Pathophysiology of gas exchange and pulmonary perfusion in pneumonococcal lobar pneumonia in dogs. J Appl Physiol 50: 524–530, 1983.

53. Lippton HL, Hauth TA, Summer WR, Hyman AL: Endothelin produces pulmonary vasoconstriction and systemic vasodilation. J Appl Physiol 66: 1008–1012, 1989.

54. Lloyd TC Jr: Influence of blood pH on hypoxic pulmonary vasoconstriction. J Appl Physiol 21: 358–364, 1966.

55. Longmore WJ, Mourning JT: Lactate production in isolated perfused rat lung. Am J Physiol 231: 351–354, 1976.

56. Lonigro AJ, Sprague RS, Stephenson AJ, Dahms TE: Relationship of leukotriene C_4 and D_4 to hypoxic pulmonary vasoconstriction in dogs. J Appl Physiol 64: 2538–2543, 1988.

57. Madden JA, Dawson CA, Harder DR: Hypoxia-induced activation in small isolated pulmonary arteries from the cat. J Appl Physiol 59: 113–118, 1985.

58. Magno MG, Fishman AP: Origin, distribution and blood flow of bronchial circulation in anesthetized sheep. J Appl Physiol 53: 272–279, 1982.

59. Malik AB, Kidd BSL: Independent effects of changes in H^+ and CO_2 concentrations on hypoxic pulmonary vasoconstriction. J Appl Physiol 34: 318–324, 1973.

60. Marshall C, Lindgren L, Marshall BE: Metabolic and respiratory hydrogen ion effects on hypoxic pulmonary vasoconstriction. J Appl Physiol 57: 545–550, 1984.

61. Marshall BE, Marshall C: A model for hypoxic constriction of the pulmonary circulation. J Appl Physiol 64: 68–77, 1988.

62. Marshall C, Marshall BE: Influence of perfusate P_{O_2} on hypoxic pulmonary vasoconstriction in rats. Circ Res 52: 691–696, 1983.

63. Mazmanian G-M, Baudet B, Brink C, Cerrina J, Kirkiacharian S, Weiss M: Methylene blue potentiates vascular reactivity in isolated rat lungs. J Appl Physiol 66 : 1040–1045, 1989.

64. McMurtry IF: Angiotensin is not required for hypoxic constriction in salt solution-perfused rat lungs. J Appl Physiol 56 : 375–380, 1984.

65. McMurtry IF: Bay K 8644, a Ca^{++} channel facilitator, potentiates hypoxic vasoconstriction in isolated rat lungs. Fed Proc 44 : 2389, 1985.

66. McMurtry IF: Humoral control, in Bergofsky EH (ed), *Abnormal Pulmonary Circulation*. New York, Churchill Livingstone, 1986, pp 83–126.

67. McMurtry IF, Hookway B, Roos S: Red blood cells play a crucial role in maintaining vascular reactivity to hypoxia in isolated rat lungs. Chest 71(Suppl) : 253–256, 1977.

68. McMurtry IF, Morris KG: Platelet activating factor causes pulmonary vasodilation in the rat. Am Rev Respir Dis 133:A227, 1986.

69. McMurtry IF, Raffestin B: Potential mechanisms of hypoxic pulmonary vasoconstriction, in Will JA, Dawson CA, Weir EK, Buckner CK (eds), *Potential Mechanisms of Hypoxic Pulmonary Vasoconstriction*. New York, Academic Press, 1987,pp 455–485.

70. McMurtry IF, Stanbrook HS, Rounds S: The mechanism of hypoxic pulmonary vasoconstriction: A working hypothesis, in Loeppky JA, Riedesel ML (eds), *Oxygen Transport to Human Tissues*. New York, Elsevier North-Holland, 1982, pp 77–87.

71. Mecham RP, Whitehouse LA, Wrenn DS, Parks WC, Griffin GL, Senior RM, Crouch EC, Stenmark KR, Voelkel NF: Smooth muscle-mediated connective tissue remodeling in pulmonary hypertension. Science 237 : 423–426, 1987.

72. Moore LG, Reeves JT: Pregnancy blunts pulmonary vascular reactivity in dogs. Am J Physiol 239:H297-H301, 1980.

73. Morganroth ML, Reeves JT, Murphy RC, Voelkel NF: Leukotriene synthesis and receptor blockers block hypoxic pulmonary vasoconstriction. J Appl Physiol 56 : 1340–1346, 1984.

74. Morganroth ML, Stenmark KR, Morris KG, Murphy RC, Mathias M, Reeves JT, Voelkel NF: Diethylcarbamazine inhibits acute and chronic hypoxic pulmonary hypertension in awake rats. Am Rev Respir Dis 131 : 488–492, 1985.

75. Naeije R, Hallemans R, Mols P, Melot C: Hypoxic pulmonary vasoconstriction in liver cirrhosis. Chest 80 : 570–574, 1981.

76. Nagasaka Y, Bhattacharya J, Nanjo S, Gropper MA, Staub NC: Micropuncture measurement of lung microvascular pressure profile during hypoxia in cats. Circ Res 54 : 90–95, 1984.

77. Newman JH, Loyd JE, English K, Ogletree ML, Fulkerson WJ, Brigham KL: Effects of 100% oxygen on lung vascular function in awake sheep. J Appl Physiol 54 : 1379–1386, 1983.

78. Orchard CH, Sanchez de Leon RS, Sykes MK: The relationship between hypoxic pulmonary vaso-

constriction and arterial oxygen tension in the intact dog. J Physiol (Lond) 338 : 61–74, 1983.

79. Porcelli RJ, Bergofsky EH: Effect of pH on pulmonary pressor responses to humoral agents. J Appl Physiol 31 : 679–685, 1971.

80. Porcelli RJ, Cutaia MV: Pulmonary vascular reactivity to biogenic amines during acute hypoxia. Am J Physiol 255 : H329–H334, 1988.

81. Rabinovitch M, Mullen M, Rosenberg HC, Maruyama K, O'Brodovich H, Olley PM: Angiotensin II prevents hypoxic pulmonary hypertension and vascular changes in rat. Am J Physiol 254 : H500–H508, 1988.

82. Raffestin B, McMurtry IF: Effects of intracellular pH on hypoxic vasoconstriction in rat lungs. J Appl Physiol 63 : 2524–2531, 1987.

83. Reid LM: The pulmonary circulation: Remodelling in growth and disease. The 1978 J. Burns Amberson Lecture. Am Rev Respir Dis 119 : 531–546, 1979.

84. Rendas A, Branthwaite M, Lennox S, Reid L: Response of the pulmonary circulation to acute hypoxia in the growing pig. J Appl Physiol 52 : 811–814, 1982.

85. Romaldini H, Rodriguez-Roisin R, Wagner PD, West J: Enhancement of hypoxic pulmonary vasoconstriction by almitrine in the dog. Am Rev Respir Dis 128 : 288–293, 1983.

86. Rounds S, McMurtry IF: Inhibitors of oxidative ATP production cause transient vasoconstriction and block subsequent pressor responses in rat lungs. Circ Res 48 : 393–400, 1981.

87. Rudolph AM, Yuan S: Response of the pulmonary vasculature to hypoxia and H$^+$ ion concentration changes. J Clin Invest 45 : 399–411, 1966.

88. Schumacker PT, Newell JC, Saba TM, Powers SR: Ventilation-perfusion relationships with high cardiac output in lobar atelectasis. J Appl Physiol 50 : 341–347, 1981.

89. Schuster DP, Dennis DR: Leukotriene inhibitors do not block hypoxic pulmonary vasoconstriction in dogs. J Appl Physiol 62 : 1808–1813, 1987.

90. Scott MP, Coburn RF: Effects of elevation of phosphorylcreatine on force and metabolism in rabbit aorta. Circ Res. In Press.

91. Shirai M, Sada K, Ninomiya I: Effects of regional alveolar hypoxia and hypercapnia on small pulmonary vessels in cats. J Appl Physiol 61 : 440–448, 1986.

92. Sibley DR, Benovic JL, Caron MG, Lefkowitz RJ: Regulation of transmembrane signaling by receptor phosphorylation. Cell 48 : 913–922, 1987.

93. Suzuki H, Twarog BM: Membrane properties of smooth muscle cells in pulmonary hypertensive rats. Am J Physiol 242 : H907–H915, 1982.

94. Sykes MK, Arnot RN, Jastrzebski J, Gibbs JM, Obdrzalek J, Hurtig JB: Reduction of hypoxic pulmonary vasoconstriction during trichloroethylene anesthesia. J Appl Physiol 39 : 103–108, 1975.

95. Sylvester JT, Gottlieb JE, Rock P, Wetzel RC:

Acute hypoxic responses, in Bergofsky EH (ed), *Abnormal Pulmonary Circulation*. New York, Churchill Livingstone, 1986, pp 127–166.

96. Sylvester JT, McGowen C: The effects of agents that bind to cytochrome P-450 on hypoxic pulmonary vasoconstriction. Circ Res 43:429–437, 1978.

97. Teisseire BP, Soulard CD: Pulmonary vasoconstrictor response to acute decrease in blood P_{50}. J Appl Physiol 56:370–374, 1984.

98. Tolins M, Weir EK, Chesler E, Nelson DP, From AH: Pulmonary vascular tone is increased by a voltage-dependent calcium channel potentiator. J Appl Physiol 60:942–948, 1986.

99. Tucker A, Weir EK, Reeves JT, Grover RF: Failure of histamine antagonists to prevent hypoxic pulmonary vasoconstriction in dogs. J Appl Physiol 40:496–500, 1976.

100. van Breemen C, Leijten P, Yamamoto H, Aaronson P, Cauvin C: Calcium activation of vascular smooth muscle. State of the art lecture. Hypertension 8(Suppl II):II89–II95, 1986.

101. Vanhoutte PM, Miller VM: Heterogeneity of endothelium-dependent responses in mammalian blood vessels. J Cardiovasc Pharmacol 7:S12–S23, 1985.

102. Vanhoutte PM, Rubanyi GM, Miller VM, Houston DS: Modulation of vascular smooth muscle contraction by the endothelium. Annu Rev Physiol 48:307–320, 1986.

103. Vender RL, Clemmons DR, Kwock L, Friedman M: Reduced oxygen tension induces pulmonary endothelium to release a pulmonary smooth muscle cell mitogen(s). Am Rev Respir Dis 135:622–627, 1987.

104. Voelkel NF: Mechanisms of hypoxic pulmonary vasoconstriction. Am Rev Respir Dis 133:1186–1195, 1986.

105. Voelkel NF, Gerber JG, McMurtry IF, Nies AS, Reeves JT: Release of vasodilator prostaglandin PGI_2 from isolated rat lung during vasoconstriction. Circ Res 48:207–213, 1981.

106. von Euler US, Liljestrand G: Observations on the pulmonary arterial blood pressure in the cat. Acta Physiol Scand 12:301–320, 1946.

107. Wagner EM, Mitzner WA: Effect of hypoxia on the bronchial circulation. J Appl Physiol 65:1627–1633, 1988.

108. Walker BR, Voelkel NF, McMurtry IF, Adams EM: Evidence for diminished sensitivity of the hamster pulmonary vasculature to hypoxia. J Appl Physiol 52:1571–1574, 1982.

109. Watanabe M, Rosenblum WI, Nelson GH: In vivo effect of methylene blue on endothelium-dependent and endothelium-independent dilations of brain microvessels in mice. Circ Res 62:86–90, 1988.

110. Weir EK, McMurtry IF, Tucker A, Reeves JT, Grover RF: Inhibition of prostaglandin synthesis or blockade of prostaglandin action increases the pulmonary pressor response to hypoxia, in Samuelsson B, Paoletti R (eds), *Advances in Prostaglandin and Thromboxane Research, Vol 2*. New York, Raven Press, 1976, pp 914–915.

111. Weir EK, Tucker A, Reeves JT, Grover RF: Increased pulmonary vascular pressor response to hypoxia in highland dogs. Proc Soc Exp Biol Med 154:112–115, 1977.

112. Weir EK, Will DM, Alexander AF, McMurtry IF, Looga R, Reeves JT, Grover RF: Vascular hypertrophy in cattle susceptible to hypoxic pulmonary hypertension. J Appl Physiol 46:517–521, 1979.

113. Wetzel RC, Zacur HA, Sylvester JT: Effect of puberty and estradiol on hypoxic vasomotor response in isolated sheep lungs. J Appl Physiol 56:1199–1203, 1984.

114. Wilson DF, Erecinska M: Effect of oxygen concentration on cellular metabolism. Chest 4(suppl):229S–232S, 1985.

115. Yanagisawa M, Kurihara H, Kimura S, Tomobe Y, Kobayashi M, Mitsui Y, Yazaki Y, Goto K, Masaki T: A novel potent vasoconstrictor peptide produced by vascular endothelial cells. Nature 332:411–415, 1988.

Walker A. Long, M.D.
D. Leslie Brown, Ph.D.

10

Central Neural Regulation of the Pulmonary Circulation

The classical view maintains that the pulmonary circulation is entirely locally regulated. It is indeed well established that hypoxia, acidosis, and certain humoral mediators cause pulmonary vasoconstriction by direct effects on the pulmonary vessels, and that oxygen, alkalosis, and certain other humoral mediators cause pulmonary vasodilatation by similar direct effects. However, the existence of easily demonstrable local regulation of the pulmonary circulation does not mean that there are no other important mechanisms by which the pulmonary circulation is regulated. Moreover, local factors such as alveolar oxygen tension and blood pH cannot account for many forms of unexplained pulmonary hypertension.

The possible role of the central nervous system in regulation of the pulmonary circulation (and in the genesis of pulmonary hypertension) has received little attention, largely because there are substantial technical difficulties in separating local effects from central neural effects. Nevertheless, a number of imaginative and persistent investigators (4,7,8,12,18–21,24,36–38,40–45,49,52,56–59) have explored the question of central neural regulation of the pulmonary circulation and have reached the same conclusion—such regulation does exist. The question remaining is not whether the brain can influence pulmonary vascular tone but, instead, whether the brain has an important role in either normal or disordered regulation of the pulmonary circulation. It is our belief that the brain does have important influences on physiologic regulation of the pulmonary circulation, particularly during fetal and neonatal life, and that central neural mechanisms contribute to or are responsible for various forms of unexplained pulmonary hypertension.

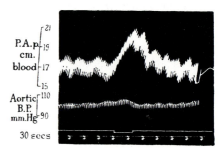

Figure 1: The response of the pulmonary circulation to bilateral electrical stellate gan-glion stimulation in a controlled flow preparation is shown. (Reproduced from Daly and von Euler [14].)

HISTORICAL PERSPECTIVE

Convincing evidence demonstrating that the central nervous system can influence the pulmonary circulation via the autonomic nervous system has existed for over 100 years (21). Citing 59 references from as early as 1822, Daly and von Euler observed:

After reviewing the experimental evidence there can be no doubt that the functional ac-tivity of the pulmonary vasomotor nerves has been definitely established in spite of state-ments to the contrary. It is true that in the more rigidly controlled experiments the alterations in pulmonary blood flow and pressure response have not been very large, but this is in part due to the difficulties encountered in keeping all perfused preparations in good condition. The point at issue appears to be not whether the pulmonary vasomotor nerves are functionally active but whether they are able to exert a powerful enough control to produce significant changes in the pulmonary blood flow and arterial pressure, and per-haps in the redistribution of blood within the lungs (21).

Daly and von Euler clearly demonstrated that electrical stimulation of the *thoracic* vagosympathetic nerves caused strong sympathetically mediated pul-monary vasoconstriction (Fig. 1) and weak parasympathetically mediated pulmo-nary vasodilatation. Forty percent increases in mean pulmonary arterial pressure were observed when the thoracic vagosympathetic nerves were stimulated. Daly and von Euler also showed that electrical stimulation of the cervical vagi or *cer-vical* vagosympathetic nerves could cause pulmonary vasoconstriction or weak pulmonary vasodilatation, and that the vasodilatation was parasympathetically mediated.

In the 57 years since publication of Daly and von Euler's paper, many different reports have appeared which continue to confirm the fact that the pulmonary vasomotor nerves can vasoconstrict (and vasodilate) the pulmonary circulation (4,12,18,19–21,36–38,40–45,49,52,56–59), but the question of whether neural regulation of the pulmonary circulation is important in either normal homeostasis or in disease states largely remains unanswered (26,28,33).

SPECIES CONSIDERATIONS

In comparing the results of physiological experiments, it is important to keep species differences in mind. For example, alveolar hypoxia causes very little pulmonary vasoconstriction in the cat and substantial pulmonary vasoconstriction in the sheep. Such species differences may play a large role in the outcome of a given series of experiments. Thus, inability to document a major autonomic contribution to hypoxic pulmonary vasoconstriction in the dog (47,60) does not invalidate observations that autonomic sectioning in the sheep (4) and alpha blockade in the cat (52) substantially reduce hypoxic pulmonary vasoconstriction in those species.

DEVELOPMENTAL CONSIDERATIONS

Similarly, it is important to recall that normal pulmonary vascular physiology is quite different in the fetus, neonate, and adult, and that physiological mechanisms responsible for regulation of the pulmonary circulation may be quite different at different stages of development. For example, hypoxic pulmonary vasoconstriction in newborn lambs is stronger than in adult sheep (17); it can be markedly inhibited by chemical sympathectomy in newborn lambs, but not in adult sheep (18). Also, beta blockade has no effect on hypoxic pulmonary vasoconstriction in the sheep during fetal life (33), but markedly inhibits hypoxic pulmonary vasoconstriction in newborn lambs (43). Similarly, PGD_2 is a potent pulmonary vasodilator in the sheep both prior to birth (33) and immediately after birth (33,55), but becomes a potent pulmonary vasoconstrictor after several days of postnatal life (55).

ANATOMICAL CONSIDERATIONS

Brain-Lung Connections

The mechanisms by which the central nervous system could influence the pulmonary vascular bed include direct neural connections via sympathetic pathways, parasympathetic pathways, or nonsympathetic spinal pathways, as well as release of humoral substances into the circulation either from the brain itself or from brain-controlled peripheral neural organs such as the adrenal glands. As considered further below, both sympathetic (37,59) and parasympathetic (37) influences on the pulmonary circulation are well established. Also, fibers originating from C2 through C5 cause pulmonary hypertension when stimulated directly and carry the efferent impulses responsible for pulmonary hypertension caused by electrical stimulation of the medulla (8). Whether other such nonsympathetic spinal pathways from the brain to the pulmonary circulation exist, or whether the brain releases humoral substances which also influence the pulmonary circulation, remains to be determined.

Pulmonary Vascular Innervation

SPECIES DIFFERENCES

Species differences in both the type and distribution of motor innervation of the pulmonary vessels are substantial (32), but virtually all mammalian species studied have at least some cholinergic or adrenergic innervation of either the pulmonary arteries or pulmonary veins. Most mammalian species have substantial cholinergic and adrenergic innervation of pulmonary arteries; in some species, such as the cat and sheep, this innervation extends into small vessels ($<70\ \mu$) (32). Most mammalian species also have substantial adrenergic innervation of pulmonary veins including some small vessels; cholinergic innervation of pulmonary veins is less pronounced, but is present in larger vessels. In the pig (see below), both the large and medium-sized (70 to 200 μ) pulmonary arteries and veins have cholinergic and adrenergic innervation, but the small vessels do not appear to be innervated (32).

DEVELOPMENTAL DIFFERENCES

Presumably, there are functional as well as anatomical changes in pulmonary vascular innervation during development, but little information is available concerning either. For example, most aspects of postnatal development of the lung circulation in the piglet were well characterized by Rendas et al. (53), but the innervation of the pulmonary circulation and its functional significance were not mentioned. It seems probable that the pulmonary vascular beds of most mammals are well innervated at birth since the sympathetic nervous system can substantially alter hypoxic pulmonary vasoconstriction at that time (18,43). It also seems likely that pulmonary vascular innervation, like pulmonary vascular smooth muscle, extends distally into the pulmonary vascular bed during postnatal development. Whether the density of innervation in vessels innervated at birth changes during postnatal development is difficult to predict.

Site of Pulmonary Vasoconstriction

Small pulmonary arterioles are generally considered to be responsible for pulmonary vascular resistance, but it is important to recall that pulmonary veins also contribute to pulmonary vascular resistance. Moreover, it cannot be assumed that a given stimulus affects the arterial and venous sides of the pulmonary circulation in the same way; for example, PGE_1 dilates pulmonary arterioles but constricts pulmonary veins (2). Similarly, hypothermia constricts pulmonary veins much more than pulmonary arteries (25,56,57).

DIRECT AUTONOMIC INFLUENCES

Sympathetic Stimulation

Electrical stimulation of the sympathetic nerves supplying the lungs can either increase or decrease pulmonary vascular tone, depending upon the preexisting tone and whether alpha or beta stimulation predominates (37). Using constant pulsatile flow through an isolated left lower lobe in the dog, Szidon and Fishman found that electrical stimulation of the left stellate ganglion caused increments in systolic pulmonary artery pressure but not in diastolic or mean pulmonary artery pressures; calculated pulmonary vascular resistance did not change (59). Szidon and Fishman concluded that the distensibility and tension of the large pulmonary vessels were altered by sympathetic stimulation, but that the small resistance vessels were largely unaffected (59). In a similar cat model with continuous rather than pulsatile constant left lower lobe flow, Hyman and colleagues found that stellate ganglion stimulation activates pulmonary vascular alpha receptors predominantly but also beta receptors; pulmonary vascular resistance increases (37). Beta blockade with propranolol increases the pulmonary vasoconstriction caused by stellate ganglion stimulation, and alpha blockade with phenoxybenzamine changes the effect of stellate ganglion stimulation from pulmonary vasoconstriction to pulmonary vasodilatation (37). Sympathetic nerve-induced pulmonary vasodilatation may be a result of enhanced prostacyclin production (61). Sympathetic stimulation constricts canine pulmonary veins as well as arteries (40).

Vagal Stimulation

The vagus nerve has been stimulated in a variety of studies as a test for parasympathetic innervation of the pulmonary vascular tree.

EFFERENT STIMULATION

Electrical stimulation of the left cervical vagosympathetic nerve has been used to investigate the effects of vagal stimulation on pulmonary vascular tone (37). However, as its name makes clear, the vagosympathetic nerve carries both vagal and sympathetic fibers. In their cat model with continuous rather than pulsatile constant left lower lobe flow, Hyman and colleagues found that under basal conditions left cervical vagosympathetic nerve stimulation causes modest elevations in pulmonary vascular resistance which are blockable by phenoxybenzamine, but after increase in pulmonary vascular tone with the alpha agonist U-46619 or with $PGF_{2\alpha}$, left cervical vagosympathetic nerve stimulation causes pulmonary vasodilatation (37). This neurally mediated pulmonary vasodilatation was blocked with atropine but not propranolol, indicating that cholinergic nerves were responsible (37). Like sympathetic nerve-induced pulmonary vasodilatation, parasympathetic nerve-induced pulmonary vasodilatation may be a result of increased prostacyclin production (9).

AFFERENT STIMULATION

Bradford and Dean demonstrated in 1894 that electrical stimulation of the cut *central* end of the vagus caused pulmonary arterial pressure to increase (8). This phenomenon has received very little subsequent attention, although Weber confirmed its existence in 1910 (cited by Daly and von Euler [21]).

BARORECEPTOR INFLUENCES

Baroreceptors in the carotid arteries, aorta, and pulmonary artery could play a role in the reflex regulation of the pulmonary circulation.

Carotid Baroreceptors

In 1957, Daly and Daly showed that stimulation of the carotid baroreceptors caused substantial reflex increases in pulmonary artery pressures in a constantly perfused isolated left lower lobe preparation (19). Daly and Daly were unable to demonstrate conclusively the efferent limb of carotid baroreceptor-induced pulmonary vasoconstriction, but in at least one animal it appeared that the sympathetic nerves supplying the lungs were responsible (19). In 1978, Pace could not confirm Daly and Daly's findings (51). Evidence supportive of the results of Daly and Daly may be adduced from the observations that electrical stimulation of the superior laryngeal nerve causes reflex pulmonary hypertension in neonatal piglets (44), and that baroreceptor fibers run in the superior laryngeal nerve. Moreover, Shoukas et al. have convincingly demonstrated that carotid baroreceptors do influence pulmonary vascular tone in adult dogs (54).

Whether the aortic baroreceptors have reflex effects on the pulmonary circulation remains unexplored.

Pulmonary Baroreceptors

Pulmonary artery baroreceptors have been demonstrated by several investigators (5,10,14,50), but whether pulmonary artery baroreceptors have any role in regulation of the pulmonary circulation remains controversial. Some investigators have demonstrated what appears to be reflex pulmonary hypertension caused by pulmonary artery distention (39,42). However, the possibility of artifact has not been entirely excluded.

UPPER AIRWAY INFLUENCES

Injecting small volumes of fresh water or salt water into the trachea causes apnea and pulmonary hypertension in both adult dogs (13,31) and newborn sheep (29). Whether pulmonary hypertension is secondary only to apnea and respiratory acidosis is unclear from these experiments, but the increments in pulmonary arterial pressure in the adult dogs were thought to be quicker, larger, and more sustained than could be easily explained by the accompanying hypoxemia and respiratory acidosis (13). The administration of supplemental oxygen during the tracheal water injections lessened, but did not abolish, the increases in pulmonary arterial pressure in the adult dogs (13). In the newborn sheep, oxygen and mechanical ventilation did counteract the hypoxia and respiratory acidosis that accompanied water-induced apnea and did reduce the systemic effects, but whether the increases in pulmonary arterial pressures observed earlier were altered was not reported (29).

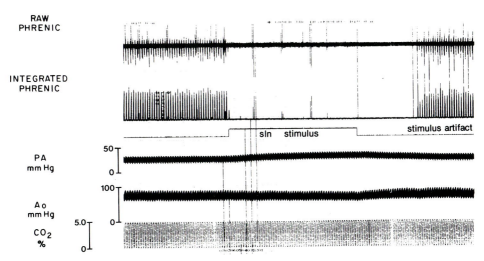

Figure 2: The effects of electrically stimulating the superior laryngeal nerve in a 1-day-old anesthetized, paralyzed, mechanically ventilated piglet. Top line: amplified phrenic neural activity (raw phrenic). Second line: full-wave rectified phrenic neural activity (integrated phrenic); each deflection is a breath, and the height of each deflection is proportional to tidal volume. Third line: the electrical superior laryngeal nerve stimulus is indicated (sln stimulus); the stimulation lasted 3 min. Fourth, fifth, and sixth lines: pulmonary arterial pressure (PA), aortic pressure (Ao), and end-tidal carbon dioxide (CO_2), respectively. Superior laryngeal nerve stimulation caused prolonged apnea, increased pulmonary artery pressure, and decreased systemic arterial pressure. By design, end-tidal CO_2 was held constant.

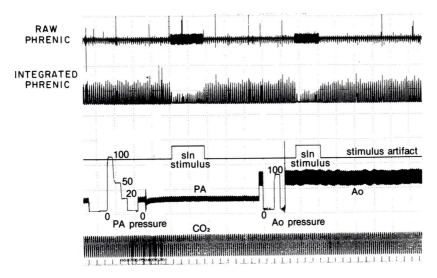

Figure 3: Electrical stimulation of the superior laryngeal nerve in a 24-day-old anesthetized, paralyzed, mechanically ventilated piglet. Stimulation of the superior laryngeal nerve inhibited phrenic neural activity but had no effect on either pulmonary or aortic pressure. By design, end-tidal CO_2 concentration was held constant.

TABLE 1 EFFECTS OF SUPERIOR LARYNGEAL NERVE ELECTRICAL STIMULATION ON MEAN PULMONARY ARTERIAL PRESSURE IN NEWBORN PIGLETS

	Younger (n = 12)	Older (n = 6)
Age	3 ± 0.6 days (range 1–7)	22 ± 2.0 days (range 14–30)
Weight	1.5 ± 0.1 kg (range 1.0–2.0)	3.4 ± 0.5 kg (range 2.3–5.4)
Baseline PA	24 ± 1 mmHg (range 18–30)	17 ± 2 mmHg (range 12–26)
Effects of SLN stimulation	10/12 increased*	1/6 increased*

*$p < 0.01$, Fischer's exact test.

Colebatch and Halmagyi found that tracheal installation of tetracaine and intravenous administration of hexamethonium in adult dogs diminished the tracheal water-induced increases in pulmonary artery pressure and that atropine blocked the response (13). Vagotomy had no effect on freshwater-induced pulmonary hypertension in adult dogs, but the site of vagal sectioning was not mentioned (13). Colebatch and Halmagyi concluded that a "local" intrapulmonary reflex was responsible for tracheal freshwater-induced pulmonary hypertension but did not identify its origin (13). Similar pharmacologic blocking experiments were done by Grogaard et al. in neonatal sheep. Although systemic changes in response to tracheal instillation of water were lessened after adrenergic blockade and atropine, pulmonary arterial pressures were not reported (29).

The possibility that the central nervous system could play a role in the pulmonary hypertension caused by tracheal fluid administration was not considered by Colebatch and Halmagyi (13) or by Grogaard et al. (29). However, as the data below will demonstrate, it seems likely that the explanation for tracheal-fluid induced pulmonary hypertension (unaccounted for by hypoxia and respiratory

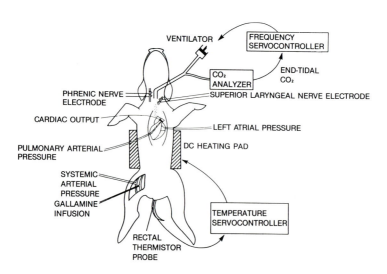

Figure 4: Preparation used to determine pulmonary vascular resistance during electrical stimulation of the superior laryngeal nerve. (Reproduced with permission from Long WA (ed), *Fetal and Neonatal Cardiology.* Philadelphia, W. B. Saunders, 1990, p. 88.)

acidosis) lies in stimulation of laryngeal chemoreceptors. Colebatch and Halmagyi probably sectioned the vagi below the level of the superior laryngeal nerves. Had they sectioned the vagus above the superior laryngeal nerves, Colebatch and Halmagyi would probably have abolished reflex pulmonary hypertension caused by tracheal water administration.

A more recent series of experiments explored whether the brain not only can influence pulmonary vascular tone, but actually does so after afferent input from the cranial nerves (44). Pulmonary arterial pressures were measured during electrical stimulation of a superior laryngeal nerve in 18 anesthetized, paralyzed piglets mechanically ventilated with 100% O_2 at constant end-tidal CO_2. In piglets less than 7 days of age (Fig. 2), but not in older piglets (Fig. 3), pulmonary arterial pressures increased consistently during the stimulation (Table 1). Cutting of the vagi below the superior laryngeal nerve had no effect on the superior laryn-

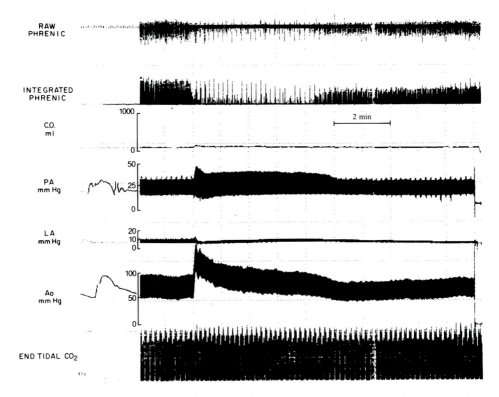

Figure 5: Electrical stimulation of the superior laryngeal nerve in an 18-day-old anesthetized, paralyzed, mechanically ventilated piglet. The cardiac output is also shown. The 5-min electrical superior laryngeal nerve stimulus (10 H, 4v) was begun at the time systemic and pulmonary artery pressures suddenly increased and phrenic neural activity decreased. Stimulation of the superior laryngeal nerve caused prolonged inhibition of phrenic activity and increased pulmonary artery pressure and systemic arterial pressure substantially. Left atrial pressure decreased slightly. Cardiac output increased slightly initially, but then returned to baseline while pulmonary and systemic pressures remained elevated. These observations indicate the occurrence of neurally mediated pulmonary and systemic vasoconstriction.

geal nerve-induced increases in pulmonary arterial pressures. The fact that systemic arterial pressure fell while pulmonary artery pressure increased (Fig. 2) suggested that the changes in pulmonary artery pressure were not simply passive.

Subsequently, the effects of electrical stimulation of the superior laryngeal nerve were explored in young (less than 7 days) anesthetized, paralyzed piglets as shown in Figure 4 (44). The piglets were mechanically ventilated with oxygen and a servo-controlled system adjusted ventilator rate to maintain end-tidal CO_2 constant. Phrenic neural output was recorded from a C5 root of the right phrenic nerve and the right superior laryngeal nerve was prepared for central stimulation. Once the preparation was stable and baseline phrenic neural activity, pulmonary arterial pressure, left atrial pressure, and pulmonary flow had been recorded, electrical stimulations of the superior laryngeal nerve (for 3 min each at 10 to 20 Hz, 2 to 4 v) were carried out (Fig. 5). During stimulation, phrenic neural activity was inhibited in each animal while pulmonary arterial pressure increased; end-tidal CO_2 concentration remained constant. Left atrial pressure, cardiac output, and systemic arterial pressure did not change significantly. Both total pulmonary resistance and pulmonary vascular resistance increased significantly (44). Sectioning of the vagi distal to the superior laryngeal nerve had no effect on the superior laryngeal nerve-induced pulmonary vasoconstriction. These observations demonstrated that afferent input from the upper airway can cause pulmonary hypertension, and that the central nervous system is responsible. The efferent limb of this reflex is as yet unproven but is probably the sympathetic nervous system.

CHEMORECEPTOR INFLUENCES

In 1927, Heymans proved the existence of the aortic chemoreceptors (34), and 4 years later proved de Castro's hypothesis (24) that the carotid body was also a chemosensory organ. Heymans' experiments were technical feats in which he determined the ventilatory response to supplying hypoxic blood from one animal to the isolated aorta or carotid artery of another, well-oxygenated animal. In 1946, von Euler and Liljestrand demonstrated that alveolar hypoxia increases pulmonary arterial pressure in cats (62). Subsequently, Daly and Daly (20), Aviado et al. (4), and Campbell et al. (12) demonstrated that hypoxia restricted to the aortic and carotid bodies causes reflex pulmonary vasoconstriction. These observations have been confirmed in less complicated preparations by subsequent investigators (56,58,59). Similarly, isolated systemic hypoxia (while alveolar P_{O_2} remains normal) causes reflex pulmonary vasoconstriction (63) whereas hypoxia of the isolated brain does not (49), all consistent with the idea that the peripheral chemoreceptors are the afferent pathways for the *reflex* pulmonary vasoconstriction induced by acute hypoxia.

The aortic and carotid chemoreceptors seem to exert different effects on the systemic and pulmonary circulations. For example, stimulation of the aortic chemoreceptors increases systemic vascular resistance whereas stimulation of the carotid chemoreceptors has little effect on systemic vascular resistance (15,23). Carotid chemoreceptor stimulation causes bradycardia (22), and appar-

A   B

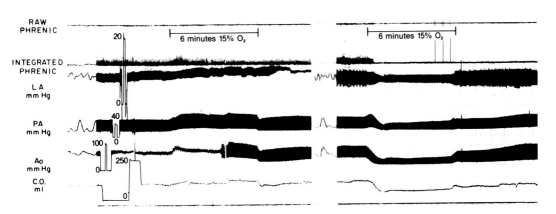

Figure 6: The effects of 15% O_2 in a 3-day-old anesthetized, paralyzed, mechanically venti-lated, ductus-ligated, otherwise intact piglet. A: before chemodenervation; B: after chemo-denervation. Abbreviations as in previous figures. In the intact animal before chemode-nervation (A), 15% O_2 increased phrenic neural activity, pulmonary artery pressure, and aortic pressure. (The aortic catheter was flushed halfway through the first exposure when it was realized that the tracing was damped.) Left atrial pressure increased slightly, and cardiac output was largely unaffected. After chemodenervation (B), phrenic neural activity decreased during repeat exposure to 15% O_2 (indicating successful chemodenervation), and left atrial pressure, pulmonary artery pressure, aortic pressure, and cardiac output fell. These observations indicate that the peripheral chemoreceptors contribute substantially to hypoxic pulmonary vasoconstriction in newborns.(Reproduced with permission from Long WA (ed), *Fetal and Neonatal Cardiology.* Philadelphia, W. B. Saunders, 1990, p. 84.)

ently aortic chemoreceptor stimulation does not. Aortic chemoreceptor stimula-tion predominantly constricts pulmonary veins (56), whereas presumably carotid chemoreceptor stimulation predominantly constricts pulmonary arteries. Carotid chemoreceptor stimulation greatly increases ventilation, whereas aortic chemo-receptor stimulation has modest effects on ventilation (23). Explanations for these differences are obscure but probably have something to do with defense of the fetus against hypoxia. There are few reports dealing with developmental dif-ferences in the site and magnitude of aortic versus carotid chemoreceptor contri-bution to hypoxic pulmonary vasoconstriction. However, Custer and Hales have shown that chemical sympathectomy markedly inhibits hypoxic pulmonary vaso-constriction in newborn sheep but has little effect in adult sheep (18).

To study the role of the chemoreceptors in hypoxic pulmonary vasoconstric-tion, total pulmonary resistance (pulmonary artery pressure/cardiac output) and pulmonary vascular resistance (pulmonary artery pressure minus left atrial pres-sure/cardiac output) were measured during hypoxia before and after denervating the peripheral chemoreceptors (45). The model used was identical to that used in the superior laryngeal nerve experiments described above (Fig. 4), except that instead of isolating the right superior laryngeal nerve, the carotid sinus nerves were isolated bilaterally. Once the preparation had become stable and records were made of baseline phrenic neural activity, pulmonary arterial pressure, left atrial pressure, and cardiac output, 6-min exposures to 12% O_2 were carried out. Exposure to the hypoxic inspired mixtures caused pulmonary arterial pressure, total pulmonary resistance, and pulmonary vascular resistance to increase in each piglet (Fig. 6A). Section of the carotid sinus nerves abolished the increase in pulmonary arterial pressure upon subsequent exposure to 12% O_2 (Fig. 6B), and total pulmonary vascular resistance increased less. After sectioning the carotid sinus nerves and vagi, 2 of the 6 piglets died acutely upon reexposure to 12% O_2; total pulmonary resistance did not increase significantly during hypoxia in the four survivors (45). Hypoxic exposure after chemodenervation has also been reported to be fatal in neonatal rats (35); in contrast, hypoxia is not fatal in adult rats after chemodenervation (41). These observations demonstrate that the peripheral chemoreceptors contribute significantly to hypoxic pulmonary hypertension in newborn animals.

DIRECT BRAIN INFLUENCES

Hypothalamus

Direct stimulation of the brain can also influence pulmonary vasomotor tone. In 1967, Anderson and Brown (3) found that electrically stimulating the hypothalamus in cats caused marked increases in pulmonary arterial pressure. Cardiac output increased as well, but the increases in pulmonary arterial pressure began before blood flow changed (3). Pulmonary vascular resistance increased modestly (6 to 8 percent) but significantly (3). The responses of the pulmonary vascular bed to hypothalamic stimulation could be blocked by hexamethonium and sectioning of the stellate ganglion, but not by vagotomy (3). Atropine exacerbated the changes in pulmonary arterial pressure (3). Thus, the sympathetic nervous system appears to mediate hypothalamic-induced pulmonary vasoconstriction.

Szidon and Fishman observed similar increases in pulmonary arterial pressure and cardiac output from electrical stimulation of the hypothalamus in intact dogs, but went a step further and repeated hypothalamic stimulation in an isolated left lower lobe preparation designed to permit constant pulsatile blood flow (59). Considerable increases in pulmonary systolic pressure were observed, and pulmonary diastolic pressures either remained unchanged or increased slightly (59). Hypothalamic stimulation was also shown to improve the distribution of pulmonary blood flow (59), a role predicted for pulmonary vasomotor nerves 38 years earlier by Daly and von Euler (21). Phenoxybenzamine blocked changes in pulmonary artery pressure induced by the hypothalamus (59). These observations suggested that hypothalamic stimulation affected the distensibility of large pulmonary vessels more than the resistance of small pulmonary blood vessels, that the hypothalamus might have a role in maintaining homogeneous pulmonary perfusion, and that the sympathetic nervous system mediates hypothalamic influences on the pulmonary circulation (59).

Brainstem

In 1894, Bradford and Dean described increases in pulmonary arterial pressure caused by electrical stimulation of the high medulla in an area they termed a vasomotor center (8). Bradford and Dean were able to demonstrate that section-

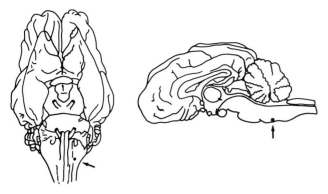

Figure 7: The location of the brainstem vasomotor center. (Reproduced with permission from Long WA (ed), *Fetal and Neonatal Cardiology*. Philadelphia, W. B. Saunders, 1990, p. 89.)

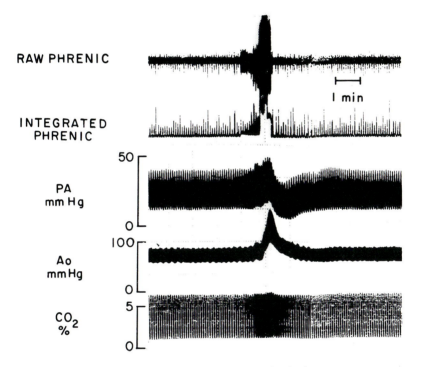

Figure 8: The effects of electrically stimulating the brainstem vasomotor center in an anesthetized, paralyzed, mechanically ventilated piglet. The electrical stimulus is indicated by the bar; the stimulation lasted for 30 sec. Electrical stimulation of the brainstem vasomotor center caused marked increases in aortic pressure and modest increases in pulmonary artery pressure. Since cardiac output and left atrial pressure were not determined, it is unclear whether the changes in pressure were passive or due to neurally induced vasoconstriction. However, the rapidity and magnitude of the changes in pulmonary and systemic pressures suggest that neurally mediated vasoconstriction took place in both the pulmonary and systemic circulations.

ing of the spinal cord at C7 largely abolished accompanying increases in systemic arterial pressure, but had no effect on the increases in pulmonary artery pressure caused by electrical stimulation of the high medulla. Bradford and Dean also showed that sectioning of the spinal cord at C2 abolished the effects of medullary

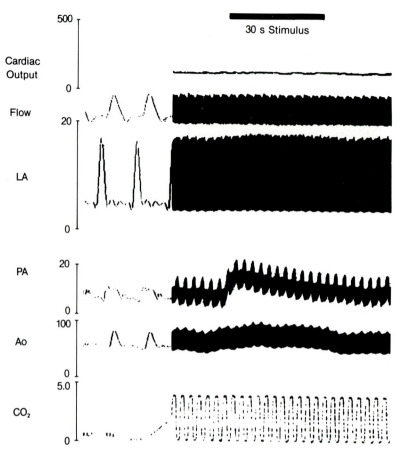

Figure 9: The effects of electrically stimulating the brainstem vasomotor center in an anesthetized, paralyzed, mechanically ventilated piglet. The electrical stimulus is indicated by the bar; the stimulation lasted 30 sec. Flow: instantaneous pulmonary blood flow. Other abbreviations as in previous figures. Electrical stimulation of the brainstem vasomotor center caused marked increases in pulmonary artery pressure and modest increases in aortic pressure without changing cardiac output, instantaneous pulmonary flow, or left atrial pressure. These observations indicate the occurrence of neurally mediated pulmonary and systemic vasoconstriction. (Reproduced with permission from Long WA (ed), *Fetal and Neonatal Cardiology*. Philadelphia, W. B. Saunders, 1990, p. 89.)

electrical stimulation on pulmonary artery pressure. They further demonstrated that similar effects on pulmonary artery pressure could be demonstrated by electrical stimulation of the spinal roots of C2, C3, and C4, and that accompanying changes in the systemic circulation could largely be abolished by sectioning of the splanchnic nerves.

Unaware of Bradford and Dean's discoveries, we began a series of preliminary experiments to investigate the effects of electrical brainstem stimulations on the pulmonary circulation. These experiments were based on recent developments in identifying the brainstem "vasomotor center" (11). This center (in rats, a 0.5-mm³ area located in the rostral brainstem in the area of the nucleus paragigantocellularis [Fig. 7]) is the hub of sympathetic circulatory control and is capable of causing tremendous changes in the systemic circulation (Fig. 8), but the effects of stimulating this area on the pulmonary circulation are unexplored. The basic preparation is the same as the superior laryngeal nerve (Fig. 4) and chemoreceptor models described above, but ventral exposure of the brainstem is added. Brief (10 to 30 sec) electrical stimulations (10 to 50 Hz, 50 to 100 milliamps) were applied to various parts of the brainstem vasomotor center using a fine monopolar stimulating electrode and areas of the vasomotor center from which hemodynamic changes of interest were elicited marked by application of direct current destruction for subsequent histologic examination. In some young piglets (2 to 3 days of age), pulmonary vasoconstriction occurred (Fig. 9), without changes in cardiac output and relatively small changes in the systemic resistance. These observations raise the possibility that a specific pulmonary vasoconstrictor area does exist within the brainstem "vasomotor center."

CLINICAL PERSPECTIVE

The concept that the nervous system may have a role in eliciting pulmonary hypertension is not new; in 1959, Halmagyi tallied evidence for and against a neural component to pulmonary hypertension in mitral stenosis, left ventricular failure, congenital heart disease, chronic cor pulmonale, and primary ("idiopathic") pulmonary hypertension, and concluded that neurogenic components were sometimes present, particularly in mitral stenosis, but that patient to patient variability was great (30). Our own experiments seem pertinent to at least three forms of unexplained pulmonary hypertension: the syndrome of persistent pulmonary hypertension of the newborn, pulmonary hypertension associated with transposition of the great vessels, and primary pulmonary hypertension.

Persistent Pulmonary Hypertension of the Newborn Syndrome

The syndrome of persistent pulmonary hypertension of the newborn is a poorly understood form of pulmonary hypertension that afflicts newborn infants. Many predisposing factors have been identified (46), but many instances remain idiopathic. Meconium aspiration is probably the single most common predisposing factor. Infants with persistent pulmonary hypertension of the newborn syndrome exhibit persistent postnatal right-to-left atrial shunting, right-to-left shunting through the ductus arteriosus, or both. Supplemental oxygen and mechanical ventilation are the mainstays of treatment, which too often is unsuccessful.

It is possible that laryngeal irritation may either predispose to, or exacerbate, pulmonary hypertension and consequent right-to-left shunting in newborn infants. Possible mechanisms of laryngeal irritation in newborn infants include meconium aspiration into the airways, mechanical abrasion by endotracheal tubes, use of tracheal suction catheters, endotracheal administration of distilled water, or 0.9% NaCl to loosen airway secretions (low or high chloride concentrations cause superior laryngeal nerve discharge [6]). Despite the preliminary data presented above suggesting that reflex laryngeal pulmonary hypertension diminishes after birth, reflex pulmonary hypertension elicited by upper airway stimulation may contribute to pulmonary hypertension in older children and adults.

For example, the abnormal mucus in cystic fibrosis could cause chronic laryngeal irritation and reflex pulmonary hypertension. Similarly, cigarette smoke could cause laryngeal irritation and reflex pulmonary hypertension.

Transposition of the Great Vessels

Early and severe pulmonary hypertension develops in infants with transposition of the great vessels, despite the fact that alveolar oxygen content is normal, blood pH is normal, and pulmonary arterial saturations are quite high. Pulmonary blood flow is increased in infants with transposition of the great vessels, but infants with atrial septal defects often have equal or greater pulmonary blood flows and yet do not develop pulmonary vascular disease for at least 20 or 30 years. Infants with transposition of the great vessels can develop irreversible pulmonary vascular disease in the second year of life. Moreover, although polycythemia frequently develops in infants with transposition of the great vessels, neither the time course of its development nor its magnitude suggest that polycythemia is likely to account for early and severe pulmonary hypertension in transposition infants.

It is possible that obligatory profound systemic hypoxia in infants with transposition of the great vessels causes marked chemoreceptor discharge, and that resulting reflex pulmonary vasoconstriction is responsible for the unexplained early and severe pulmonary hypertension seen in infants with transposition.

Primary Pulmonary Hypertension

Primary pulmonary hypertension is an unexplained form of pulmonary hypertension which occurs largely in young adult females. In all likelihood a number of different, as yet unrecognized, diseases cause primary pulmonary hypertension. It seems likely that endothelial disorders, clotting derangements, and enzyme deficiencies will eventually be found to account for various subtypes of the disease now known as primary pulmonary hypertension.

The brain certainly has a very important role in the regulation of the systemic circulation, and the experimental evidence reviewed in this chapter clearly demonstrates that the brain can influence the pulmonary circulation as well. Pertinent to this point, recent studies have demonstrated that patients with essential systemic hypertension often also have elevated pulmonary arterial pressures (1,27); similarly, in patients with primary pulmonary hypertension, systemic vascular resistance is often increased before cardiac output is compromised (Long et al., unpublished observations). Pulmonary vasoconstriction occurs in many patients with primary pulmonary hypertension: in 77 of a series of 100 patients with primary pulmonary hypertension, prostacyclin caused a decrease in pulmonary vascular resistance that exceeded 20 percent of control values (Long et al., unpublished observations). It is possible that abnormal central neural pulmonary vasoconstriction initiates some forms of primary pulmonary hypertension and exacerbates others.

CONCLUSION

The central nervous system can alter pulmonary vascular tone at all stages of development, but appears to be particularly important during the neonatal period. It is possible that further advances in the laboratory will provide new explanations for unexplained forms of pulmonary hypertension, and eventually to new treatments that are based on altering central neurotransmission rather than vasodilator-induced direct relaxation of pulmonary vascular smooth muscle.

ACKNOWLEDGMENTS

The experiments described in this chapter were supported by grants from the Physicians New Orleans Foundation, the North Carolina Affiliate of the American Heart Association, and the Wellcome Research Laboratories.

REFERENCES

1. Alpert MA, Bauer JH, Parker BM, Sanfelippo JF, Brooks CS: Pulmonary hemodynamics in systemic hypertension. South Med J 78 : 784–789, 1985.

2. Altura BM, Chand N: Differential effects of prostaglandins on canine intrapulmonary arteries and veins. Br J Pharmacol 73 : 819–827, 1981.

3. Anderson FL, Brown AM: Pulmonary vasoconstriction elicited by stimulation of the hypothalamic integrative area for defense reactions. Circ Res 21 : 747–756, 1967.

4. Aviado DM Jr, Ling JS, Schmidt CF: Effects of anoxia on pulmonary circulation: Reflex pulmonary vasoconstriction. Am J Physiol 289 : 253–262, 1957.

5. Bianconi R, Green JH: Pulmonary baroreceptors in the cat. Arch Ital Biol 97 : 305–315, 1959.

6. Boggs DF, Bartlett D Jr: Chemical specificity of a laryngeal apneic reflex in puppies. J Appl Physiol 53 : 455–462, 1982.

7. Bradford JR, Dean HP: On the innervation of the pulmonary vessels. J Physiol (Lond) 10 : Pi–iv, 1889.

8. Bradford JR, Dean HP: The pulmonary circulation. J Physiol (Lond) 16 : 34–96, 1894.

9. Brandt R, Dembinska-Kiec A, Korbut R, Gryglewski RJ, Nowak J: Release of prostacyclin from the human pulmonary vascular bed in response to cholinergic stimulation. Naunyn-Schmied Arch Pharmacol 325 : 69–75, 1984.

10. Brofman BL, Charms BL, Kohn PM, Elder J, Newman R, Rizika M: Unilateral pulmonary artery occlusion in man. J Thorac Surg 34 : 206–227, 1959.

11. Brown DL, Guyenet PG: Electrophysiological study of cardiovascular neurons in the rostral ventrolateral medulla of rats. Circ Res 56 : 359–369, 1985.

12. Campbell AGM, Cockburn F, Dawes GS, Milligan JE: Pulmonary vasoconstriction in asphyxia during cross-circulation between twin foetal lambs. J Physiol (Lond) 192 : 111–121, 1967.

13. Colebatch HJH, Halmagyi DFJ: Reflex pulmonary hypertension of fresh-water aspiration. J Appl Physiol 18 : 179–185, 1963.

14. Coleridge JCG, Kidd C: Reflex effects of stimulating baroreceptors in the pulmonary artery. J Physiol 166 : 197–210, 1963.

15. Comroe JH: The location and function of the chemoreceptors of the aorta. Am J Physiol 27 : 176–191, 1939.

16. Cox RH, Peterson LH, Detweiler DK: Hemodynamic responses to stellate ganglion stimulation in mongrels and greyhounds. Am J Physiol 231 : 1062–1067, 1976.

17. Custer JR, Hales CA: Influence of alveolar oxygen on pulmonary vasoconstriction in newborn lambs versus sheep. Am Rev Respir Dis 132 : 326–331, 1985.

18. Custer JR, Hales CA: Chemical sympathectomy decreases alveolar hypoxic vasoconstriction in lambs but not sheep. J Appl Physiol 60 : 32–37, 1986.

19. Daly I de Burgh, Daly M de Burgh: Observations on the changes in resistance of the pulmonary vascular bed in response to stimulation of the carotid sinus baroreceptors in the dog. J Physiol 137 : 427–435, 1957.

20. Daly I de Burgh, Daly M de Burgh: The effects of stimulation of the carotid body chemoreceptors on the pulmonary vascular bed in the dog: The 'vaso-

sensory controlled perfused living animal' preparation. J Physiol 148 : 201–219, 1959.

21. Daly I de Burgh, von Euler V: The functional activity of the vasomotor nerves to the lungs in the dog. Proc Roy Soc Lond B 110 : 92–111, 1932.

22. Daly M de Burgh, Scott MJ: The effects of stimulation of the carotid body chemoreceptors on heart rate in the dog. J Physiol 144 : 148–166, 1958.

23. Daly M de Burgh, Ungar A: Comparison of the reflex responses elicited by stimulation of the separately perfused carotid and aortic body chemoreceptors in the dog. J Physiol (Lond) 182 : 379–403, 1966.

24. de Castro F: Sur la structure et l'innervation du sinus carotidien de l'homme et des mammifères. Nouveaux faits sur l'innervation et la fonction du glomus caroticum. Trab Lab Invest Biol Univ Madrid 25 : 331–384, 1928.

25. De Pasquale NP, Burch GE, Hyman AL: Pulmonary venous response to immersion hypothermia and hyperthermia. Am Heart J 70 : 486–493, 1965.

26. Downing SE, Lee JC: Nervous control of the pulmonary circulation. Annu Rev Physiol 42 : 199–210, 1980.

27. Fiorentini C, Barbier P, Galli C, Loaldi A, Tamborini G, Tosi E, Guazzi MD: Pulmonary vascular overreactivity in systemic hypertension: A pathophysiological link between the greater and lesser circulation. Hypertension 7 : 995–1002, 1985.

28. Fishman AP: Hypoxia on the pulmonary circulation: How and where it acts. Circ Res 38 : 221–231, 1976.

29. Grogaard J, Lindstrom DP, Stahlman MT, Marchal F, Sundell H: The cardiovascular responses to laryngeal water administration in young lambs. J Dev Physiol 4 : 353–370, 1982.

30. Halmagyi DFJ: Role of the autonomous nervous system in the genesis of pulmonary hypertension in heart disease. J Chronic Dis 9 : 525–535, 1959.

31. Halmagyi DFJ, Colebatch HJH: Ventilation and circulation after fluid aspiration. J Appl Physiol 16 : 35–40, 1961.

32. Hebb C: Motor innervation of the pulmonary blood vessels of mammals, in Fishman AP, Hecht HH (eds), *The Pulmonary Circulation and Interstitial Space.* Chicago, University of Chicago Press, 1969, pp 195–222.

33. Heymann MA: Control of the pulmonary circulation in the perinatal period. J Dev Physiol 6 : 281–290, 1984.

34. Heymans J-F, Heymans C: Sur les modifications directes et sur la regulation reflexe de l'activité du centre respiratoire de la tête isolée du chien. Arch Intern Pharmacodyn 33 : 272–370, 1927.

35. Hofer MA: Lethal respiratory disturbance in neonatal rats after arterial chemoreceptor denervation. Life Sci 34 : 489–496, 1984.

36. Hyman AL, Kadowitz PJ: Enhancement of alpha- and beta-adrenoreceptor responses by eleva-

tions in vascular tone in pulmonary circulation. Am J Physiol 250 : H1109–H1116, 1986.

37. Hyman AL, Lippton HL, Kadowitz PJ: Autonomic regulation of the pulmonary circulation. J Cardiovasc Pharmacol 7S : S80–S95, 1985.

38. Ingram RH, Szidon JP, Skalak R, Fishman AP: Effects of sympathetic nerve stimulation on the pulmonary arterial tree of the isolated lobe perfused in situ. Circ Res 22 : 801–815, 1968.

39. Juratsch CE, Jengo JA, Laks MM: Role of the autonomic nervous system and pulmonary artery receptors in production of experimental pulmonary hypertension. Chest 71S : 265–269, 1977.

40. Kadowitz PJ, Joiner PD, Hyman AL: Influence of sympathetic stimulation and vasoactive substances on the canine pulmonary veins. J Clin Invest 56 : 354–365, 1975.

41. Lagneaux D: Relation between peripheral chemoreceptor stimulation and pulmonary arterial pressure in rats. Arch Int Physiol Biochim 94 : 127–134, 1986.

42. Laks MM, Juratsch CE, Garner D, Beazell J, Criley JM: Acute pulmonary artery hypertension produced by distention of the main pulmonary artery in the conscious dog. Chest 68 : 807–813, 1975.

43. Lock JE, Olley PM, Coceani F: Enhanced beta-adrenergic function in fetal sheep. Am J Obstet Gynecol 112 : 1114–1121, 1981.

44. Long WA: Superior laryngeal nerve-induced reflex pulmonary hypertension in neonatal piglets. Am Rev Respir Dis 135 : A299, 1987.

45. Long WA: Effects of chemoreceptor sectioning on hypoxia induced pulmonary hypertension. Am Rev Respir Dis 135 : A520, 1987.

46. Long WA: Persistent pulmonary hypertension of the newborn syndrome, in Long WA (ed), *Fetal and Neonatal Cardiology.* Philadelphia, W.B. Saunders, in press.

47. Malik AB, Kidd BSL: Adrenergic blockade and the pulmonary vascular response to hypoxia. Respir Physiol 19 : 96–106, 1973.

48. Nishi K, Sakanashi M, Takenaka F: Afferent fibres from pulmonary arterial baroreceptors in the left cardiac sympathetic nerve of the cat. J Physiol (Lond) 240 : 53–66, 1974.

49. Olson NC, Robinson NE, Scott JB: Effects of brain hypoxia on pulmonary hemodynamics. J Surg Res 35 : 21–27, 1983.

50. Osorio J, Russek M: Reflex changes on the pulmonary and systemic pressures elicited by stimulation of the baroreceptors in the pulmonary artery. Circ Res 10 : 664–667, 1962.

51. Pace JB: Influence of carotid occlusion on pulmonary vascular resistance in anesthetized dog. Proc Soc Exp Biol Med 158 : 215–219, 1978.

52. Porcelli RJ, Bergofsky EH: Adrenergic receptors in pulmonary vasoconstrictor responses to gaseous and humoral agents. J Appl Physiol 34 : 483–488, 1973.

53. Rendas A, Branthwaite M, Reid L: Growth of the pulmonary circulation in normal pig—structural analysis and cardiopulmonary function. J Appl Physiol 45:806–817, 1964.

54. Shoukas AA, Brunner MJ, Frankle AE, Kallman CH: Carotid sinus baroreceptor reflex control and the role of autoregulation in the systemic and pulmonary arterial pressure-flow relationships of the dog. Circ Res 54:674–682, 1984.

55. Soifer SJ, Morin FC III, Kaslow DC, Heymann MA: The developmental effects of prostaglandin D2 on the pulmonary and systemic circulations in the newborn lamb. J Dev Physiol 5:237–250, 1983.

56. Stern S, Braun K: Effect of chemoreceptor stimulation on the pulmonary veins. Am J Physiol 210:535–539, 1965.

57. Stern S, Braun K: Pulmonary arterial and venous response to cooling: Role of alpha-adrenergic receptors. Am J Physiol 219:982–985, 1970.

58. Stern S, Ferguson RE, Rappaport E: Reflex pulmonary vasoconstriction due to stimulation of the aortic body by nicotine. Am J Physiol 206:1189–1195, 1964.

59. Szidon JP, Fishman AP: Autonomic control of the pulmonary circulation, in Fishman AP, Hecht HH (eds), *The Pulmonary Circulation and Interstitial Space*. Chicago, University of Chicago Press, 1969, pp 239–268.

60. Thilenius OG, Candiolo BM, Beug JL: Effect of adrenergic blockade on hypoxia-induced pulmonary vasoconstriction in awake dogs. Am J Physiol 213:990–998, 1967.

61. Tong EY, Mathe AA, Tisher PW: Release of norepinephrine by sympathetic nerve stimulation from rabbit lungs. Am J Physiol 235:H803–H808, 1978.

62. von Euler US, Liljestrand G: Observations on the pulmonary arterial blood pressure in the cat. Acta Physiol Scand 12:301–320, 1946.

63. Wilcox BR, Autin WG, Bender HW: Effect of hypoxia on pulmonary artery pressure in dogs. Am J Physiol 207:1314–1318, 1964.

Michael Magno, Ph.D.

11 ————————————

Bronchial Circulation

Most studies on the bronchial circulation were done in cats, dogs, and sheep. Similarities in the behavior of the bronchial circulation in these species and humans suggests extrapolation of these studies to humans. For example, Charan et al. (6) have shown in sheep that the bronchial circulation proliferates during disease (lung abscess). We have found that in sheep with pneumonia, pleural adhesions form within which the bronchial circulation proliferates from the intercostal arteries via the parietal pleura (16).

The extrinsic regulation of the bronchial circulation is mediated by the autonomic nervous system. McLean (19) has summarized the literature on the neural control of the lung vasculature: the blood vessels of all the three animal species and human receive adrenergic, cholinergic, and peptidergic innervation. The only apparent exception is that the human bronchial circulation is not innervated by acetylcholine esterase-positive neurons. Whether peptidergic nerves exist in the sheep lung is uncertain since such studies have not been conducted. However, Sheller and Brigham (20) have presented physiological evidence suggesting the presence of nonadrenergic, noncholinergic (possibly peptidergic) nerves in the extra- and intrapulmonary airways of the sheep.

RESPONSES TO HYPOXIA

The bronchial circulation vasodilates during hypoxia. This response is mediated by both intrinsic, or locally mediated mechanisms, and by extrinsic, or reflex mechanisms.

Intrinsic Regulation

Using anesthetized dogs, Warren and Powell (22) demonstrated that alveolar hypoxia caused vasodilation in the bronchial circulation. This response was intrinsically mediated because the hypoxic stimulus was confined to the alveoli by virtue of a biventricular bypass. The use of the bypass enabled these investigators to maintain hyperoxic gas tensions in systemic arterial blood; the blood perfusing the bronchial arteries was also hyperoxic. The vasodilation was blocked by cyclooxygenase inhibitors indicating that the bronchial vasodilation is mediated by prostaglandins.

Charan et al. (5) reported similar findings using the isolated perfused left lower lobe in anesthetized dogs: hypoxia caused a bronchial vasodilation in the bronchial circulation that was blocked by prostaglandin synthesis inhibitors. Whereas Warren and Powell restricted the hypoxic stimulus to the alveoli (while systemic arterial blood was normoxic), Charan et al. maintained the P_{O_2} of the test lung normoxic while producing systemic hypoxemia by ventilating the rest of the pulmonary system with hypoxic gas, i.e., they tested the response to perfusing the bronchial artery with hypoxic blood in the presence of alveolar normoxia in the test lobe. Their results support the conclusion that hypoxia causes vasodilation in the bronchial circulation. However, it is not possible to judge whether the vasodilator was produced within the bronchial circulation in response to perfusion with hypoxic blood or whether it was produced in the other lung and transported by the blood.

In contrast, Baile and Paré (3), using a radiolabeled microsphere technique in anesthetized dogs, reported that hypoxia caused bronchial vasoconstriction. Their preparation was carefully controlled to avoid artifacts due to trapping radiolabeled microspheres that passed through systemic arteriovenous shunts. Their protocol called for 30 min of ventilation with 15% O_2 immediately followed by another 30 min of ventilation with 10% O_2: 15% O_2 failed to elicit any vasomotor response whereas bronchial vasoconstriction occurred after the second period during which 10% O_2 was administered.

The longer duration of their experiments relative to those of Warren and Powell (22) and of Charan et al. (5) may explain the different responses. Wagner et al. (21) recently reported that the bronchial vascular response to breathing hypoxic gas mixtures was biphasic. They used an anesthetized sheep preparation in which the common bronchial artery was pump-perfused at constant flow with blood drawn from a systemic artery. Hypoxia was induced by ventilating the sheep with a hypoxic gas mixture: initial vasodilation was succeeded by vasoconstriction. The findings of both Wagner et al. and Baile and Paré also raise the possibility that severe hypoxic stress, which may cause cerebral anoxia and a strong sympathetic nervous discharge, can ultimately override the dilator response (see chapter by Long/Brown).

Extrinsic Regulation

In the studies cited above, only that of Warren and Powell (22) restricted the hypoxic stimulus to the alveoli. In the other studies, systemic hypoxemia was present as well. Since systemic hypoxemia stimulates the chemoreceptors,

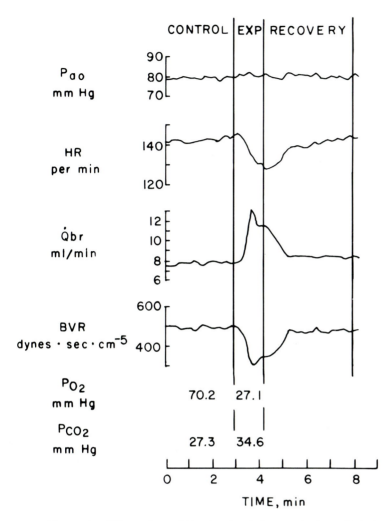

Figure 1: Effect of carotid body stimulation on the bronchial circulation. Blood gas values refer to those perfusing the carotid body. The systemic arterial blood gas values were the same as those shown during the control period. Pao = aortic pressure; HR = heart rate; Q̇br = bronchial blood flow; BVR = bronchial vascular resistance.

it would be expected, as in other systemic arterial beds, to evoke bronchial vasoconstriction.

Systemic Arterial Chemoreceptors

Alsberge et al. (1) reported that stimulation of the carotid body chemoreceptor in chloralose anesthetized sheep caused bronchial vasodilation (Fig. 1). Subsequent studies in the same laboratory have shown that the carotid body chemoreceptor is the source of this response; section of the carotid sinus nerve abolished the bronchial vascular response to carotid body stimulation. That the bronchial vasodilation was the direct effect of stimulating the carotid body was ensured by keeping both alveolar gas and systemic blood normoxic by mechanical ventilation of the paralyzed sheep while the carotid body perfusate was rendered hypoxic (unpublished observations).

Efferent Pathways

The systemic vascular responses to chemoreceptor stimulation are mediated by the autonomic nervous system. Stimulation of the stellate ganglion and vagus nerve are ways of experimentally engaging the autonomic nervous system.

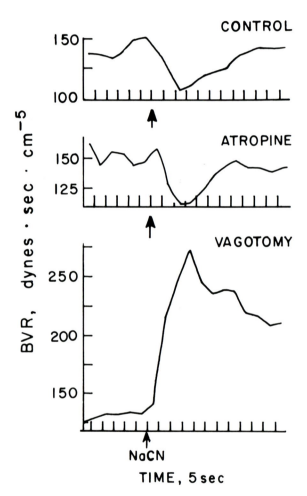

Figure 2: Effect of atropine and vagotomy on the bronchial vascular resistance response to cyanide stimulation of the carotid artery. At the arrows, NaCN (0.005 mg/kg) was injected into the carotid artery. The dose of atropine was 0.40 mg/kg, IV. BVR = bronchial vascular resistance; time marks = 5 sec.

SYMPATHETIC NERVES

Bruner and Schmidt (4) demonstrated that stimulation of the stellate ganglion in anesthetized dogs caused bronchial vasoconstriction. Hence, carotid body stimulation, which normally activates the sympathetic division of the autonomic nervous system, should cause a vasoconstriction of the bronchial circulation. However, Alsberge et al. failed to elicit vasoconstriction by stimulating the carotid body in the anesthetized sheep (1). Therefore, the role of the sympathetic vasomotor nerves in the control of the bronchial circulation is unclear.

Vagus Nerve

In the intact sheep, the bronchial vasodilation induced by stimulating the carotid body is not affected by atropine (0.40 mg/kg, IV), but it is affected by bilateral cervical vagotomy (Fig. 2). The finding that the bronchial vasodilation was not blocked by atropine suggests that this response is mediated by noncholinergic vagal fibers.

Moreover, after vagotomy, carotid body stimulation caused bronchial vasoconstriction. This vasoconstriction is probably mediated by sympathetic nerves as is the vasoconstriction in other systemic vascular beds caused by stimulation of the chemoreceptors. The results also indicate that noncholinergic fibers may be capable of overriding the effect of sympathetic vasoconstrictor nerves.

Using anesthetized dogs, Bruner and Schmidt (4) have shown that stimulation of the caudal stump of the cervical vagi caused bronchial vasodilation which was not blocked by atropine. Martling et al. (17) have shown a similar response in anesthetized cats. They also reported that the vasodilation was reduced by ganglionic blocking agents suggesting that some atropine resistant vasodilator was released by postganglionic nerves.

PEPTIDERGIC NERVES

Dey et al. (9) have reported that vagal neurons containing vasoactive intestinal peptide (VIP) and peptide histidine isoleucine (PHI) immunoreactive substances are associated with pulmonary and bronchial arteries as well as with airway smooth muscle. VIP has been shown to cause relaxation of pulmonary and systemic arterial smooth muscle as well as of airway smooth muscle. Martling et al. (17) have proposed that electrical stimulation of the vagus nerve causes bronchial vasodilation by releasing VIP and/or substance P, the former being released primarily from postganglionic fibers and the latter from sensory fibers.

Prostaglandins

As noted above, Charan et al. (5) and Warren and Powell (22) reported that the bronchial vasodilation was blocked by cyclooxygenase inhibitors. Because the experiments of Charan et al. (5) entailed systemic hypoxemia, it is likely that the carotid body chemoreceptors were stimulated and contributed to the bronchial vascular response. Since the response was blocked by cyclooxygenase inhibitors, it is possible that vasodilator prostaglandins play an essential role in the reflex vasodilation, as well as in the locally mediated response, to hypoxia.

In support of this possibility are the findings of Kulik et al. (13). They reported that VIP infusions into the pulmonary artery of sedated lambs caused pulmonary vasodilation and that this vasodilation was blocked by cyclooxygenase inhibitors. Therefore, it is possible that carotid body stimulation leads to release of VIP which, in turn, initiates the synthesis of vasodilator prostaglandins. It appears then that vasodilator prostaglandin synthesis is key to both the extrinsic and intrinsic regulatory mechanisms.

What still remains to be determined is the exact sequence of events that leads to the reversal of the local and reflex vasodilation to vasoconstriction. Also to be determined is whether the vasoconstriction observed by Baile and Paré (3) and by Wagner et al. (21) is mediated solely by the sympathetic nerves or whether the same mechanism(s) that cause pulmonary vasoconstriction is (are) involved.

FUNCTIONAL SIGNIFICANCE

Kelly et al. (12) have provided evidence that the bronchial circulation participates in washing mediators out of the bronchial tree. Using anesthetized dogs, they induced bronchoconstriction by histamine aerosol and observed the time constant for recovery before, and after, obstruction of the bronchial blood flow. Obstruction of bronchial blood flow increased the time for the airway to relax after histamine aerosol. Therefore, the bronchial circulation may also remove other biologically active substances from the airways.

Regulation of the Pulmonary Circulation

The suggestion has also been made that the bronchial circulation may deliver mediators to the tissues it perfuses (2). These mediators could be humoral agents (e.g., epinephrine released from the adrenal glands), locally produced substances (e.g., prostaglandins and leukotrienes), or neurotransmitters. Since the bronchial circulation also perfuses the vasa vasorum of the pulmonary circulation, it can clearly affect the pulmonary vascular bed. Moreover, substances can be delivered via the vasa vasorum to the lumen of the pulmonary arterial tree (11), raising the possibility that mediators formed in the bronchial vasculature, or released into the bronchial arterial blood, may be delivered to smooth muscle located in the periphery of the lung where the density of innervation is less than for the larger arteries (19).

Transport of Vasodilator Mediators

Daly and Daly (7) tested the effect of selectively stimulating the carotid body chemoreceptors on pulmonary vascular resistance in anesthetized dogs. By using a multicircuit perfusion system, they were able to maintain normal P_{O_2} values in the systemic circulation and in the alveoli. They found that carotid body stimulation caused pulmonary vasodilation provided the bronchial circulation was intact. This vasodilation became vasoconstriction if the bronchial circulation was obstructed.

They interpreted their results as indicating hemodynamic interaction between the bronchial and pulmonary circulations. They further assumed that vasoconstriction occurred in the bronchial circulation since it is a systemic vascular bed and because perfusion pressure increased in the segment of aorta giving rise to the bronchial arteries. However, this segment of aorta also gave rise to other systemic vascular beds that underwent vasoconstriction, thereby masking the bronchial vasodilation. That their assumption of bronchial vasoconstriction is incorrect is indicated by the findings of Alsberge et al. (1) who actually measured the change in bronchial vascular resistance.

The failure of Daly and Daly (7) to find a vasodilation in the pulmonary circulation after reducing bronchial flow to zero is consistent with the possibility that a vasodilator mediator is transported via the vasa vasorum of the pulmonary circulation. The question then arises as to whether the vasodilator that is transported into the pulmonary circulation is the same as that which regulates the response of the bronchial circulation to carotid body stimulation. Could vasodilator "spill over" (i.e., diffuse) from the bronchial arterial wall into the bronchial arterial blood and be transported via the vasa vasorum of the pulmonary circulation? If the vasodilator were a relatively small molecule, such as a prostaglandin, then this spill over would not be difficult to accept. VIP could also be the vasodilator that enters bronchial arterial blood by diffusion.

Goadsby and McDonald (10) have reported that stimulation of the pterygopalatine ganglion caused vasodilation in both common carotid arteries of spinalized cats. Infusion of VIP antibodies into one common carotid artery blocked vasodilation in that carotid artery when the ganglion was stimulated (during the infusion); contralateral carotid blood flow still increased. The blockade of the carotid artery vasodilation by VIP antibodies was not a nonspecific effect because sham antiserum (raised against the same source of rabbit albumin as used to conjugate the VIP) did not affect the vasodilation caused by stimulating the ganglion; nor did antibodies raised against bradykinin and substance P. These findings indicate that the VIP antibodies, which are guinea pig IgG proteins, are able to reach the neuroeffector junction where they bind the neurotransmitter. If proteins as large as IgG can diffuse out of the blood, then smaller molecules such as VIP can also gain access into bronchial arterial blood.

Matsuzaki et al. (18) showed that electric field stimulation of guinea pig trachealis in vitro caused release of measurable amounts of VIP immunoreactive-like substance into the tissue bath. Both the amount of VIP-like material released and the relaxation of the trachealis muscle increased as the stimulus intensity increased. Since measurable amounts of VIP-like material (2.5 to 7.5 picograms) can diffuse into the muscle bath, then it seems possible for VIP to diffuse into the arterial blood.

Blunting Hypoxic Pulmonary Vasoconstriction

If regional alveolar hypoxia is sufficiently widespread so that systemic arterial hypoxia and stimulation of arterial chemoreceptors occur, then hypoxic pulmonary vasoconstriction is attenuated. This attenuation is mediated by systemic arterial chemoreceptors. Denervation of these chemoreceptors restores the hypoxic pulmonary vasoconstriction (15). The bronchial circulation may play a key role in this chemoreceptor attenuation of the hypoxic pulmonary vasoconstriction. Daly and Daly (7), using anesthetized dogs with alveolar normoxia, reported that selective carotid body stimulation caused a vasodilation in the pulmonary circulation when the bronchial circulation was perfused, but not when bronchial blood flow was arrested. These data suggest that the bronchial circulation plays a key role in the reflex modulation of the locally mediated hypoxic pulmonary vasoconstriction.

Possible Adverse Effect of the Bronchial Circulation on the Regulation of the Pulmonary Circulation

It might be argued that the delivery of a vasodilator to the pulmonary circulation via the bronchial circulation would have a negative homeostatic value since it would oppose maintenance of ventilation/perfusion relationships normally achieved by hypoxic pulmonary vasoconstriction. However, this stimulus to pulmonary vasodilation would only be expected to occur when the systemic arterial chemoreceptors are stimulated. In clinical disorders in which regional alveolar hypoxia is unaccompanied by severe systemic hypoxemia, the arterial chemoreceptors are not apt to be strongly stimulated. Hence, the reflex vasodilator mechanism will not be activated and vasoconstriction in the hypoxic alveoli will be not affected.

Bronchial vasodilation would be apt to cause engorgement and swelling of the mucosa of the airways. Bronchial vasodilation would also be expected to increase capillary filtration and further promote mucosal edema. In keeping with these propositions, vagal stimulation in anesthetized dogs causes hyperemia and swelling of the tracheal mucosa (4): tracheal mucosa increased in thickness by as much as 50 μ.

SUMMARY AND CONCLUSIONS

A synthesis has been presented of the mechanisms regulating the normal bronchial circulation. How these mechanisms apply to the expanded bronchial circulation that accompanies intrinsic lung disease (8) or pulmonary hypertension is unknown. The possibility is raised that a significant contribution of the bronchial circulation is the generation and transport of vasodilators into the pulmonary circulation. Since the pulmonary vasodilator response is mediated by the carotid body chemoreceptors, it is apt to be triggered only when pulmonary disease is so severe that there is considerable arterial hypoxemia. Therefore, in the more usual run of patients with intrinsic lung disease who have neither severe arterial hypoxemia nor hypoxic pulmonary hypertension, the impact of bronchial arterial blood on ventilation/perfusion relationships is apt to be minimal. The possibility is raised that bronchial vasodilation during systemic arterial hypoxia could promote mucosal swelling and aggravate obstructive disease. Whether the bronchial vasodilation evoked by hypoxia exerts an overall beneficial, or an adverse, effect in humans is not known.

ACKNOWLEDGMENTS

This work was supported in part by grant number HL29861 and a grant from the Hahnemann University Graduate School.

REFERENCES

1. Alsberge M, Magno M, Lipschutz M: Carotid body control of bronchial circulation in sheep. J Appl Physiol 65 : 1152–1156, 1988.

2. Baier H, Long WM, Wanner A: Bronchial circulation in asthma. Respiration 48 : 199–205, 1985.

3. Baile EM, Paré PD: Response of the bronchial circulation to acute hypoxemia and hypercarbia in the dog. J Appl Physiol 55 : 1474–1479, 1983.

4. Bruner HD, Schmidt CF: Blood flow in the bronchial artery of the anesthetized dog. Am J Physiol 148 : 647–666, 1947.

5. Charan NB, Lakshminarayan S, Albert RK, Kirk W, Butler J: Hypoxia and hypercarbia increase bronchial blood flow through bronchopulmonary anastomoses in anesthetized dogs. Am Rev Respir Dis 134 : 89–92, 1986.

6. Charan NB, Turk GM, Dhand R: The role of the bronchial circulation in lung abscess. Am Rev Respir Dis 131 : 121–124, 1985.

7. Daly I de Burgh, Daly M de Burgh: The effects of stimulation of the carotid body chemoreceptors on the pulmonary vascular bed in the dog: The 'vasosensory controlled perfused living animal' preparation. J Physiol (Lond) 148 : 201–219, 1959.

8. Deffebach ME, Charan NB, Lakshminarayan S, Butler J: The bronchial circulation. Am Rev Respir Dis 135 : 463–481, 1987.

9. Dey RD, Shannon WA Jr, Said SI: Localization of VIP-immunoreactive nerves in airways and pulmonary vessels in dogs, cats, and human subjects. Cell Tissue Res 220 : 231–238, 1981.

10. Goadsby PJ, McDonald GJ: Extracranial vasodilation mediated by vasoactive intestinal polypeptide (VIP). Brain Res 329 : 285–288, 1985.

11. Hyman AL, Knight DS, Joiner PD, Kadowitz PJ: Bronchopulmonary arterial shunting without anatomic anastomosis in the dog. Circ Res 37 : 285–298, 1975.

12. Kelly L, Kolbe J, Mitzner W, Spannhake EW, Bromberger-Barnea B, Menkes H: Bronchial blood flow affects recovery from constriction in dog lung periphery. J Appl Physiol 60 : 1954–1959, 1986.

13. Kulik TJ, Johnson DE, Elde RP, Lock JE: Pulmonary vascular effects of vasoactive intestinal peptide in conscious newborn lambs. Am J Physiol 246 : H716–H719, 1984.

14. Laitinen LA, Laitinen MV, Widdicombe JG: Parasympathetic nervous control of tracheal vascular resistance in the dog. J Physiol (Lond) 385 : 135–146, 1987.

15. Levitzky MG: Chemoreceptor stimulation and hypoxic pulmonary vasoconstriction in conscious dogs. Respir Physiol 37 : 151–160, 1979.

16. Magno MG, Fishman AP: Origin, distribution, and blood flow of bronchial circulation in anesthetized sheep. J Appl Physiol 53 : 272–279, 1982.

17. Martling CL, Anggard A, Lundberg JM: Noncholinergic vasodilation in the tracheobronchial tree of the cat induced by vagal nerve stimulation. Acta Physiol Scand 125 : 343–346, 1985.

18. Matsuzaki Y, Hamasaki Y, Said SI: Vasoactive intestinal peptide: A possible transmitter of nonadrenergic relaxation of guinea pig airways. Science 210 : 1252–1253, 1980.

19. McLean JR: Pulmonary vascular innervation, in Bergofsky EH (ed), *Abnormal Pulmonary Circulation* (Contemporary Issues in Pulmonary Disease Series: Vol 4). New York, Churchill Livingstone, 1986, pp 27–81.

20. Sheller JR, Brigham KL: Bronchomotor responses of isolated sheep airways to electric field stimulation. J Appl Physiol 53 : 1088–1093, 1982.

21. Wagner EM, Mitzner WA, Bleecker ER: Effects of airway pressure on bronchial blood flow. J Appl Physiol 62 : 561–566, 1987.

22. Warren RL, Powell WJ Jr: Acute alveolar hypoxia increases bronchopulmonary shunt flow in the dog. J Clin Invest 77 : 1515–1524, 1986.

Sidney Cassin, Ph.D.

12

Tone and Responsiveness in the Fetal and Neonatal Pulmonary Circulation

Understanding of the factors responsible for the dramatic changes which occur in the pulmonary circulation with the onset of ventilation is still incomplete despite years of intense investigation. The factors involved in regulating blood flow through the perinatal pulmonary circulation include (1) mechanical, i.e., lung expansion; (2) oxygen tension; (3) carbon dioxide tension and acid-base balance; (4) local factors; (5) reflexes or neural mechanisms; and (6) the effects of vasoactive substances.

CHANGES IN THE PERINATAL PULMONARY CIRCULATION

In the fetal state, the exchange of CO_2 and O_2 occurs in the placenta. Therefore, pulmonary blood flow is quite low, perhaps providing only nutritional requirements for lung maturation and/or subserving some metabolic function. A large pulmonary blood flow would constitute an unnecessary demand on the developing cardiovascular system. A large arteriovenous shunt between the two sides of the heart would divert a large fraction of right ventricular output to the left heart. This diversion of blood would be of little value to the fetus; it would only increase the workload of the left heart. Normally, most of the right ventricular output passes through the ductus arteriosus and down the descending aorta to the placental circulation for gas exchange. In the unanesthetized fetal sheep approaching term, the pulmonary blood flow is approximately 30 to 40 ml/min per kg body weight (approximately 8 to 10 percent of the total combined ventricular output).

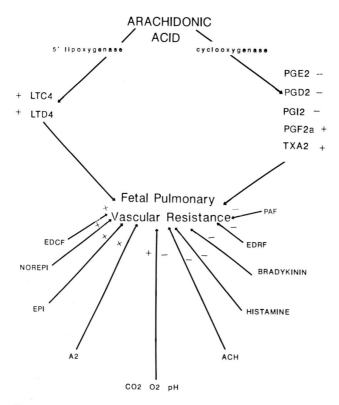

Figure 1: Interaction of vasoactive materials in controlling pulmonary vascular resistance. Arachidonic acid is metabolized to primary prostaglandins, thromboxanes, and leukotrienes. PAF = platelet activating factor; EDRF = endothelium-dependent relaxing factor; ACH = acetylcholine; A_2 = angiotensin II; EDCF = endothelium-dependent contracting factor; + = vasoconstriction; − = vasodilatation.

The very high resistance of the pulmonary vascular bed in the fetal lamb may be due to (1) small-lumen arterioles that generally have a thick smooth muscle layer; (2) vasoconstriction in utero of the pulmonary vessels which are chronically exposed (normal pulmonary arterial P_{O_2}, 18 to 20 mmHg) to low oxygen tensions; and/or (3) marked reactivity of the pulmonary vessels to small changes in pH, blood gas tensions, and circulating vasoactive materials.

Postnatal survival of the fetus depends on rapid establishment of pulmonary blood flow and alveolar ventilation with an appropriate balance achieved between the two. To accomplish this remarkable transformation at birth, the course of the circulation through the heart rearranges to resemble that of the adult system in which the ventricles work in series rather than in parallel and the lungs become the organ of gas exchange. In the transition from a liquid-breathing fetus to an air-breathing newborn (lamb or kid), pulmonary blood flow increases 5- to 10-fold. In term lambs and goats, the pulmonary arterial blood pressure decreases in several hours almost to adult levels whereas in humans the decrease in mean pulmonary arterial blood pressure is more gradual, often reaching only half of the aortic pressure within the first 60 hr after birth.

Many influences interact to cause pulmonary vasodilatation at birth: expansion of the alveoli with gas and/or an increase in arterial P_{O_2}, a decrease in arterial P_{CO_2}, and an increase in arterial pH could activate the synthesis and/or release of vasoactive substances, e.g., eicosanoids, bradykinin, endothelium-dependent relaxing factor, platelet activating factor, or other vasoactive materials. The operation of these influences in concert could conceivably account for the decrease in pulmonary vascular resistance that occurs when breathing starts and for the subsequent maintenance of pulmonary vascular resistance at low levels (Fig. 1).

THE EFFECTS OF EXPANSION OF THE LUNGS WITH GASES

Close to term, regardless of whether fetal lamb lungs are expanded with air, O_2, or N_2, pulmonary vasodilatation results. Lungs of fetal lambs that are rebreathed periodically with a gas mixture containing 3% O_2 and 7% CO_2 in nitrogen ("fetal gas," i.e., approximately equivalent in composition to the gas mixture that would be in equilibrium with fetal arterial P_{O_2} and P_{CO_2}) undergo marked pulmonary vasodilatation even though the change in arterial blood gas tension is insignificant (5). Substitution of a 21% O_2 with 7% CO_2 mixture evokes a greater dilatation. Finally, ventilation of fetal lamb lungs with ambient air elicits a dilatation that is almost maximal. The decrease in pulmonary vascular resistance that accompanies ventilation of the lungs with "fetal gas" is probably due to surface tension at the alveolar air-liquid interfaces which decreases perivascular pressures. Ventilation of fetal lungs with liquid results in pulmonary vasoconstriction due to compression of pulmonary capillaries. However, ventilation of the lungs with fluid rich in oxygen elicits pulmonary vasodilatation.

Changing the composition of arterial blood supplying the unventilated fetal lungs also changes pulmonary vascular resistance. For example, ventilation of one lung with a gas mixture that increased the pulmonary arterial P_{O_2} or decreased its P_{CO_2} or both caused pulmonary vasodilatation in the nonventilated lung. In contrast, a decrease in the P_{O_2} or an increase in the P_{CO_2} in the ventilating gas mixture caused pulmonary vasoconstriction in the unventilated lung. These experiments suggest that changes in the blood gases are responsible for either vasoconstriction or vasodilatation. They do not indicate whether the responses are reflex (chemoreceptors) in nature or due to direct effects on the vascular smooth muscle. Nor do they settle whether the final common pathway involves humoral agents that are released locally. Subsequent experiments of Campbell et al. extended these observations by resorting to cross-circulation techniques in fetal lambs (1). They demonstrated that variation of the blood gas composition in fetal lambs exerted a direct local effect and also raised the possibility of the reflex control of the pulmonary vasculature in animals 100 days of age or older. To date, this reflex mechanism has not been explored systematically.

LOCALIZATION OF PULMONARY VASCULAR RESISTANCE

Little has been reported about the sites of change in pulmonary vascular resistance in fetal and neonatal lungs exposed to changes in ventilation, to changes in blood gas tensions, or to drugs. Using a model involving Starling resistors (13), Gilbert et al. found that the average pressure surrounding the Starling resistors in the fetal lung of a goat is about 21 mmHg (11). Ventilation of the lungs with fetal gas (3% O_2, 7% CO_2) decreased this pressure to 16 mmHg. Subsequent ventilation with air decreased the surrounding pressure to 13 mmHg. In the fetus, pulmonary vascular resistance proximal to the Starling resistor proved to be 4 to 5 times greater than the resistance distal to it. Although location of the precise sites at which the equivalents of Starling resistors in the pulmonary circulation is uncertain, they are believed to be in both the pre- and post-capillary vessels: the proximal resistance has been estimated to be about 87 percent of the total vascular resistance across the lungs and to be located on the arterial side of the capillaries whereas distal vascular resistance, which contributes only about 11 percent of the total resistance, seems to be located in the venules (11).

THE EFFECTS OF ALTERATIONS IN ARTERIAL CO_2 AND pH

The demonstration by von Euler and Liljestrand in 1946 that hypoxia and hypercarbia in adult cats cause an increase in pulmonary arterial pressure (20) was of great interest to those concerned with the fetal circulation since the vessels of fetal lungs are usually exposed to a low P_{O_2} (i.e., 18 to 22 mmHg). Dawes and Mott subsequently demonstrated that hypoxia produced in ewes by compression of the umbilical cord produced profound pulmonary vasoconstriction in fetal lambs (9). Furthermore, they also showed that relief of ischemia produced by occlusion of pulmonary arterial inflow for 2 minutes elicited reactive hyperemia. This appears to be the only evidence for reactive hyperemia in fetal lungs.

With respect to the effects of increasing inspired P_{CO_2}, Cook et al., using fetal lambs in which the pulmonary arterial pressure was maintained constant and flow was allowed to vary, showed that increasing the inspired P_{CO_2} or decreasing inspired P_{O_2} caused a diminution in flow (8). In these experiments, no attempt was made to keep arterial pH constant. Subsequent observations by Rudolph and Yuan in newborn calves suggest that changes attributed to increased P_{CO_2} could be due to changes in pH of the blood (16). Moreover, when arterial P_{O_2} exceeded 100 mmHg, pulmonary vascular resistance barely increased over a range of arterial pH from 7.39 to 7.18; however, over the same range of pH values, a decrease in arterial P_{O_2} to 42 mmHg evoked a dramatic increase in pulmonary vascular resistance. These observations indicated an interaction between acidemia and hypoxemia in increasing pulmonary vascular resistance.

NEURAL CONTROL OF THE FETAL PULMONARY CIRCULATION

Although the pulmonary vessels of the fetal animal are innervated by both sympathetic and parasympathetic nerves, changes in pulmonary vascular resistance can be elicited in surgically denervated or isolated vascular preparations, suggesting that the autonomic nervous system is not essential for mediating changes in vascular tone. In fetal and newborn lambs, Colebatch et al. demonstrated that electrical stimulation of the peripheral stump of the vagus nerve causes pulmonary vascular dilatation; stimulation of cardiac sympathetic nerves to the fetal lung causes vasoconstriction. Following bilateral thoracic sympathectomy (T1–T8), the pulmonary vascular conductance increases (7). However, even in the denervated state, ventilation of lungs with "fetal gas" further decreases pulmonary vascular resistance. These observations are in keeping with those of the cross-circulation experiments in twin fetal lambs which showed that in mature fetal lambs, the induction of systemic hypoxia without pulmonary hypoxia triggers reflexes (perhaps involving the carotid and aortic bodies) that increase pulmonary vascular tone.

THE EFFECTS OF CERTAIN NATURALLY OCCURRING AND SYNTHETIC VASOACTIVE SUBSTANCES ON THE FETAL PULMONARY CIRCULATION

The fetal pulmonary circulation of sheep and goats is reactive not only to changes in its blood gases but also to a variety of endogenous and exogenous vasoactive materials: in the isolated lung preparation of the mature fetal lamb, acetylcholine and histamine are powerful vasodilators. Small doses of histamine, acetylcholine, isoproterenol, and nanogram quantities of bradykinin elicit marked, transient pulmonary vasodilatation in the immature, as well as the mature, isolated lung preparation. Finally, similar results have been obtained in unanesthetized fetal lambs with indwelling catheters (15). Moreover, at increasing gestational ages of fetal lambs in utero, comparable doses of acetylcholine (based on the fetal body weight) elicit progressively greater reductions in pulmonary vascular resistance (15). Injections of norepinephrine and epinephrine directly into the pulmonary arteries of immature fetal lambs (0.5 to 0.6 term) produce reversible vasoconstriction (6).

In the immature fetal lamb, the injection of norepinephrine often evokes a short-lived vasoconstriction that is followed by vasodilatation; the vasoconstrictor response can be abolished by the administration of the alpha-receptor antagonist, Dibenamine, after which vasodilatation persists (6). This observation indicates that there are both functional alpha- and beta-adrenergic receptors in the fetal pulmonary vasculature.

THE EFFECTS OF EICOSANOIDS ON THE PERINATAL PULMONARY CIRCULATION PROSTAGLANDIN PRECURSORS

In fetal and neonatal goats, infusion of arachidonic acid into the pulmonary artery consistently causes an increase in pulmonary vascular resistance along with a decrease in systemic arterial pressure. Similar results were obtained with di-homo-gamma-linolenic acid. These results differ from those reported for the effects of arachidonic acid in adults in which these precursors have elicited either an increase or a decrease in pulmonary vascular resistance. To explain the increase in pulmonary vascular resistance, it has been proposed that arachidonic acid is metabolized to PGE_2 and $PGF_{2\alpha}$, both of which are vasoconstrictors of the adult pulmonary circulation. In contrast, a decrease in pulmonary vascular resistance could be explained by an increase in the production of prostacyclin-like (PGI_2) material.

The pulmonary vascular responses of fetal and neonatal animals to primary prostaglandins are also often different from those of the adult animals. For example, PGE_2, a constrictor of the adult pulmonary circulation, is a dilator of the fetal pulmonary circulation. Ventilation appears to exert a powerful influence on the effects of primary prostaglandins on the perinatal pulmonary circulation: dilator agents (e.g., PGI_2) could be synthesized after ventilation and constrictor agents before ventilation. Moreover, the effects of primary prostaglandins on vascular smooth muscle may depend on antecedent vascular tone. Finally, it seems evident that the effects of infusing arachidonic acid can vary with age, species, and initial tone, depending on the pathways and products that predominate at different stages of development (2–4).

E-Series Prostaglandins

Prostaglandin E_1 (PGE_1), infused into the pulmonary artery of fetal goats close to term as well as in newborn goats, decreases pulmonary vascular resistance. PGE_1 is about ten times as potent as PGE_2. PGEs are effective in preventing the hypoxic pressor response of mature fetal goats (135 to 145 days gestation); however, the same relative potencies exist (i.e., PGE_1 is more powerful than PGE_2) (3). Systemic hypotension does not occur during the infusion of PGE_1 presumably because PGE_1 is metabolized avidly by fetal goat lungs (2,3). The effects of PGE_2 on the pulmonary circulation of perinatal goats contrast sharply with their effects in adult animals: in adult goats and sheep, PGE_2 causes pulmonary vasoconstriction. The difference may reflect the greater amount of smooth muscle, the greater tone of the perinatal pulmonary circulation, and age-related differences in the numbers, types, and affinities of PGE_2 receptors.

The Effects of Prostacyclin and Thromboxanes

TXA_2 stimulates platelet aggregation and vascular constriction, whereas PGI_2 is an inhibitor of platelet aggregation and a vascular dilator. Two lines of evidence suggest that PGI_2 may play an important role in controlling the perinatal pulmonary circulation: (1) PGI_2 is a pulmonary vasodilator in the adult dog and cat; and (2) when fetal lungs are ventilated, endogenous dilator prostaglandins (probably of the E- and I-series) are released into pulmonary blood (2–4). In keeping with these observations, the infusion of PGI_2 directly into the left pulmonary arterial circulation causes dose-dependent decreases in pulmonary vascular resistance and mean systemic arterial pressure. Two-minute infusions produced more pronounced decreases in pulmonary vascular resistance than did one-minute infusions. The responses appear to be species dependent, the depressor response in fetal goats being greater than that in fetal lambs. Since PGI_2 is not metabolized well by fetal or adult lungs, it is not surprising that systemic hypotensive responses and increases in heart rate occurred in both species. PGI_2 proved to be a more powerful vasodilator of the fetal pulmonary circulation than PGE_1 and PGE_2 (2,4).

No information is as yet available concerning the effects of TXA_2 and TXB_2 on the perinatal pulmonary vasculature. Little has even been done on the adult pulmonary circulation with TXA_2 because of its instability. However, in the adult cat pulmonary circulation, TXB_2 appears to be a weak pulmonary vasoconstrictor, approximately 1,000 times less powerful than $PGF_{2\alpha}$ (2,4).

The Effects of Prostaglandins PGD_2 and PGD_3 on the Perinatal Pulmonary Circulation

PGD_2 constricts the adult canine pulmonary circulation. However, the administration of PGD_2 to an experimentally dilated fetal pulmonary circulation elicits further dilatation (3). Subsequent experiments using PGD_2 in the fetal, neonatal, and adult pulmonary circulation of sheep and goats demonstrated that the responses of the pulmonary circulation to PGD_2 are age-related. Parenthetically, systemic hypotension did not occur in response to the administration of PGD_2 to fetal animals.

The mechanisms responsible for the age-related differences in the pulmonary vascular responses to PGD_2 have not been elaborated. However, several explanations seem tenable: (1) the larger smooth muscle mass and the greater tone of the perinatal pulmonary circulation; (2) variability in the numbers, types, and affinities of prostaglandin receptors in the perinatal and adult lung; and (3) variation in the rate and amount of conversion of PGD_2 to $PGF_{2\alpha}$ in perinatal and adult peripheral blood (2,4).

Recently PGD_3, a metabolite of eicosapentanoic acid, has been shown to be an inhibitor of platelet aggregation and a constrictor of the adult pulmonary circulation. In the fetal circulation, PGD_3 seems to behave qualitatively like PGD_2 as a vasodilator; however, quantitatively it is much more powerful than PGD_2. Moreover, in the fetus, PGD_3, like PGD_2, does not decrease systemic pressure when injected into the pulmonary circulation (2,4).

Leukotrienes and Antagonists

Evidence was provided in 1982 that lipoxygenase activity is present in human fetal lungs 12 to 18 weeks of gestational age (17). More recently, Stenmark et al. showed that leukotrienes (C_4 and D_4) are present in lung lavage fluid of human neonates with persistent pulmonary hypertension (19). In contrast, these substances were not found in the fluid obtained from infants without neonatal pulmonary hypertension. Leukotriene D_4 (LTD_4) has also proved to be a powerful vasoconstrictor of the pulmonary and systemic circulations of newborn lambs and piglets. In the isolated perfused rat lung (14), the pressor response to hypoxia was blocked by three structurally unrelated antagonists of leukotriene synthesis or receptors (diethylcarbamazine citrate, U-60257, and FPL 55712) (Fig. 2). BW755C, an antioxidant that blocks both cyclooxygenase and lipoxygenase pathways, also inhibits the pressor response to hypoxia in the isolated perfused rat lung preparation (4). However, similar antagonists were ineffective in blocking the hypoxic pressor response in mechanically ventilated newborn piglets (12). The possibility remains that the concentration of antagonist was not large enough to block the pressor response to hypoxia. Indeed, Soifer et al. used a putative

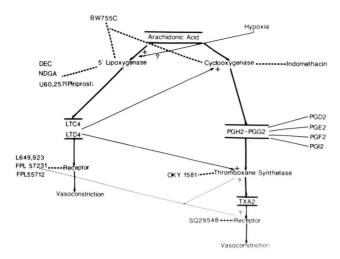

Figure 2: Arachidonic acid cascade with sites of action of inhibitors. Solid lines indicate stimulation of system; dotted lines indicate inhibition. There are suggestions that hypoxia stimulates release of leukotrienes. If this is so, the pressor response to hypoxia should be blocked by 5′ lipoxygenase as well as leukotriene receptor antagonists. See body of paper for controversy.

leukotriene receptor antagonist, FPL 57231, in newborn unanesthetized lambs (3 to 7 days old) subjected to hypoxia while breathing spontaneously. They found that the agent did block the pressor response to hypoxia, suggesting that the leukotrienes do play a role mediating the hypoxic pressor response (18). However, observations since then indicate that the putative blocking agent, FPL 57231, is not a specific blocker of the hypoxic pressor response (10). At present, there are no convincing data to indicate that the leukotrienes are involved in the pulmonary hypoxic pressor response of the fetus.

Finally, the pressor effect of LTD_4 on the fetal pulmonary circulation appears to involve the cyclooxygenase pathway (via thromboxane A_2)(10).

EPILOGUE

The fetal pulmonary circulation is characterized by a high degree of tone. The fetal pulmonary circulation has more tone than the newborn which in turn has more tone than the adult. Remarkable circulatory adjustments occur at birth which include pulmonary vasodilatation, along with constriction of umbilical vessels and the ductus arteriosus. Although the basic mechanism(s) for these changes is still not entirely clear, it is clear that a single factor is not responsible.

A complex interaction of mechanical, hormonal vasoactive, physical (gases) and morphological factors is responsible for the transitional period and maintenance of these changes in the newborn period. Vasoactive eicosanoids, by direct action and interaction with other systems, may play an important regulatory role in rearrangement of the circulation. Responsiveness of the pulmonary vasculature is not only species dependent but also age dependent. Some views are presented to explain these differences.

REFERENCES

1. Campbell AG, Cockburn F, Dawes GS, Milligan JE: Pulmonary vasoconstriction in asphyxia during cross-circulation between twin foetal lambs. J Physiol (Lond) 192:111–121, 1967.

2. Cassin S: Role of prostaglandins and thromboxanes in the control of the pulmonary circulation in the fetus and newborn. Semin Perinatol 4:101–107, 1980.

3. Cassin S: Arachidonic acid metabolites and the pulmonary circulation of the fetus and newborn, in MacLeod S, Okey A, Spielberg S (eds), *Progress in Clinical and Biological Research, Vol 135: Developmental Pharmacology.* New York, Alan R. Liss, 1983, pp 227–250.

4. Cassin S: Role of prostaglandins, thromboxanes and leukotrienes in the control of the pulmonary circulation in the fetus and newborn. Semin Perinatol 11:53–63, 1987.

5. Cassin S, Dawes GS, Mott JC, Ross BB, Strang LB: The vascular resistance of the foetal and newly ventilated lung of the lamb. J Physiol (Lond) 171:61–79, 1963.

6. Cassin S, Dawes GS, Ross BB: Pulmonary blood flow and vascular resistance in immature foetal lambs. J Physiol (Lond) 171:80–89, 1964.

7. Colebatch HJ, Dawes GS, Goodwin JW, Nadeau RA: The nervous control of the circulation in the foetal and newly expanded lungs of the lamb. J Physiol (Lond) 178:544–562, 1965.

8. Cook CG, Drinker PA, Jacobsen HW, Levison H, Strang LB: Control of pulmonary blood flow in the foetal and newly born lamb. J Physiol (Lond) 169:10–29, 1963.

9. Dawes GS, Mott JC: The vascular tone of the foetal lung. J Physiol (Lond) 164:465–477, 1962.

10. Gause GE, Baker R, Cassin S: Specificity of FPL 57231 for leukotriene D_4 receptors in the fetal pulmonary circulation? Am J Physiol 254:H120–H125, 1988.

11. Gilbert RD, Hessler JR, Eitzman DV, Cassin S: Site of pulmonary vascular resistance in fetal goats. J Appl Physiol 32:47–53, 1972.

12. Leffler CW, Mitchell JA, Green RS: Cardiovascular effects of leukotrienes in neonatal piglets: Role in hypoxic pulmonary vasoconstriction? Circ Res 55:780–787, 1984.

13. McDonald IG, Butler J: Distribution of vascular resistance in the isolated perfused dog lung. J Appl Physiol 23:463–474, 1967.

14. Morganroth ML, Reeves JT, Murphy RC, Voelkel NF: Leukotriene synthesis and receptor blockers block hypoxic pulmonary vasoconstriction. J Appl Physiol 56:1340–1346, 1984.

15. Rudolph AM: Fetal and neonatal pulmonary circulation. Annu Rev Physiol 41:383–395, 1979.

16. Rudolph AM, Yuan S: Response of the pulmonary vasculature to hypoxia and H^+ ion concentration changes. J Clin Invest 45:399–411, 1966.

17. Saeed SA, Mitchell MD: Arachidonate lipoxygenase activity in human fetal lung. Eur J Pharmacol 78:385–391, 1982.

18. Soifer SJ, Schreiber MD, Leitz RD, Roman C, Heymann MA: The effects of leukotriene inhibition on the perinatal pulmonary circulation in the lamb, in Jones C, Nathanielsz P (eds), *The Physiological Development of the Fetus and Newborn.* London, Academic Press, 1985, pp 451–455.

19. Stenmark KR, James SL, Voelkel NF, Toews WH, Reeves JT, Murphy RC: Leukotriene C_4 and D_4 in neonates with hypoxemia and pulmonary hypertension. N Engl J Med 309:77–80, 1983.

20. von Euler US, Liljestrand G: Observations on the pulmonary arterial blood pressure in the cat. Acta Physiol Scand 12:301–320, 1946.

PART TWO

Vascular Injury

Alice R. Johnson, Ph.D.

13 ⎯⎯⎯⎯⎯⎯⎯⎯⎯⎯⎯⎯⎯⎯

Endothelial Injury
Studied in Cell Culture

Damage to the pulmonary vasculature is a common feature of lung injury from various causes. Often it is one of the earliest events in the adult respiratory distress syndrome and other diseases involving alveolar-capillary dysfunction. Acute endothelial injury is commonly manifest by passage of fluid into the alveolar space (24) and by the accumulation of inflammatory cells within the lung (5). Experimental studies show that a number of endothelial functions are altered early in the course of injury, including hemostatic balance (45), metabolic functions, and influence on smooth muscle vasoreactivity (15).

Even when the pulmonary endothelium is not the primary target of injury, its strategic location between blood and the alveolar space exposes it to alveolar macrophages, leukocytes sequestered within the lungs, and circulating inflammatory mediators. Leukocyte-derived proteases and oxidants are thought to play a prominent role in some forms of endothelial injury (5). In addition, mediators such as platelet-activating factor (PAF) (22) or cytokines may contribute indirectly to endothelial injury or modify endothelial functions. Our studies with cultured endothelial cells explore some of the mechanisms through which these agents interact at the endothelium.

The endothelial substratum is an important determinant for the extent and the ultimate response to injury. Endothelial and epithelial surfaces share a composite basal lamina composed of components contributed by cells from each (23). The deposition of connective tissue components and inflammatory cells within the interstitium can affect not only gas exchange but also the composition of the subendothelial environment. Studies by a number of investigators showed that the composition of the substratum influences growth characteristics, migration, and morphology of endothelial cells (35), as well as biochemical properties, such as the synthesis and secretion of glycoproteins (19). Deposition of fibrin and fibronectin within the vascular lumen and beneath the endothelium enhances vascular permeability and stimulates endothelial cell migration and replication (11). Although these processes are important for wound healing, inappropriate or prolonged deposition combined with activation of inflammatory cells may result in abnormal vascular functions, including development of fibrosis following injury.

MEDIATORS FROM ENDOTHELIUM

Despite the original concept that endothelium is a relatively inert tissue, it is now appreciated that metabolically active endothelial cells serve a variety of regulatory functions. Prostacyclin generated by release of arachidonic acid from the endothelium helps to maintain blood flow as well as prevent intravascular platelet aggregation (39). The enhanced release of arachidonic acid in response to membrane-active stimuli may be, in part, a protective response of endothelium.

Recent studies with cultured endothelial cells suggest that the endothelium has an active role in generation of pro-inflammatory mediators, such as PAF (8,36) or cytokines (32,38). Growth factors, such as PDGF (10,18) and granulocyte-macrophage colony-stimulating factor (6), are also produced by endothelial cells under certain conditions. Although the exact role of these mediators is still unknown, they could influence several aspects of the inflammatory response, including leukocyte adherence, migration, or activation.

ENDOTHELIAL INJURY STUDIED IN VITRO

Because of complexity of in vivo animal models of lung injury, a number of investigators use isolated tissues and cultured cells to determine functional changes in response to injury. In general, cell cultures have proven superior to isolated lung preparations for certain types of injury studies. For example, cultures of endothelial cells can be used to determine the link between a specific cytotoxic or genotoxic signal and alteration of a particular function. Culture systems are particularly appropriate for determining receptor-mediated phenomena or the expression of regulatory molecules.

The primary goal of cultured cell models is to isolate and preserve specific cell activities that account for phenomena observed in vitro. The immediate cell environment can be manipulated through varied culture conditions, gas composition, and extracellular matrix components; homogeneous cell cultures eliminate factors such as blood flow, mechanical stress, and neural signals that complicate in vitro systems. Some of the properties commonly measured in these highly differentiated cells include the enzymatic activity of angiotensin I converting enzyme (ACE), the generation of prostacyclin, and the barrier function of endothelial monolayers. In addition, immunologic (helper) function, procoagulant and fibrinolytic activities can be measured in cultured endothelial cells.

Even within well-defined culture systems, however, endothelial cells differ in their basic properties and in their response to injurious agents. ACE activity differs in endothelial cells cultured from various vascular sites, and conditions for its release also vary with the vascular source of the cell and the animal species from which it comes. Despite significant differences in enzyme activity at different stages of cell growth and age in culture, release of ACE activity can be used to assess injury (25,29).

Several studies indicate differences in the release and metabolism of arachidonic acid by cells from different vascular sites. For example, umbilical venous cells, but not those from either human pulmonary arteries or veins, respond to thrombin with enhanced release of prostacyclin. All of these human endothelial cells, however, release prostacyclin when treated with melittin (25). Histamine, bradykinin, and thrombin stimulate prostacyclin formation in either bovine coronary artery cells or human umbilical venous cells, but bovine aortic endothelial cells respond only to bradykinin (40).

These varied responses may reflect differences in agonist receptors between diverse cell preparations. Lollar and Owen (34) showed that thrombin interacts with at least two populations of receptors on endothelial cells. Low affinity sites are linked to arachidonate release, but high affinity sites might serve other functions, such as mitogenesis or inactivation of plasminogen activator (34). Alternatively, differences in the response to agonists such as thrombin or bradykinin might be due to diverse mechanisms regulating arachidonate release and metabolism. Comparison of human and porcine endothelial cells revealed a species difference in the phospholipid pools from which arachidonic acid is released and provided evidence for participation of a phospholipase C-mediated pathway in addition to the primary phospholipase A_2-induced release of arachidonic acid (20). Studies with microvessel preparations from bovine and rat tissues suggest that an alternate pathway of PGH_2 metabolism results primarily in formation of PGE_2. These findings might account, in part, for the predominance of PGE_2 over PGI_2 in microvascular endothelial cell preparations (14).

A recent review of the heterogeneous properties of cultured endothelial cells emphasizes that the structural and functional features of endothelium are probably not a result of terminal differentiation but of signals from the immediate environment (14). A growing body of evidence indicates that the behavior of endothelial cells in situ depends upon the influence of other vascular cells as well as the subcellular matrix. The interplay between endothelium, subcellular matrix, and smooth muscle is lost in culture systems, but co-cultures and application of cells to selected matrices can approximate the in vivo environment. Matrix components can influence the phenotypic expression of basement membrane constituents by endothelial cells as well as their proliferation and structural organization (35). The extracellular matrix also influences the response to injury (19,25).

Microvessels have been used by many investigators to study various endothelial functions and properties. These preparations, which are commonly made from brain and adipose tissue, preserve some of the cellular interactions and retain the influence of the endothelial matrix. Thus, when vascular reactivity and cellular interactions are of primary interest, isolated microvessels may prove more valuable than isolated cells. There are, however, some distinct differences in the properties of large vessel and microvascular endothelium (14). Comparison of these properties within the lung would be of considerable interest, but despite efforts of several laboratories, microvessels have not been successfully isolated from lung tissue.

MECHANISMS OF INJURY

Mechanisms of injury to the pulmonary vascular endothelium may be as varied as the number of causal agents. Injury of endothelium can cause detachment or lysis of individual cells, alteration of metabolic properties, exposure of subendothelial surfaces, or disruption of intercellular communication. Aside from cytolysis, which results in cell death, quantitation of endothelial injury depends upon measuring some alteration of specific cell functions. Although endothelial cells produce a finite number of measurable responses, some of these can be used to monitor receptor-mediated events or the expression of specific molecules. Several laboratories contributed elegant studies of receptor-mediated mechanisms for prostacyclin generation in endothelial cells (1–3,34). Others emphasized signal-induced expression of IgG and C3 receptors (9), expression of procoagulant molecules, such as tissue factor (42) and prothrombin (41), growth factors (6,10,18), or inflammatory mediators, such as PAF (8,36). Several recent publications examined gene expression of factors such as interleukin-1 (32) or PDGF (10) to determine how these factors influence pathologic responses of the endothelium.

Gap junctional communication may be important for functional coupling of cells within the vascular wall (30). Experiments done by Larson and colleagues using bovine brain microvessels indicate that endothelial cells communicate with smooth muscle cells and pericytes through specialized membrane sites. Gap junctions have been implicated in such diverse processes as growth control (33), metabolic interactions (44), and hormonal stimulation (31). Although it is not yet known if these structures participate in intercellular communication within pulmonary vessels, altered gap junctional transfer would be one mechanism through which acute or subacute injury could affect pulmonary vascular functions. For example, hypoxia and other forms of injury cause increased muscularization of pulmonary arterioles in humans and experimental animals; this phenomenon is thought to contribute to development of pulmonary hypertension (28). A recent report of elastogenic factors from cultured smooth muscle cells emphasizes the importance of communication between vascular cells. Mecham and colleagues (37) found that a factor produced by smooth muscle cells cultured from pulmonary arteries of hypoxic calves stimulated elastin production by adventitial cells. Since this material from altered smooth muscle cells influenced both the secretory phenotype and the responsiveness of the adventitial cells, it might affect the pathogenesis of pulmonary hypertension.

CELL-MEDIATED ENDOTHELIAL INJURY

Many studies have been devoted to the mechanism of injury to endothelium by adherent granulocytes. Adherence of activated polymorphonuclear leukocytes (PMN) occurs early in acute lung injury, and experiments in animals clearly implicate the activated neutrophil as a contributor, if not the cause, of pulmonary edema (5,7,24,46). Inflammatory mediators were shown to increase granulocyte adherence to the endothelium, and acute inflammatory changes within the lungs are associated with pulmonary vascular injury (5).

Many different experimental conditions can generate toxic oxygen radicals to damage endothelium (46). Although there is a wealth of evidence that oxidants from PMN can injure endothelium in vivo and in vitro, it is apparent that PMN may cause other, more subtle changes in endothelial function.

Several laboratories used endothelial cell cultures in experiments designed to mimic in vivo lung injury. Bowman and colleagues (4) found that hyperoxic injury to bovine pulmonary arterial endothelial cells correlated with enhanced PMN adherence and suggested that, in addition to extrinsic damage by PMN, hyperoxia stimulates production of oxygen radicals by the endothelium. Alternatively, subtle injury to the endothelium might amplify recruitment and attachment of PMN through expression of adherence molecules.

Based upon experiments with selected inhibitors and PMN that lack oxidant pathways, other investigators found that oxygen radicals could alter functions of cultured endothelial cells without necessarily injuring them. Using endothelial cells cultured from bovine and human vessels, Harlan and Callahan (16) showed that hydrogen peroxide produced by adherent PMN stimulated prostaglandin generation by endothelium but did not lyse the cells. This mechanism could amplify edema formation in acute inflammation through vasodilation and increased permeability caused by prostacyclin.

ENDOTHELIAL BARRIER FUNCTION

Other investigators measured oxidant- or PMN-induced changes in the barrier function of endothelial monolayers. This technique involves application of intact monolayers of endothelial cells to one side of a gelatin-coated porous filter positioned to separate the luminal and abluminal sides. Radiolabeled macromolecules are applied in a specified volume to the luminal side, and the rate of passage across the filter is measured under carefully controlled conditions of pressure and volume. Shasby and co-workers (43) used this method to show that oxygen radicals reversibly increased the permeability of porcine endothelial monolayers to albumin. Increased permeability was associated with reversible change in cell shape, and the oxidant-induced changes were related to changes in intracellular calcium and to contraction of actin filaments within the cells.

Studies by Garcia et al. (13) with bovine pulmonary arterial endothelial cells showed that thrombin increased permeability of monolayers to albumin through contraction and formation of intercellular gaps. This alteration was not linked to either fibrinogen recognition or serine protease active sites. As indicated by a lack of lactic dehydrogenase release, structural changes with increased permeability were not cytotoxic. These authors noted, in addition, an interesting interaction between neutrophils and activating agents. Figure 1, taken from their publication (13), shows how the macromolecular clearance technique can be used to quantitate functional changes in endothelial cells. Since neither PMN nor PMA applied directly to endothelial cells on the filter enhanced the clearance of albumin, the combined effect must involve activation on or near the endothelial surface. These experiments show that permeability changes in endothelium can be produced by activated PMN as well as by oxidants or thrombin. Moreover, such changes observed in vivo (edema) can be studied and quantitated using an in vitro system.

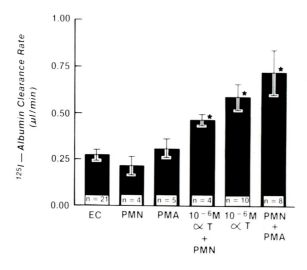

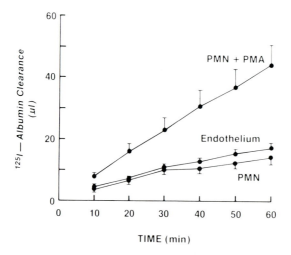

Figure 1: The heights of the bars in the top graph indicate the clearance of albumin through a monolayer of endothelial cells following several experimental interventions. Although neither PMN alone nor PMA altered the barrier properties of the cells, addition of alpha thrombin alone or with PMN significantly enhanced clearance. The effect of combined PMN and PMA is even greater. The bottom graph shows how the clearance of albumin is increased by activated PMN over 60 min. (Data from Garcia et al. [13].)

The phenomenon of endothelial retraction and formation of gaps through which filtration occurs is probably a common response to various types of stimuli. We find that antigen-antibody reaction, as well as melittin or thrombin, cause distinct morphological changes, including contraction (see below). A similar effect was described for ethchlorvynol, an anesthetic agent that causes pulmonary edema in experimental animals. The findings of Wysolmerski and Lagunoff (49) suggest that cytoskeletal proteins are essential for retention of an intact endothelial monolayer. These investigators showed that ethchlorvynol stimulated reversible retraction of pulmonary arterial endothelial monolayers without detachment or lysis of the cells, but F-actin was lost from the normally dense peripheral band of actin filaments. They proposed that actin filaments maintain the spreading of the cells; when this band is disrupted, the cells retract to form gaps that might account for edema formation in vivo (49).

Changes in macromolecular filtration, regardless of the initiating stimulus, are probably very important for extension of the inflammatory process and its eventual resolution. The transendothelial passage of fibrinogen and fibronectin provides a stroma on which wound healing occurs. If, as proposed by Dvorak (11), the continued filtration of these macromolecules stimulates cell replication and motility, the increase in permeability could ultimately contribute to the injurious process. The chronic stimulation of adventitial cells to produce matrix components or the stimulated mitogenesis of smooth muscle cells are potential pathogenic mechanisms in fibrosis and in pulmonary hypertension.

In vitro models of injury, including cultured cells, will help to define the relationships between endothelial cell activation, injury, and altered function in vivo. The filtration technique provides a valuable tool for such studies. Co-cultures of endothelial cells with smooth muscle cells or fibroblasts as well as studies of gap junctions will help to determine how vascular cells communicate and how altered communication affects the response to injury. More extensive studies of cytoskeletal elements and the phenomena of cell contraction and mobility are clearly indicated. Several laboratories are already committed to these goals, and interesting new findings should soon unravel the events linking changes in specific cytoskeletal elements to edema formation.

INFLAMMATORY MEDIATORS AND CYTOTOXICITY

It is generally accepted that sublethal cytotoxicity alters properties such as the integrity of the endothelial cell membrane and the generation of prostacyclin. One way to quantitate injury is to measure release of ^{51}Cr from previously labeled endothelial cells. Enhanced release of radioactivity signals disruption of the cell membrane. This technique enabled us to determine that potent vasoactive mediators, such as bradykinin, histamine, leukotrienes, and PAF, do not damage the endothelial membrane, even in concentrations as high as 10^{-6}M. Similarly, thrombin, which causes both morphological and functional changes in cultured endothelial cells, is not cytotoxic as determined by ^{51}Cr release. In contrast, data in Table 1 show that either antibody to endothelial surface antigens or melittin, a proinflammatory polypeptide from bee venom, disrupts the cells during a brief incubation.

Although this approach is useful for determining which agents are acutely cytotoxic, release of radioactivity alone is insufficient for discriminating mechanisms of cell injury. Concomitant measurement of some other property helps to determine how loss of cellular integrity relates to altered function. Figure 2 shows that treatment with an antibody alone does not alter the morphology of endothelial cells examined by scanning electron microscopy, but when complement (20 percent serum) is added, there is a change in cell shape and formation

TABLE 1 RELEASE OF ⁵¹Cr BY INFLAMMATORY MEDIATORS

Treatment	Percent release of ^{51}Cr
None (medium)	4.3 + 1.0
PAF (10^{-7} M)	6.8 + 1.8
Histamine (10^{-6} M)	2.8 + 0.2
Bradykinin (10^{-6} M)	4.9 + 0.7
LTB$_4$ (10^{-6} M)	4.5 + 1.1
Thrombin (5 U/ml)	7.7 + 1.2
Antibody + Complement*	36.0 + 7.3
Melittin (10^{-6} M)	34.8 + 3.0

^{51}Cr-labeled endothelial cells were incubated with medium or with the various mediators for 30 min at 37°. The amount of radioactivity released into the supernatant medium is expressed as a percent of the total cell radioactivity. Values are means of 3 to 5 separate determinations.

* Anti-HLA serum was a gift from Dr. Peter Stastny, Department of Medicine, University of Texas Health Science Center at Dallas.

of gaps between adjoining cells. These changes are similar to those reported for thrombin (13) or ethchlorvynol (49).

Bradykinin, histamine, thrombin, and melittin are all potent stimuli for arachidonate release and the subsequent conversion to prostacyclin (1,2,20,25,26). The lack of ⁵¹Cr release by bradykinin, histamine, or thrombin indicates that release of arachidonic acid can occur without cytolysis. Presumably, these agents act through receptor-mediated mechanisms to promote a regulated activation of

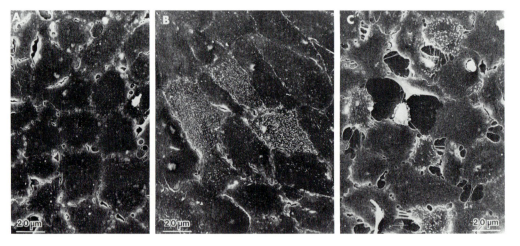

Figure 2: The three panels are scanning electron micrographs of cultured endothelial cells following treatment with medium alone (A), medium plus an antibody to endothelial surface antigens (B), or antibody applied in combination with complement (20 percent serum) (C). Antibody was applied to cells plated on coverslips and the preparations were incubated for 15 min. Serum or medium was added and incubation was continued for 15 min longer. The cells were fixed with glutaraldehyde and processed for microscopy. Antibody alone does not alter the appearance of the cells, and they remain closely joined in a monolayer. The morphological changes caused by antibody-complement include retraction of the cells or formation of gaps between them. (Courtesy of Dr. Werner Schulz, Department of Pathology, University of Texas Health Center, Dallas, TX.)

phospholipase. Even when low concentrations of melittin are applied to the cells, however, prostaglandin formation and cytolysis occur in parallel. Release of arachidonic acid by melittin or by complement probably occurs as the result of the primary injury and not through a receptor-mediated mechanism.

PAF is an inflammatory mediator of particular interest in acute lung injury. Although PAF does not harm the endothelium directly, it is a potent activator of polymorphonuclear leukocytes. Because PAF promotes adherence of circulating PMN to the pulmonary endothelium and causes pulmonary edema in animal models (7), it might injure endothelium via products from activated PMN.

We found that PAF increases adherence of human PMN to endothelial cells by interaction with specific endothelial receptors (12). Although PAF alone does not alter the permeability of endothelial monolayers, in combination with PMN it increases the clearance of radiolabeled albumin, as shown in Figure 3.

As reported by Garcia et al. (13), nonactivated PMN in contact with endothelial monolayers do not alter permeability, but after activation with PMA, they increase clearance of labeled albumin through a nonlytic mechanism. This was confirmed in experiments with PAF-activated PMN using ^{51}Cr release as an index of cytotoxicity (Table 2).

Endothelial "injury" measured in these experiments is cell lysis. Sublethal injury resulting from PMN activation may not be detected under these conditions. A cumulative effect or subtle changes caused by adherence of PMN is, perhaps, a more realistic concept of the situation in vivo, and possibly cooperation between oxidants and PMN proteases might be required for full expression of cell injury.

The idea that activated PMN might promote cytotoxicity from another stimulus was the basis for addition experiments with ^{51}Cr-labeled endothelial cells.

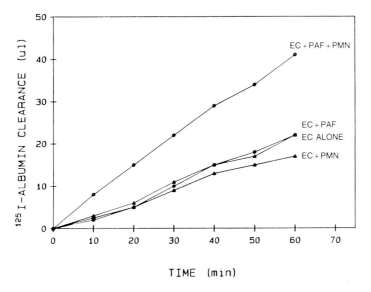

Figure 3: The graph of albumin clearance by monolayers of bovine pulmonary arterial endothelial cells shows effects of PAF and PMN on the barrier function of endothelium in vitro as described previously. (Data from Garcia et al. [13].)

TABLE 2 ACTIVATED PMN DO NOT INJURE ENDOTHELIAL CELLS

Treatment	Percent release of ^{51}Cr
PMN alone (untreated)	6.2 + 0.3
PAF alone (10^{-7} M)	6.4 + 0.7
PMA alone (10^{-6} M)	5.5 + 0.6
PMN treated with PAF	5.0 + 0.6
PMN treated with PMN	6.8 + 1.0
Triton X-100 (0.1%)	95.3 + 6.2

Labeled endothelial cells were incubated 60 min at 37° with PMN, PAF, or PMA alone or with a combination of the mediators and PMN. Radioactivity released into the media is expressed as percent of total. Treatment with Triton X-100 causes almost complete lysis. Data are means ± SEM of four separate determinations.

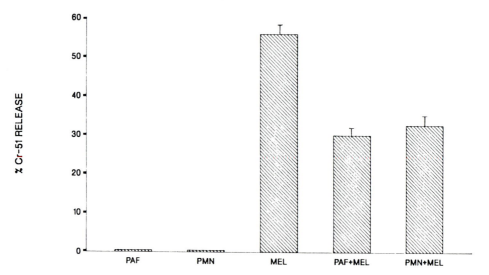

Figure 4: Human endothelial cells were labeled with ^{51}Cr as described in the text. PAF (10^{-6}M) or PMN (10^5 cells) were applied to cells in multi-well plates and incubated for 30 min. The medium was removed, and fresh medium containing 2×10^{-6}M melittin was added to each well. The percent release of radioactivity was determined by comparison of the amount of media from each well with the total released activity (the amount released by lysis with Triton X-100). Each bar represents the mean ± SEM of four experiments. (Data from Dr. A. Azghani)

Figure 4 shows that, contrary to our expectations, the cytotoxic effect of melittin was blunted when the endothelial cells were incubated first with either PAF alone or with PAF-activated PMN. In these experiments, PAF or PMN were applied to the cells during a 30-min incubation and then either melittin or buffer was added for an additional 30 min. The mechanism of this "protection" is not obvious. Since we did not measure oxidant production in these experiments, an antioxidant effect cannot be excluded. Since melittin is a potent activator of phospholipase A_2, possibly either PAF or activated PMN influences activation of this enzyme and subsequent formation of eicosanoids.

Arachidonate metabolites from either endothelial cells or PMN could affect the membrane response. Our hypothesis was that release of endothelial prostaglandins could protect the cells from additional harmful stimuli. The observations of Harlan and Callahan (16) that PMN stimulated to adhere to endothelial cells increase release of prostacyclin but do not injure the cells are compatible with this idea. Data obtained with an inhibitor of cyclooxygenase support the prostacyclin hypothesis (Table 3).

Since inhibition of cyclooxygenase promotes the cytotoxicity of melittin or antibody, cyclooxygenase products from endothelium might affect the stability of the cell membrane. In additional experiments, media that was removed from cultures in which cells were stimulated to release prostacyclin had a similar protective effect. Despite these observations which appear to support our hypothesis, the picture remains somewhat cloudy. First, direct application of prostacyclin had little or no effect on melittin-induced cytotoxicity. Even though prostacyclin is short-lived, it can elevate cyclic AMP in endothelial cells for as long as 30 to 60 min (21). Second, later studies revealed that even high concentrations of PAF (10^{-6}M) did not stimulate prostacyclin release (12). Possibly prostacyclin is not the protective agent. We reported in a previous publication, however, that the other cyclooxygenase products from endothelium (HETEs) did not protect cells from melittin cytotoxicity (26), and although PAF is reported to stimulate leukotriene formation in lung tissue (47), endothelial cells do not produce leukotrienes (27). Thus, the mechanism of PAF- or PMN-induced "protection" of endothelium remains uncertain. These simple experiments are reported here to illustrate how cultured cells can be used to explore cellular interactions and the actions of inflammatory mediators in vitro. Future experiments with selected inhibitors could be used to dissect relevant regulatory pathways and to establish whether eicosanoids have a significant effect on endothelial injury.

Clearly, viable endothelial cells interact in a variety of ways with activated inflammatory cells and mediators to counter potentially injurious agents. Antioxidant defense mechanisms, including the glutathione redox cycle, are operative in cultured cells (17) as well as in vivo. A recent observation that the cytokines, tumor necrosis factor and interleukin-1, decrease lung injury in a hyperoxic animal model (48) suggests that the endothelium is capable of responding to a chronic

TABLE 3 EFFECT OF INDOMETHACIN ON CYTOTOXICITY

Treatment	Percent release of ^{51}Cr	6-keto $PGF_{1\alpha}$
Medium alone	2.9 + 0.2	3.4 + 0.3
Antibody + Complement (C)	25.0 + 5.2	14.7 + 2.1
Melittin (10^{-6} M)	21.0 + 2.8	12.7 + 1.0
Indomethacin (10^{-6} M)	2.3 + 0.1	1.2 + 1.0
Antibody + C + Indomethacin	41.8 + 4.3	1.2 + 0.3
Melittin + Indomethacin	39.4 + 4.4	1.3 + 0.0

^{51}Cr-labeled endothelial cells were treated first with medium alone or with indomethacin for 30 min at 37°. Antibody-complement or melittin was added and incubation was continued for 30 min. Radioactivity released into the supernatant media is expressed as percent of total. In parallel experiments, unlabeled cells were treated as above and the media were assayed by RIA for 6-keto $PGF_{1\alpha}$, the stable metabolite of prostacyclin. PG data are ng/well (approximately 10^5 cells). All data are means ± SEM of 3 to 5 separate determinations.

injurious stimulus. This particular aspect of endothelial cell biology is still in its infancy, but with the advent of molecular biology and attendant technologies, protective pathways, as well as injurious ones, can be explored.

ACKNOWLEDGMENTS

The author wishes to thank Drs. Ali Azghani and Joe G.N. Garcia of the University of Texas Health Center at Tyler for contributing data on endothelial interactions with activated neutrophils. Dr. Werner W. Schulz of the University of Texas Health Science Center in Dallas kindly provided the photomicrographs of cells, and Dr. Peter Stastny provided the antibody to human endothelial antigen. Ms. Sue Jean Tsai performed the radioimmunoassays for prostacyclin, and Ms. Laurie Davis helped with the cytotoxicity studies. The published work from our laboratories as well as unpublished data reported here was supported by grants from the National Heart, Lung, and Blood Institute of the National Institutes of Health (HL 36549, HL 36538, and HL 36545).

REFERENCES

1. Alhenc-Gelas F, Tsai SJ, Callahan KS, Campbell WB, Johnson AR: Stimulation of prostaglandin formation by vasoactive mediators in cultured human endothelial cells. Prostaglandins 24 : 723–742, 1982.

2. Baenziger NL, Fogerty FJ, Mertz LF, Chernuta LF: Regulation of histamine-mediated prostacyclin synthesis in cultured human vascular endothelial cells. Cell 24 : 915–923, 1981.

3 Benjamin CW, Hopkins NK, Oglesby TD, Gorman RR: Agonist specific desensitization of leukotriene C_4-stimulated PGI_2 biosynthesis in human endothelial cells. Biochem Biophys Res Commun 117 : 780–787, 1983.

4. Bowman CM, Butler EN, Repine JE: Hyperoxia damages cultured endothelial cells causing increased neutrophil adherence. Am Rev Respir Dis 128 : 469–472, 1983.

5. Brigham KL, Meyrick B: Interactions of granulocytes with the lungs. Circ Res 54 : 623–635, 1984.

6. Broudy VC, Kaushansky K, Segal GM, Harlan JM, Adamson JW: Tumor necrosis factor type alpha stimulates human endothelial cells to produce granulocyte/macrophage colony-stimulating factor. Proc Natl Acad Sci USA 83 : 7467–7471, 1986.

7. Burhop KE, Garcia JG, Selig WM, Lo SK, van der Zee H, Kaplan JE, Malik AB: Platelet-activating factor increases lung vascular permeability to protein. J Appl Physiol 61 : 2210–2217, 1986.

8. Camussi G, Aglietta M, Malavasi F, Tetta C, Piacibello W, Sanavio F, Bussolino F: The release of platelet-activating factor from human endothelial cells in culture. J Immunol 131 : 2397–2403, 1983.

9. Cines CB, Lyss AP, Bina M, Corkey R, Kefalides NA, Friedman HM: Fc and C3 receptors induced by herpes simplex virus on cultured human endothelial cells. J Clin Invest 69 : 123–128, 1982.

10. Daniel TO, Gibbs VC, Milfay DF, Garovoy MR, Williams LT: Thrombin stimulates c-*sis* gene expression in microvascular endothelial cells. J Biol Chem 261 : 9579–9582, 1986.

11. Dvorak HF: Tumors: wounds that do not heal. N Engl J Med 315 : 1650–1659, 1986.

12. Garcia JG, Azghani A, Callahan KS, Johnson AR: Effect of platelet activating factor on leukocyte-endothelial cell interactions. Thromb Res 51 : 83–96, 1988.

13. Garcia JG, Siflinger-Birnboim A, Bizios R, Del Vecchio PJ, Fenton JW, Malik AB: Thrombin-induced increase in albumin permeability across the endothelium. J Cell Physiol 128 : 96–104, 1986.

14. Gerritsen ME: Functional heterogeneity of vascular endothelial cells. Biochem Pharmacol 36 : 2701–2711, 1987.

15. Gruetter CA, Lemke SM: Comparison of endothelial-dependent relaxation in bovine intrapulmonary artery and vein by acetylcholine and A23187. J Pharmacol Exp Ther 238 : 1055–1062, 1986.

16. Harlan JM, Callahan KS: Role of hydrogen peroxide in the neutrophil-mediated release of prostacyclin from cultured endothelial cells. J Clin Invest 74 : 442–448, 1984.

17. Harlan JM, Levine JD, Callahan KS, Schwartz BR, Harker LA: Glutathione redox cycle protects cultured endothelial cells against lysis by extracellularly generated hydrogen peroxide. J Clin Invest 73 : 706–713, 1984.

18. Harlan JM, Thompson PJ, Ross RR, Bowen-Pope DF: α-thrombin induces release of platelet-derived growth factor-like molecule(s) by cultured human endothelial cells. J Cell Biol 103 : 1129–1133, 1986.

19. Heifetz A, Johnson AR: Sulfated glycoproteins and extracellular matrix of cultured human pulmonary endothelial cells. J Supramol Struct Cell Biochem 15 : 359–367, 1981.

20. Hong SL, Deykin D: Activation of phospholipases A_2 and C in pig aortic endothelial cells synthesizing prostacyclin. J Biol Chem 257 : 7151–7154, 1982.

21. Hopkins NK, Gorman RR: Regulation of endothelial cell cyclic nucleotide metabolism by prostacyclin. J Clin Invest 67 : 540–546, 1981.

22. Huang TW: Composite epithelial and endothelial basal laminas in human lungs. Am J Pathol 93 : 681–692, 1978.

23. Humphrey DM, McManus LM, Hanahan DJ, Pinckard RN: Morphologic basis of increased vascular permeability induced by acetyl glyceryl ether phosphorylcholine. Lab Invest 50 : 16–25, 1984.

24. Johnson A, Tahamont MV, Kaplan JE, Malik AB: Lung fluid balance after pulmonary embolization: Effect of thrombin vs. fibrin aggregates. J Appl Physiol 52 : 1565–1570, 1982.

25. Johnson AR, Callahan KS, Tsai SC, Campbell WB: Prostacyclin and prostaglandin biosynthesis in human pulmonary endothelial cells. Bull Eur Physiopathol Respir 17 : 531–551, 1981.

26. Johnson AR, Revtyak G, Campbell WB: Arachidonic acid metabolites and endothelial injury: Studies with cultures of human endothelial cells. Fed Proc 44 : 19–24, 1985.

27. Johnson AR, Revtyak GE, Ibe BO, Campbell WB: Endothelial cells metabolize but do not synthesize leukotrienes, in Lefer AL, Gee MH (eds), *Leukotrienes in Cardiovascular and Pulmonary Function*. Philadelphia, Alan R. Liss, Inc., 1986, pp 185–196.

28. Jones R, Langleben D, Reid LM: Patterns of remodeling of the pulmonary circulation in acute and subacute lung injury, in Said S (ed), *The Pulmonary Circulation and Acute Lung Injury*. New York, Futura Publishing Co., Inc., 1985, pp 137–188.

29. Krulewitz AH, Fanburg BL: The effect of oxygen tension on the in vitro production and release of angiotensin-converting enzyme by bovine pulmonary artery endothelial cells. Am Rev Respir Dis 130 : 866–869, 1984.

30. Larson DM, Carson MP, Haudenschild CC: Junctional transfer of small molecules in cultured bovine brain microvascular endothelial cells and pericytes. Microvasc Res 34 : 184–199, 1987.

31. Lawrence TS, Beers WH, Gilula NB: Transmission of hormonal stimulation by cell-to-cell communication. Nature 272 : 501–506, 1978.

32. Libby P, Ordovas JM, Auger KR, Robbins AH, Birinyi LK, Dinarello CA: Endotoxin and tumor necrosis factor induce interleukin-1 gene expression in adult human vascular endothelial cells. Am J Pathol 124 : 179–186, 1986.

33. Loewenstein WR: Junctional intercellular communication and the control of growth. Biochim Biophys Acta 560 : 1–65, 1979.

34. Lollar P, Owen WG: Evidence that the effects of thrombin on arachidonate metabolism in cultured human endothelial cells are not mediated by a high affinity receptor. J Biol Chem 255 : 8031–8034, 1980.

35. Madri JA, Williams SK: Capillary endothelial cell cultures: phenotypic modulation by matrix components. J Cell Biol 97 : 153–165, 1983.

36. McIntyre TM, Zimmerman GA, Prescott SM: Leukotrienes C_4 and D_4 stimulate human endothelial cells to synthesize platelet-activating factor and bind neutrophils. Proc Natl Acad Sci USA 83 : 2204–2208, 1986.

37. Mecham RP, Whitehouse LA, Wrenn DS, Parks WC, Griffin GL, Senior RM, Crouch EC, Stenmark KR, Voelkel NF: Smooth muscle-mediated connective tissue remodeling in pulmonary hypertension. Science 237 : 423–426, 1987.

38. Miossec P, Cavender D, Ziff M: Production of interleukin 1 by human endothelial cells. J Immunol 136 : 2486–2491, 1986.

39. Moncada S, Vane JR: The role of prostacyclin in vascular tissue. Fed Proc 38 : 66–71, 1979.

40. Revtyak GE, Johnson AR, Campbell WB: Prostaglandin synthesis in bovine coronary endothelial cells: Comparison with other commonly studied endothelial cells. Thromb Res 48 : 671–683, 1987.

41. Rodgers GM, Shuman MA: Prothrombin is activated on vascular endothelial cells by factor Xa and calcium. Proc Natl Acad Sci USA 80 : 7001–7005, 1983.

42. Schorer AE, Kaplan ME, Rao GH, Moldow CF: Interleukin 1 stimulates endothelial cell tissue factor production and expression by a prostaglandin-independent mechanism. Thromb Haemost 56 : 256–259, 1986.

43. Shasby DM, Lind SE, Shasby SS, Goldsmith JC, Hunninghake GW: Reversible oxidant-induced increases in albumin transfer across cultured endothelium: Alterations in cell shape and calcium homeostasis. Blood 65 : 605–614, 1985.

44. Sheridan JD, Finbow ME, Pitts JD: Metabolic interactions between animal cells through permeable intercellular junctions. Exp Cell Res 123 : 111–117, 1979.

45. Stern D, Nawroth P, Handley D, Kisiel W: An endothelial-cell dependent pathway of coagulation. Proc Natl Acad Sci USA 82 : 2523–2527, 1985.

46. Taylor AE, Martin D, Parker JC: The effects of oxygen radicals on pulmonary edema formation. Surgery 94 : 433–438, 1983.

47. Voelkel NF, Worthen S, Reeves JT, Henson PM, Murphy RC: Nonimmunologic production of leukotrienes induced by platelet-activating factor. Science 218:286–288, 1982.

48. White CW, Ghezzi P, Dinarello CA, Caldwell SA, McMurtry IF, Repine JE: Recombinant tumor necrosis factor/cachectin and interleukin 1 pretreatment decreases lung oxidized glutathione accumulation, lung injury, and mortality in rats exposed to hyperoxia. J Clin Invest 79:1868–1873, 1987.

49. Wysolmerski R, Lagunoff D: The effect of ethchlorvynol on cultured endothelial cells. A model for the study of the mechanism of increased vascular permeability. Am J Pathol 119:505–512, 1985.

William E. Benitz, M.D.

14 ———————————

Inhibition of Proliferation of Vascular Smooth Muscle Cells by Heparin

The observation that heparin blocks intimal smooth muscle cell proliferation following denudation of the arterial endothelium (10) stimulated numerous investigations of the effects of heparin upon smooth muscle proliferation in vivo and in vitro. Although most of these studies have been designed primarily to address the problem of atheroma formation in systemic arteries, there are now several reports which have focused upon a potential role for heparin or heparin-like materials in regulation of smooth muscle cell growth and medial remodeling in the pulmonary arteries.

HEPARIN BIOCHEMISTRY

Heparin is a member of the closely related group of endogenous sulfated polysaccharides known as heparan sulfates. Heparan sulfate glycosaminoglycan chains consist of alternating residues of glucosamine and uronic acid, which may be either glucuronic acid or its epimer, iduronic acid (Fig. 1). Sulfate residues may be found on the 2-hydroxyl group of the iduronic acids, at the 6-hydroxyl group of the glucosamines, and occasionally at the 3-hydroxyl group of a glucosamine. These potential variations in the relative contents of iduronic and glucuronic acid and in sulfation at several sites in each disaccharide allow for great heterogeneity amongst the various heparan sulfates, and even within single heparan sulfate chains. For example, many heparan sulfate chains include heavily sulfated iduronic acid-rich regions interspersed with regions with little iduronic acid and

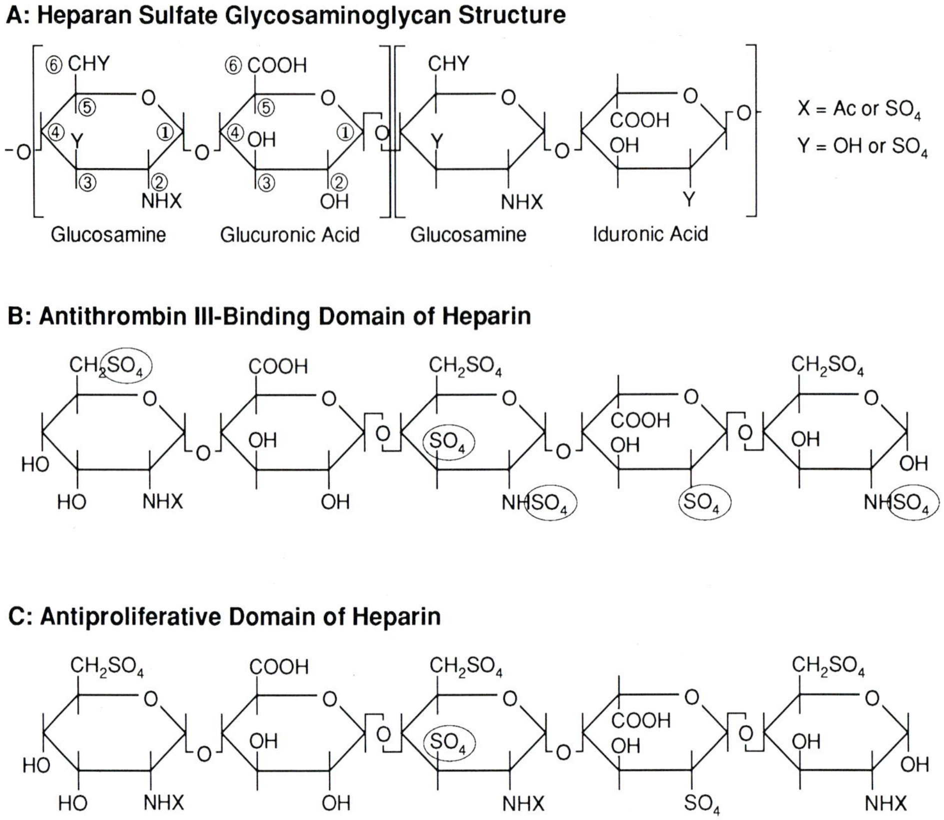

A: Heparan Sulfate Glycosaminoglycan Structure

Glucosamine   Glucuronic Acid   Glucosamine   Iduronic Acid

X = Ac or SO_4
Y = OH or SO_4

B: Antithrombin III-Binding Domain of Heparin

C: Antiproliferative Domain of Heparin

Figure 1:

A. Heparan sulfate glycosaminoglycans are complex sulfated polysaccharides consisting of alternating glucosamine and uronic acid residues. The uronic acid residues may be either glucuronic acid or its epimer, iduronic acid. The glucosamine residues may be modified by sulfation of the hydroxyl group at the 6-carbon or, less frequently, at the 3-carbon; the amine groups are substituted with either an acetyl or sulfate moiety. Iduronic acid may be sulfated at the hydroxyl group of the 2-carbon. Taking all of these structural variants into account, there are potentially 24 different disaccharides, such as those indicated in the large brackets, in heparan sulfate, allowing tremendous heterogeneity in the structure of these molecules. Heparin is distinguished from other heparan sulfate glycosaminoglycans by its extensive sulfation and high iduronic acid content. The number of the carbons in the sugar skeletons is indicated by the small circled numerals.

B. The anticoagulant effects of heparin are mediated by the specific pentasaccharide diagrammed here. The circled sulfate groups have been demonstrated to be essential for antithrombin III-binding. 3-O-sulfation of the middle glucosamine residue is a distinctive feature of this binding domain.

C. The antiproliferative effects of heparin also require 3-O-sulfation of the middle glucosamine residue, but N-sulfation is not essential. It is not known whether 6-O-sulfation of the glucosamines or 2-O-sulfation of the iduronic acid residue are required, but it is likely that at least some of these sulfate groups are necessary.

sparse sulfation. N-sulfation of the glucosamine residues is unique to the heparan sulfates and confers the specificity of both heparinase and nitrous acid digestions, which selectively cleave the glycosidic bonds adjacent to these residues in heparan sulfate but do not cleave other glycosaminoglycans. In vivo, heparan sulfate glycosaminoglycan chains are found only as constituents of proteoglycans, in which they are linked to a core protein. The polysaccharide chains are linked to the core protein by xylose-serine linkages, which are readily broken under alkaline conditions. Heparan sulfate proteoglycans are highly variable in size and structure and are virtually ubiquitous in distribution, being found intracellularly, at the cell surface, and in the extracellular matrix, including the basement membrane.

Heparin is a pharmaceutical product, which consists of polysaccharide fragments of molecular weight 5,000 to 15,000 daltons. These polysaccharide fragments are prepared from a distinctive heparan sulfate proteoglycan found within mast cells. The core protein of this proteoglycan has a relative mass of approximately 20,000 daltons and carries several glycosaminoglycan chains of 50,000 to 100,000 daltons. Heparin is distinguished from other heparan sulfate glycosaminoglycans because of extensive N-sulfation and a relatively high content of iduronic (as compared to glucuronic) acid. The anticoagulant effects of heparin are mediated by activation of antithrombin III, which binds only those heparin chains which contain the oligosaccharide sequence shown in Figure 1. The most distinctive feature of this pentasaccharide is the 3-O-sulfate on the glucosamine residue at position 3; N-sulfation of the glucosamines at positions 4 and 6 also is required for antithrombin binding. Due to the great heterogeneity of heparin structure, only about a third of the molecules in commercial heparin preparations include this sequence and have anticoagulant activity. The antiproliferative effects of heparin on vascular smooth muscle depend on a pentasaccharide which also contains a 3-O-sulfoglucosamine residue (Fig. 1); however, these effects do not require N-sulfation of the glucosamines (4,5).

EFFECTS OF HEPARIN UPON VASCULAR SMOOTH MUSCLE CELL GROWTH

Heparin Inhibits Proliferation of Vascular Smooth Muscle Cells in Vivo

In their initial report, Clowes and Karnovsky (10) demonstrated that anticoagulant doses of heparin were sufficient to inhibit intimal smooth muscle proliferation in rat carotid arteries following injury by intimal desiccation. Following this injury, the endothelium was sloughed from the desiccated segment and was rapidly replaced by a layer of adherent platelets. Over the next 14 days, there was marked intimal thickening due to smooth muscle proliferation in the denuded segment, as the endothelium slowly regenerated from the ends of the injured segment. Treatment with heparin, beginning 24 hr after injury, in doses sufficient to prolong the clotting time three to eight times normal, had no effect upon platelet attachment to the subendothelium of the denuded segment but significantly reduced intimal smooth muscle cell proliferation. Subsequently, heparin deleted of its anticoagulant components by affinity chromatography on antithrombin-Sepharose (12) was also found to inhibit myointimal proliferation, indicating that the growth inhibiting effects of heparin were not mediated by effects on the co-agulation system. These studies also demonstrated no effect of heparin upon en-dothelial regeneration in the injured vessels, suggesting that the heparin might act directly upon the smooth muscle cells. More recently, Clowes and Clowes (9) have shown that administration of heparin after intimal arterial injury both inhib-its migration of smooth muscle cells from the media into the intima and reduces the number of smooth muscle cells that initiate mitosis. These results support the hypothesis that heparin may act directly upon smooth muscle cells in injured systemic arteries to inhibit their migration and proliferation in response to arte-rial injury.

The effects of heparin upon pulmonary arterial remodeling have been less exten-sively studied. In experiments in mice subjected to chronic hypoxia (FI_{O_2} 0.1), administration of heparin in anticoagulant doses resulted in significant reduction in remodeling of the pulmonary arteries (13). In treated animals, the increment in the medial thickness of the small pulmonary arteries was only 36 percent of that in controls, and the decrement in the number of small arteries was only 33 percent of that in control animals. These structural effects on the pulmonary ar-teries was only 36 percent of that in controls and the decrement in the number of small arteries was only 33 percent of that in control animals. These structural effects on the pulmonary arteries were associated with significant reductions in right ventricular pressures and right ventricular hypertrophy. The mechanism by which heparin exerts these effects is unknown. However, proliferation of smooth muscle cells or their precursors appears to be an important feature of pulmonary arterial remodeling in chronically hypoxic animals, suggesting that factors which inhibit proliferation of smooth muscle cells, such as heparin, may be able to block the development of pulmonary hypertension. These experiments also suggest that heparin-like materials may be involved in maintenance of nor-mal pulmonary arterial anatomy, implying a significant role for such materials in regulation of pulmonary arterial morphogenesis.

Heparin Inhibits Proliferation of Smooth Muscle Cells in Vitro

EFFECTS ON SYSTEMIC ARTERIAL SMOOTH MUSCLE CELLS

Because the early in vivo studies suggested that heparin might affect vascular smooth muscle cell proliferation via a direct interaction with those cells, a number of investigators have studied the effects of heparin on growth of these cells in vitro. As expected, heparin was found to inhibit proliferation of smooth muscle cells cultured from the aortas of calves or mature rats (3,15). The growth inhib-iting effects of heparin were dependent upon both the concentration of heparin used and the growth state of the cells. Smooth muscle cells which were growth-arrested by serum deprivation for 72 hr exhibited growth inhibition in response to heparin concentrations as low as 10 ng/ml; progressively greater effects were apparent at concentrations up to 10 μg/ml. Effects on exponentially proliferating smooth muscle cells were smaller in magnitude at all heparin concentrations, and reduced growth was apparent only with heparin in concentrations at or exceeding 1 μg/ml. Other polysaccharides, including dermatan sulfate, chondroitin sulfate, heparan sulfate, hyaluronic acid, and protamine, had little or no inhibitory effect upon smooth muscle cell growth. Only low molecular weight dextran sulfate (MW

25,000) mimicked heparin in these experiments. As in vivo, anticoagulant and non-anticoagulant heparins were equally effective inhibitors of smooth muscle cell growth in vitro. Heparin was also equally effective in medium depleted of anti-thrombin and in medium supplemented with antithrombin after depletion by heparin-Sepharose affinity chromatography (15). These results supported the argument that heparin does not act through effects upon an intermediary cell or the coagulation system, suggesting that heparin may act through a direct interaction with the smooth muscle cells themselves.

EFFECTS ON PULMONARY ARTERIAL SMOOTH MUSCLE CELLS

Because it was not certain that these observations could be applied to the pulmonary arteries, we investigated the effects of heparin on proliferation of smooth muscle cells cultured from the pulmonary arteries of near-term bovine fetuses (2). In these experiments, we demonstrated reversible inhibition of smooth muscle cell proliferation in the presence of heparin (Fig. 2). Growth inhibition was modest at 48 hr but was readily apparent by 96 hr. Inhibition of smooth

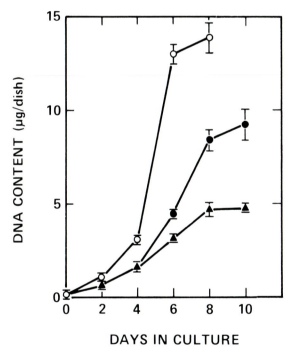

Figure 2: Effect of heparin (100 μg/ml) on proliferation of smooth muscle cells from the fetal calf pulmonary artery. Smooth muscle cell cultures exposed to heparin (▲) grew more slowly and achieved a lower final cell density than control cultures (○). In the recovery limb of this experiment (●), cells were exposed to heparin only during the first 4 days in culture. Cell proliferation was measured as the DNA content of each 35-mm tissue culture dish. The initial DNA content for all dishes was 0.32 μg. All pairs of samples for any day are significantly different (p < 0.001). (Reproduced from Benitz et al. [2].)

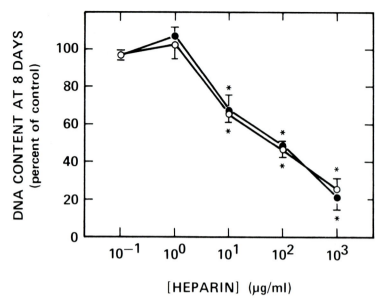

Figure 3: Dose-response relationship for effects of heparin on proliferation of pulmonary arterial (●) and aortic (○) smooth muscle cells. The DNA content of cultures at 8 days is expressed as a percentage of the DNA content of control cultures, which was 16.5 ± 0.6 μg/dish for pulmonary artery and 18.6 ± 1.2 μg/dish for aortic smooth muscle cell cultures (mean $\pm$ SE). Samples indicated with an asterisk are significantly different from controls ($p < 0.005$). (Reproduced from Benitz et al. [2].)

muscle cell growth was dose-dependent (Fig. 3). Heparin concentrations at or below 1 μg/ml did not inhibit proliferation of the exponentially growing smooth muscle cells used in our growth inhibition assay. However, inhibition of smooth muscle cell growth at heparin concentrations of 10 to 100 μg/ml was similar in magnitude to that reported for rat aortic smooth muscle cells (3). As for rat aortic cells (3,15), growth was not inhibited by dermatan sulfate, chondroitin sulfate, or hyaluronic acid, but was reduced by low molecular weight (MW 8,000) dextran sulfate. Thus, growth of pulmonary arterial smooth muscle cells, as well as that of smooth muscle cells from systemic arteries, is inhibited by heparin. In fact, we found that the effects of heparin on growth of smooth muscle cells from the fetal aorta were identical to those on cells from the pulmonary arteries (Fig. 3).

MECHANISMS OF ANTIPROLIFERATIVE EFFECTS

Reduced growth of pulmonary arterial smooth muscle cells was also evident in medium prepared by affinity chromatography on heparin-Sepharose (2). Treatment with heparinase reversed the inhibitory effects of heparin but not those of heparin-Sepharose chromatography, implying that the growth-inhibiting effects of heparin might result from interactions between heparin and soluble mitogens in the medium. Because platelet-derived growth factor (PDGF), a major serum mitogen for smooth muscle cells, was known to bind to heparin, we further assessed the potential role of interactions between heparin and PDGF. To do so, we prepared serum from fetal calf plasma, in which PDGF could not be detected by a sensitive radioreceptor assay (Table 1). Smooth muscle cell growth in this serum was comparable to growth in serum prepared from whole blood, in which PDGF was relatively abundant. The growth-inhibiting effects of heparin were indistinguishable in cultures grown in media prepared with these two sera (Table 1). Thus, inhibition of smooth muscle cell growth by heparin is not mediated solely by decreased availability or activity of exogenous PDGF. Reilly and colleagues (21) further demonstrated that heparin retains its capacity to inhibit smooth muscle cell growth in medium which has been depleted of heparin-binding mitogens by heparin-Sepharose chromatography, and showed that heparin does not inhibit binding of PDGF to its receptor on the smooth muscle cell surface (22). However, binding of epidermal growth factor to smooth muscle cells is reduced after 48 hr of exposure to heparin, but not after 2 hr of heparin exposure. These experiments indicate that heparin does not act by interfering with binding of mitogens to their receptors.

Reilly and colleagues found that the addition of heparin to quiescent smooth muscle cell cultures 2 hr prior to stimulation by serum was associated with a decrease in cell numbers that was not apparent until 48 to 72 hr after growth stimulation; the number of cells that initiated mitosis after stimulation fell by 27 percent. In cultures continuously exposed to heparin beginning 48 hr prior to serum stimulation, reduction in cell proliferation was reflected in a lower cell count in heparin-treated cultures 24 hr after stimulation and correlated with a 74 percent reduction in the number of cells initiating mitosis after serum stimulation (21). In cultures treated with heparin only during the 48 hr prior to serum stimulation (but not thereafter), growth inhibition was apparent in the first 24 hr after stimulation; the cells in these cultures subsequently proliferated at a rate identical to that of control cells.

The above experiments suggest that growth inhibition depends upon a direct interaction between heparin and the smooth muscle cells. Castellot et al. have shown that heparin does bind to specific, high affinity binding sites on the surface of smooth muscle cells (7). Therefore, it appears likely that the antiproliferative effects of heparin are mediated by binding of heparin to specific receptors, but that these effects are maximal only after several hours of heparin exposure. Al-

TABLE 1 THE ROLE OF PLATELET-DERIVED GROWTH FACTOR (PDGF) IN HEPARIN-INDUCED INHIBITION OF SMOOTH MUSCLE CELL PROLIFERATION

Medium	PDGF in medium (pg/ml)*	DNA content at 6 days (μg/dish)*	p
FCS 10%	114 ± 5	11.1 ± 0.2	<0.001
FCS 10% + Heparin	114 ± 5	2.4 ± 0.2	
FCPDS 10%	<5	10.3 ± 1.7	<0.002
FCPDS 10% + Heparin	<5	1.9 ± 0.6	

*Mean ± standard deviation
FCS = Fetal calf serum
FCPDS = Fetal calf platelet-derived serum

though this delay in achievement of maximal growth inhibition could be explained by slow intracellular accumulation of heparin, with levels eventually reaching a critical level needed to block progression into mitosis (21), it has not been established that internalization of heparin is necessary, although this clearly does occur (7).

IMPLICATIONS OF IN VITRO STUDIES

We found that the effects of heparin on growth of aortic smooth muscle cells in vitro were identical to those on growth of cells from the pulmonary artery. In contrast, abnormal pulmonary arterial morphogenesis in infants with persistent pulmonary hypertension and arterial remodeling induced by chronic hypoxia selectively affect the pulmonary arteries. If heparin-like materials are involved in regulation of pulmonary arterial morphogenesis or maintenance of normal pulmonary arterial structure, as suggested by experiments in mice (13), these observations suggest that these growth regulators are produced and act locally within the lungs (2), because remote production and action as a systemic hormone would be expected to have similar effects on the systemic and pulmonary arteries in these conditions. This conclusion is strengthened by in vitro experiments demonstrating that heparin acts through a direct interaction with the smooth muscle cells. Such interactions would clearly be facilitated by local production and deposition of heparin-like materials in the arterial wall itself. It is less likely that heparin-like materials in the pulmonary arterial blood would be able to cross an intact endothelium and its basement membrane to gain access to the medial smooth muscle cells. We, therefore, hypothesized that pulmonary arterial endothelial cells might produce a heparin-like inhibitor of smooth muscle cell proliferation, as had been described for endothelial cells from systemic vessels (3).

ENDOGENOUS SOURCES OF HEPARIN-LIKE GROWTH REGULATORS

Postconfluent Smooth Muscle Cells Produce an Antiproliferative Heparan Sulfate

To determine whether smooth muscle cells in the arterial media might themselves produce an antiproliferative heparan sulfate, Fritze et al. prepared heparan sulfate from the medium, cell surface, and cell pellet of postconfluent and exponentially proliferating smooth muscle cells cultured from bovine aortas (11). Only modest growth inhibition was achieved using heparan sulfate obtained from exponentially proliferating cells or from the cell pellet or medium of postconfluent cultures. However, potent growth inhibition (approximately 40-fold greater activity than commercial heparin) was obtained using heparan sulfate proteoglycan fragments released from the cell surfaces of postconfluent smooth muscle cells by treatment with diluted trypsin. These growth-inhibiting proteoglycan fragments contained heparan sulfate chains of MW 35,000 to 40,000 daltons, which could be partially degraded by platelet heparitinase. Growth inhibiting activity was retained by fragments of MW greater than 2,600 daltons. Smooth muscle cells were not able to degrade this heparan sulfate. Therefore, postconfluent vascular smooth muscle cells produce an antiproliferative heparan sulfate, which is present on the surface of these cells.

However, the role of heparan sulfate of the smooth muscle cell surface in maintaining arterial structure remains indeterminate. If this heparan sulfate must be released from the cell surface before it can inhibit growth of adjacent smooth muscle cells, it may be of little significance in uninjured vessels, because neither proteolytic enzymes nor platelet heparitinase are present in the intact arterial media. On the other hand, if inhibitory effects are realized without its release from the cell surface, it could have an important function in maintenance of medial smooth muscle cells in the contractile, nonproliferating state. In this case, increased catabolism and removal of this material from the arterial media after intimal injury, due to exposure of medial smooth muscle cells to platelet heparitinase and proteolytic enzymes, could enable medial smooth muscle cell proliferation in response to mitogens released from platelets, macrophages, endothelium, or other sources (6). Decreased expression of cell surface heparan sulfate by these proliferating smooth muscle cells (if this occurs in vivo as it does in vitro) could provide another mechanism by which the level of this tonic growth inhibitor is reduced, permitting further recruitment of smooth muscle cells into the proliferative state.

Pulmonary Arterial Endothelial Cells Produce an Antiproliferative Heparan Sulfate

Castellot et al. have shown that medium conditioned by endothelial cells cultured from the aortas of calves contains a heparin-like inhibitor of smooth muscle cell proliferation (3). This growth inhibitor has not been extensively characterized. However, it is soluble in trichloroacetic acid, insoluble in ethanol, and susceptible to digestion with heparinase. Release of this heparin-like material into culture medium requires a platelet heparitinase, which cleaves specific glycosidic bonds in heparan sulfate glycosaminoglycans (6). These properties suggest that this endothelial cell-derived inhibitor of smooth muscle cell growth may be a heparan sulfate glycosaminoglycan.

To determine whether a similar growth inhibitor might be produced by endothelial cells from the pulmonary arteries, we assessed smooth muscle cell growth in medium conditioned by pulmonary arterial endothelium (1). After 6 days, the DNA content of sparsely plated smooth muscle cell cultures grown in medium conditioned by endothelial cells was only 53 percent of that in control cultures grown in unconditioned medium. Repletion experiments indicated that these effects were not due to depletion of medium or serum components. The growth inhibiting activity of endothelium-conditioned medium was not reduced after treatment with *Streptomyces* protease (Pronase®) and resisted digestion by chondroitinase, which digests chrondroitin sulfate and dermatan sulfate glycosaminoglycans, but does not affect heparan sulfate glycosaminoglycans, including heparin (Fig. 4). Growth inhibition was markedly reduced after treatment of protease-digested conditioned medium with heparinase or with nitrous acid, which both selectively cleave heparan sulfate glycosaminoglycans at glycosidic

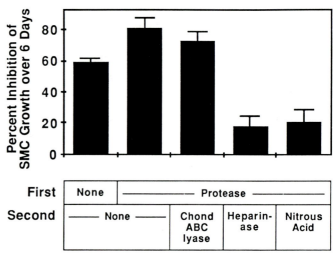

Treatment of EC-Conditioned Medium

Figure 4: The endothelial cell-derived growth inhibitor resists destruction by protease, boiling, and chondroitin ABC lyase, but is destroyed by nitrous acid. The upper panel shows the percent inhibition of smooth muscle cell (SMC) growth (as defined in Methods and Materials) by media prepared as indicated in the lower panel. SMC growth in conditioned medium is indicated by solid bars; growth in control medium is indicated by open bars. The inhibitory effects of EC-conditioned medium on SMC growth were increased by protease digestion ($p < 0.01$) and reduced by treatment with either heparinase ($p < 0.005$) or nitrous acid ($p < 0.005$). Treatment with chondroitin ABC lyase did not alter the effects of protease-treated conditioned medium on SMC growth.

bonds adjacent to sulfaminoglucose residues. Therefore, endothelial cells cultured from the pulmonary arteries of near-term bovine fetuses produce a heparin-like inhibitor of smooth muscle cell growth.

To characterize this growth inhibitor, conditioned medium was fractionated by cesium chloride buoyant density gradient ultracentrifugation under dissociative conditions (Fig. 5). This procedure allows separation of free glycosaminoglycan chains, which have a buoyant density greater than 1.6 g/ml, from glycosaminoglycans that are constituents of proteoglycans, in which they are attached to a low buoyant density core protein that confers a lower overall density upon the molecule. Thus, if the heparin-like growth inhibitor produced by cultured endothelium is a free heparan sulfate chain, it should be recovered only from the highest density fractions (pool I, Fig. 5) from the buoyant density gradient. When the fractions from these gradients are pooled and reconstituted for assay for growth inhibiting activity, only the *lowest* density fractions (pool IV) inhibited smooth muscle growth (Fig. 5). This result implies that the heparan sulfate chains that are responsible for the growth-inhibiting activity of medium conditioned by endothelial cells are present only as constituents of a low density proteoglycan, and few, if any, are present as free glycosaminoglycan chains.

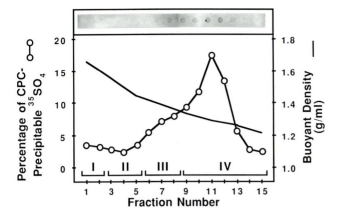

Figure 5: Buoyant density fractionation of endothelial cell-conditioned medium. EC-conditioned medium was fractionated by cesium chloride gradient ultracentrifugation, which yielded fractions ranging in buoyant density (—) from 1.2 to 1.7 g/ml. Cetylpyridinium chloride (CPC)-precipitable radioactivity (○) in conditioned medium was recovered predominantly in a peak of median buoyant density 1.3 g/ml. Little radioactivity was recovered in the high density fraction s(>1.6 g/ml), indicating that little free glycosaminoglycan was present. Immunodot assay of these fractions (upper panel) demonstrated that material which reacts with antiserum against low density basement membrane heparan sulfate proteoglycan of the Englebreth-Holm-Swarm tumor codistributed with the radiosulfate-labelled material of modal buoyant density 1.3 g/ml.

The low density pool prepared from the cesium chloride gradients (pool IV) was then digested with chondroitinase to remove contaminating chondroitin sulfates. Gel filtration chromatography on Sepharose CL-4B indicated that the remaining heparan sulfate had a relative mass of approximately 1 million daltons. After alkaline treatment under reducing conditions, which cleaves the xylose-serine linkage that attaches the glycosaminoglycan chains to the core protein, the free heparan sulfate chains were found to have a relative mass of 60,000 to 70,000 daltons, confirming our suspicion that the inhibitory material was a proteoglycan. These glycosaminoglycan chains were extensively digested by treatment with nitrous acid, indicating that this material was, in fact, heparan sulfate. These results indicate that the heparin-like inhibitor of smooth muscle cell proliferation which is produced by endothelial cells from the pulmonary arteries is a heparan sulfate proteoglycan of low buoyant density (1.3 g/ml) and overall MW approximately 10^6 daltons, with heparan sulfate chains of MW 60,000 to 70,000.

The characteristics of this heparan sulfate proteoglycan are quite similar to those of the prototypic basement membrane heparan sulfate proteoglycan produced by the Englebreth-Holm-Swarm tumor (14), which is also of low buoyant density, has an overall MW of approximately 750,000 daltons and heparan sulfate chains of MW 60,000 to 70,000. In addition, antibody raised against the prototypic basement membrane proteoglycan (provided by Dr. John Hassell, National Institutes of Dental Research) reacted with the proteoglycan in the low density fractions of endothelium-conditioned medium (Fig. 5). These results indicate that the growth inhibitor produced by the pulmonary arterial endothelium has the characteristics of a basement membrane heparan sulfate proteoglycan. The location of this putative endogenous heparin-like inhibitor of smooth muscle cell proliferation in the endothelial basement membrane places it in a strategic position to act as a regulator of the behavior of medial smooth muscle cells.

Regulation of Production of Heparan Sulfate by Endothelial Cells

It is well established that heparan sulfate proteoglycans are produced by endothelial cells in vitro and are present in the arterial intima and media in vivo. Material which stains with antibody raised against the Englebreth-Holm-Swarm tumor basement is present in the endothelial basement membrane and extracellular matrix of the arterial media in vivo, and has been identified in the matrix produced by cultured endothelial cells. However, the factors which might affect production of this material have been less extensively studied. Kinsella and Wight (17) have shown that postconfluent monolayers of bovine aortic endothelial cells produce predominantly (approximately 80 percent of total proteoglycan) heparan sulfate proteoglycan. After these monolayers are wounded, they produce more chondroitin sulfate proteoglycan (up to 60 percent of the total). This increased production of chondroitin sulfate proteoglycan has been associated with migration of the endothelial cells into the wounded areas of the dish. Humphries et al. (16) have found that pulmonary arterial endothelial cells release only 62 percent as much heparan sulfate into culture medium when grown in 3 percent oxygen ($P_{O_2} \approx 22$ mmHg) as when cultured in 20 percent oxygen ($P_{O_2} \approx 145$ mmHg), suggesting that hypoxia might reduce production of the heparan sulfate inhibitor of smooth muscle cell growth which we identified in medium conditioned by pulmonary arterial cells. Production of heparan sulfate by these cells is markedly reduced after these cells undergo a phenotypic change from the "cobblestone" monolayer typical of early passage cultures to the "sprouting" morphology of late passage cultures, in which the cells become elongated, overlap, and fail to form the close lateral adhesions typical of early passage cultures (18). These observations suggest that reduced synthesis of heparan sulfate proteoglycan, which may be accompanied by increased production of chondroitin proteoglycan, may be a characteristic endothelial cell response to injury.

THE ROLE OF HEPARIN-LIKE COMPOUNDS IN PULMONARY HYPERTENSION

A Proposed Model

Endothelial cell swelling and disruption of the endothelial basement membrane are prominent features of the pulmonary arterial injury induced by hypobaric hypoxia (380 mmHg; Pa_{O_2} 40 mmHg) (20). The latter may result in loss of basement membrane heparan sulfate proteoglycan from the arterial intima. If endothelial cell injury is associated with decreased production of the basement membrane heparan sulfate proteoglycan as the reports of others (16,17) and our preliminary results suggest, replacement of this material may also be impaired. In the absence of this growth-inhibiting material, medial smooth muscle cells would readily respond to mitogens and chemotactic agents present in the plasma or released locally by adherent platelets, endothelial cells, monocytes, or perhaps other cells. The resulting migration of smooth muscle cells into smaller, normally nonmuscular arteries and proliferation of smooth muscle cells in those vessels, as well as in the larger, muscular arteries, would lead to the increased muscularity of the pulmonary arteries which is typical of chronic pulmonary hypertension. The observations that heparin, presumably acting in the stead of the missing or deficient basement membrane heparan sulfate, can inhibit both the pulmonary arterial remodeling and the hemodynamic effects of chronic hypoxia in mice (13) indicates that such a scenario is at least plausible. Pulmonary hypertension due to causes other than chronic hypoxia might also be mediated, at least in part, by altered production of the growth-inhibiting basement membrane proteoglycan by endothelial cells.

Clinical Implications

The most immediate clinical implications of the observation that heparin inhibits proliferation of pulmonary arterial smooth muscle cells both in vitro (2) and in vivo (13), and that this is associated with amelioration of the hemodynamic consequences of chronic hypoxia (13), relate to the promise of effective therapy for this condition. However, a number of problems must be resolved before this becomes a reality. First, it is obviously impractical to subject patients with pulmonary hypertension to long-term treatment with anticoagulant doses of heparin. If non-anticoagulant heparin is also effective in inhibiting pulmonary arterial remodeling, as would be predicted if the effects on pulmonary arterial structure are mediated by effects on smooth muscle cell proliferation, this problem could be avoided by use of non-anticoagulant heparins for this treatment. Preparation of non-anticoagulant heparin by affinity chromatography on antithrombin III columns may be difficult to adapt for preparation of the large quantities of heparin which would be required. Fortunately, Castellot et al. (4) have shown that N-desulfation followed by N-acetylation of porcine intestinal heparin results in complete loss of anticoagulant activity, while reducing antiproliferative activity only slightly. Because these are chemical procedures, they promise to be more readily adaptable to preparation of non-anticoagulant heparins on a pharmacologic scale. In addition, problems in drug delivery and potential adverse effects of long-term treatment remain to be addressed.

Perhaps the most difficult issue raised by the potential development of non-anticoagulant heparin therapy is one of timely diagnosis. Presently, pulmonary hypertension is rarely, if ever, diagnosed before pulmonary arterial remodeling is already advanced. It is not known whether treatment with antiproliferative heparin would be able to reverse these changes even partially. Therefore, appropriate strategies will have to be developed for anticipatory treatment of patients in whom the development of pulmonary hypertension is predictable, such as those with uncorrectable cyanotic heart disease or cystic fibrosis, with the objective of preventing or ameliorating this complication. However, for patients with primary pulmonary hypertension, the strategy will have to rest on early diagnosis, if possible, and pharmacologic therapy to prevent or retard progression of the disease.

The greatest clinical benefits to come from these studies may be less direct. If additional work should establish the validity of the etiopathogenetic model outlined above, or of a similar model based upon the cellular and biochemical processes that mediate the structural changes that accompany pulmonary hypertension, a fresh conceptual framework will have been provided for reorganizing our understanding and management of pulmonary arterial hypertension.

REFERENCES

1. Benitz WE, Kelley RT, Bernfield M: The endothelial cell-derived inhibitor of smooth muscle cell growth is a basement membrane heparan sulfate proteoglycan. J Cell Biol (Abstract, in press).

2. Benitz WE, Lessler DS, Coulson JD, Bernfield M: Heparin inhibits proliferation of fetal vascular smooth muscle cells in the absence of platelet-derived growth factor. J Cell Physiol 127:1–7, 1986.

3. Castellot JJ, Addonizio ML, Rosenberg R, Karnovsky MJ: Cultured endothelial cells produce a heparinlike inhibitor of smooth muscle cell growth. J Cell Biol 90:372–379, 1981.

4. Castellot JJ, Beeler DL, Rosenberg RD, Karnovsky MJ: Structural determinants of the capacity of heparin to inhibit the proliferation of vascular smooth muscle cells. J Cell Biol 102:315–320, 1984.

5. Castellot JJ, Choay J, Lormeau JC, Petitou M, Sache E, Karnovsky MJ: Structural determinants of the capacity of heparin to inhibit the proliferation of vascular smooth muscle cells. II. Evidence for a pentasaccharide sequence that contains a 3-O-sulfate group. J Cell Biol 102:1979–1984, 1986.

6. Castellot JJ, Favreau LV, Karnovsky MJ, Rosenberg R: Inhibition of vascular smooth muscle cell growth by endothelial cell-derived heparin: Possible role of a platelet-derived endoglycosidase. J Biol Chem 257:11256–11260, 1982.

7. Castellot JJ, Wong K, Herman B, Hoover RL, Albertini DF, Wright TC, Caleb BL, Karnovsky MJ: Binding and internalization of heparin by vascular smooth muscle cells. J Cell Physiol 124:13–20, 1985.

8. Choay J, Lormeau JC, Petitou M, Sinay P, Fareed J: Structural studies of a biologically active hexasaccharide obtained from heparin. Ann NY Acad Sci 370:644–649, 1981.

9. Clowes AW, Clowes MM: Kinetics of cellular proliferation after arterial injury IV. Heparin inhibits rat smooth muscle mitogenesis and migration. Circ Res 58:839–845, 1986.

10. Clowes AW, Karnovsky MJ: Suppression by heparin of smooth muscle cell proliferation in injured arteries. Nature 256:625–626, 1977.

11. Fritze LMS, Reilly CF, Rosenberg RD: An antiproliferative heparan sulfate species produced by postconfluent smooth muscle cells. J Cell Biol 100:1041–1049, 1985.

12. Guyton JR, Rosenberg RD, Clowes AW, Karnovsky MJ: Inhibition of rat arterial smooth muscle cell proliferation by heparin: In vivo studies with anticoagulant and nonanticoagulant heparin. Circ Res 46:624–634, 1980.

13. Hales CA, Kradin RL, Brandstetter RD, Zhu YJ: Impairment of hypoxic pulmonary artery remodeling by heparin in mice. Am Rev Respir Dis 128:747–751, 1983.

14. Hassell JR, Leyshon WC, Ledbetter SR, Tyree B, Suzuki S, Kato M, Kimata K, Kleinman HK: Isolation of two forms of basement membrane proteoglycans. J Biol Chem 260:8098–8105, 1985.

15. Hoover RL, Rosenberg RD, Haering W, Karnovsky MJ: Inhibition of rat smooth muscle cell proliferation II: In vitro studies. Circ Res 47:578–583, 1980.

16. Humphries DE, Lee SL, Fanburg BL, Silbert JE: Effect of hypoxia and hyperoxia on proteoglycan production by bovine pulmonary artery endothelial cells. J Cell Physiol 126:249–253, 1986.

17. Kinsella MG, Wight TN: Modulation of sulfated proteoglycan synthesis by bovine aortic endothelial cells during migration. J Cell Biol 102:679–687, 1986.

18. Oohira A, Wight TN, Bornstein P: Sulfated proteoglycans synthesized by vascular endothelium in culture. J Biol Chem 258:2014–2021, 1983.

19. Poole AR: Proteoglycans in health and disease: Structures and functions. Biochem J 236:1–14, 1986.

20. Reid L, Meyrick B: Hypoxia and pulmonary vascular endothelium, in *Metabolic Activities of the Lung* (Ciba Foundation Symposium 78). Amsterdam, Excerpta Medica, 1980, pp 37–61.

21. Reilly CF, Fritze LMS, Rosenberg RD: Heparin inhibition of smooth muscle cell proliferation: A cellular site of action. J Cell Physiol 129:11–19, 1986.

22. Reilly CF, Fritze LMS, Rosenberg RD: Antiproliferative effects of heparin on vascular smooth muscle cells are reversed by epidermal growth factor. J Cell Physiol 131:140–157, 1987.

Steven M. Albelda, M.D.

15

Role of Growth Factors in Pulmonary Hypertension

Pulmonary hypertension is the end result of a large group of diseases that affect the pulmonary circulation and the lungs (16). Regardless of cause, sustained pulmonary hypertension is associated with proliferative lesions in the distal arterial tree. The proliferative lesions affect intima or media, often both, almost invariably in the small to medium-sized arterial resistance vessels of the lung. A common denominator in these proliferative lesions is an increase in the numbers of cells in the vessel walls. Although medial hypertrophy involves primarily smooth muscle cells, the identities of the cells that comprise the intimal lesions are less clear and probably include endothelial cells and fibroblasts as well as smooth muscle cells. Since an increase in the number of vessel wall cells is such a prominent part of the pathology of pulmonary hypertension, an understanding of the factors that regulate the proliferation of these cells is central to an understanding of the pathogenesis of this syndrome.

The process of cellular proliferation begins when a cell is stimulated to move from a resting state into the reproductive cell cycle. Although the regulation of this process is complex and not completely understood, some of the factors that control cell proliferation have been identified: neural signals, contacts with other cells, interaction with the cell's underlying substratum, and a variety of soluble chemical messages that can both stimulate (growth factors) or inhibit (growth inhibitors) cell proliferation (22). This chapter deals with the possible role of soluble agents in the development of pulmonary hypertension.

GROWTH FACTORS

Two major categories of growth factors relevant to pulmonary hypertension are currently under investigation: polypeptide growth factors and the cytokines. Although other growth factors may also be involved, less is known about these agents.

Polypeptide Growth Factors

The polypeptide growth factors represent the largest and best understood group of mediators that stimulate cell proliferation. They are a rather diverse group of small proteins that share the ability to trigger cellular division by transmitting signals from the extracellular environment into the cell nucleus (22). All of the polypeptide growth factors exert their effects by binding tightly to highly specific receptors for growth factors on the surface of target cells. This growth factor-receptor complex triggers a complicated, and only partially understood, system of amplifiers and second messsages. The cellular transduction pathways are similar for many of the growth factors; specificity in the system is provided by the initial interaction of the growth factor with its receptor. Another common feature of the polypeptide growth factors is that they are ultimately internalized into the cell after binding to their receptors and thereby inactivated.

Among the first polypeptide growth factors to be discovered and characterized were epidermal growth factor and nerve growth factor. In more than 30 years since these discoveries, a large number of other polypeptide growth factors with a wide variety of cellular specificities have been discovered and characterized.

TABLE 1 POLYPEPTIDE GROWTH FACTORS POTENTIALLY IMPORTANT IN PULMONARY HYPERTENSION

Growth factor	Size (kD)	Sources	Actions	Vascular target cells
Platelet-derived growth factor (PDGF)	30	Platelets Endothelial cells Macrophages	↑ Proliferation Chemotactic	Smooth muscle cells Fibroblasts
Fibroblast growth factors (FGFs)	16	Pituitary Brain	↑ Proliferation Angiogenic	Endothelial cells Smooth muscle cells Fibroblasts
Insulin-like growth factor-1 (IGF-1)	7.6	Plasma Liver Fibroblasts Macrophages	↑ Proliferation	Endothelial cells Smooth muscle cells Fibroblasts
Epidermal growth factor	5.7	Salivary glands Platelets	↑ Proliferation Chemotactic Vasoconstriction	Endothelial cells Smooth muscle cells Fibroblasts
Transforming growth factor-α (TGF-α)	5–20	Transformed cells Macrophages Epithelial cells	↑ Proliferation Chemotactic Vasoconstriction	Endothelial cells Smooth muscle cells Fibroblasts
Transforming growth factor-β (TGF-β)	25	Platelets Bone	Variable effect on proliferation depending on cell type (see text)	Endothelial cells Smooth muscle cells Fibroblasts

Among these are peptides that stimulate the proliferation of myeloid cells (colony stimulating factors), lymphoid cells (interleukin 1 and 2), and neural cells (nerve growth factor).

The polypeptide growth factors that are most likely to be important in the development of pulmonary hypertension are those with an ability to influence proliferation of the cells of the vessel wall, i.e., endothelial cells, smooth muscle cells, and fibroblasts. The most important members of this group include (1) platelet-derived growth factor (PDGF), (2) the fibroblast growth factors (FGFs), (3) insulin-like growth factor 1 (IGF-1), (4) epidermal growth factor (EGF), (5) transforming growth factor alpha (TGF-α), and (6) transforming growth factor beta (TGF-β) (see Table 1).

MECHANISM OF ACTION OF THE POLYPEPTIDE GROWTH FACTORS

Even though the detailed mechanism of action of each growth factor probably differs slightly, platelet-derived growth factor (PDGF), which causes the proliferation of smooth muscle cells and fibroblasts (see below), is a prototypical example of how the polypeptide growth factors might exert their effects (33). Like all the polypeptide growth factors, PDGF must first bind to a specific receptor on an appropriate target cell. The activated PDGF receptor then triggers a number of cellular events which include changes in intracellular pH and activation of the arachidonic acid cascade (34) (Fig. 1). Although these responses undoubtedly play a role in signal transduction, it appears that the most powerful mitogenic signals

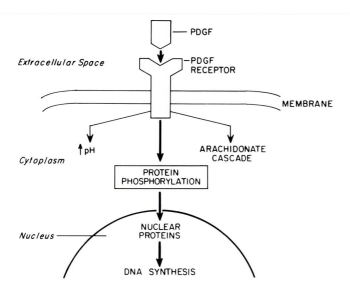

Figure 1: The mechanism of action of polypeptide growth factors. The polypeptide growth factor, platelet-derived growth factor (PDGF), exerts its mitogenic effects by first binding to a specific membrane bound receptor. This complex then triggers a number of intracellular events including a fall in cytoplasmic pH, activation of the arachidonate cascade, and phosphorylation of certain cytoplasmic proteins. These phosphorylated proteins appear to carry signals into the nucleus where specific nuclear regulatory proteins are quickly produced. The nuclear proteins then direct the new DNA synthesis required for cellular proliferation.

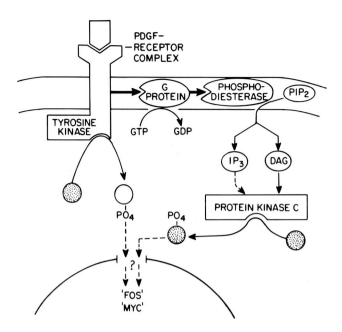

Figure 2: Phosphorylation pathways triggered in polypeptide growth factor action. Two main pathways for protein phosphorylation are triggered by the binding of a polypeptide growth factor such as platelet-derived growth factor (PDGF) to its receptor. First, the receptor, itself, undergoes a conformational change so that it becomes capable of phosphorylating proteins containing tyrosine residues (tyrosine kinase activity). Second, the receptor activates a membrane bound GTP-binding (G) protein which, in turn, activates a membrane bound phosphodiesterase. This enzyme cleaves a membrane lipid, phosphatidylinositol bisphosphate (PIP_2), into two molecules, diacylglycerol (DAG) and inositol 1,4,5-trisphosphate (IP_3). DAG, in conjunction with calcium ions released by IP_3, activates protein kinase C. The yet to be identified phosphorylated cytoplasmic proteins trigger the production of nuclear regulatory proteins such as 'fos' and 'myc' which then bind to specific regions of DNA and thus regulate gene transcription.

are generated by the activation of two enzymes called protein kinases (20). Protein kinases function by adding phosphate groups to the serine, threonine, or tyrosine residues of proteins. These phosphorylation reactions are important regulators of a variety of cytoplasmic protein functions. Some of these phosphorylated cytoplasmic proteins appear to carry into the nucleus the signals required for cell division.

The first kinase pathway involves the phosphorylation of tyrosine residues. After growth factor is bound at the cell surface, a change occurs in the conformation of the receptor and the cytoplasmic portion of the molecule becomes an enzymatically-active tyrosine kinase. This activated enzyme then phosphorylates the cytoplasmic protein(s) that communicates the growth signal to the nucleus (20). Identification of the proteins that are phosphorylated and how they act is currently an area of intense research. In addition, the PDGF receptor also phosphorylates a tyrosine residue on itself (autophosphorylation) that may play a role in the subsequent internalization and inactivation of the receptor.

The other important kinase pathway involves protein kinase C, an enyzme that also phosphorylates cytoplasmic proteins which, in turn, trigger a wide variety of effects including cell division, cell differentiation, the release of various cell products, cell contraction, and modulation of cellular ion pumps (25). Tumor-promoting phorbol esters act by directly stimulating protein kinase C. In contrast to the intrinsic tyrosine kinase activity demonstrated by the activated growth factor receptor, stimulation of protein kinase C involves the generation of second messages. After binding growth factor, the receptor activates a regulatory protein that requires binding of guanosine triphosphate (GTP); this protein has been designated a G protein (a similar G protein is involved in the signal transduction pathway of the beta adrenergic receptor). The activated G protein then triggers a membrane-bound phosphodiesterase to cleave the membrane lipid phosphatidylinositol bisphosphate into two molecules, one of which, diacylglycerol, in conjunction with calcium ions, activates protein kinase C (Fig. 2).

The cytoplasmic events that occur after the activation of tyrosine kinase and protein kinase C are not well understood. However, something is known about some of the early nuclear events that are triggered by these phosphorylation reactions. A number of nuclear proteins seem to be critical for the ability of the cell to replicate. The two best understood are named the "myc" protein and the "fos" protein after the oncogenes which led to their identification (13). The messenger RNA which codes for these proteins appears inside the cell within minutes after stimulation by an appropriate growth factor. Although the precise function of these proteins is not known, they appear to bind to DNA and, somehow, to regulate gene transcription.

In summary, growth factors are external messages that are transduced to signals that trigger cell proliferation (Fig. 2). They work by binding to specific receptors on the cell surface. These growth factor-receptor complexes either phosphorylate directly the tyrosine residues of certain cytoplasmic proteins or activate GTP-binding proteins which initiate the cleavage of membrane phosphatidylinositols; the latter, in turn, increase the intracellular concentration of calcium and activate protein kinase C. The phosphorylated cytoplasmic proteins trigger synthesis of certain regulatory proteins in the nucleus which then direct the cell to replicate.

SPECIFIC POLYPEPTIDE GROWTH FACTORS POTENTIALLY INVOLVED IN PULMONARY HYPERTENSION

A variety of growth factors could be involved in the pathogenesis of pulmonary hypertension (Table 1).

Platelet-Derived Growth Factor (PDGF). Platelet-derived growth factor is a highly cationic polypeptide with a molecular weight of about 30 kilodaltons. It consists of two chains (an A and B chain) and is active either as a homo- or heterodimer. PDGF is a major mitogen for connective tissue cells (i.e., smooth muscle cells and fibroblasts) but has no effect on endothelial cells that lack the PDGF receptor (33). PDGF displays a variety of effects that suggest it may also be important as an inflammatory mediator (12). In addition to its ability to stimulate the proliferation of mesenchymal cells, PDGF is chemotactic for fibroblasts, smooth muscle cells, neutrophils and monocytes, can stimulate collagen and collagenase production by fibroblasts, and is a potent vasoconstrictor (3).

The primary source of PDGF is the platelet, where it is released from granules after platelet stimulation. Therefore, PDGF is of major importance in vascular injury that is associated with thrombosis. In addition to its release by platelets, PDGF or PDGF-like molecules can also be released by macrophages and endothelial cells (12,33). The regulation of PDGF secretion by endothelial cells appears to be complex, but secretion can be stimulated by mediators such as endotoxin, interleukin 1, and thrombin or inhibited by agents such as beta-adrenergic agonists or fish oils (1). Perhaps important with respect to the development of pulmonary hypertension is the hypothesis that almost any form of endothelial cell "injury" can trigger release of PDGF-like molecules (33).

Fibroblast Growth Factors (FGFs). The FGFs are protein mitogens with a molecular weight of 16 kD that induce proliferation of a wide range of cells in culture (2,36). One important property of this group of growth factors is their ability to bind tightly to heparin (17,41). There are two distinct forms of FGFs, differentiated by their isoelectric points: one has a pI of 9 to 10 and is called basic FGF; the other has a pI of 5 and is called acidic FGF. The amino acid sequences of these two FGFs are about 55 percent homologous. However, they bind to the same high affinity receptor.

The designation "fibroblast growth factor" is somewhat of a misnomer because, in addition to their mitogenic effects on fibroblasts, these polypeptides are powerful stimulators of most nonterminally differentiated cells including endothelial cells, smooth muscle cells, epithelial cells, chondrocytes, osteoblasts, and glial cells (19,36). Moreover, they appear to be important in embryonic development and angiogenesis. Both FGFs form complexes with heparin or the naturally occurring, basement membrane component, heparan sulfate. Although this association has little effect on the activity of basic FGF, the activity of acidic FGF is enhanced 30- to 100-fold by heparin binding, apparently due to the ability of heparin to prevent the rapid inactivation of acidic FGF that would otherwise occur (36).

The physiological role of the FGFs remains somewhat of a mystery. They are present in high concentration in brain and pituitary extracts but are not detectable in blood or in platelets (2). The mRNAs coding for the FGFs have been found widely distributed among tissues, most notably in capillary endothelial cells. The significance of these findings is clouded by the fact that the FGFs lack the classical hydrophobic leader sequences for cellular excretion. Therefore, the mechanism by which these proteins are released from cells is not obvious. Interestingly, basic FGF binds to the extracellular matrix (ECM) of endothelial cells. It is postulated that the FGFs are released by injured and/or dying cells and then bind to the underlying ECM where they stimulate the proliferation of other cells (2).

Insulin-like Growth Factor 1 (IGF-1). Insulin-like growth factor 1 (also called somatomedin C) is a 7.6-kD, single-chain, nonglycosylated polypeptide composed of 70 amino acids (35). Unlike many of the other growth factors, it is present in significant quantities in plasma and is released from the liver under the control of growth hormone: IGF-1 levels are low in hypopituitarism and increased in acromegaly. At high concentrations, insulin can bind to and activate the IGF-1 receptor, thus accounting for some of its growth stimulatory properties. IGF-1 stimulates the proliferation of a variety of mesenchymal cell types including fibroblasts, smooth muscle cells, and endothelial cells (19,39).

In addition to the circulating form of IGF-1, other higher molecular mass forms of IGF-1, the so-called "tissue IGF-1s," also exist (8,32). These molecules are released from fibroblasts after stimulation by growth factors such as PDGF and by alveolar macrophages after stimulation by particulates or cytokines.

Epidermal Growth Factor (EGF). Epidermal growth factor is a small (5.7 kD) protein that was one of the first growth factors isolated. It is identical to the gastric acid-inhibiting beta-urogastrone and is related to the tumor produced TGF-α (see below) (9). EGF is mitogenic for most cell types including epithelial cells, endothelial cells, smooth muscle cells, and fibroblasts (9,19,39). Like many of the other growth factors, it is a chemoattractant for leukocytes. In addition, EGF may also function as a vasoconstrictor for smooth muscle cells (4).

EGF was originally isolated from salivary glands where it is present in high concentrations. EGF is also found in high concentrations in platelet granules along with PDGF and TGF-β (26). Levels in the plasma are low and arise from this platelet source.

Transforming Growth Factor-α (TGF-α). Transforming growth factor-α is a secreted mitogen originally detected in the culture supernatants of transformed rodent fibroblasts (11,24). Secreted TGF-α exists as multiple species ranging from 5 to 20 kD. The smallest form (50 amino acids) shares about 30 percent structural homology with EGF. All forms of TGF-α bind the same cell-surface receptor as epidermal growth factor and, therefore, stimulate the proliferation of epithelial cells, fibroblasts, smooth muscle cells, and endothelial cells.

TGF-α has been identified in the culture supernatants of virally transformed cells, human tumor cell lines, human keratinocytes, and activated human macrophages (11).

Transforming Growth Factor-β (TGF-β). This is a homodimeric peptide with a molecular weight of 25 kD. Originally isolated by virtue of its ability to induce the phenotypic transformation of normal indicator cells (in combination with TGF-α), its activities have proved to be protean (31). One interesting feature of the action of TGF-β is the multifunctional nature of its effects; depending on ambient conditions, TGF-β can act either to stimulate or to inhibit cellular proliferation, differentiation, and function. Therefore, the activity of the peptide is not intrinsic to the factor but dependent on the cellular environment.

In terms of blood vessels, TGF-β is generally growth inhibitory toward endothelial cells in vitro (18,19). However, the peptide is strongly angiogenic in vivo (31). The ability of TGF-β to attract macrophages, which in turn release a number of angiogenic factors, may account for the differences observed in the in vitro versus in vivo activities. TGF-β has only a slight stimulatory effect (10 to 15 percent) on the proliferation of smooth muscle cells (19) but can markedly stimulate proteoglycan synthesis in these cells. The effect on fibroblasts is multifaceted: even though TGF-β is a chemotactic for fibroblasts and increases the accumulation of matrix proteins, such as collagen and fibronectin, it seems to be growth inhibitory (31). Sorting out a physiologic importance has proved to be more complex for TGF-β than for any other growth factor.

The primary sources of TGF-β are platelets and bone. Most of the TGF-β released from platelet granules is in a biologically inactive form that must be activated for it to interact with its receptor; this activation can be accomplished by changes in pH or by limited proteolysis. Since the TGF-β receptor is essentially universally expressed, in vivo activation at sites of inflammation may represent an important control mechanism (38).

Cytokines

Stimulation of immune cells in a variety of ways causes them to release soluble proteins called "cytokines." Although many of the cytokines are not growth factors in the traditional sense, they do effect cell proliferation, either directly or by attracting and stimulating the release of growth factors from other cells. With respect to the vascular wall, the three best characterized cytokines are interleukin-1 (IL-1), tumor necrosis factor (TNF), and gamma-interferon.

INTERLEUKIN-1 (IL-1)

Interleukin-1 was originally described as a T-cell co-stimulator molecule. However, this molecule has proved to have multiple pro-inflammatory effects including endogenous pyrogen activity, stimulation of neutrophils from bone marrow, promotion of acute phase reactants in the blood, and activation of white blood cells (27). IL-1 triggers the expression of procoagulant activity on endothelial cells as well as promoting the synthesis of proteins that make the endothelial cell more "sticky" for circulating leukocytes (10). In addition, after the confounding effects of IL-1 stimulated release of inhibitory prostaglandins is blocked, IL-1 stimulates the growth of smooth muscle cells and fibroblasts in vitro (23).

TUMOR NECROSIS FACTOR (TNF)

Tumor necrosis factor-α (also known as "cachectin") is a 17-kD polypeptide released from macrophages, that possesses a wide range of pro-inflammatory activities (5). A molecule with similar activities, called TNF-β or lymphotoxin, is secreted by activated lymphocytes. In addition to their ability to inhibit the growth of certain tumor cells, these cytokines also exert profound effects on lipid metabolism and are endogenous pyrogens, activators of leukocytes, and stimulators of endothelial cell-mediated adhesion of white blood cells. The effects of TNF on normal cells in culture depends on the cell type: by itself, TNF is a weak stimulator of fibroblast proliferation; however, the combinations of TNF and gamma-interferon or TNF and interleukin-1 act synergistically to inhibit lung fibroblast proliferation (14). TNF is a potent inhibitor of endothelial cell growth in vitro, although it is angiogenic in vivo. As in the case of TGF-β, this is probably a result of an intense inflammatory response induced by TNF that causes the release of angiogenic factors from the newly recruited, activated leukocytes.

GAMMA-INTERFERON

Gamma-interferon is a small glycopeptide released from lymphocytes stimulated by antigens or plant lectins. It has a broad range of immunomodulatory and antiproliferative effects (6). In general, gamma-interferon inhibits the proliferation of a number of cell types in vitro, including fibroblasts and endothelial cells; however, culture conditions can modify this effect. Although the mechanism responsible for the inhibition is unknown, it does not appear to be due to the induction of the production of cellular prostaglandins by the cells. The in vivo effects of gamma-interferon on cell proliferation are again complicated by its powerful immune stimulatory activity which results in the concomitant release of a number of macrophage products.

Other Growth Factors

A number of other factors that stimulate the growth of mesenchymal cells may play a role in the development of pulmonary hypertension. The protease thrombin, produced in the activation of the coagulation cascade, can serve as a mitogen for both fibroblasts and endothelial cells (29,39). This activity does not appear to be linked to its protease activity since enzymatically inactive forms of thrombin still induce cell proliferation (39). The action of thrombin establishes another link between coagulation and proliferation.

Although angiotensin II, a powerful vasoconstrictor, has been found by some to be mitogenic for smooth muscle cells, others are not convinced. The concept that angiotensin is also a growth factor received support from the discovery that the "mas" oncogene, which can cause transformation of 3T3 cells and tumors in nude mice, encodes an angiotensin receptor (21).

The effects of arachidonic acid metabolites on cell proliferation are complex. While the direct effect of most prostaglandins (including PGE_1, PGE_2, and prostacyclin) are inhibitory to cell growth in vitro (15), the effect of these compounds in vivo is angiogenic (17). Again, this is likely due to recruitment of other inflammatory cells which then release a number of growth factors. In contrast to the inhibitory effects of prostaglandins, the possibility has been raised that leukotrienes stimulate proliferation of smooth muscle cells (28).

Some corticosteroids, such as dexamethasone, play an important permissive role in cell proliferation, at least in serum-free cell culture systems (29). In contrast, other steroids, such as tetrahydrocortisol, a naturally occurring metabolite of cortisone, inhibit angiogenesis, especially in conjunction with heparin (17). In addition to these relatively well-described factors, there are probably many other important mediators of vascular cell wall proliferation that have yet to be characterized. For example, Vender et al. (37) have described a smooth muscle cell mitogen that is released by hypoxic endothelial cells and seems to be unrelated to other known agents that stimulate smooth muscle cell proliferation. As advances are made in cellular and molecular biology, other vascular mitogens will doubtlessly be uncovered.

GROWTH INHIBITORS

Less is known about agents that inhibit proliferation of cells in the vascular wall than about those that stimulate proliferation. As discussed above, a number of mediators that are angiogenic in vivo because of their ability to cause the release of growth factors from other cells are, per se, growth inhibitory. These include TGF-β, tumor necrosis factor, and the prostaglandins.

The best studied inhibitor of vascular growth is heparin (see chapter by Benitz). Heparin can inhibit the proliferation of vascular smooth muscle cells in cell culture and in animal models (7). Under certain culture conditions, heparin can also inhibit the growth of endothelial cells and fibroblasts. These inhibitory effects are shared by naturally occurring heparan sulfate proteoglycan. It has been postulated that heparan sulfate in the subendothelial basement membrane is important in keeping the underlying smooth muscle cells in a quiescent state (7). Loss of this membrane may allow smooth muscle cell proliferation. However, the effects of heparin may not be so straightforward: as mentioned above, heparin is very important in stabilizing the effects of acidic FGF; in this capacity, it is mitogenic for all vessel wall cells (36,41).

INTERACTIONS AMONG GROWTH FACTORS

A wide array of soluble factors can affect cell proliferation. Although some of the effects of these agents have been demonstrated in simplified tissue culture models, how these factors interact in vivo is far from clear.

A number of important types of interactions warrant consideration. To begin with, the progression of a cell from its resting (G_0) state into active mitosis is a multistep process that requires multiple activation signals. This process has been best studied using immortalized mouse 3T3 cells (a fibroblast-like cell) (30). These cells first seem to need a "competence" signal to move out of the resting G_0 state to a premitotic G_1 state; this signal could be provided by a number of growth factors such as PDGF, EGF, or FGF. After the action of the competence signal, a second signal or "progression" factor is required for the cell to move into a mitotic state; agents such as IGF-1 and insulin are progression factors. However, this paradigm is probably not strictly valid in normal human diploid cells. For example, human fibroblasts can be made to proliferate in the presence of only PDGF. This may be due to the ability of many cells to produce their own "progression" type factor (8). Nonetheless, certain combinations of growth factors are synergistic and optimal cell growth requires representatives from a number of classes of growth factors (29).

Another important consideration is that many growth factors behave differently depending on their environment. The best studied growth factor with this bifunctional type of behavior is TGF-β which can either stimulate or inhibit cell proliferation (31). Another example of the bifunctional activity of a growth regulating factor is that of heparin: although heparin, per se, is antimitogenic and leads to the inhibition of cell proliferation (best described for smooth muscle cells) (7), it can be extremely promitogenic in its capacity to bind and to stabilize acidic FGF (36).

One major theme that has appeared many times in this chapter is the balance between the direct action of a growth factor and its indirect effects. TGF-β and tumor necrosis factor provide good examples of this type of interaction. Although the direct effect of both TGF-β and TNF on endothelial cell growth is inhibitory, these factors are markedly angiogenic in vivo, probably due to their ability to recruit inflammatory cells which then release stimulatory factors (41).

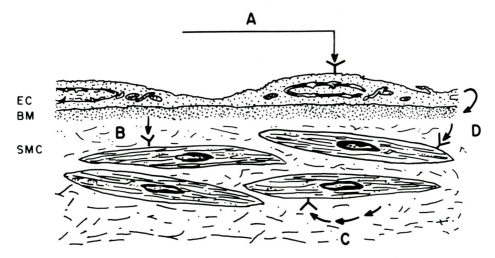

Figure 3: Delivery and sources of growth factors. There are four potential routes by which growth factors can be delivered to their vascular target cells: (A) Endocrine, (B) Paracrine, (C) Autocrine, and (D) "Crinopexy." EC = endothelial cell; BM = basement membrane; SMC = smooth muscle cell.

DELIVERY AND SOURCES OF GROWTH FACTORS

Many effects of a growth factor depend on how it is presented to its target tissue. Four potential mechanisms for growth factor delivery have been proposed (Fig. 3). For example, the growth factor, IGF-1, can be delivered by an endocrine route, i.e., the factor can be secreted at a distant site, enter the bloodstream, and be carried to a target cell. Certain other growth factors, such as PDGF, TGF-β, and EGF, are delivered by a paracrine system where they are released by one cell and act on another in close proximity. Recently, two other sources of growth factors have been described: "autocrine secretion" and "crinopexy." Autocrine secretion refers to the ability of a cell to secrete growth factors that cause auto-stimulation. This process may be relatively common in tumor cells and provide at least one explanation for their uncontrolled growth state. In addition, autocrine secretion of growth factors may also occur in normal, nonmalignant cells (33), e.g., under certain circumstances, smooth muscles cells seem to be able to secrete PDGF. "Crinopexy" (2) refers to a process that accounts for secretion and adherence of soluble factors into the extracellular matrix for stabilization and storage and may be most applicable in the case of basic FGF.

The role of the inflammatory process and the coagulation system in the delivery of growth factors should also be emphasized. Two of the most important sources of growth factors which act on the vascular wall are macrophages and platelets (41). Activated macrophages, a prominent part of the inflammatory response, have been shown to release a host of growth factors and growth regulating cytokines including interleukin-1, TGF-α, TNF, PDGF, FGF, and IGF-1 (32). Platelets are a rich source of PDGF, TGF-β, and EGF. In addition, the coagulation cascade generates thrombin which, along with its enzymatic actions, has growth promoting activity.

ROLE OF GROWTH FACTORS IN PULMONARY HYPERTENSION: A HYPOTHESIS

It is difficult to construct a hypothesis about the mechanism of development of pulmonary hypertension because pulmonary hypertension is not one disease, but a response to a variety of etiologies (16). One could conceive of at least three possible starting points (Fig. 4): (1) a mechanical stimulus to the vessel wall, as in high-pressure or flow-states; (2) a circulating factor or toxin that interacts with the pulmonary endothelial cell; and (3) an intrinsic change in the pulmonary endothelial cell that predisposes to a thrombotic or inflammatory reaction. All of these possibilities place major emphasis on the role of the pulmonary endothelial cell (Fig. 4).

A severe mechanical or toxic injury could cause frank endothelial cell damage leading to actual loss of vascular integrity (Fig. 4, pathway 1). Lysis of endothelial cells could lead to release of fibroblast growth factors; this damage would also expose the subendothelial matrix to circulating blood elements and result in platelet aggregation, thrombosis and/or the adhesion of white blood cells, and a subsequent inflammatory response. As discussed above, platelet aggregation and subsequent degranulation would release large amounts of PDGF, TGF-β, EGF, IGF-1, and thrombin close to the underlying pulmonary vascular smooth muscle cells, perhaps triggering intimal proliferation (41). The adherence of monocytes and lymphocytes to the exposed basement membrane and the movement of these cells into the vessel wall would provide another source of vascular growth factors. In addition, the activated white blood cells could release enzymes which might degrade the heparan sulfate proteoglycan present in the basement membrane resulting in a release of growth inhibition (7).

A more likely scenario may be a milder form of "injury" that does not actually disrupt the endothelial cell, but leads to a number of more subtle biological changes (Fig. 4, pathways 2 and 3). A number of agents, such as endotoxin, IL-1, and TNF, cause the normally inert endothelial cell to become "activated" (1,10,33). These activated cells express receptors for immunoglobulins, produce surface proteins that promote the adhesion of white blood cells and procoagulant activity, and secrete at least one growth factor, PDGF. Therefore, endothelial cell activation can be accompanied by an inflammatory response in which growth factors are secreted by the newly recruited white blood cells (pathway 2); or endothelial cell activation may be unaccompanied by any sort of inflammation (pathway 3). In the latter case, PDGF and other growth factors could be secreted as a direct response to perturbation. It is interesting to note that endothelial cells have been shown to respond to stimuli such as shear stress, stretch, and hypoxia.

Another way by which a similar cascade of events could be initiated is by some sort of intrinsic defect or abnormality of the endothelial cell. Patients with primary pulmonary hypertension may have pulmonary endothelial cells with a defect that predisposes toward thrombosis. This abnormality could result in microthrombus deposition in the pulmonary circulation, excessive release of platelet growth factors, and subsequent proliferative thrombotic lesions. Alternatively, there could be some sort of excess production of endothelial cell-derived growth factors, a tendency for white blood cells to adhere excessively, or a defect in heparan sulfate proteoglycan biosynthesis.

In any case, the end result of any of these pathways would be the excessive

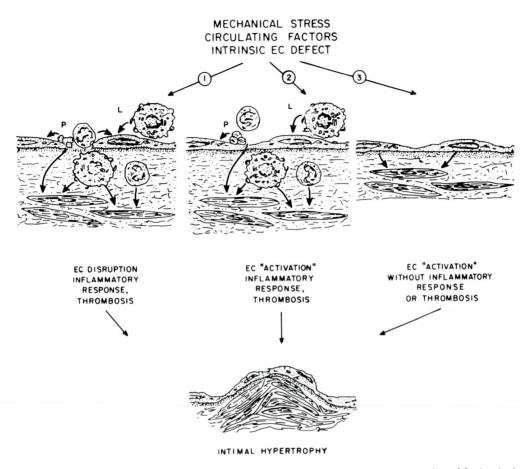

Figure 4: A hypothesis for the development of pulmonary hypertension. Mechanical stress, some sort of circulating factor, or an intrinsic endothelial cell defect begins the pathogenetic process. These perturbations can lead to endothelial cell (EC) and basement membrane (BM) disruption with subsequent adhesion of leukocytes (L) and platelets (P) (Pathway 1) or more subtle endothelial cell "activation". The activated endothelial cell either initiates a thrombotic and/or inflammatory response (Pathway 2) or releases growth factors without inflammation (Pathway 3). These growth factors stimulate the proliferation of EC and smooth muscle cells (SMC) ultimately leading to intimal hypertrophy.

release of growth factors. The proper combination of mitogens could then lead to a proliferation of smooth muscle cells, endothelial cells, and perhaps fibroblasts, ultimately leading to vascular wall hyperplasia.

CONCLUSIONS

It is potentially misleading to postulate etiology from histology because so many processes can lead to a final common pathologic pathway. Unfortunately, in the case of pulmonary hypertension, most of our information about the pathology of the disorder arises from such "end-stage" lungs. A number of other approaches may be helpful. Factors that activate or damage endothelial cells could be searched for in the serum of patients with primary pulmonary hypertension. Growth factor mRNAs could be identified in pulmonary vascular tissue by in situ hybridization techniques as has been described for atherosclerotic tissue (40). It would be extremely interesting to culture endothelial cells from patients with early primary disease to see if these cells have intrinsic abnormalities.

This chapter has reviewed a number of growth factors that might be involved in the proliferative responses that characterize pulmonary hypertension. The role played by each of these factors in the pathogenesis of pulmonary hypertension remains to be clarified.

REFERENCES

1. Albelda SM, Elias JA, Levine EM, Kern JA: Endotoxin stimulates platelet-derived growth factor-like production from cultured human adult pulmonary endothelial cells. Am J Physiol:Lung Cellular and Molecular Physiology, in press.

2. Baird A, Ueno N, Esch F, Ling N: Distribution of fibroblast growth factors (FGFs) in tissues and structure-function studies with synthetic fragments of basic FGF. J Cell Physiology 5: 101–106, 1987.

3. Berk BC, Alexander RW, Brock TA, Gimbrone MA Jr, Webb RC. Vasoconstriction: A new activity for platelet-derived growth factor. Science 232: 87–90, 1986.

4. Berk BC, Brock TA, Webb RC, Taubman MB, Atkinson WJ, Gimbrone MA Jr, Alexander RW: Epidermal growth factor, a vascular smooth muscle mitogen, induces rat aortic contraction. J Clin Invest 75: 1083–1086, 1985.

5. Beutler B, Cerami A: Cachectin: More than a tumor necrosis factor. N Engl J Med 316: 379–385, 1987.

6. Bonnem EM, Oldham RK: Gamma-interferon: Physiology and speculation on its role in medicine. J Biol Response Mod 6: 275–301, 1987.

7. Castellot JJ Jr, Rosenberg RD, Karnovsky MJ: Endothelium, heparin, and the regulation of vascular smooth muscle cell growth, in Jaffe EA (ed), *Biology of Endothelial Cells*. Boston, Martinus Nijhoff Publishers, 1984, pp 118–128.

8. Clemmons DR, Shaw DS: Purification and biologic properties of fibroblast somatomedin. J Biol Chem 261: 10293–10298, 1986.

9. Cohen S: Epidermal growth factor. In Vitro Cell Dev Biol 23: 239–246, 1987.

10. Cotran RS: New roles for the endothelium in inflammation and immunity. Am J Pathol 129: 407–413, 1987.

11. Derynck R: Transforming growth factor α. Cell 54: 593–595, 1988.

12. Deuel TF, Senior SM: Growth factors in fibrotic diseases. N Engl J Med 317: 236–237, 1987.

13. Eisenman RN, Thompson CB: Oncogenes with potential nuclear function: myc, myb and fos. Cancer Surv 5: 309–327, 1986.

14. Elias JA: Tumor necrosis factor interacts with interleukin-1 and interferons to inhibit fibroblast proliferation via fibroblast prostaglandin-dependent and -independent mechanisms. Am Rev Respir Dis 138: 652–658, 1988.

15. Elias JA, Zurier RB, Schreiber AD, Leff JA, Daniele RP: Monocyte inhibition of lung fibroblast growth: Relationship to fibroblast prostaglandin production and density-defined monocyte subpopulations. J Leukocyte Biol 37: 15–28, 1985.

16. Fishman AP: Pulmonary hypertension and cor pulmonale, in Fishman AP (ed), *Pulmonary Diseases and Disorders*, 2/e. New York, McGraw-Hill, 1988, pp 999–1048.

17. Folkman J, Klagsburn M: Angiogenic factors. Science 235: 442–447, 1987.

18. Heimark RL, Twardzik DR, Schwartz SM: Inhibition of endothelial regeneration by type-beta transforming growth factor from platelets. Science 233: 1078–1080, 1986.

19. Hoshi H, Kan M, Chen J-K, McKeehan WL: Comparative endocrinology-paracrinology-autocrinology of human adult large vessel endothelial and smooth muscle cells. In Vitro Cell Dev Biol 24: 309–320, 1988.

20. Hunter T: The proteins of oncogenes. Sci Am 251: 70–79, 1984.

21. Jackson TR, Blair LAC, Marshall J, Goedert M, Hanley MR: The mas oncogene encodes an angiotensin receptor. Nature 335: 437–440, 1988.

22. James R, Bradshaw RA: Polypeptide growth factors. Annu Rev Biochem 53: 259–292, 1984.

23. Libby P, Warner SJC, Friedman GB: Interleukin 1: A mitogen for human vascular smooth muscle cells that induces the release of growth-inhibitory prostanoids. J Clin Invest 81: 487–498, 1988.

24. Madtes DK, Raines EW, Sakariassen KS, Assoian RK, Sporn MB, Bell BI, Ross R: Induction of transforming growth factor-α in activated human alveolar macrophages. Cell 53:285–293, 1988.

25. Nishizuka Y: Studies and perspectives of protein kinase C. Science 233:305–312, 1986.

26. Oka Y, Orth DN: Human plasma epidermal growth factor/β- urogastrone is associated with blood platelets. J Clin Invest 72:249–259, 1983.

27. Oppenheim JJ, Kovacs EJ, Matsushima K, Durum SK: There is more than one interleukin 1. Immunology Today 7:45–55, 1986.

28. Palmberg L, Claesson H-E, Thyberg J: Leukotrienes stimulate initiation of DNA synthesis in cultured arterial smooth muscle cells. J Cell Sci 88:151–159, 1987.

29. Phillips PD, Cristofalo VJ: Classification system based on the functional equivalency of mitogens that regulate WI-38 cell proliferation. Exp Cell Res 175:396–403, 1988.

30. Pledger WJ, Stiles CD, Antoniades HN, Scher CD: Induction of DNA synthesis in BALB/c3T3 cells by serum components. Re-evaluation of the commitment process. Proc Natl Acad Sci USA 74:4481-4485, 1977.

31. Roberts AB, Thompson NL, Heine U, Flanders C, Sporn MB: Transforming growth factor-β: Possible roles in carcinogenesis. Br J Cancer 57:594–600, 1988.

32. Rom WN, Basset P, Fells GA, Nukiwa T, Trapnell BC, Crystal RG: Alveolar macrophages release an insulin-like growth factor I-type molecule. J Clin Invest 82:1685–1693, 1988.

33. Ross R, Raines EW, Bowen-Pope DF: The biology of platelet-derived growth factor. Cell 46:155–169, 1986.

34. Rozengurt E: Early signals in the mitogenic response. Science 234:161–166, 1986.

35. Spencer EM, Skover G, Hunt TK: Somatomedins: Do they play a pivotal role in wound healing?, in Barbul A, Pines E, Caldwell M, Hunt TK (eds), *Growth Factors and Other Aspects of Wound Healing: Biological and Clinical Implications*. New York, Alan R. Liss, Inc., 1988, pp 103–116.

36. Thomas KA: Fibroblast growth factors. FASEB J 1:434–440, 1987.

37. Vender RL, Clemmons DR, Kwock L, Friedman M: Reduced oxygen tension induces pulmonary endothelium to release a pulmonary smooth muscle cell mitogen(s). Am Rev Respir Dis 135:622–627, 1987.

38. Wakefield LM, Smith DM, Flanders KC, Sporn MB: Latent transforming growth factor-β from human platelets: A high molecular weight complex containing precursor sequences. J Biol Chem 263:7646–7654, 1988.

39. Weinstein R, Wenc K: Growth factor responses of human arterial endothelial cells in vitro. In Vitro Cell Dev Biol 22:549–556, 1986.

40. Wilcox JN, Smith KM, Williams LT, Schwartz SM, Gordon D: Platelet-derived growth factor mRNA detection in human atherosclerotic plaques by in situ hybridization. J Clin Invest 82:1134–1143, 1988.

41. Zetter BR: Angiogenesis: State of the art. Chest 93:159S–166S, 1988.

Susan L. Lindsay, M.B.B.S
Bruce A. Freeman, Ph.D.

16

Oxygen Radicals and Vascular Injury

For the past two decades, it has been recognized that toxic oxygen metabolites can be released from certain biological systems. Properties possessed by free radicals include chemical instability, reactivity, and cytotoxicity. There are a series of intracellular enzymic and nonenzymic antioxidants, such as catalase, superoxide dismutase (SOD), glutathione peroxidase and ascorbate and α-tocopherol, which provide a measure of protection against oxidative stress. The vascular endothelium, in particular that lining the pulmonary microvasculature, is frequently exposed to reactive oxygen species derived from activated inflammatory cells, xenobiotics, or hyperoxia; a high rate of generation of endogenous reactive oxygen species by endothelium also occurs. Therefore, endothelial response to injury induced by reactive oxygen metabolites has important implications in the understanding of various pulmonary pathophysiological processes.

THE NATURE OF FREE RADICALS

The most common type of covalent bond consists of a pair of electrons with opposite spins sharing a single molecular orbital. A free radical is a molecule which contains an odd number of electrons. The odd electron can be considered as a half-bond only, which makes the molecule more chemically reactive. The formation of a free radical is termed initiation, one of a series of reactions in which free radicals can participate. Reactions can proceed further via intermediates of reactive O_2

species, known as propagation reactions, whereby cell damage may occur. Most commonly, radicals abstract univalent atoms such as hydrogen atoms or halides:

$$R\cdot + XH \rightarrow HR + X\cdot \tag{1}$$

Radical addition to unsaturated bonds such as those present in free fatty acids or aromatic rings can also occur (15).

These reactions can occur indefinitely or be terminated by a wide variety of scavenging agents, some of which are essential to cellular integrity and, if depleted, predispose to cytotoxicity.

Biochemical defenses against partially reduced oxygen species include low molecular weight scavengers and complex enzyme systems. These defenses serve to reduce the steady state concentration of partially reduced oxygen species, which would otherwise be injurious to the cell. Scavenger systems are also a useful tool for in vivo and in vitro study systems to identify the nature of toxic O_2 metabolites.

In the absence of catalysts, molecular O_2 is relatively nonreactive because it is thermodynamically unfavorable for O_2 to combine with additional spin-paired electrons. This barrier is bypassed by the univalent addition of electrons to molecular O_2 which gives rise to a series of reactive intermediates as shown below:

No. of electrons	At pH 7.0	Name
0	O_2	Oxygen
1	$O_2\cdot$	Superoxide
2	H_2O_2	Hydrogen peroxide
3	$\cdot OH + H_2O$	Hydroxyl radical + H_2O
4	$H_2O + H_2O$	Water

Superoxide ($O_2^-\cdot$) undergoes dismutation either spontaneously or enzymically via superoxide dismutase to give H_2O_2:

$$O_2^-\cdot + O_2^-\cdot + 2H^+ \rightarrow O_2 + H_2O_2 \tag{2}$$

Superoxide dismutase is detectable in extracellular fluids (EC SOD) but is mainly an intracellular enzyme. All cells are equipped with this enzyme as part of their armamentarium against the production of $O_2^-\cdot$ which occurs physiologically in minute amounts (less than 10^{-11} M).

Superoxide is a good reducing agent with mild oxidant properties, which can initiate chain reactions. It is less reactive than $\cdot OH$, but still exerts significant toxicity, partly because it can diffuse to areas distal to the sites of generation.

The formation of the hydroxyl radical ($\cdot OH$) occurs indirectly from the reaction between H_2O_2 and $O_2^-\cdot$, known as the Fenton reaction, which is catalyzed by a transition metal, usually Fe^{2+}, although sometimes by Cu^{2+}.

$$Fe^{3+} + O_2^-\cdot \rightarrow Fe^{2+} + O_2 \tag{3}$$
$$Fe^{2+} + H_2O_2 \rightarrow Fe^{3+} + OH^- + \cdot OH \tag{4}$$

The hydroxyl radical is a much more potent oxidant than either $O_2^-\cdot$ or H_2O_2 and is capable of producing broad nonspecific oxidative damage, as well as participating in chain reactions. The reactivity of hydroxyl radical is so high and nonspecific that the site of target reaction is confined to within a few molecular radii of the site of $\cdot OH$ generation (15). There are no direct enzymatic scavenging systems present in vivo for this radical. However, superoxide dismutase, catalase, and glutathione peroxidase collaborate to reduce levels of $O_2^-\cdot$ and H_2O_2 which serve as precursors of $\cdot OH$. And iron binding proteins such as transferrin serve to keep free Fe^{+2} levels low. In vitro, the presence of hydroxyl radical is revealed by the inhibition of its formation by the scavenging action of mannitol.

Hydrogen peroxide is not a classically defined free radical in that it has no unpaired electrons, but it is included in the generic sense. It possesses considerable oxidative properties, participates in chain reactions, and is the precursor of $\cdot OH$. It is less reactive than either $O_2^-\cdot$ or $\cdot OH$, but it can exert toxic effects more distal than either $O_2^-\cdot$ or $\cdot OH$.

Under normal oxygen tensions in humans, approximately 98 percent of oxygen reduction is catalyzed by mitochondrial cytochrome oxidase, yielding 2 mol H_2O after a 4-electron reduction. Reactive O_2 species are not produced by cytochrome c oxidase during reduction of O_2 to $2\ H_2O$; however, the NADPH dehydrogenase complex and the ubiquinone-cytochrome b region of the electron transport chain have been shown to reduce O_2 to $O_2^-\cdot$ in lung, heart, and liver mitochondria.

Reactive O_2 species are generated in vivo as by-products of normal metabolism, but excessive production of reactive O_2 species may occur secondarily to various phenomena including ionizing radiation, trauma, acute inflammation, sepsis, and O_2 toxicity. The pulmonary vascular endothelium is both a significant source of reactive O_2 species and a critical target for tissue injury due to overproduction of toxic O_2 metabolites.

SOURCES OF REACTIVE OXYGEN SPECIES

The abundance of molecular O_2 in aerobic organisms and the ability of O_2 to univalently accept electrons means that partially reduced O_2 species are often mediators of cellular free radical reactions. The catalytic action of many cellular enzymes and electron-transport processes frequently involves one-electron transfers, and can inadvertently form toxic O_2 intermediates.

Antineoplastic agents such as adriamycin, daunorubicin, doxorubicin, and antibiotics which depend on quinoid groups or bound metals for activity are able to generate reactive O_2 metabolites. Many of the therapeutic actions and cytotoxic side effects of these drugs have been ascribed to their ability to reduce O_2 to $O_2^-\cdot$, H_2O_2, and OH^-.

Electromagnetic and particulate radiation generate primary radicals by transferring energy to cellular components such as H_2O. Secondary reactions can then occur with dissolved O_2 or cellular solutes to yield H_2O_2 and $O_2^-\cdot$.

Environmental agents, including photochemicals, air pollution, hyperoxia, pesticides, tobacco smoke, solvents, and anesthetics, also cause reactive O_2 damage to cells.

Intracellular Sources

AUTOOXIDATION OF SMALL MOLECULES

Thiols, hydroquinones, catecholamines, flavins, and tetrahydropterins all produce $O_2^-\cdot$ as the primary radical by reducing molecular O_2.

Chelated ferric iron is reduced to ferrous iron by a variety of agents including $O_2^-\cdot$, thiols, and ascorbate. Ferrous iron can then be autooxidized producing $O_2^-\cdot$. H_2O_2 can always be a secondary product of $O_2^-\cdot$ formation, produced either spontaneously or via enzymatically catalyzed dismutation: the latter reaction has a much faster rate constant than the former by a factor of 10^4.

ENZYMES AND PROTEINS

Probably the most studied reactive O_2 intermediate-producing enzyme is xanthine oxidase, which generates $O_2^-\cdot$ during the reduction of O_2 to H_2O_2. In vivo, it is present as an NAD^+-requiring dehydrogenase and produces no reactive O_2 intermediates. During in vivo ischemia or during purification, the dehydrogenase form converts to the oxidase form by limited proteolysis or sulfhydryl oxidation. Other enzymes include aldehyde oxidase, dihydroorotate-dehydrogenase, and flavoprotein dehydrogenase.

MITOCHONDRIA

The majority of, if not all, mitochondrial H_2O_2 is derived from the dismutation of $O_2^-\cdot$. Mitochondrial cytochrome c reduces O_2 and H_2O by a 4-electron transfer, without toxic oxygen intermediate generation. Superoxide production by mitochondria is greatest when the respiratory chain carriers on the inner membrane are highly reduced. Endogenous factors that regulate respiration also regulate the production of $O_2^-\cdot$, which include availability of various substrates of O_2 (6). If mitochondrial PO_2 is low enough to limit the reduction of O_2 and H_2O by cytochrome oxidase (on the order of 1 to 3 mmHg PO_2), then the increase in respiratory chain reduction and the accumulation of reduced cofactors in cells may enhance $O_2^-\cdot$ produced by the electron transport carrier components in ischemic cells.

Hydroxyl radical production by mitochondria has also been reported which requires iron and reacts with $O_2^-\cdot$ as in the Fenton reaction. $O_2^-\cdot$ reduces iron which, in turn, reduces H_2O_2 to $\cdot OH$ and OH^-. Superoxide is not always essential for this reaction to take place, as strong reducing agents such as ascorbic acid can also reduce Fe^{3+} (6).

Extracellular Sources

PULMONARY ALVEOLAR MACROPHAGES (PAMS)

Oxygen dependent cytotoxicity is the major microbicidal mechanism of PAM. Phagocytosis triggers an increased rate of O_2 consumption and generation of partially reduced O_2 species. PAMs generate H_2O_2 in the resting state, which is then augmented during phagocytosis. The mechanism of H_2O_2 production is not clearly established, but evidence exists for the presence of NADPH oxidase in PAMs (11) that may be responsible for the process. Superoxide is primarily generated, which then by dismutation yields H_2O_2. There is also evidence that NADPH oxidases directly or indirectly via glutathione dependent peroxidative pathway may provide a link between the stimulation of respiration and the hexose monophosphase shunt pathway. It has been demonstrated that O_2^- generation is augmented after phagocytosis (2). The oxidases may sit on the cell surface as ectoenzymes and become incorporated into the vacuole during particle ingestion, thus generating high intravacuolar concentrations of O_2 and H_2O_2 (11).

Human PAMs may contain peroxidase, distinct from neutrophil myeloperoxidase, which under certain circumstances functions in an antimicrobial system.

POLYMORPHONUCLEAR LEUKOCYTES (PMNLs)

The respiratory burst which occurs in activated neutrophils is one of the characteristics of the acute inflammatory response. This phenomenon includes increased O_2 consumption and the production of H_2O_2 and $O_2^-\cdot$. The respiratory burst has important implications for normal host defense mechanisms through microbicidal and tumoricidal activities, and also through inflammatory and immunological changes following tissue injury. The quantity of $O_2^-\cdot$ and H_2O_2 produced by PMNL is both species- and stimulus-specific, and will also vary with experimental conditions.

A variety of particulate and soluble mediators have been shown to induce metabolic activation by PMNL and include bacteria, opsonized zymosan, immunoglobulins, and immune complexes C5a and C5 as well as phorbol myristate acetate (PMA)—a synthetic nonspecific stimulator. The most potent of these agents are PMA and opsonized phagocytic particles. Most of the O_2 consumed by PMNL after the initiation of respiratory burst can be accounted for by $O_2^-\cdot$ production. The enzyme responsible for the increased O_2 consumption has been identified as a membrane-associated NADPH oxidase (18).

In vitro studies have demonstrated that PMNL-derived $O_2^-\cdot$ itself has little bactericidal effect. Current evidence would suggest that the primary means of microbicidal activity lies with the metabolism of H_2O_2 in the presence of halides. Hydrogen peroxide has significant bactericidal activity on its own, which is augmented by ascorbic acid and some metals. The most potent microbicidal combination is H_2O_2 with myeloperoxidase and halide system. The active product of this combination is likely to be hypochlorous acid (5). The mechanism of action is probably halogenation $\pm$ oxidation of the surface of the microorganism. Additional evidence suggests that $\cdot OH$ may also play an important part in the killing of bacteria (5).

The effects of the bactericidal activity of the phagocytes are not confined to within the phagolysozyme. In vitro studies have demonstrated that O_2 metabolites, released from activated phagocytes, may be toxic to a wide variety of eukaryotic cells, including erythrocytes, endothelial cells, fibroblasts, and leukocytes. These toxic effects appear to be mediated analogous to bactericidal effects. All reactive O_2 metabolites have been implicated in extracellular cytolysis of host cells. The ability to kill specific cells depends on various factors including species of effector cells, target cells, and the activating stimulus.

ENDOTHELIAL CELLS

With the exception of physiological shunts, the entire cardiac output from the right side of the heart passes through the pulmonary microvasculature. The pulmonary vascular endothelium is exposed to and metabolizes a variety of biologically active substances either by interiorizing the material via specific plasma membrane transport processes or by enzymatic activity at the plasma membrane.

It is technically difficult to isolate and subculture pulmonary microvascular endothelial cells; therefore, most work has been performed on subcultures of aortic and pulmonary arterial endothelial cells together with isolated and perfused lung preparations.

Endothelial cells are able to generate and secrete $O_2^-\cdot$ (19). The vascular endothelium is extremely sensitive to oxidative damage mediated by reactive O_2 metabolites either released from inflammatory cells or those produced within the cell. Hydrogen peroxide is often an important mediator of such acute cell injury. Oxidative damage may also play a role in the endothelial cell-associated mechanisms of pathogenesis of atherosclerosis. Unfortunately, traditional methods of assessing cell injury often rely on relatively crude measurements such as ^{51}Cr release, cell detachment from plates, and lactate dehydrogenase (LDH) release. Earlier indices of nonlethal cellular dysfunction include loss of PGI_2 synthetic activity (23), K^+ efflux (1), release of cytoplasmic purines from endothelial cells (1), and decrease in membrane fluidity (7). Loss of PGI_2 has been observed in aging phenomena and may be mediated at least in part by the overproduction of toxic O_2 species. Both cyclooxygenase activity and PGI_2 synthesis have been shown to be extremely sensitive to oxidative metabolites generated during arachidonic acid metabolism.

At much lower concentrations than those usually seen for cell lysis, exogenous H_2O_2 can block PGI_2 synthesis by inhibition of cyclooxygenase. Although $O_2^-\cdot$ is the primary radical species generated by polymorphonuclear leukocytes (PMNL), the dismutation product H_2O_2 can induce target cell injury as well. Endothelial cells have been shown to be important in the detoxification of $O_2^-\cdot$, due to the intracellular presence of SOD (12). Activated granulocytes must be closely applied to endothelial cells both in order to mediate the increase in permeability caused by toxic O_2 metabolites (3,22) and in order to limit the injurious effects of such toxic species (12). Further endogenous endothelial antioxidant defense mechanisms include the glutathione redox cycle (9).

SMOOTH MUSCLE ARTERIAL CELLS

Extracellular $O_2^-\cdot$ has been detected recently from human arterial smooth muscle cells (10). Unlike the burst of activity seen with activated granulocytes, $O_2^-\cdot$ production is continuous and progressively accumulates. Superoxide production by smooth muscle arterial cells reacts with lipids to give lipids peroxides, which may contribute to modification of low density lipoproteins (LDL) with consequent foam cell formation and atherogenesis (10).

TARGETS OF FREE RADICAL DAMAGE

Intracellular Sites of Damage

PROTEINS

Proteins having amino acids with unsaturated bonds or containing sulphur are at risk from free radical damage because of the reactivity of such bonds and sulphur; examples include tryptophan, tyrosine, phenylalanine, and cysteine. Enzymes which depend on these proteins for reactivity will also be inhibited, such as glyceraldehyde 3-phosphate dehydrogenase (G3PD). Strongly reactive O_2 species such as OH· can react with protein constituents commonly regarded as resistant to modification such as peptide bonds, or amino acids such as proline or lysine. The susceptibility of proteins to free radical damage depends upon the amino acid composition; the importance and location of susceptible amino acids, which mediate protein conformation and activity; and cellular distribution of the protein and whether the damaged protein can be repaired. An example of this is in the re-reduction of radical induced disulfide bonds.

NUCLEIC ACIDS AND DNA

Cell mutation and death from ionizing radiation is primarily the result of reactions of toxic O_2 metabolites with DNA. Hydroxyl radical has been implicated as the agent responsible for the majority of radiation-induced cytolysis in both eukaryotic and prokaryotic cells. Cytotoxicity is generally a consequence of chromosomal damage arising from nucleic acid base modifications or DNA strand scission, which results from radical reaction with the sugar phosphate backbone.

MEMBRANE LIPIDS

The unsaturated bonds on membrane cholesterol and free fatty acids can readily react with partially reduced O_2 species and undergo peroxidation. This mechanism has three phases. Initially, when a reactive O_2 species reacts with a fatty acid, a fatty acid radical is formed by electron removal. The radical then reacts with O_2 to form a fatty acid peroxyradical, which then reacts with other lipids, proteins, and radicals, thereby setting up chain reactions, all involving oxidation. This process can become autocatalytic after initiation and will yield lipid peroxide, lipid alcohol, and aldehyde by-products. Plasma membrane and organelle lipid peroxidation can be stimulated by toxic O_2 species and is potentiated by the presence of metals which can either serve as redox catalysts or catalyze the conversion of $O_2^-·$ and H_2O_2 to more potent oxidants. Lipid peroxides and lipid peroxy-radicals can exert toxicity by reacting with many of the same cellular components as reactive O_2 species. Peroxidation can be terminated in one of several ways. Glutathione peroxidase reduces lipid peroxides to nonreactive hydroxy fatty acids. Rearrangement of bonds may cause formation of diene conjugates or degradation products such as malonyldialdehyde. Antioxidants such as α-tocopherol or enzymic scavengers can also terminate chain reactions by reducing the level of peroxide radicals. The hydrophobic nature of lipid radicals means that most of the reactions will take place with membrane-associated molecules, which may significantly alter membrane permeability and microviscosity.

Malondialdehyde, which is a product of peroxidation of free fatty acids containing three or more double bonds, can cause cross-linking and polymerization of membrane components. This can alter intrinsic membrane properties such as deformability, ion transport, enzyme activity, and the aggregation state of cell surface determinants. Malondialdehyde is diffusable and, therefore, will react with nitrogenous bases of DNA, which may explain why malondialdehyde is mutagenic.

CYTOSOLIC EFFECTS

Reactive O_2 species produced extracellularly and which diffuse into cells, or those produced intracellularly, can react with many of the previously mentioned cytosolic targets. Another important intracellular reaction involves erythrocytes. Hemoproteins such as oxygenated hemoglobin can react with either $O_2^-\cdot$ or H_2O_2 to oxidize ferrous to ferric iron, forming methemoglobin. A variety of hemoproteins can be damaged by reactive O_2 species.

EXTRACELLULAR EFFECTS

Toxic O_2 species play an important role in modulating the extent of an inflammatory response and consequent tissue damage. Tissue components which are especially at risk from inflammatory cell-mediated free radical damage include collagen and hyaluronic acid, which are both affected in inflammatory osteoarthritis. Extracellular fluids have very little SOD and catalase activities, therefore, there is great potential for extensive damage in this fluid compartment.

Toxic O_2 metabolites can react with plasma membrane lipid component to generate chemotactic factors, causing further inflammatory cell infiltration. Diffusion of H_2O_2 and $O_2^-\cdot$ from the endothelium exposes macromolecular serum components to free radical damage. Lipid peroxides can also exert toxicity by reacting with many of the same cellular components as toxic O_2 metabolites. An example of this is the generation of an albumin-bound lipid neutrophil chemoattractant (which can be inhibited by SOD) (16), secondary to the reaction of $O_2^-\cdot$ with a plasma component. A further example is the modification of LDL to cytotoxic species by free radicals.

REACTIVE O_2 MODULATION OF PROSTAGLANDIN (PG) SYNTHESIS

In mammals, the majority of prostaglandins are of the 2 series (dienoic), with very small amounts present from the 1 or 3 series. These derive from eicosatetraenoic acid, commonly known as arachidonic acid, which is biosynthesized from a polyunsaturated fatty acid linoleic acid, one of the essential fatty acids. The importance of the eicosanoids derive from their mediation of a wide variety of pathophysiological disorders.

Arachidonate reacts with cyclooxygenase to form the PG endoperoxide PGH_2. This enzyme is membrane bound, is found in the endoplasmic reticulum and the nuclear membrane, and requires heme as a cofactor. The normal rate of synthesis of prostaglandins represents 1/100,000 of the maximal potential. Overproduction of prostaglandins by cyclooxygenase is prevented by a self-destruct mechanism on the enzyme which operates after 15 to 30 sec of reaction. Cyclooxygenase is

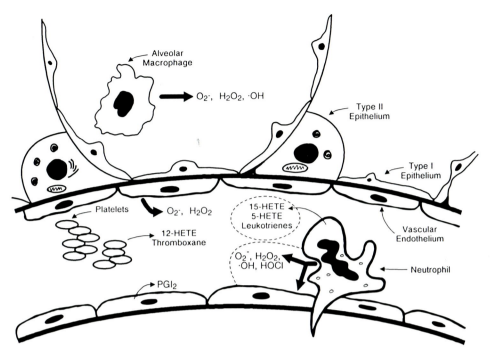

Figure 1: Schematic diagram of alveolar-capillary region, showing sources of free radicals and prostaglandin production. Complex interrelationships exist, together with positive and negative feedback loops between prostaglandin biosynthesis and toxic O_2 metabolites.

reversibly inhibited by aspirin and irreversibly inhibited by indomethacin and ibuprofen.

There are at least five different types of enzymes collectively known as PG synthase, each manufacturing a different type of prostaglandin. These act on PGH_2 to convert it to the various species of prostaglandins. The mixture of prostaglandins released by the cell depends on the synthases contained within. For example, PGI_2 is the main product of vascular endothelial cell, while thromboxane is the main product of platelets (Fig. 1).

Arachidonic acid can also give rise to another group of regulatory compounds known as leukotrienes. The initial step in leukotriene synthesis is the addition of a hydroperoxy group to arachidonic acid by lipoxygenase.

Platelets contain 12-lipoxygenase (12-LPO) which acts on arachidonate to give 12-hydroperoxy-eicosatetraenoic acid (HPETE) which reduces to 12-hydroxy-eicosatetraenoic acid (HETE), and does not seem to undergo any further transformations. The role of these substances in platelet function is unknown. Leukocytes contain 15-LPO which acts on arachidonate to give 15-HPETE and, subsequently, 15-HETE. These are chemoattractant and inhibit other lipoxygenase and prostaglandin production. Leukocytes also contain 5-LPO which forms 5-HPETE and then leukotriene A_4 (LTA$_4$) which can be converted enzymatically by hydration to LTB$_4$ and by the addition of glutathione to LTC$_4$. LTD$_4$ and LTE$_4$ are biosynthesized from LTC$_4$ by the successive elimination of glutamyl residue and glycine (20). Leukotrienes function in relation to inflammation and allergic reactions. LTC$_4$ and D$_4$ are the active components of slow releasing substance of anaphy-

laxis-A. They are 1,000 times more potent than histamine in causing bronchoconstriction. They also cause an increase in permeability of small blood vessels and
constrict pulmonary arterioles (20). LTB$_4$ is one of the most potent agents known
for serving as a chemoattractant of neutrophils and eosinophils.

The linkage between pulmonary production of toxic O$_2$ species and eicosanoid
synthesis occurs at the fatty acid oxygenases, in that both cyclooxygenase and
lipoxygenase require hydroperoxide for activity (14). It has been proposed that
normal vascular endothelial cells possess a certain low basal level of peroxide and
a basal level of production of PGI$_2$.

If the basal level of hydroperoxide is exceeded, then increased cyclooxygenase
activity is triggered. Thus, hydroperoxide is amplified and serves as a positive
feedback loop on cyclooxygenase until the level of hydroperoxide reaches a critical level, when peroxidase activity present in the prostaglandin intermediate
PGH$_2$ is activated, thereby reducing peroxides to alcohol (14). The glutathione
redox cycle is the key regulator of reactive O$_2$ species by its effect on the peroxide
tone of the cell (9). Vascular endothelial cells are very sensitive to damage by
H$_2$O$_2$, which has been shown to inhibit PGI$_2$ synthesis presumably by cyclooxygenase. Cyclooxygenase especially is sensitive to inhibition by toxic O$_2$ species. Exogenous lipid peroxides seem to selectively inhibit PGI$_2$ synthase (13).
The mechanism for these effects is unknown.

The enzymatic reduction of PGG$_2$ to PGH$_2$ by the peroxidase component of
cyclooxygenase has been shown to produce a radical which is destructive to this
enzyme. Although not positively identified, ·OH has been implicated (4). Hydroxyl radical may also be involved in the inactivation of cyclooxygenase by H$_2$O$_2$.
It is possible that the polarity of the peroxide involved dictates which enzyme is
inactivated by radical attack. For example, polar peroxides such as H$_2$O$_2$ may
selectively inhibit cyclooxygenase whereas lipophilic peroxides inhibit PGI$_2$ synthase, especially at low levels (23).

ENDOTHELIAL-DERIVED RELAXING FACTOR (EDRF)

Acetylcholine-induced vascular relaxation is dependent on the presence of an intact endothelium (8). Endothelial cells stimulated by acetylcholine release a factor
which diffuses to the underlying smooth muscle and causes relaxation. Vascular
relaxation can be induced by a variety of agents which use endothelial-derived
relaxing factor (EDRF) as a mediator. Such agents include adenine nucleotides,
thrombin, substance P, vasoactive intestinal peptide, and bradykinin. Agents
which cause endothelium-independent relaxations include nitrovasodilators such
as glyceryl trinitrate, nitroprusside, atrial natriuretic factor, and prostacyclin.
Other properties of EDRF include inhibition of platelet aggregation and the reversal of aggregated platelets. The mechanism by which vasodilatation and inhibition of platelet aggregation acts is by increasing the levels of GMP in smooth
muscle cells and platelets.

One component of EDRF activity has been identified as being nitric oxide
(NO·) (17). Superoxide adds to the instability of NO·, and redox compounds generally inhibit NO· by the generation of O$_2^-$. Nitric oxide has been confirmed as
an endogenous nitrate acting as a second messenger, mediating vasodilatation

caused by a variety of compounds. Evidence is accumulating showing that NO· synergizes with PGI_2 to inhibit platelet aggregation, and also that in contrast to PGI_2, NO· is a very effective inhibitor of platelet adhesion to vessel endothelium. The future implications of NO· lie toward a better understanding of the pathogenesis of atherosclerosis and hypertension.

LIPOXIN

Lipoxin is one of a new series of oxygenated derivatives of arachidonate. Interactions between the 5- and 15-lipoxygenase pathways from activated leukocytes give rise to this class of compound. Currently, there are two known subtypes of lipoxin termed lipoxin A and B (LXA and LXB). They have been shown to have a pattern of activity distinct from that of prostaglandins, thromboxane, and leukotrienes. LXA has been shown to have chemotactic and spasmogenic properties independent of cyclooxygenase, norepinephrine, histamine, or acetylcholine products. When added to neutrophils, LXA provokes O_2^- generation but no aggregation. Lipoxins are an additional means by which oxygenation of arachidonic acid can exert effects on the inflammatory process and host defense (21).

IMPLICATIONS OF PULMONARY MICROVASCULAR FREE RADICAL PROCESSES IN MEDICINE

Numerous laboratory models using in vitro and in vivo preparations have provided strong evidence for toxic oxygen metabolites as mediators of pulmonary dysfunction. Most of the evidence relating to humans is inferential and, therefore, must be interpreted with caution in view of interspecies differences. As a consequence, the therapeutic use of free radical scavengers in ameliorating diffuse lung injury remains largely experimental.

The clinical manifestations of adult respiratory distress syndrome and its multiple etiologies are well recognized. Evidence, largely derived from experimental models, has suggested an important role for toxic oxygen metabolites in their pathogenesis along with neutral proteases released from neutrophils and arachidonic acid metabolites.

A number of cell types within the lung possess biochemical mechanisms which can result in the generation and release of toxic O_2 metabolites which, if produced in quantities that overwhelm local scavenging systems, will result in pulmonary microvascular damage.

By virtue of their location, PAMs are vulnerable to activation by inhaled agents. Neutrophils, following activation by circulating complement, opsonized bacteria, or immune complexes, are known to sequestrate within the pulmonary microvasculature one of the features of diffuse lung injury. Experimentally, neutrophil depletion is protective to lung in animal models following exposure to PAM. Prior administration of scavengers such as SOD further ameliorates this damage, implicating a role for toxic oxygen metabolites.

Clinical examples of PMNL-independent metabolic oxygen injury include radiation damage, whereby absorbed radiant energy leads to generalized radiolysis of cellular water and the formation of ionized water molecules with the subsequent formation of toxic oxygen metabolites. Following exposure to paraquat, selective reduction within the pulmonary parenchymal cell occurs with the production of stable radical intermediates which react with oxygen to form O_2^- and H_2O_2.

The macrophage has been cited as the key effector cell in the generation and maintenance of granulomatous inflammation. The prior administration of free radical scavengers in vitro has been shown to cause a reduction in the size of granulomata.

In a variety of stress conditions, such as diabetes mellitus and trauma, the profile of circulating free fatty acids alters. These have been shown to cause changes in pulmonary microvascular permeability both directly and by stimulating the formation of toxic O_2 metabolites, probably derived from macrophages.

Heart-lung transplantation provides many exciting possibilities for elucidating the effects of toxic O_2 metabolites in the transient pulmonary dysfunction occurring after a period of ischemia and subsequent reperfusion. Additionally, the pulmonary microvasculature is exposed to the insult of cardiopulmonary bypass which itself causes intrapulmonary neutrophil sequestration following complement activation with the further release of toxic O_2 metabolites. The inclusion of mannitol by some centers as a component of the pulmonary perfusate when using a single cold flush preservation technique may exert a beneficial effect by virtue of its scavenging properties.

Concepts developed from both in vitro and animal models implicate a key role for reactive O_2 species in ischemic tissue injury. Extrapolation to the human case is difficult because of interspecies differences in key aspects of tissue processes of metabolic O_2 generation. Much more work is necessary to broaden our current knowledge in order to develop models with greater application to the clinical situation. However, the current potential is enormous for clarifying pathophysiological mechanisms and for developing therapeutic interventions.

ACKNOWLEDGMENTS

We gratefully acknowledge the skillful secretarial assistance of Ms. Yvonne Lambott in the preparation of this manuscript.

REFERENCES

1. Ager A, Gordon JL: Differential effects of hydrogen peroxide on indices of endothelial cell function. J Exp Med 159:592–603, 1984.

2. Boxer LA, Ismail G, Allen JM, Baehner RL: Oxidative metabolic responses of rabbit pulmonary alveolar macrophages. Blood 53:486–491, 1979.

3. Del Maestro RF, Bjork J, Arfors KE: Increase in microvascular permeability induced by enzymatically generated free radicals. I. In vivo study. Microvasc Res 22:239–254, 1981.

4. Egan RW, Paxton J, Kuehl FA Jr: Mechanism of irreversible self-deactivation of prostaglandin synthetase. J Biol Chem 251:7329–7335, 1976.

5. Fantone JC, Ward PA: Role of oxygen-derived

free radicals and metabolites in leukocyte-dependent inflammatory reactions. Am J Pathol 107:397–418, 1982.

6. Freeman BA, Crapo JD: Biology of disease: Free radicals and tissue injury. Lab Invest 47:412–426, 1982.

7. Freeman BA, Rosen GM, Barber MJ: Superoxide perturbation of the organization of vascular endothelial cell membranes. J Biol Chem 261:6590–6593, 1986.

8. Furchgott RF, Zawadzki JV: The obligatory role of endothelial cells in the relaxation of arterial smooth muscle by acetylcholine. Nature 288:373–376, 1980.

9. Harlan JM, Levine JD, Callahan KS, Schwartz BR, Harker LA: Glutathione redox cycle protects cultured endothelial cells against lysis by extracellularly generated hydrogen peroxide. J Clin Invest 73:706–713, 1984.

10. Heinecke JW, Baker L, Rosen H, Chait A: Superoxide-mediated modification of low density lipoproteins by arterial smooth muscle cells. J Clin Invest 77:757–761, 1986.

11. Hocking WG, Golde DW: The pulmonary alveolar macrophage. N Engl J Med 301:580–587; 639–645, 1979.

12. Hoover RL, Robinson JM, Karnovsky MJ: Adhesion of polymorphonuclear leukocytes to endothelium enhances the efficiency of detoxification of oxygen-free radicals. Am J Pathol 126:258–268, 1987.

13. Kent RS, Kitchell BB, Shand DG, Whorton AR: The ability of vascular tissue to produce prostacyclin decreases with age. Prostaglandins 21:483–490, 1981.

14. Lands WE: Interactions of lipid hydroperoxides with eicosanoid biosynthesis. J Free Radic Biol Med 1:97–101, 1985.

15. McCord JM: *Therapeutic Approaches to Myocardial Infarct Size Limitation.* New York, Raven Press, 1984, pp 209–218.

16. McCord JM, Wong K, Stokes S, Petrone W, English D: Superoxide and inflammation: A mechanism for the anti-inflammatory activity of superoxide dismutase. Acta Physiol Scand 492:25–30, 1980.

17. Palmer RM, Ferrige AG, Moncada S: Nitric oxide release accounts for the biological activity of endothelial derived relaxing factor (Letter). Nature 327:524–526, 1987.

18. Patriarca P, Cramer R, Moncalvo S, Rossi F, Romeo D: Enzymatic basis of metabolic stimulation in leukocytes during phagocytosis: the role of activated NADPH oxidase. Arch Biochem Biophys 145:255–262, 1971.

19. Rosen GM, Freeman BA: Detection of superoxide generated by endothelial cells. Proc Natl Acad Sci USA 81:7269–7273, 1984.

20. Samuelsson B: Leukotrienes: mediators of immediate hypersensitivity reactions and inflammation. Science 220:568–575, 1983.

21. Samuelsson B, Dahlen S-E, Lindgren JA, Rouzer CA, Serhan CN: Leukotrienes and lipoxins: structures, biosynthesis and biological effects. Science 237:1171–1176, 1987.

22. Shasby DM, Shasby SS, Peach MJ: Granulocytes and phorbol myristate acetate increase permeability to albumin of cultured endothelial monolayers and isolated perfused lungs. Am Rev Respir Dis 127:72–76, 1983.

23. Whorton AR, Montgomery ME, Kent RS: Effect of hydrogen peroxide on prostaglandin production and cellular integrity in cultured porcine aortic endothelial cells. J Clin Invest 76:295–302, 1985.

Katherine A. Hajjar, M.D.
Ralph L. Nachman, M.D.

17 ⎯⎯⎯⎯⎯⎯⎯⎯⎯⎯⎯⎯⎯⎯

Endothelial Cell Modulation of Coagulation and Fibrinolysis

Traditionally, the endothelium has been considered a static barrier which prevented contact between clotting factors and the thrombogenic subendothelium. It is now clear that the endothelial cell participates in a variety of highly regulated anticoagulant and profibrinolytic mechanisms which serve to limit the formation and propagation of a clot, thereby maintaining the fluidity of blood. Upon activation, the endothelial cell acquires a new set of properties which favor its participation in procoagulant and antifibrinolytic reactions (Fig. 1).

CHARACTERISTICS OF "QUIESCENT" ENDOTHELIAL CELLS

Under normal conditions, the procoagulant properties of the endothelial cell— appear to be expressed to a minimal degree, while their anticoagulant and profibrinolytic functions predominate (Fig. 1A). Resting human endothelial cells synthesize and secrete a variety of clotting factors including von Willebrand factor (37), tissue factor (46), and Factor V (15), but these are produced either in inactive form or in such small quantities as to represent a rather minor contribution to total cell function. These cells also possess potential binding sites for additional clotting factors including Factor IX/IXa (64,72,75), Factor X (65,74), thrombin (2,43), and possibly fibrinogen (18), but the system is regulated in such a way that intravascular clotting is precluded. On the other hand, two important anticoagulant systems, the heparin-antithrombin III system and the thrombomodulin-thrombin-protein C system, appear to play a key role in preventing

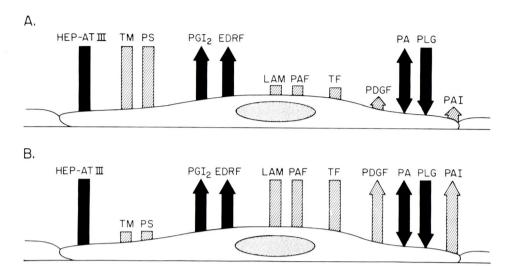

Figure 1: Endothelial cell modulation of coagulation and fibrinolysis.
A. "Quiescent" endothelial cell. In the absence of endothelial cell activators, prominent anticoagulant mechanisms include inactivation of factors II_a, IX_a, and X_a by heparin-associated antithrombin III (HEP-AT III), inactivation of factors V_a and VIII_a by the thrombomodulin (TM)-protein C-protein S (PS) system, and inhibition of platelet aggregation by prostacyclin (PGI_2) and endothelium-derived relaxing factor (EDRF). Baseline profibrinolytic components include elaboration and surface binding of plasminogen activator (PA), and surface binding of plasminogen (PLG) with potential enhancement of fibrinolytic activity.
B. In the "activated" state, the modulated coagulant systems include impairment of thrombomodulin (TM) and protein S (PS) expression, synethesis of leukocyte adhesion molecules (LAM) and platelet-activating factor (PAF), enhanced expression of tissue factor (TF), and elaboration of platelet-derived growth factor (PDGF). In addition, synthesis of plasminogen activator inhibitor (PAI) is enhanced in the activated state.

intravascular clotting. In addition, the endothelial cell may also impede clot formation by expressing surface binding sites to which fibrinolytic proteins bind in a highly functional fashion.

Anticoagulant Mechanisms

HEPARIN-ANTITHROMBIN III

Under baseline conditions, the endothelial cell possesses two distinct surface-oriented anticoagulant mechanisms. The first involves surface-associated heparin-like molecules which function to enhance the inactivation of clotting factors by the protease inhibitor antithrombin III. Endothelial cells synthesize and secrete heparin, heparan sulfate, and other related glycosaminoglycans (13). In experiments involving bovine aortic segments, heparinase-sensitive molecules facilitate binding of antithrombin III to the endothelium, thereby allowing for inactivation of clotting factors IXa and Xa (76). Inactivation of these clotting factors is relatively vessel-dependent and requires the presence of heparin-like moieties on the endothelial cell surface. Antithrombin III also inactivates thrombin by a mechanism which is much more efficient in the presence of endothelium (14).

THROMBIN-THROMBOMODULIN-PROTEIN C

The second cell surface anticoagulant mechanism involves the intrinsic membrane protein, thrombomodulin (24). Thrombomodulin is a MW 74,000 thrombin-binding glycoprotein which is present on the surface of all endothelial cells (approximately 50,000 sites per cell) except those in the microcirculation of the human brain (36,45). Once thrombin complexes with thrombomodulin, there is a 1000-fold increase in activation of protein C, a MW 62,000 anticoagulant protein (38,58). At the same time, the procoagulant activity of thrombin is reversibly impaired (23). Once protein C has been activated, it must interact with a membrane surface to function (34,73,82). Its high affinity interaction with membranes requires the presence of protein S which, like protein C, is a vitamin K-dependent protein. Protein S binding to membranes is mediated by at least one MW 138,000 protein S binding protein (82) and could involve others as well. Activated protein C in the presence of protein S can then assemble on the cell (endothelial or platelet) surface and inactivate factors Va or VIIIa (34,73). These are the two nonenzymatic regulatory proteins of the coagulation cascade which serve as cofactors for protease factors Xa and IXa, respectively.

PROSTACYCLIN AND ENDOTHELIUM-DERIVED RELAXING FACTOR

The endothelial cell also possesses intracellular mechanisms which retard clot formation. In response to a vessel wall injury, vasospasm is followed by platelet activation, aggregation, and recruitment, processes required for the formation of an effective hemostatic plug. Endothelial cells synthesize and secrete basal levels of prostacyclin and PGD_2, both of which inhibit platelet activation and promote vasodilatation through a cyclic AMP-dependent mechanism (84). Synthesis of prostacyclin is enhanced by stimulation with thrombin or calcium ionophore A23187 (83). Recently, endothelial cells have been found to produce a labile humoral agent, endothelium-derived relaxing factor (EDRF), which mimics the action of nitrovasodilators (26). It has been proposed that EDRF is related to nitric oxide, an equally unstable vasodilator whose action is inhibited by hemoglobin and enhanced by superoxide dismutase (59). In addition, EDRF from porcine aortic endothelial cells has been shown to inhibit platelet aggregation induced by collagen or a thromboxane-like agent (U46619) through a cyclic GMP-dependent mechanism (63).

PLASMIN

Plasmin is the catalytically active product of plasminogen activation whose major function appears to be the degradation of fibrin. However, recent evidence suggests that plasmin may also represent a physiologically important anticoagulant. Plasmin has recently been shown to inactivate Factor Va by cleaving both the heavy and light chains of this MW 168,000 species (57). This inactivation is lipid-dependent, suggesting that it might be oriented on cell surfaces, such as the endothelial cell (31), in vivo. The reaction results in a series of plasmin-specific proteolytic cleavages which are distinguishable from those produced by protein C. In addition, both prothrombin and Factor Xa, critical factors in the Va-mediated generation of thrombin, protect Va from inactivation by plasmin. Plasmin can also inactivate Factor VIIIa, another nonenzymatic cofactor which bears

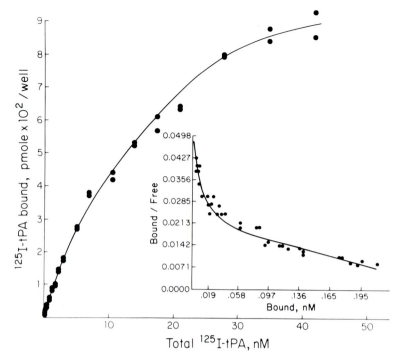

Figure 2: Binding of ^{125}I-tissue plasminogen activator to human vascular endothelial cells (HUVEC). HUVEC, grown to confluency in plasminogen depleted medium, were washed and exposed to ^{125}I-t-PA (specific activity 149,000 cpm/pmole), diluted in various ratios with unlabeled t-PA for 30 min at 4°C. Unbound radioactivity from a 100-μl aliquot was sampled prior to emptying and washing each well rapidly five times (total wash time 45 sec). Bound radioactivity was recovered in the washed cell reaction solubilized in 1 percent SDS/0.5 M NaOH/0.01 M EDTA and counted as a 100-μl aliquot. Inset: Scatchard plot. (Reproduced from Hajjar et al. [30].)

substantial structural homology with Va (47). Whether these plasmin-mediated anticoagulant mechanisms operate on cell surfaces in vivo is not yet known.

Endothelial Cell Fibrinolytic System

Cultured endothelial cells synthesize and secrete plasminogen activators, as well as the fast-acting antiactivator, plasminogen activator inhibitor (PAI-1) (39,40,79,80). They also provide binding sites for the surface assembly of plasminogen, tissue plasminogen activator, and urokinase (30–32). This binding may serve to support the catalytic efficiency of plasmin generation while also protecting these activators from circulating inhibitors.

PLASMINOGEN ACTIVATORS

The major physiological activators of plasminogen are tissue plasminogen activator (t-PA) and urokinase (u-PA). Urokinase has been demonstrated to bind to several cell types including the monocytic U937 cell line (1,17,77,81), A431 epidermoid carcinoma cell line (25,78), fibroblasts (3,4,19), mouse spermatozoa (35), and possibly cultured bovine corneal endothelial cells (69) as well as Friend eryth-roleukemia cells (20). Binding of urokinase and its inactive precursor prourokinase to U937 cells has been well characterized and is dose-dependent, saturable, and of high affinity (K_d ~0.5 nM) (17,81). The relevant U937 binding site is a MW 55,000–60,000 which accepts u-PA, proenzyme u-PA, and ATF but not t-PA or unrelated proteins (56). It appears to be mediated via the epidermal growth factor domain-containing amino terminal fragment (ATF) of urokinase (1). Interestingly, binding of ^{125}I-ATF to U937 cells is enhanced 10- to 20-fold upon differentiation of these cells into a macrophage-like species through stimulation with phorbol ester (77). Urokinase binding to A431 cells also requires the noncatalytic ATF-containing "A chain" (25). Once u-PA is synthesized by these cells, it appears to be secreted and immediately to saturate surface binding sites in an "autocrine" fashion (78). In addition, human fibroblasts express high affinity "cryptic" or "latent" u-PA binding sites on their surface which also appear to be saturated in the resting state but do not permit efficient internalization of the ligand (3,4,19).

Tissue plasminogen activator (t-PA) was previously thought to function efficiently only on a fibrin clot or on a thrombospondin- or histidine-rich glycoprotein-coated surface (70). However, it has recently been shown that t-PA can bind to and function on the surface of cultured human endothelial cells (7,30). The binding isotherm describes a specific, reversible, high affinity interaction consisting of two saturable sites (K_d 19 pM and 18 nM; B_{max} 3,700 and 815,000 sites per cell,

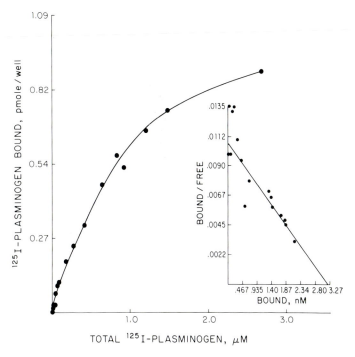

Figure 3: Binding of ^{125}I-plasminogen to HUVEC. HUVEC were prepared as described in the legend to Figure 2 and exposed to ^{125}I-plasminogen (specific activity 18,400 cpm/pmole) in the presence and absence of 10 mM EACA for 30 min at 4°C. The data are plotted as the difference between total and nonspecific binding. Inset: Scatchard plot. (Reproduced from Hajjar et al. [31].)

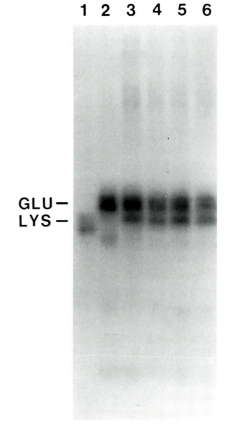

Figure 4: Recovery of ^{125}I-glu-PLG from cultured HUVEC. HUVEC, grown as described in the legend to Figure 1, were washed twice, incubated with ^{125}I-glu-PLG, form 1, and then washed and either solubilized in 1 percent SDS/0.5 M NaOH/0.01 M EDTA or surface-eluted with 10 mM EACA. Authentic ^{125}I-lys-PLG (lane 1), authentic self-incubated ^{25}I-glu-PLG (lane 2), whole cell extracts (lanes 3 and 4), and EACA eluates (lanes 5 and 6) were run on a 7.5 percent nonreducing Laemmli SDS polyacrylamide gel, fixed, dried, and exposed. A small amount of inactive plasmin was present in the authentic glu-PLG sample (lane 2, lower band). (Reproduced from Hajjar and Nachman [32].)

respectively) (30) (Fig. 2). This interaction is lysine-binding site-independent and, interestingly, is blocked in a dose-dependent fashion (I_{50} ~10 nM) by urokinase, which also binds to these cells with high affinity (K_d ~1 nM) (30). Once t-PA localizes on the surface of the endothelial cell, it appears to retain its catalytic activity and, importantly, appears to be protected from its physiological inhibitor (PAI) at up to 20-fold molar excess (30). Recent evidence suggests that t-PA interacts with PAI-1 on the surface of cultured endothelial cells (5,66) and that membrane-associated PAI may represent a storage pool of the active inhibitor (66).

PLASMINOGEN

Human glu-plasminogen is the MW 93,000 precursor of plasmin which circulates in the plasma at a concentration of approximately 1.5 uM (42). Plasminogen binds reversibly and with high affinity (K_d 310 nM) to the surface of cultured human umbilical vein endothelial cells (31) (Fig. 3). Binding to these cells is lysine-binding site specific, relatively cell-surface specific, and species specific. The interaction of plasminogen with the cell surface results in a 10-fold enhancement in the efficiency of plasmin generation by t-PA by enhancing 10-fold the enzyme-substrate affinity of this reaction. This is reflected in the markedly lower Michaelis constant (K_m) for the cell surface activation of plasminogen by t-PA. This "fibrinlike" effect has also been reported for platelets which can also bind plasminogen and enhance its activation (48,50). Plasmin, but not plasminogen, appears to bind to mini-pig aortic endothelial cells (6), but no information regarding its catalytic activity on the cell surface is presently available.

It now appears that the enhanced plasmin generation on the endothelial cell surface may be the result of conversion of circulating glu-plasminogen to lys-plasminogen as it binds to the cell surface (Fig. 4) (32). Lys-plasminogen is the plasmin-modified form of native glu-plasminogen, and displays enhanced binding affinity for fibrin as well as enhanced activation by both urokinase and tissue plasminogen activator (10- to 20-fold greater catalytic efficiency due to a decrease in K_m for the reaction). Lys-plasminogen binds to endothelial cells with greater affinity (2- to 3-fold) than glu-plasminogen. Upon interaction with endothelial cells, glu-plasminogen is partially converted to a molecular species which comigrates with lys-plasminogen and which reacts with a lys-plasminogen-specific monoclonal antibody in immunoblot analyses. This conversion is completely blocked by diisopropylfluorophosphate (DFP) but not by other protease inhibitors, suggesting that it is mediated by a surface-associated serine protease. Lys-plasminogen can also be identified in epsilon-aminocaproic acid eluates of intact umbilical veins by immunoblotting and in frozen sections from a variety of tissues by immunohistochemistry. Thus, endothelial cells appear to actively modify circulating glu-plasminogen to form lys-plasminogen which binds with high affinity to the cell surface, thereby enhancing the fibrinolytic potential of the vessel wall (32).

Since cultured human endothelial cells bind both plasminogen and its major circulating activator, t-PA (30–32), it is reasonable to suppose that there exist specific cell surface binding sites which function to enhance the activatability of plasminogen and to protect t-PA from its physiological inhibitor, thereby augmenting the fibrinolytic potential of the endothelial cell. Evidence for a similar dual binding system has also been reported for extravascular cells, namely monocyte-like U937 cells and GM1380 fetal lung fibroblasts (60).

ENDOTHELIAL CELL ACTIVATION

Elements of the endothelial cell's coagulant system which are subject to modulation by endothelial cell activators include surface expression of tissue factor, down-regulation of the thrombomodulin-thrombin-protein C system, expression of leukocyte adhesion molecules (LAM), and production of platelet-derived growth factor. In addition, the endothelial cell's profibrinolytic system may also be down-regulated as enhanced synthesis of plasminogen activator inhibitor has been well documented (Fig. 1B).

Procoagulant Modulation

TISSUE FACTOR

The monocyte-derived immunological mediator, interleukin-1 (IL-1), represents a potent "activator" of endothelial cells. This association was first suggested when it was observed that endotoxin could induce expression of tissue factor in monocytes (41) and in endothelial cells (16) and that this expression was associated with a coagulation response. Subsequently, it was shown that when endothelial cells are injured or "perturbed" by treatment with IL-1, they undergo a dramatic colchicine-sensitive shape change and acquire a new set of properties which may be described as "procoagulant" (54). Primary among these new properties is the expression of tissue-factorlike activity on the cell surface (9). Upon treatment with low levels of IL-1 (11 U/ml), for example, human vascular endothelial cells (HUVEC) express a 4- to 15-fold increase in tissue-factorlike activity (9). This induced activity peaks at 3 to 6 hr of stimulation, declines to near baseline by 24 hr, and is inhibited by prior treatment of cells with cycloheximide or actinomycin D (9). Theoretically, induction of tissue factor on the cell surface could provide binding sites for circulating VIIa, leading in turn to activation of Factor X by the IXa-VIII-X surface complex. Factors Xa and V would then activate thrombin, leading to the formation of fibrin strands on the vessel wall. Whether sufficient procoagulant activity produced by such immunological mediators is of physiological significance remains to be determined. However, it is well documented that clinical thrombosis may follow an acute infectious event, and this process may represent a vestigial defense mechanism whereby infection is physically contained.

In addition to the direct effects of exogenous IL-1, both endotoxin and alpha-thrombin (but not gamma-thrombin or prothrombin) elicit protein synthesis-dependent release of IL-1 from cultured endothelial cells (71). Tumor necrosis factor (TNF) can also interact directly with specific, high affinity (K_d ~100 pM) endothelial cell surface receptors leading to a parallel release of IL-1 (53). Since release of IL-1 by these agents has been associated with enhanced procoagulant activity, IL-1 has been said to act in an "autocrine" fashion, by targeting specific receptors on its cell of origin (71). Recombinant TNF also induced a rise in total cellular and cell surface procoagulant activity which displayed identical kinetic properties and similar inhibition by cycloheximide and actinomycin D (12). However, the effects of these two mediators were additive when used in combination, suggesting that they may operate through disparate binding sites or cause release of separate procoagulant pools (16).

THROMBIN-THROMBOMODULIN-PROTEIN C

When endothelial cells are exposed to IL-1 or related agents (endotoxin and TNF), the protein C anticoagulant system becomes significantly depressed (22). For example, in 6 to 12 hr, thrombomodulin is reduced to 20 to 50 percent of normal activity, and protein S function, as determined by binding to the cell surface, is reduced to 10 percent of normal (51,54,55). The duration of these effects far exceeds the return of tissue factor and leukocyte adherence to normal, suggesting that this inhibition of normal anticoagulant activity may be physiologically most relevant. In addition, the circulating level of C4BP—a protein which binds to protein S, rendering it unavailable for cell surface binding—is increased under these conditions (22), serving to further down-modulate the system by limiting binding of activated protein C to the endothelial cell surface.

LEUKOCYTE ADHESION

The fully developed hemostatic plug contains a variety of cell types, including red cells, platelets, and leukocytes. Another effect of IL-1 on endothelium possibly related to hemostasis is the promotion of adhesion of neutrophils to human endothelial cells by IL-1 (10 U/ml) or by recombinant TNF (1–10,000 U/ml, 5 min) (10,28). This effect, when induced by IL-1, requires protein synthesis and peaks after 4 to 6 hr of stimulation (10). TNF, on the other hand, seems to induce leukocyte adhesion after as little as 5 minutes of exposure to rTNF and does not require protein synthesis (28), again suggesting a separate mechanism of action.

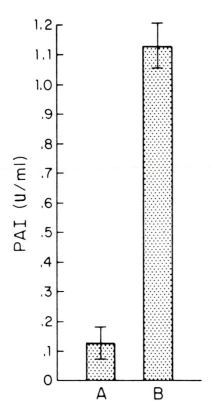

Figure 5: Effect of IL-1 on the PAI content of conditioned medium from cultured endothelial cells. Confluent HUVEC were incubated at 37°C for 18 hr with or without IL-1 (5.32 ng/ml). Postculture medium was then collected, made 0.01 percent with Triton X-100, centrifuged to remove cellular debris, and assayed for PAI activity by preincubation with t-PA (0.5 U for 1 hr at 37°C and measuring the residual t-PA activity on ^{125}I-fibrin plates containing plasminogen.
A. Postculture medium from nonstimulated cells. Mean 0.125 U/ml ± 0.042 (SEM). n = 4.
B. Postculture medium from IL-1 stimulated cells. Mean 1.13 U/ml ± 0.075 (SEM). n = 6.
(Reproduced from Nachman et al. [52].)

Endotoxin, like IL-1, also induced leukocyte adhesion to cultured endothelial cells (61,68).

Thrombin stimulated human endothelial cells produce a biologically active phospholipid called platelet-activating factor (PAF; 1-alkyl-2-acetyl-sn-glycero-3-phosphocholine) (58,79). The PAF synthesized by these cells remains surface-associated and is not released (58). PAF is a potent stimulus for activating neutrophils, as well as platelets, and also promotes the adherence of neutrophils to endothelial cell monolayers (80). It is not yet clear whether the effects described above for IL-1 and TNF on leukocyte adhesion to endothelial cells (EC) might also be mediated through release of PAF.

PLATELET-DERIVED GROWTH FACTOR

Finally, release of platelet-derived growth factor from cultured endothelial cells induced by IL-1 or its secretogogues may also impact on the coagulant properties of the endothelial cell. Stimulation with either TNF (0.5 to 3.0 nM; 18 hr) or IL-1 (70 to 250 pM; 18 hr) leads to a time- and concentration-dependent PDGF release which involves new protein synthesis (29). In similar studies, both alpha-thrombin and activation of Factor Xa on the cell surface also released PDGF from human endothelial cells (27,33). Since PDGF may act as a vasoconstrictor (8) and also a smooth muscle cell mitogen, it may act upon the vessel wall in a prothrombotic fashion. While vasoconstriction may serve to stem the flow of blood early in the course of vessel wall injury, subsequent smooth muscle cell proliferation would promote vessel healing. These findings suggest the existence of multiple levels of control through which immune mediators and cell surface coagulant function are linked. Thus, with appropriate stimulation, the endothelial cell draws upon a vast repertoire of synthetic capabilities leading to dramatic changes in cell function.

Modulation of Fibrinolysis

To the extent that synthesis of plasminogen activator inhibitor is increased during endothelial cell activation, the endothelial cell's profibrinolytic system may also be attenuated. Available evidence would indicate that surface expression of binding sites for plasminogen and its activators is modulated to only a minimal degree upon endothelial stimulation (49; K. Hajjar, unpublished data). Endothelial cell elaboration of tissue plasminogen activator does appear to be regulated during cellular activation (12,67).

PLASMINOGEN ACTIVATOR INHIBITOR

The profibrinolytic system of the human endothelial cell in culture may also be down-regulated by inflammatory mediators such as IL-1. Cultured human endothelial cells constitutively synthesize and secrete the major fast-acting inhibitor of t-PA, plasminogen activator inhibitor (PAI) (79). Following stimulation with IL-1 (5.3 ng/ml; 18 hr), PAI release increases approximately 10-fold when assayed in the presence of a nonionic detergent (52) (Fig. 5). Functional PAI was identified in this study by two methods: the ^{125}I-fibrin plate lysis assay, and reverse fibrin autography. IL-1-induced release of PAI peaks at 18 to 24 hr, requires de novo protein synthesis, and is not associated with a significant change in t-PA antigen activity (11,52). Similarly, in an in vivo rat model, infusion of endotoxin causes a rapid dose-dependent (0.01 to 1000 μg/kg) increase in plasma levels of PAI (21). Thus, immunological mediators may limit circulating plasminogen activator activity by eliciting high levels of PAI. However, on the endothelial cell surface t-PA appears to be protected from inhibition by fluid phase PAI at up to a 20-fold molar excess (31). Therefore, the cell surface may provide a protected pool of active t-PA, even in the presence of excess PAI.

TISSUE PLASMINOGEN ACTIVATOR

Upon maximal stimulation with IL-1b or TNFa, cultured human umbilical vein endothelial cells displayed a 50 percent decrease in secretion of t-PA together with a 400 percent increase in PAI-1 release (12,67). Both IL-1 and TNF acted in a dose- and time-dependent, but nonadditive fashion, suggesting a common mechanism of action.

ACKNOWLEDGMENTS

Dr. Hajjar is the recipient of Clinical Investigator Award KO8 HL01352 from the National Institutes of Health, and an Andrew W. Mellon Foundation Teacher-Scientist Award. This work was also supported by grant HL18828 (Specialized Center of Research in Thrombosis) from the National Institutes of Health and a grant from the Council for Tobacco Research—U.S.A., Inc. (#2169).

REFERENCES

1. Appella E, Robinson EA, Ullrich SJ, Stoppelli MP, Corti A, Cassani G, Blasi F: The receptor-binding sequence of urokinase. J Biol Chem 262:4437–4440, 1987.

2. Awbrey BJ, Hoak JC, Owen WG: Binding of human thrombin to cultured human endothelial cells. J Biol Chem 254:4092–4095, 1979.

3. Bajpai A, Baker JB: Cryptic urokinase binding site on human foreskin fibroblasts. Biochem Biophys Res Commun 133:475–482, 1985.

4. Bajpai A, Baker JB: Urokinase binding sites on human foreskin cells. Evidence for occupancy with endogenous urokinase. Biochem Biophys Res Commun 133:994–1000, 1985.

5. Barnathan ES, Kuo A, Van der Keyl H, McCrae KR, Larsen GR, Cines DB: Tissue-type plasminogen activator binding to human endothelial cells: Evidence for two distinct binding sites. J Biol Chem 263:7792–7799, 1988.

6. Bauer PI, Machovich R, Buki KG, Csonka E, Koch SA, Horvath I: Interaction of plasmin with endothelial cells. Biochem J 281:119–124, 1984.

7. Beebe DP: Binding of tissue plasminogen activator to human umbilical vein endothelial cells. Thromb Res 46:241–254, 1987.

8. Berk BC, Alexander RW, Brock TA, Gimbrone MA, Webb RC: Vasoconstriction: A new activity for platelet-derived growth factor. Science 232:87–90, 1986.

9. Bevilacqua MP, Pober JS, Majeau GR, Cotran RS, Gimbrone MA: Interleukin 1 (IL-1) induces biosynthesis and cell surface expression of procoagulant activity in human vascular endothelial cells. J Exp Med 160:618–623, 1984.

10. Bevilacqua MP, Pober JS, Majeau GR, Fiers W, Cotran RS, Gimbrone MA: Recombinant tumor necrosis factor induces procoagulant activity in cultured human vascular endothelium: characterization and comparison with the actions of interleukin 1. Proc Natl Acad Sci USA 83:4533–4537, 1986.

11. Bevilacqua MP, Pober JS, Wheeler ME, Cotran RS, Gimbrone MA: Interleukin 1 acts on cultured human endothelium to increase the adhesion of polymorphonuclear leukocytes, monocytes, and related leukocyte cell lines. J Clin Invest 76:2003–2011, 1985.

12. Bevilacqua MP, Schleef RR, Gimbrone MA, Loskutoff DJ: Regulation of cultured human vascular endothelium by interleukin 1. J Clin Invest 78:587–591, 1986.

13. Buonassisi V: Sulfated mucopolysaccharide synthesis and secretion in endothelial cell culture. Exp Cell Res 76:363–368, 1973.

14. Busch PC, Owen WG: Identification in vitro of an endothelial cell surface cofactor for antithrombin III. J Clin Invest 69:726–729, 1982.

15. Cerveny TJ, Fass DN, Mann KG: Synthesis of coagulation factor V by cultured aortic endothelium. Blood 63:1467–1474, 1984.

16. Colucci M, Balconi G, Lorenzet R, Pietra A, Locati D, Donati MB, Semeraro N: Cultured human endothelial cells generate tissue factor in response to endotoxin. J Clin Invest 71:1893–1896, 1983.

17. Cubellis MV, Nolli ML, Cassani G, Blasi F: Binding of single chain prourokinase to the urokinase receptor of human U937 cells. J Biol Chem 261:15819–15822, 1986.

18. Dejana P, Languino LR, Polentarutti N, Balconi G, Ryckewaert JJ, Larrieu MJ, Donati MB, Mantovani A, Marguerie G: Interaction between fibrinogen and cultured endothelial cells. Induction of migration and specific binding. J Clin Invest 75:11–18, 1985.

19. Del Rosso M, Dini G, Fibbi G: Receptors for plasminogen activator, urokinase, in normal and Rous sarcoma virus-transformed mouse fibroblasts. Cancer Res 45:630–636, 1985.

20. Del Rosso M, Pucci M, Fibbi G, Dini G: Interaction of urokinase with specific receptors abolishes the time of commitment to terminal differentiation of murine erythroleukaemia (Friend) cells. Br J Haematol 66:289–294, 1987.

21. Emeis JJ, Kooistra T: Interleukin 1 and lipopolysaccharide induce an inhibitor of tissue-type plasminogen activator in vivo and in cultured endothelial cells. J Exp Med 163:1260–1266, 1986.

22. Esmon CT: The regulation of natural anticoagulant pathways. Science 235:1348-1352, 1987.

23. Esmon CT, Esmon NL, Harris KW: Complex formation between thrombin and thrombomodulin inhibits both thrombin-catalyzed fibrin formation and factor V activation. J Biol Chem 257:7944–7947, 1982.

24. Esmon NL, Owen WG, Esmon CT: Isolation of a membrane cofactor for thrombin-catalyzed activation of protein C. J Biol Chem 257:859–864, 1982.

25. Fibbi G, Dini G, Pasquali F, Pucci M, Del Rosso M: The MW 17500 region of the A chain of urokinase is required for interaction with a specific receptor in

A431 cells. Biochim Biophys Acta 885:301–308, 1986.

26. Furchgott RF, Zawadzki JV: The obligatory role of endothelial cells in the relaxation of arterial smooth muscle by acetylcholine. Nature 288:373–376, 1980.

27. Gajdusek C, Carbon S, Ross R, Nawroth P, Stern D: Activation of coagulation releases endothelial cell mitogens. J Cell Biol 103:419–427, 1986.

28. Gamble JR, Harlan JM, Klebanoff SJ, Vadas MA: Stimulation of the adherence of neutrophils to umbilical vein endothelium by human recombinant tumor necrosis factor. Proc Natl Acad Sci USA 82:8667–8671, 1985.

29. Hajjar KA, Hajjar DP, Silverstein RL, Nachman RL: Tumor necrosis factor-mediated release of platelet-derived growth factor from cultured endothelial cells. J Exp Med 166:235–245, 1987.

30. Hajjar KA, Hamel NM, Harpel PC, Nachman RL: Binding of tissue plasminogen activator to cultured human endothelial cells. J Clin Invest 80:1712–1719, 1987.

31. Hajjar KA, Harpel PC, Jaffe EA, Nachman RL: Binding of plasminogen to cultured human endothelial cells. J Biol Chem 261:11656–11662, 1986.

32. Hajjar KA, Nachman RL: Endothelial cell-mediated conversion of glu-plasminogen to lys-plasminogen. Further evidence for assembly of the fibrinolytic system on the endothelial cell surface. J Clin Invest 82:1769–1778, 1988.

33. Harlan JM, Thompson PJ, Ross RR, Bowen-Pope DF: Alpha-thrombin induces release of platelet-derived growth factor-like molecule(s) by cultured human endothelial cells. J Cell Biol 103:1129–1133, 1986.

34. Harris KW, Esmon CT: Protein S is required for bovine platelets to support activated protein C binding and activity. J Biol Chem 260:2007–2010, 1985.

35. Huarte J, Belin D, Bosco D, Sappino AP, Vassalli JD: Plasminogen activator and mouse spermatozoa: urokinase synthesis in the male genital tract and binding of the enzyme to the sperm cell surface. J Cell Biol 104:1281–1289, 1987.

36. Ishii H, Salem HH, Bell CE, Laposata EA, Majerus PW: Thrombomodulin, an endothelial anticoagulant protein is absent from human brain. Blood 67:362–365, 1986.

37. Jaffe EA, Hoyer LW, Nachman RL: Synthesis of antihemophilic factor antigen by cultured human endothelial cells. J Clin Invest 52:2757–2764, 1973.

38. Johnson AE, Esmon NL, Laue TM, Esmon CT: Structural changes required for activation of protein C are induced by Ca^{++} binding to a high affinity site that does not contain gamma-carboxyglutamic acid. J Biol Chem 258:5554–5560, 1983.

39. Laug WE: Glucocorticoids inhibit plasminogen activator production by endothelial cells. Thromb Haemost 50:888–892, 1983.

40. Levine EG, Loskutoff DJ: Cultured bovine endothelial cells produce both urokinase and tissue-type plasminogen activators. J Cell Biol 94:631–636, 1982.

41. Levy GA, Schwartz BS, Curtiss LK, Edgington TS: Plasma lipoprotein induction and suppression of the generation of cellular procoagulant activity in vitro. J Clin Invest 67:1614–1622, 1981.

42. Lijnen HR, Collen D: Interaction of plasminogen activators and inhibitors with plasminogen and fibrin. Semin Thromb Hemost 8:2–10, 1983.

43. Lollar P, Hoak JC, Owen WG: Binding of thrombin to cultured human endothelial cells. Nonequilibrium aspects. J Biol Chem 255:10279–10283, 1980.

44. Mammen EF: Protein C, in Semin Thromb Hemost. New York, Thieme-Stratton, 1984, vol 10.

45. Maruyama I, Bell CE, Majerus PW: Thrombomodulin is found on endothelium of arteries, veins, capillaries and lymphatics and on synctiotrophoblast of human placenta. J Cell Biol 101:363–371, 1985.

46. Maynard JR, Dreyer BE, Stemerman MB, Pitlick FA: Tissue-factor coagulant activity of cultured human endothelial and smooth muscle cells and fibroblasts. Blood 50:387–396, 1977.

47. McKee PA, Andersen JC, Switzer ME: Molecular structural studies of human factor VIII. Ann NY Acad Sci 240:8–33, 1975.

48. Miles LA, Ginsberg MH, White JG, Plow EF: Plasminogen interacts with human platelets through two distinct mechanisms. J Clin Invest 77:2001–2009, 1986.

49. Miles LA, Levin EG, Plescia J, Collen D, Plow EF: Plasminogen receptors, urokinase receptors and their modulation on human endothelial cells. Blood 72:628–635, 1988.

50. Miles LA, Plow EF: Binding and activation of plasminogen on the platelet surface. J Biol Chem 260:4303–4311, 1985.

51. Moore KL, Andreoli SP, Esmon NL, Esmon CT, Bang NU: Endotoxin enhances tissue factor and suppresses thrombomodulin expression of human vascular endothelium in vitro. J Clin Invest 79:124–130, 1987.

52. Nachman RL, Hajjar KA, Silverstein RL, Dinarello CA: Interleukin 1 induces endothelial cell synthesis of plasminogen activator inhibitor. J Exp Med 163:1595–1600, 1986.

53. Nawroth PP, Bank I, Handley D, Cassimeris J, Chess L, Stern D: Tumor necrosis factor/cachectin interacts with endothelial cell receptors to induce release of interleukin 1. J Exp Med 163:1363–1375, 1986.

54. Nawroth PP, Handley DA, Esmon CT, Stern DM: Interleukin 1 induces endothelial cell procoagulant activity while suppressing cell-surface anticoagulant activity. Proc Natl Acad Sci USA 83:3460–3464, 1986.

55. Nawroth PP, Stern DM: Modulation of endothelial cell hemostatic properties by tumor necrosis factor. J Exp Med 163:740–745, 1986.

56. Nielsen LS, Kellerman GM, Behrendt N, Picone R, Dan K, Blasi F: A 55,000–60,000 M_r receptor protein for urokinase-type plasminogen activator: Identification in human tumor cell lines and partial purification. J Biol Chem 263:2358–2363, 1988.

57. Omar MN, Mann KG: Inactivation of factor Va by plasmin. J Biol Chem 262:9750–9755, 1987.

58. Owen WG, Esmon CT: Functional properties of an endothelial cell cofactor for thrombin-catalyzed activation of protein C. J Biol Chem 256:5532–5535, 1981.

59. Palmer RM, Ferrige AG, Moncada S: Nitric oxide release accounts for the biological activity of endothelium-derived relaxing factor. Nature 327:524–526, 1987.

60. Plow EF, Freaney DE, Plescia J, Miles LA: The plasminogen system and cell surfaces: Evidence for plasminogen and urokinase receptors on the same cell type. J Cell Biol 103:2411–2420, 1986.

61. Pohlman TH, Stanness KA, Beatty PG, Ochs HD, Harlan JM: An endothelial cell surface factor(s) induced in vitro by lipopolysaccharide, interleukin 1, and tumor necrosis factor-alpha increases neutrophil adherence by a CDw18-dependent mechanism. J Immunol 136:4548–4553, 1986.

62. Prescott SM, Zimmerman GA, McIntyre TM: Human endothelial cells in culture produce platelet-activating factor (1-alkyl-2-acetyl-sn-glycero-3-phosphocholine) when stimulated with thrombin. Proc Natl Acad Sci USA 81:3534–3538, 1984.

63. Radomski MW, Palmer RM, Moncada S: Comparative pharmacology of endothelium-derived relaxing factor, nitric oxide and prostacyclin in platelets. Br J Pharmacol 92:181–187, 1987.

64. Rimon S, Melamed R, Savion N, Scott T, Nawroth PP, Stern DM: Identification of factor IX/IX$_a$ binding protein on the endothelial cell surface. J Biol Chem 262:6023–6031, 1987.

65. Rodgers GM, Shuman MA: Prothrombin is activated on vascular endothelial cells by factor X$_a$ and calcium. Proc Natl Acad Sci USA 80:7001–7005, 1983.

66. Sakata Y, Okada M, Noro A, Matsuda M: Interaction of tissue-type plasminogen activator and plasminogen activator inhibitor 1 on the surface of endothelial cells. J Biol Chem 263:1960–1969, 1988.

67. Schleef RR, Bevilacqua MP, Sawdey M, Gimbrone MA, Loskutoff DJ: Cytokine activation of vascular endothelium: Effects on tissue-type plasminogen activator and type 1 plasminogen activator inhibitor. J Biol Chem 263:5797–5803, 1988.

68. Schleimer RP, Rutledge BK: Cultured human vascular endothelial cells acquire adhesiveness for neutrophils after stimulation with interleukin 1, endotoxin, and tumor-promoting diesters. J Immunol 136 : 649–654, 1986.

69. Shuman MA, Merkel CH: Urokinase binding to bovine corneal endothelial cells. Exp Eye Res 41 : 371–382, 1985.

70. Silverstein RL, Nachman RL, Leung LL, Harpel PC: Activation of immobilized plasminogen by tissue activator. Multimolecular complex formation. J Biol Chem 260 : 10346–10352, 1985.

71. Stern DM, Bank I, Nawroth PP, Cassimeris J, Kisiel W, Fenton JW II, Dinarello C, Chess L, Jaffe EA: Self-regulation of procoagulant events on the endothelial cell surface. J Exp Med 162 : 1223–1235, 1985.

72. Stern DM, Drillings M, Nossel HL, Hurlet-Jensen A, LaGamma KS, Owen J: Binding of factors IX and IX_a to cultured vascular endothelial cells. Proc Natl Acad Sci USA 80 : 4119–4123, 1983.

73. Stern DM, Nawroth PP, Harris K, Esmon CT: Cultured bovine endothelial cells promote activated protein C-protein S-mediated inactivation of factor Va. J Biol Chem 261 : 713–718, 1986.

74. Stern DM, Nawroth PP, Kisiel W, Handley D, Drillings M, Bartos J: A coagulation pathway on bovine aortic segments leading to generation of factor X_a and thrombin. J Clin Invest 74 : 1910–1921, 1984.

75. Stern DM, Nawroth PP, Kisiel W, Vehar G, Esmon CT: The binding of factor IX_a to cultured bovine aortic endothelial cells. Induction of a specific site in the presence of factors VIII and X. J Biol Chem 260 : 6717–6722, 1985.

76. Stern DM, Nawroth P, Marcum J, Handley D, Kisiel W, Rosenberg R, Stern K: Interaction of antithrombin III with bovine aortic segments. Role of heparin in binding and enhanced anticoagulant activity. J Clin Invest 75 : 272–279, 1985.

77. Stoppelli MP, Corti A, Soffientini A, Cassani G, Blasi F, Assoian RK: Differentiation-enhanced binding of the amino-terminal fragment of human urokinase plasminogen activator to a specific receptor in U937 monocytes. Proc Natl Acad Sci USA 82 : 4939–4943, 1985.

78. Stoppelli MP, Tacchetti C, Cubellis MV, Corti A, Hearing VJ, Cassani G, Appella E, Blasi F: Autocrine saturation of prourokinase receptors on human A431 cells. Cell 45 : 675–684, 1986.

79. Van Hinsbergh VW, Binnema D, Scheffer MA, Sprengers ED, Kooistra T, Rijken DC: Production of plasminogen activator and inhibitor by serially propagated endothelial cells from adult human blood vessels. Arteriosclerosis 7 : 389–400, 1987.

80. Van Mourik JA, Lawrence DA, Loskutoff DJ: Purification of an inhibitor of plasminogen activator (antiactivator) synthesized by endothelial cells. J Biol Chem 259 : 14914–14921, 1984.

81. Vassalli JD, Baccino D, Belin D: A cellular binding site for the Mr 55,000 form of the human plasminogen activator, urokinase. J Cell Biol 100 : 86–92, 1985.

82. Walker FJ: Identification of a new protein involved in the regulation of the anti-coagulant activity of activated protein C protein S-binding protein. J Biol Chem 261 : 10941–10944, 1986.

83. Weksler BB, Ley CW, Jaffe EA: Stimulation of endothelial cell prostacyclin production by thrombin, trypsin, and the ionophore A23187. J Clin Invest 62 : 923–931, 1978.

84. Weksler BB, Marcus AJ, Jaffe EA: Synthesis of prostaglandin I_2 (prostacyclin) by cultured human and bovine endothelial cells. Proc Natl Acad Sci USA 74 : 3922–3926, 1977.

85. Zimmerman GA, McIntyre TM, Prescott SM: Production of platelet-activating factor by human vascular endothelial cells: Evidence for a requirement for specific agonists and modulation by prostacyclin. Circulation 72 : 718–727, 1985.

86. Zimmerman GA, McIntyre TM, Prescott SM: Thrombin stimulates the adherence of neutrophils to human endothelial cells in vitro. J Clin Invest 76 : 2235–2246, 1985.

Robert W. Wissler, M.D., Ph.D.

Dragoslava Vesselinovitch, M.S., D.V.M.

18

Atherogenesis in the Pulmonary Artery

Progressive pulmonary artery atherosclerosis develops infrequently in adult humans. This is true even though the endothelium of the main pulmonary artery and its branches is exposed to the same blood-borne factors that are responsible, at least in part, for atherogenesis in nearby elastic and muscular arteries, including the aorta and the coronary arteries. In the vast majority of adult human autopsies, little or no gross or microscopic evidence of any degree of pulmonary artery atherosclerotic disease is observed, even though the blood lipid levels may be very high, and risk factors such as cigarette smoking, systemic hypertension, diabetes, sustained immune complex, or autoimmune disease (or other circulating endothelial damaging agents) that are known to cause endothelial injury, may have been documented.

In this chapter, the subject of pulmonary artery atherosclerosis will be utilized to demonstrate some of the current principles of atherogenesis and to pose some of the basic questions that still need investigation. This chapter may also serve to contribute to the understanding of the total subject of the pulmonary circulation—normal and abnormal.

For many years, pathologists have recognized that although progressive atherosclerosis of the main pulmonary arteries is uncommon and any significant effect on pulmonary circulation is rare, certain exceptions have been documented. In general, these exceptions are characterized by congenital or acquired diseases that raise the pulmonary artery pressure substantially and that permit survival well into adult life. These include chronic left-to-right shunt conditions that have not been surgically corrected early in life, chronic congenital or rheumatic vascular disease, especially chronic mitral stenosis and chronic obstructive or fibrosing pulmonary disease, including certain types of pulmonary neoplasms, chronic fibrosing granulomatous disease, pulmonary emphysema, and a number of miscellaneous diseases that terminate with severe interference with the pulmonary circulation and result in pulmonary hypertension.

Some of these predisposing pathological processes also result in severe obstructive disease of small pulmonary arteries. Although these narrowings of small pulmonary arteries and arterioles (see Chapter 34) are not atheromatous, they often share two features with the atheromatous lesions, namely, chronic endothelial injury and smooth muscle cell (SMC) proliferation. Moreover, they may contribute to the failure of reducing or reversing the pulmonary artery effects of a chronic left-to-right shunt or a chronic intimal stenosis when they are corrected during adult life. Therefore, there is an ongoing relationship between what happens in the wall of the small pulmonary arteries and what happens in relation to atherogenesis in the large and medium-sized pulmonary arteries.

Why devote a chapter in a monograph on pulmonary circulation to a disease process that practically never results in any functional effects in this vascular bed? When trying to understand the determining factors responsible for the development of plaques, which in many nearby arteries cause a high incidence of morbidity and mortality, studying the reasons for natural protection may lead to valuable insights into atherogenesis and about the pulmonary circulation. Unfortunately, there is as yet little work reported either in experimental animals or in the area of cell biology and molecular biology that sheds light on this remarkable protection of the pulmonary artery.

This chapter will review the current state of knowledge about pulmonary arterial atherosclerosis, most of which has resulted from repeated and confirmed clinical pathological correlations. It will also attempt to pose some of the more obvious questions which, if answered, might increase understanding of this type of relative resistance to atheromatous stimuli.

THE PULMONARY ARTERIAL SYSTEM AND THE GENERAL PRINCIPLES OF ATHEROGENESIS

One of the two major components of the fully developed atherosclerotic plaque, from which the disease is named, is the soft, lipid-rich center, which usually contains predominantly cholesterol esters along with lesser quantities of free cholesterol, triglycerides, lower density lipoproteins, and protein debris. It is usually poor in intact living cells and has the consistency of a thick paste; hence, the prefix "athero-" from the Greek word (athera) for porridge or gruel. The second component is the fibrous cap, which is composed largely of smooth muscle cells and the main products they synthesize, namely, collagen, elastin, and proteoglycans. This component of the plaque is sclerotic and contains variable amounts of lipid and intact lipoproteins, mostly BVLDL and LDL, which are usually located both intracellularly and intercellularly. There they are often bound to the SMCs fibrous products, including the proteoglycans. Variable numbers of other bloodborne cells are present in most lesions. These include monocytes, monocyte-derived macrophages, and lymphocytes. Often the monocyte-derived macrophages are filled with abundant lipid droplets so that they are enlarged, stain very deeply with fat stains, and accurately reflect their common name of "foam cells." It is probable that most developing lesions also contain SMC-derived "foam cells" recently described as deriving their large amounts of lipid by directly engulfing lipid droplets that were originally formed and released from fat-filled macrophages (19). Although this scheme of SMC foam cell formation is largely based on in vitro studies, it is an attractive way to explain the large numbers of SMC-derived foam cells seen in developing human lesions (17).

In general, other components of the advanced human plaque (i.e., calcium deposits, neovascularization, intraplaque hemorrhage, as well as ulceration and/ or fracture of the fibrous caps) are thought to be complications and not an integral part of plaque development.

The major processes of plaque development are lipid deposition and smooth muscle cell proliferation. Both processes are recognized contributors to the mass of the plaque and to its later clinical effects (16). It is also important to note that the SMCs which migrate into the intima and proliferate in the developing plaque are not the same as those in the media (3). They are modified so that they are more active as synthetic cells.

At present, two major factors thought to be responsible for progression of the atherosclerotic plaque are the degree and type of the hyperlipidemia and the condition of the intimal (endothelial) surface of the artery. In addition, many observations of human arteries indicate that there are certain sites of predilection for lesion development (4,13,15) and that these areas are more susceptible than others primarily because they are subject to certain hemodynamic forces (6). In final analysis, it appears that the low pressure in the pulmonary arterial circulation and the low tension in the artery walls, as well as the relatively small changes in these forces with each cardiac cycle, are most responsible for the low incidence and severity of atherosclerosis in this circulation.

It is also likely that certain chronic disease states such as hypertension and diabetes may increase the susceptibility of arteries to atherogenic effects by means of changes they produce in the arterial wall and the arterial endothelium. These changes, in turn, increase the facility of cholesterol carrying lipoproteins to enter the artery from the bloodstream and to be retained (14). Moreover, cigarette smoking is likely to produce its atherogenic effects at least partly by means of chemical changes induced in the intima of the artery (10). There are a number of factors that increase the progression rate of atherogenesis. These factors, which include circulating immune complexes (18), homocystinemia (7), circulating endotoxins (12), and viremia (20), may exert their effects by means of sustained endothelial injury.

The relative resistance of the pulmonary artery to atherogenesis may be largely a function of difference in hemodynamic effects. There is no direct evidence that the endothelium, intima, and media of the pulmonary arteries are fundamentally different from other arteries; therefore, one must assume that the low mean pressure (9 to 16 mmHg) during the cardiac cycle is a major factor protecting the pulmonary arterial tree from atherogenesis. Nor is there evidence that the serum or plasma constituents or the cellular components of the blood are any different as they leave the right side of the heart to enter the lungs—where the pulmonary arteries are not likely to develop atherosclerosis—than when they enter the aorta and the systemic arteries, which are much more susceptible to atherosclerosis.

The other major mechanism to be considered with respect to the natural protection of the pulmonary artery from atherosclerosis is influence of the organization of microthrombi or emboli in these arteries. This mechanism of atherogenesis has been popular in certain scientific circles for many years. Most likely, it would be of importance in the pulmonary arterial tree where the thromboemboli from the entire systemic venous side of the circulation would probably be localized. Accordingly, at face value, this formulation would seem to be at odds with the very low incidence of atherosclerosis in the pulmonary arteries.

Recently, the concept that hypoxia of the arterial wall is a significant factor in the progression of atherosclerosis has been revived. The precapillary vessels of the pulmonary circulation, naturally conveying hypoxemic blood, should be particularly vulnerable to this mechanism. Therefore, the natural resistance of this arterial bed to atherogenesis seems to belie serious consideration of arterial wall hypoxia as a pathogenetic mechanism.

SPECIAL FEATURES OF PULMONARY ARTERY ATHEROGENESIS AS INDICATED BY EXPERIMENTAL STUDIES

One of the reasons why we relate the resistance of the pulmonary artery to atherosclerosis with artery wall tension is the remarkable demonstration by Glagov and Ozoa (5). They found that pulmonary arterial disease can be artificially intensified in the rabbit by increasing the resistance of one pulmonary bed even though the pressure is presumably the same in both arteries. A similar phenomenon appears to be demonstrable in the renal arteries where pressure and artery wall tension are not synonymous (11).

The relationship of arterial mural thrombosis to atherogenesis in both humans and experimental animals has been a subject of intensive study in many laboratories. Many of these investigators have utilized the albino New Zealand rabbit with or without diet-induced hyperlipidemia. The thromboembolic materials have varied from fresh red clots to autologous thrombi formed in the veins of the same experimental animals being utilized for the study, or emboli formed mostly from condensed fibrin plugs. All of these approaches produce reactive lesions in the pulmonary arteries, but few of them contain appreciable lipid unless the animals are hypercholesterolemic. Then the lesions are largely foam cell plaques that resemble those resulting from feeding a high cholesterol ration without embolization. The major effects of the emboli are to increase the frequency and severity of the plaques and to increase the smooth muscle foam cell population of the plaques. Rarely do the plaques seem to develop into advanced plaques, and unless accompanied by sustained hypercholesterolemia, their usual fate is to regress and to form small fibrous cushions on the intima.

Interesting reactive intraluminal lesions have been reported in a number of species when the pulmonary arteries are embolized either as a part of parasitic disease or as the result of tests of materials that may be used for instrumentation or for blood sustitutes and that turn out to produce serious reactions in the artery wall. The embolization by parasites or their products may also produce immune complex modifications of the atheromatous lesion. Other risk factors that may be especially important in relation to the pulmonary artery include virus infection that is likely to be more common in this vascular bed than in many others.

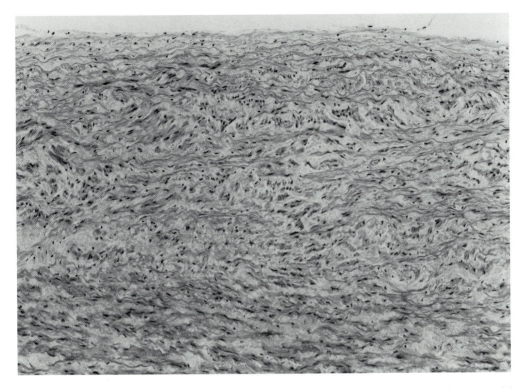

Figure 1: A representative microscopic view of the main pulmonary artery of a 6-year-old girl who had severe homozygous familial hypercholesterolemia with very high blood cholesterol levels. She suffered from severe occlusion atheroma of her coronary arteries and thoracic aorta, and had extensive myocardial infarction. Nevertheless, the main pulmonary artery was virtually free of any evidence of atherosclerosis, even though it was anatomically very near the thoracic aorta. H&E stain. X25. (Courtesy of Dr. Ronald Jaffe, Department of Pathology, Children's Hospital of Pittsburgh.)

FACTORS THAT ARE ESPECIALLY IMPORTANT IN PULMONARY ARTERY ATHEROGENESIS IN HUMANS

The few reports in the literature (9) and our own autopsy experience indicate that hyperlipidemia is a much less potent risk factor than is increased resistance and/ or elevated pressure in increasing the atherosclerotic process. Our study has indicated that even in cases of homozygous familial hypercholesterolemia, little or no atherosclerosis may develop in the pulmonary artery while the adjacent aorta has very severe disease (2) (Fig. 1). On the other hand, in cases of rheumatic heart disease with marked mitral stenosis, more advanced atherosclerosis has been observed in the pulmonary artery (Fig. 2A, B, and C) than in the nearby aorta (Fig. 2D). This accentuated pulmonary atherosclerosis is sometimes associated with thrombosis or thromboembolism (Fig. 3), which bears a striking resemblance to coronary artery atherosclerosis with superimposed thrombosis.

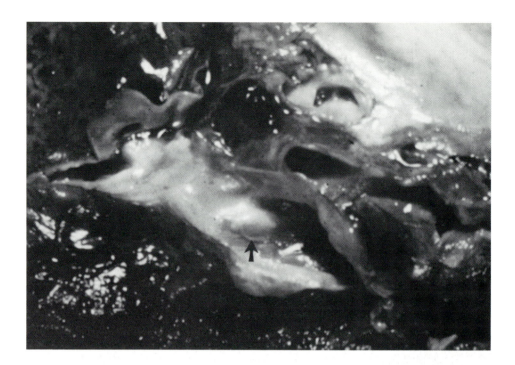

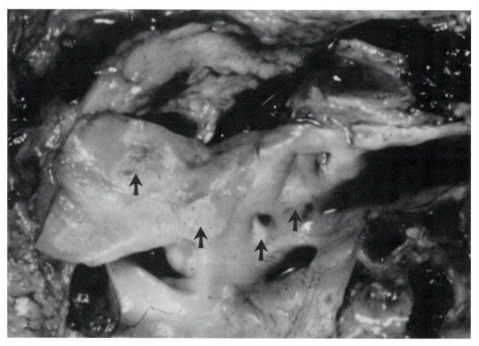

Figure 2: Severe pulmonary artery atherosclerosis found at autopsy of a 44-year-old male who had severe chronic rheumatic mitral valvulitis.

A & B: These two gross views of the pulmonary arteries show severe raised lesions typical of advanced atherosclerosis. The arrows indicate some of the more severe plaques.

C: This raised plaque in the pulmonary artery is a microscopic view of the one indicated by an arrow in Figure 2A. It shows an advanced plaque with a large necrotic cholesterol-rich center and a thick fibrous cap. H&E stain. X10.

D: The aorta adjacent to the pulmonary artery shows virtual absence of microscopic evidence of atherosclerosis. This is a representative section. H&E stain. X25.

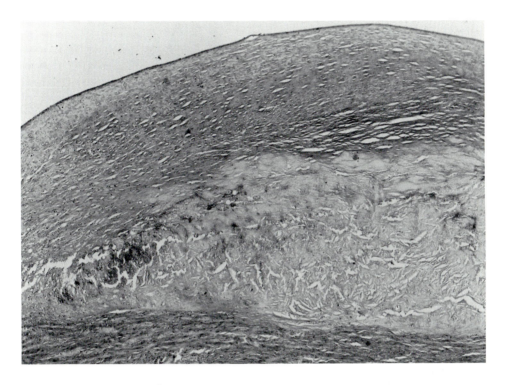

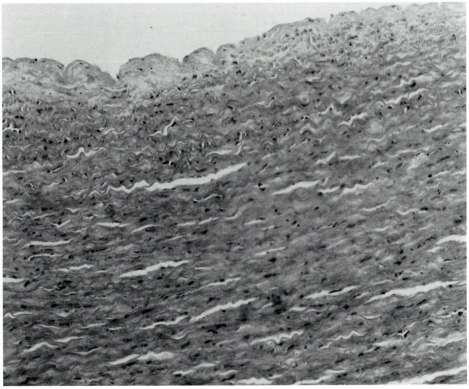

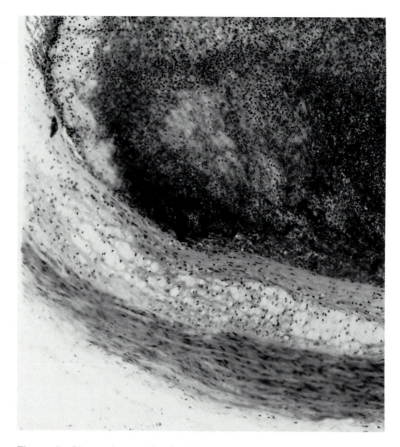

Figure 3: Photomicrograph of a histopathological section of the left lung of a 4-year-old victim of chronic rheumatic mitral valvulitis and pulmonary embolism. Severe atherosclerosis of the pulmonary artery underlies a recent thrombotic embolism in the artery lumen. The atherosclerosis probably developed over a period of months or years before the embolism occurred. Gormori Trichrome Aldehyde Fuchsin. X25.

In the autopsy survey we have conducted, as well as in a recent one from Johns Hopkins (9), one of the diseases most frequently associated with gross pulmonary arterial atherosclerosis is chronic emphysema (Fig. 4). The other remarkable association is the frequency with which notable pulmonary artery atherosclerosis is linked with severe aortic and coronary atherosclerosis, especially in patients with severe systemic hypertension (9).

Pulmonary artery atherosclerosis may be especially prominent in those rare cases of significant congenital left-to-right shunt in which the defects are not diagnosed until adult life, after years of very high pulmonary artery pressure flow and pulsating increased tension, and then only in those individuals in whom the risk factors are present for systemic atherosclerosis. In our experience as well as in published reports, there is no correlation between the carcinoid syndrome and accentuated pulmonary artery atherosclerosis even though the pulmonary valve and the proximal main pulmonary artery are severely damaged.

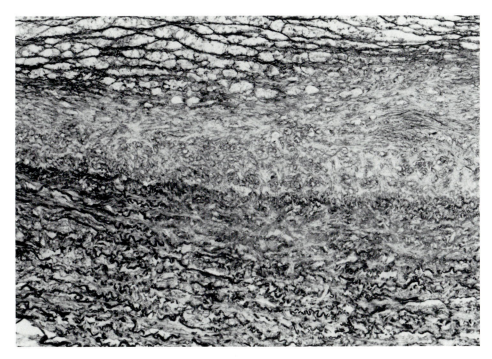

Figure 4: Pulmonary arterial atherosclerosis in a 75-year-old male with severe atherosclerosis, coronary heart disease, and cenetrilobular emphysema. Although atherosclerosis of the pulmonary artery was evident grossly, it was much less severe than the atherosclerosis of the aorta and coronary arteries. H&E stain. X33.

SUMMARY AND REMAINING PROBLEMS

Pulmonary artery atherosclerosis, like atherosclerosis in the systemic arterial system, is mainly limited to the large elastic pulmonary arteries and the first order branches of these arteries, i.e., the major muscular arteries to the lungs.

Pulmonary hypertension, especially when accompanied by restricted blood flow through the pulmonary arterial system, has been shown both clinically and experimentally to be a serious risk factor that favors the development of unusually marked pulmonary atherosclerosis; sometimes pulmonary atherosclerosis is more severe than the usually severe atherosclerosis of the aorta or coronary arteries. One question that needs further exploration is the somewhat paradoxical finding that these pressure and flow abnormalities seem to be more significant for the development of pulmonary artery atherosclerosis than is severe hyperlipidemia.

Another unsettled question is the role of immunological factors in the development of severe pulmonary artery atherosclerosis—especially in chronic rheumatic valvular disease and in severe emphysema caused by cigarette-smoking.

Both of these conditions are likely to be associated with inflammatory vascular disease (1,8). The fact that severe hyperlipidemia, such as that seen in homozygous familial hypercholesterolemia (FH), does not necessarily lead to pulmonary artery atherosclerosis underscores that considerable protection against atherogenesis is afforded by low vascular pressures.

There are numerous reports of experimental animal research, especially involving rabbits, on the role of thromboembolism in the formation of pulmonary atherosclerosis. However, it is very difficult to find convincing evidence that this pathogenetic mechanism is operative in human disease. Although thromboembolism is certainly associated at times with atherosclerotic lesions (Fig. 4), these seem to be two independent factors that, when associated, represent atherosclerosis preceding thrombosis. The multiple reports in rabbits of pulmonary arterial thromboemboli developing into atherosclerotic plaques probably reflects, on the one hand, the sluggish cholesterol catabolism of this species and, on the other, the greater proportion of monocyte-derived foam cells in these atheromatous lesions than in the lesions of most humans and of most nonhuman primates.

In view of evidence implicating the lung as a final resting place for platelets as well as monocytes, it is conceivable that endothelial damage resulting from the release of biologically active substances by morbid platelets could augment pulmonary atherogenesis. Cigarette smoking may also promote atherogenesis, not only by immunologic mechanisms but also by the release of endogenous substances, such as norepinephrine and serotonin. Susceptibility to the harmful effects of endogenous substances, as well as of exogenous materials, can vary from time to time and in different individuals. Pulmonary atherogenesis affords an opportunity to explore these and other mechanisms under controlled experimental conditions.

ACKNOWLEDGMENTS

The authors appreciate the contributions of Mrs. Gertrud Friedman who acted as editorial assistant in preparing this chapter, and Ms. Blanche Berger and Mr. Gordon Bowie who helped in preparing the illustrations.

REFERENCES

1. Becker CG, Dubin T, Wiedemann HP: Hypersensitivity to tobacco antigen. Proc Natl Acad Sci USA 73: 1712–1716 1976.

2. Buja LM, Kovanen PT, Bilheimer DW: Cellular pathology of homozygous familial hypercholesterolemia. Am J Pathol 97: 327–358, 1979.

3 Campbell GR, Chamley-Campbell JH: The cellular pathobiology of atherosclerosis. Pathology 13: 423–440, 1981.

4. Cornhill JH, Herderick EE: Topography of human aortic sudanophilic lesions. International Symposium on Biofluid Mechanics, Palm Springs, California, 1988.

5. Glagov S, Ozoa AK: Significance of the relatively low incidence of atherosclerosis in the pulmonary, renal, and mesenteric arteries. Ann NY Acad Sci 149: 940–955, 1968.

6. Glagov S, Zarins CK, Giddens D, Ku DN, Beere P: Localization of atherosclerosis in man. Biorheology 23: 197, 1986.

7. Harker LA, Ross R, Slichter SJ, Scott CR: Homocystine-induced arteriosclerosis. The role of endothelial cell injury and platelet response in its genesis. J Clin Invest 58 : 731–741, 1976.

8. Kaplan MH: Autoimmunity in rheumatic fever: Relationship to streptococcal antigens cross-reactive with valve fibroblasts, myofibres, and smooth muscle, in Dumonde DC (ed), *Infection and Immunology in the Rheumatic Diseases.* Oxford, Blackwell, 1976, pp 113–118.

9. Moore GW, Smith RRL, Hutchins GM: Pulmonary artery atherosclerosis: Correlation with systemic atherosclerosis and hypertensive pulmonary vascular disease. Arch Pathol Lab Med 106 : 378–380, 1982.

10. Mustard JF, Murphy EA: Effect of smoking on blood coagulation and platelet survival in man. Br Med J 1 : 846–849, 1963.

11. Ozoa AK, Glagov S: Induction of atheroma in renal arteries of rabbits. Arch Pathol Lab Med 76 : 667–676, 1963.

12. Reidy MA, Schwartz SM: Endothelial injury and regeneration. IV. Endotoxin: A nondenuding injury to aortic endothelium. Lab Invest 48 : 25–34, 1983.

13. Stary HC: Comparison of the morphology of atherosclerotic lesions in the coronary arteries of man with the morphology of lesions produced and regressed in experimental primates, in Malinow MR, Blaton VH (eds), *Regression of Atherosclerotic Lesions: Experimental Studies and Observations in Humans.* New York, Plenum Press, 1984, pp 235–254.

14. Steinberg D: Lipoproteins and atherosclerosis: A look back and a look ahead. Arteriosclerosis 3 : 283–301, 1983.

15. Svindland A: The localization of sudanophilic and fibrous plaques in the main left coronary bifurcation. Atherosclerosis 48 : 139–145, 1983.

16. Wissler RW: The evolution of the atherosclerotic plaque and its complications, in Connon WE, Bristow JD (eds), *Coronary Heart Disease: Prevention, Complications, and Treatment.* Philadelphia, J.B. Lippincott, 1985, pp 193–214.

17. Wissler RW, Vesselinovitch D, Davis HR: Cellular components of the progressive atherosclerotic process, in Olsson AG (ed), *Atherosclerosis: Biology and Clinical Science.* Edinburgh, Churchill Livingstone, 1987, pp 57–73.

18. Wissler RW, Vesselinovitch D, Davis HR, Lambert PH, Bekermeier M: A new way to look at atherosclerotic involvement of the artery wall and the functional effects. Ann NY Acad Sci 454 : 9–22, 1985.

19. Wolfbauer G, Glick JM, Minor LK, Rothblat GH: Development of the smooth muscle foam cell: Uptake of macrophage lipid inclusions. Proc Natl Acad Sci USA 83 : 7760-7764, 1986.

20. Yamashiroya HM, Ghosh L, Yang R, Robertson AL: Herpes-viridae in the coronary arteries and aorta of young trauma victims. Am J Pathol 130 : 71–79, 1988.

PART THREE

Pulmonary Hypertension

Lynne M. Reid, M.D.

19

Vascular Remodeling

Clinical pulmonary hypertension is a restrictive, not a constrictive, vascular disease. Remodeling of the lung's vascular structure is the critical abnormality in the various types of pulmonary hypertension. Some structural changes represent the cause of the hypertension, others an adaptation to its presence: but, whatever the original injury, hypertension of itself causes additional vascular damage. Constriction, sometimes added to structural remodeling, is clinically important since it is a component that is perhaps reversible with treatment: but, it is a safe generalization that once pulmonary hypertension is a recognizable clinical problem, its basis is structural.

The causes of pulmonary hypertension are numerous and varied, a fact blurred by the physiological denominator of raised pulmonary hypertension. The widespread emphasis on vasoconstriction as the cause of the disease implies that vasodilators prevent or cure—a misplaced hope. Focus on restriction helps identify critical differences between the pulmonary hypertensions (28,44,45). The causes of restriction are numerous, the pathogenetic pathways by which these causes produce their effect are also varied, and even a single injury causes restriction in a variety of ways. The various vascular segments are affected differently by a given injury. Vascular cell injury, recovery or adaptation to the new environment, and repair, including scar, all change the structure and reactivity of the vascular bed (4,17). This must be recognized in order to distinguish the critical features of the various diseases and formulate appropriate treatment. As the vascular bed is structurally remodeled, the vessel wall cells change their metabolism and their reactivity.

The study of mediators of cell injury and tissue restructuring is currently one of the most active fields of biomedical research. It offers an embarrassingly wide array of candidates for the cellular events described here (46). And yet, a large gap exists between our knowledge of cell behavior in vitro and its relevance to homeostasis in the intact tissue or to its disturbance in disease.

The normal structure of the lung's vascular bed holds the key to its remodeling. The cast of cells is similar at all levels of the pulmonary vascular bed, yet the various segments of the vascular loop between right ventricle and left atrium have special features and different patterns of response. And, at the various levels, response to injury varies with the injury. While cell types are similar in pulmonary and systemic systems, behavior of the lung's vascular cells cannot be deduced from that of systemic cells. Studies of systemic cell-cell interactions are largely driven by interest in atheroma, a disease of large arteries. In most forms of pulmonary hypertension, it is injury or restructuring of the microcirculation that is key. While signals and receptors may be conserved throughout both systems, it is likely that they do not transduce to the same message. The variations in structure of the pulmonary vascular segments make it prudent to consider them different as well as separate from the systemic bed.

In this chapter, patterns of structural remodeling leading to restriction are described for hypoxia: changed metabolic conditions cause a hypertrophic or reactive cell response, with intriguing changes in cell function that lend themselves to exploration in vitro (21,35,36,42). Hyperoxia, by contrast, produces necrosis, an injury that leads to restriction first by obliteration and then by restructuring in the residual but restricted bed (25,26,29,30). To each of these injuries the vessels adapt—that which was abnormal becomes normal. In fact, return to ambient air after hyperoxia produces an additional injury of weaning or recovery.

The primary or idiopathic form of pulmonary hypertension, while rare, can affect mainly the arterial or venous segment (1,2,9,34). It offers special restructuring localized to a particular segment of the vascular loop. Persistent pulmonary hypertension of the newborn is yet another disease (16,19,40,41). The obvious cause to invoke is failure of adaptation at birth. Normally at birth the hypertension that is present in the fetus rapidly drops to low adult pressures. While dilatation and a change in compliance of the small resistance arteries is the basis of this normal adaptation (28), in virtually all fatal cases of persistent pulmonary hypertension of the newborn, it is a disease of structure. Remodeling points to abnormal growth and differentiation of the microcirculation before birth. Arteries in the alveolar wall that are normally free of muscle are heavily muscularized (19,40,41): the normal resistance arteries are smaller in size and their adventitial sheath thicker because of dense collagen.

Sepsis and endotoxin can be associated with obliterative changes of the vascular bed (27,31,32). In the experimental models we have studied, it seems that only the intermittent administration of endotoxin produces pulmonary hypertension. In addition to obliteration and major vascular damage, some "tenderizer" seems to thin vessel walls, causing dilatation of the patent circulation. This interaction of factors that cause a rise in resistance with those that would lower could explain some of the clinical variations seen in these conditions.

Characteristically, high flow lung injuries are seen in patients with increased total cardiac output, as with congenital heart lesions (12,43,46). Such lesions are also a feature of any condition involving restriction of the pulmonary vascular bed. The residual patent bed receives either the normal or increased cardiac output: depending on the degree of restriction, localized flow is increased.

NORMAL VASCULAR BED

Double Circulation

Both hemodynamically and metabolically, the lung provides important interaction between the right and left heart. The total systemic venous return is 'processed' by the lung which adds its own metabolic products before blood is recirculated. The lung receives blood from each ventricle and returns blood to each. The double circulations overlap, which further enhances the possibility of interaction between right and left heart (28). The pulmonary artery supplies the capillary bed of the alveolar wall and of most of the pleura. The bronchial artery supplies the hilar structures as well as the capillary bed in the wall of intrapulmonary airways (bronchi and bronchioli). The capillary bed from these intrapulmonary airways, like the capillary bed of the alveoli, drains to the pulmonary veins: only the region around the hilum drains to the true bronchial veins and returns to the azygos system. In this way, products of large airways are circulated next to the lung periphery, and products of intrapulmonary airways and alveoli are circulated to the large airways as well as to the systemic organs. An interface between the capillary beds lies in the region of the terminal bronchiolus and respiratory bronchioli.

Normal Pulmonary Artery System

This account concentrates on the pulmonary artery/pulmonary vein vascular loop. The cast of cells that comprises the vessel wall is small, its repertoire is large. In each vessel, be it large or small, three layers or coats can be distinguished: each has a single cell type which is responsible for its organization, including production of extracellular matrix. For the intima, it is the endothelial cell; for the adventitia, the vascular fibroblast; and for the media or 'muscle layer', the contractile cell. Depending on the segment, the contractile cell is either smooth muscle or a precursor smooth muscle cell, namely, the intermediate cell or pericyte (8). The numerous vascular pathways that pass through the lung from right ventricle to left atrium can be relatively long or short. For example, pathways near the hilum are short; those that supply the diaphragmatic lung region are long. Long or short, each includes the same succession of segments. Artery passes to capillary through a special precapillary segment; capillary passes to vein through a special postcapillary segment (Fig. 1). These pre- and postcapillary segments have a peculiar arrangement. Although superficially they appear to have similar structures, they do not always restructure in the same way in response to injury.

The large arteries, as they decrease in size, change from an elastic to a muscular structure. Each has an external and internal elastic lamina with, in between, additional, but progressively fewer, central elastic laminae. The pre- and postcapillary segments and the smaller muscular arteries represent segments of major significance in the structural remodeling that causes and is caused by pulmonary hypertension. In a recent study combining microdissection with transmission electron microscopy, the transition from the small muscular or resistance artery to the thin-walled arteries of the precapillary unit has been analyzed

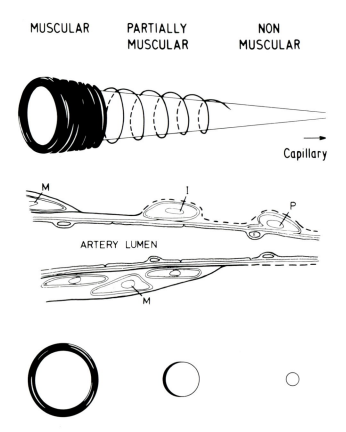

MUSCULAR   PARTIALLY   NON
               MUSCULAR   MUSCULAR

Capillary

ARTERY LUMEN

Figure 1: Diagrammatic representation of the end of any arterial pathway. Top drawing shows appearance by light microscopy: middle drawing additional features shown by electron microscopy. In the muscle-free region of the wall, a pericyte (P) is found in the nonmuscular artery and an intermediate cell (I) in the nonmuscular part of the partially muscular artery. These are precursor smooth muscle cells. E = endothelial cell; M = x (Reproduced from Reid L, Fried R, Greggel R, Langleben D: Anatomy of pulmonary hypertensus stated in Bergofsky EH [ed], *Abnormal Pulmonary Circulation. Contemporary Issues in Pulmonary Disease,* Vol 4. New York, Churchill Livingstone, 1986, Fig. 7-2, pp 221–263. Reprinted by permission.)

within the rat acinus. This provides important normal data that explain the changes seen so rapidly in injury and adaptation (Fig. 2) (5).

Accompanying the terminal bronchiolus is a muscular artery with four to six layers of obliquely arranged muscle. At the level of the respiratory bronchiolus, the wall reduces relatively abruptly to one to three layers of circumferentially arranged muscle. As the artery runs distally with one or two more distal generations of respiratory bronchioli, the media thins, so that by light microscopy the artery now appears only partially muscular or nonmuscular. Electron microscopy reveals around at least part of the wall a thin layer of cytoplasm of either a smooth muscle cell or an intermediate cell. This layer is so thin that it lacks the organelles typical of the smooth muscle cell: but it cannot be assumed that such organelles, notably the dense bodies, are not present somewhere within the cell.

Further distally, at the second generation of alveolar ducts, and then beyond, the medial or contractile layer is represented ultrastructurally by a single cell layer consisting of either an intermediate cell or pericyte. The distinction between these cells can be difficult when the cytoplasmic layer is thin. The pericyte is a solitary cell and lies within the single elastic lamina that demarcates the vessel. The endothelial cell has a basement membrane, but through numerous gaps the endothelial cell and pericyte lie immediately adjacent.

From muscular artery to capillary, the external diameter of the artery falls steadily so that there is good correlation between arterial diameter and the number of layers of medial cells. This ultrastructural serial reconstruction of the ultimate precapillary vascular segment demonstrates that precursor smooth muscle cells are present in the normal vessel and that they lie within the single elastic lamina of these small vessels. Using these techniques, we have also analyzed the structure of this segment in animals after exposure to hypoxia. Changes within the precursor smooth muscle cells are seen as are the stages by which these cells hypertrophy, divide, and then transform their phenotype so that the artery comes to resemble a muscular artery. This study confirms the essential features in the microcirculation identified by light microscopy on serial sections and by electron microscopy on randomly selected sections (35).

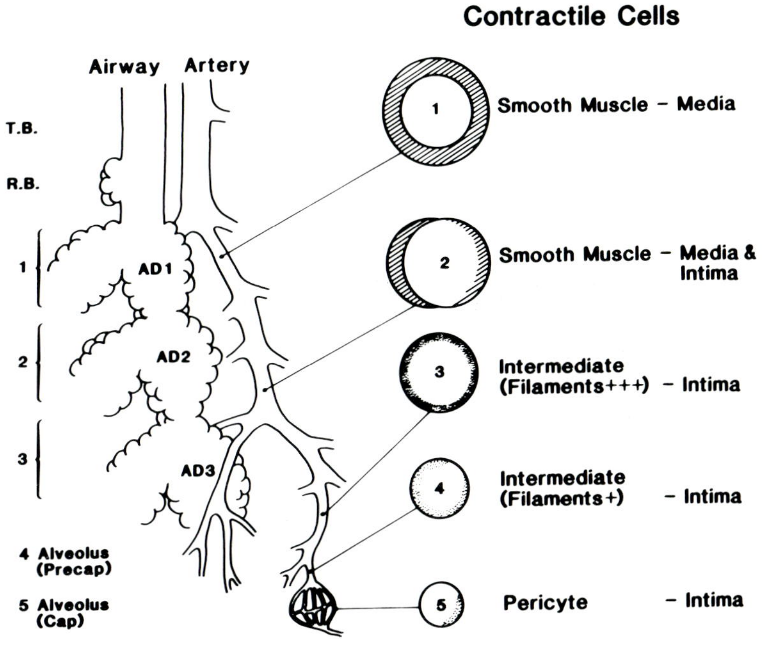

Figure 2: Diagrammatic reconstruction of axial arterial pathway within an acinus of adult rat lung to demonstrate distribution of contractile cells. At level of AD_2, the internal elastic lamina becomes incomplete so muscle cells are apparent in both the media and the intima. Beyond this level, only a single elastic lamina is present: the contractile cells, now of intermediate cell type, at first surround the artery and then only part of the circumference before being replaced by a pericyte. In the adult human lung, these transitions occur within the alveolar wall; in the fetal and newborn human lung, distribution is similar to the adult rat. T.B. = terminal bronchiolus; R.B. = respiratory bronchiolus; AD = alveolar duct; Precap = precapillary; Cap = capillary. (Courtesy of Dr. Rosemary Jones.)

The special pre- and postcapillary segments are present in all mammalian lungs we have examined. In the adult human lung, these segments lie within the alveolar wall, that is within the respiratory unit. Muscular arteries also are found in the alveolar wall: at least some have connective tissue sheaths, are alveolar angle vessels, and can be considered resistance arteries.

In the fetal and newborn lung, the structure of the vascular segments is similar but their relation to airway segments is different (28). The resistance arteries are all upstream from the alveolar surface and the muscular veins downstream. The size distribution of the partially muscular and nonmuscular arteries is similar to the adult: relating size to structure, the adult, fetal and newborn lungs are similar. The differences lie within the acinus. In the fetus, this is about a millimeter in diameter compared with a centimeter for the adult. In the newborn, the resistance arteries run with the terminal bronchiolus or more proximally; they are not within the acinus as in the adult.

In childhood as the acinus increases in volume and alveoli multiply, intra-acinar arteries increase in size and density, but muscularization lags, meaning that larger arteries than in the adult have virtually a nonmuscular wall. The increase in vessel number and size is necessary for the volume of the vascular bed to keep up with alveolar multiplication. Multiplicatory branching of arteries is probably possible because of the nonmuscular structure of the pre- and postcapillary vessels. When this wall is remodeled and becomes muscular, as in high flow congenital heart disease (43), the density of the vascular bed does not achieve normal levels. It seems that a partially or nonmuscular structure is necessary for branching to occur.

Species differences need to be taken into account in interpreting experimental studies. In the rat, the acinus is about 1 mm in diameter and resistance arteries are upstream to it, as they are in the fetal human. The sheep has a large acinus at birth and has a burst of alveolar multiplication just before birth; in this regard, the sheep is unlike the rat, human, or pig (48). Also at birth, the sheep has hardly any muscularized arteries within the alveolar region.

GENERAL FEATURES OF REMODELING

Restriction of the vascular bed can occur by reduction in vessel number or by wall thickening that encroaches on the lumen. Each of the coats of the pulmonary vessels can contribute to lumen narrowing.

Necrosis of endothelial cells leads to obliteration, an obvious and irreversible form of pulmonary vascular restriction. Encroachment on the lumen occurs from endothelial cell hypertrophy, hyperplasia, edema, or the production of new intimal matrix. In pulmonary hypertension, the medial or contractile cell coat commonly increases in thickness. Muscle cells show hypertrophy and often hyperplasia, but this is usually not as striking as the hyperplasia of precursor smooth muscle cells or of the adventitial fibroblast. In animal models of pulmonary hypertension, the smooth muscle cell is usually in the synthetic rather than the contractile phase, and increase in intercellular matrix contributes more to the medial hypertrophy than increase in the number of smooth muscle cells (46).

In the precapillary segment, where the intermediate cell and pericyte are present (although not obvious by light microscopy), narrowing of the lumen from hypertrophy and hyperplasia of these cells is the critical factor in vascular bed restriction from structural remodeling. Hypertrophy of the pericyte and sometimes hyperplasia is a striking response to a variety of injuries: the cell changes in phenotype and comes to resemble a smooth muscle cell. Even at the stage of hypertrophy, the cell increases the production of matrix. The intermediate cell also shows hypertrophy, hyperplasia with change in phenotype toward a typical smooth muscle cell, and a striking increase in matrix production.

The adventitial fibroblasts often show hyperplasia and increased collagen production. Commonly, an increase in adventitial thickness and mass is associated with reduction in the external diameter of the artery (measured internal to the external elastic lamina). This represents contracture, i.e., the reduced diameter is not 'corrected' or overcome by distention of the artery. It is not clear whether this contracture arises because the artery constricts and the collagen 'sets' in this new state, or whether the collagen contracts against the transluminal pressure, thereby reducing the lumen size of the artery. Within the alveolar wall, the vascular fibroblast calls for further study: by its position, it can be distinguished from the myofibroblast.

VARIOUS TYPES OF PULMONARY HYPERTENSION—PATTERNS OF VASCULAR REMODELING AND POSSIBLE MEDIATORS

Hypoxia

Hypoxia is a common cause of pulmonary hypertension in man, both as an acute and transient change or as a chronic and persistent one. From experimental studies, we can trace the mild and mainly functional response to the severe and persistent form. In chronic airways obstruction in man, as occurs within chronic bronchitis or cystic fibrosis, chronic hypoxia/hypoxemia causes the right ventricular hypertrophy of cor pulmonale. Living at altitude also produces the pulmonary hypertension of chronic hypoxia. In the simulated climb of Mt. Everest recently conducted at Natick, Massachusetts, healthy young volunteers virtually doubled their pulmonary artery pressure, an elevation that was not reversed on breathing oxygen (18). This suggests that the structural changes described in the experimental model occurred in the human subject in this vicarious experiment.

Acute challenge with hypoxia causes a pulmonary vasoconstrictor response. In any species, there are some individuals that seem to be nonresponders. To find the mediator responsible for this response has been a tantalizing challenge to physiologists. And yet, typically, this rise in pressure is small—several millimeters of mercury—and is rapidly reversible on return to air or breathing oxygen. This constrictor response is not necessary to the development of the structural remodeling described below. Even after exposure to chronic hypoxia, with restructuring of the vascular bed, nonresponders to acute hypoxic challenge can still be identified (23). As exposure continues, pulmonary artery pressure rises steadily to levels well above that caused by vasoconstriction. The ultimate pressure level reflects the acute constriction and polycythemia as well as restructuring of vessel wall (13).

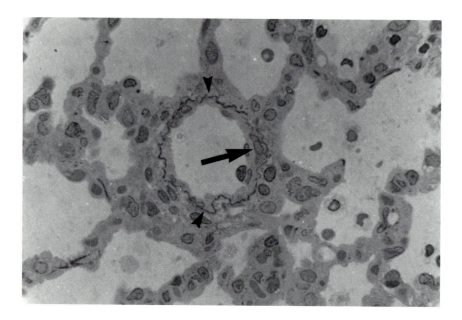

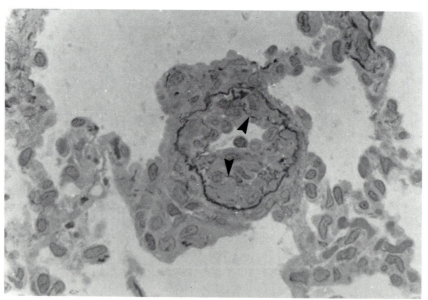

Figure 3: Light photomicrograph of nonmuscular arteries at alveolar duct level from a rat chronically exposed to hypoxia.

A. The artery shows the mildest degree of structural remodeling with a hypertrophied precursor cell (arrow) apparent between the endothelium and single elastic lamina (arrowheads). In the normal artery, the precursor cells are not visible.

B. In a well-developed lesion, the precursor cells have proliferated to form a new medial layer and have laid down a network of additional elastic fibers (arrowheads) (× 1000).

(Reproduced from Davies et al. [8].)

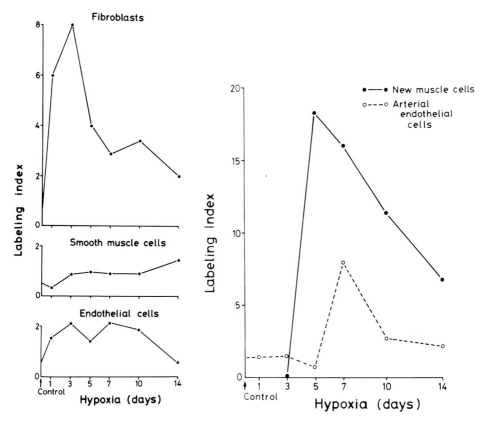

Figure 4: Labeling index of vascular cells after exposure to hypoxia.
A. Adventitial fibroblasts, medial smooth muscle cells, and endothelial cells of the hilar muscular artery.
B. Intraacinar new muscle cells (solid circles) and arterial endothelial cells (open circles) of intraacinar arteries.
(Reproduced from Meyrick and Reid [36].)

   This structural remodeling is an example of remodeling, mainly from metabolic shift, since necrosis is not obvious as it is in the acute injury of hyperoxia (29,30) or monocrotaline (20,38). Hypoxia causes structural changes, reflecting changed cell activity in large and small arteries and in the precapillary segment where they are particularly striking (8,21,22,35,36) (Fig. 3A and B). The veins and postcapillary segments, however, seem largely spared. The large preacinar arteries show early and striking changes. The intra-acinar changes are described first, since the chronic pressure rise is independent of the acute constrictive component and most closely follows the remodeling of the microcirculation (42).
   In the rat, exposure to hypobaric hypoxia (half atmospheric pressure) causes rapid structural remodeling (Fig. 4A and B). In the partially and nonmuscular arteries, the pericyte and intermediate cell rapidly hypertrophy and, using light microscopy, are obvious by day 3. By day 5, 20 percent of the cells are labeled with radioactive thymidine—a burst of mitosis (36). Even by day 14, 8 percent of cells are labeled. At this time, the endothelial cell is closely associated with the precursor smooth muscle cells. It lies internal to a single elastic lamina with either the intermediate cell or pericyte as neighbor: in the case of the pericyte, they share the basement membrane. The peak of division of the endothelial cell

is at day 7. As the pericyte multiplies and develops into a smooth muscle cell, it distances itself from the endothelial cell by the development of a thicker basement membrane and additional elastic laminae. Each new muscle cell virtually creates a corset of elastic fibers for itself. In the normally muscular arteries that run with the terminal bronchioli, modest increase in labeling of both muscle cell and fibroblast occurs; in the case of the fibroblast, this labeling is less than at the hilum.

In the large arteries, both the media and the adventitia increase in tissue mass and thickness, but there is a reduction in the external diameter of the artery (as measured from the external elastic lamina). During the first 3 days, the adventitia doubles in thickness, and after 1 week, it is more than three times its original thickness. The response by the media lags somewhat. Endothelial cells are swollen and show an interesting form of injury. While the cells remain tethered to the basement membrane at their periphery and at some points centrally, most of the base of the cell is separated from the basement membrane by fluid. Increased extracellular matrix is laid down within this pocket of fluid.

In the hilar arteries (37) after 24 hr of hypoxia, the labeling index of the adventitial fibroblast already shows a 6-fold increase that rises to an 8-fold increase by day 3 (Fig. 4A). While it drops somewhat from this height, increased activity is maintained over the 14 days of study. Both endothelial cells and smooth muscle cells show a modest rise in mitotic activity, which is virtually maintained throughout the period of study. Medial thickening owes much to increase of extracellular matrix. The smooth muscle cells show relatively greater increase in organelles that synthesize protein than in those that represent contractile elements (35). The mitotic response of the smooth muscle cell is much more modest than that of either the fibroblast or precursor smooth muscle cells or, usually, of the endothelial cell.

CONTROL OF STRUCTURAL REMODELING

Among the numerous growth factors now identified in vitro, none is the obvious candidate for the different patterns of mitotic activity seen for each cell type and at the various arterial levels (46). Some cells show a short-lived burst, others an increased activity that is maintained, and others a minimal but maintained response. While their absence does not exonerate inflammatory cells, it does encourage us to focus on the resident cells as the cause of shift in homeostasis.

Circulating substances from systemic organs could be the stimulus or at least the modulator of the level of cell response in the lung's blood vessels: hypoxic organs could lead to increase in circulating levels of hormones, notably from the suprarenal or sympathetic nerves. Serotonin and histamine released from mast cells have, under other circumstances, been shown to promote replication of smooth muscle and endothelial cells, respectively. Released heparin would be expected to potentiate endothelial growth but reduce smooth muscle proliferation (6).

Anoxic endothelial cells from large pulmonary arteries produce a factor that stimulates growth-arrested normoxic smooth muscle cells (50). Our own studies show that smooth muscle cells obtained from normal large arteries of rat grow more slowly than those from hypoxic rats. If the anoxic endothelial factor operates, it could account for the somewhat elevated mitotic level in the smooth muscle cell from the start of hypoxia.

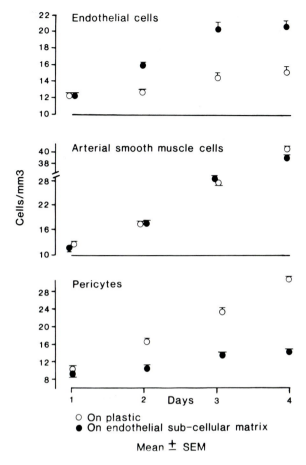

Figure 5: The effect on pulmonary vascular cell growth in vitro of substrate derived from rat lung microvascular endothelial cells. The endothelial cells were grown to postconfluence and treated with 0.5% aqueous Triton-X. Filled circles indicate cells plated on substrate; open circles indicate cells plated on plastic. (Each point is the mean ± SEM.) The pericyte multiplication is inhibited, that of muscle cell unaffected, and that of endothelial cells enhanced. (Reproduced from Davies et al. [10]. Reprinted by permission.)

Because of the small increase in smooth muscle division, it does not seem to represent the biological key to the response in pulmonary hypertension. The intriguing question is the cause of the adventitial fibroblast's rapid and large response to hypoxia maintained over several days. Originally, we thought this might reflect increased transmural pressure, but this seems relatively unimportant. The striking mitotic activity while pressure levels are still low favors it being a metabolic response. The modest rise in endothelial cell mitosis has returned to baseline by the time pressure rise is well established.

A mediator such as platelet-derived growth factorlike protein (PDGFc), produced by resident cells, would stimulate fibroblasts and also smooth muscle cells. In the hypoxic rat, however, the difference in the response between these two cells is so wide that it does not offer a simple answer. Hypoxia itself emerges as

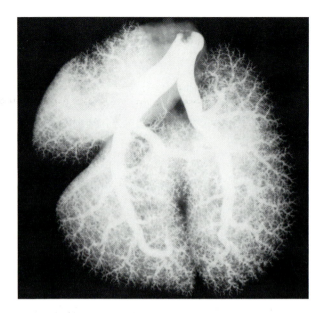

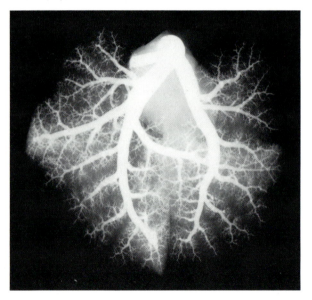

Figure 6: Exposure to hyperoxia causes pulmonary hypertension by widespread obliteration of small arteries. Rat pulmonary arteriogram (original magnification X2.5):
A. Normal.
B. Showing narrowing of main axial pathways and loss of filling of small branches after 87% O_2 for 28 days.
(Reproduced from Jones et al. [30].)

a candidate, perhaps as a modulator. It could be that it acts through cellular metabolic pathways so that the sensitivity of a cell to mitogens is altered. In this case, the emphasis is on the receptor state of the dividing cell, rather than on the production of a mitogen.

In the microcirculation, a different series of agents probably operates (6,7). The endothelial cell of the microcirculation produces a substrate that inhibits the pericyte (10) (Fig. 5). This is likely to be important in homeostasis. The striking proliferation of the pericyte during hypoxia suggests failure of this inhibiting control. Does the hypoxic endothelial cell no longer produce the appropriate substance, or does hypoxia remove the pericyte's susceptibility? The fact that this inhibitory mechanism is mediated by the endothelial cell substrate and that the pericyte distances itself from the endothelial cell so effectively suggests that loss of contact is an early stage in the remodeling. This also could be the effect of hypoxia on one or both cell types. Perhaps loss of contact removes the inhibition of endothelium by the pericyte, a property demonstrated in systemic cells (46).

Matrix-bound basic fibroblast growth factor (bFGF) is possibly released from subendothelial matrix by hypoxia. This mediator is a likely mitogen for the endothelial cell, and perhaps for the pericyte. The delay in response of the endothelial cell is difficult to explain. A change in sensitivity of this cell by hypoxia could be the critical factor rather than the release of the mediator.

A simple explanation of the burst of pericyte activity is that liberation from the inhibitory control of the endothelial cell (10) leads to hypertrophy which is premitotic. However, hypertrophy can occur independently of mitosis, as in the monocrotaline injury (38). If hypoxia is sensed in the alveolar and small airway region, the possibility that a mediator is produced here and then in its next circulation goes to the bronchial arteries and vaso vasorum of large arteries to stimulate the fibroblasts is not unreasonable.

Hyperoxia

Clinically, the potentially toxic nature of hyperoxia is well recognized and can be studied experimentally at an FI_{O_2} of 0.8. While this level causes severe injury, the animals survive so that the evolution of injury, adaptation, and repair can be followed (29,30). Necrosis is important, vasoconstriction is not. Weaning from oxygen does cause constriction—vide infra. The considerable cell debris apparent within the first 24 to 48 hr of exposure clears rapidly, but necrosis is still apparent and continuing. In this model, the intra-alveolar wall veins are affected, as well as the intra-alveolar wall capillaries and precapillary arteries. An early feature is necrosis with collapse of small vessels and ultimately their obliteration (Fig. 6). In the capillaries as well as in adjacent patent segments, upstream and downstream, endothelial cell hypertrophy is striking and sometimes sufficient to occlude the lumen. This is a functional block but is probably reversible, unlike the obliterative lesion.

Hypertrophy is also striking in the subendothelial precursor smooth muscle cells, principally the pericyte. Since one third to one half of arteries seen in sections are effectively obliterated in this model, the residual circulation with narrowed lumen is effectively a high flow system. The local increase in velocity of blood flow is an additional stimulus to structural remodeling (Fig. 7). The down-

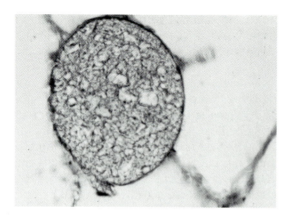

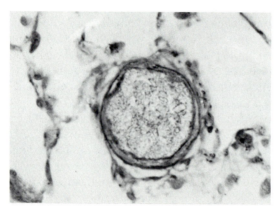

Figure 7: Rat intra-acinar arteries (4-μm sections, Miller's elastic van Gieson[99]). The lumen of each vessel was distended with barium gelatin.
A. Control showing normal thin-walled vessel with a single elastic lamina (external diameter 72 μm, original magnification X640).
B. 87% O_2 for 28 days showing a muscular artery with a well-developed media (that stains for muscle) between an internal and external elastic lamina (external diameter, 53 μm; X640).
(Reproduced from Jones et al. [30].)

stream veins (i.e., those between the acinus and the heart) seem relatively spared (24). The cross section of these vessels is normal.

In this injury, an inflammatory cell response is striking. At certain levels in 100% O_2, for example, platelets first sequester in the pulmonary vessels, followed by polymorphonuclear leukocytes. At 87% O_2 (the level we have studied), such widespread and acute inflammatory infiltrate is rarely seen, but by day 7, monocytes are seen in the vessel wall and alveolar space; these increase in number as exposure continues. The plasma levels of 6-keto-PGF$_{1\alpha}$ are increased.

The small arteries at alveolar duct and alveolar wall level remodel: they develop an internal and external elastic lamina, and a media of precursor smooth muscle cells is obvious. Unlike hypoxia, these cells do not change their phenotype. It is only when these animals are weaned back to air, i.e., are exposed to relative hypoxia, that change in phenotype is seen.

The mechanical properties of the pulmonary arteries injured by hyperoxia are different from those injured by hypoxia, although in each case there is medial hypertrophy and increase in adventitial collagen (4,17,45).

RECOVERY FROM HYPEROXIA

Return to air does not immediately produce regression of these lesions; in fact, it is associated with an additional and different injury caused by change in oxygen tension (30). For the animal to survive, weaning to air is necessary; but this very process of weaning and then normoxia causes further damage and a different structural adaptation (Fig. 8). It seems that a drop from high oxygen is sensed as relative hypoxia; vasoconstriction occurs. More precapillary arteries develop a media-like layer of cells derived from a subendothelial precursor cell, and an increasing amount of elastin is deposited abluminal to the endothelial cell. This effectively separates the precursor cells from the endothelium.

The patterns of cell multiplication are very different in the hyperoxic from the hypoxic injury (25). The return to air that is associated with a constrictor response and change in phenotype of the precursor smooth muscle cells is associated with a different pattern of cell multiplication from that produced by a first exposure to hypoxia. In the early days of exposure to hyperoxia, pulmonary artery pressure does not rise; it is only when the obliterative lesion is well developed that pressure is elevated. An elevation from the normal of about 17 to 26 mmHg can be detected after 7 days. In larger arteries, contracture and wall thickening encroach on the lumen.

At present, results for thymidine labeling during hyperoxia are available only from the small arteries (25,26). The smooth muscle cells do not increase their thymidine labeling until day 28. At day 4, the endothelial cell, pericyte, and ad-

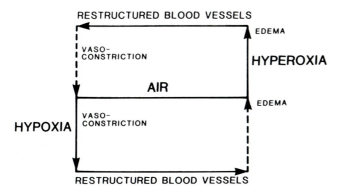

Figure 8: The effects of hypoxic and hyperoxic alveolar tensions on the pulmonary vascular bed. Both types of change in alveolar P_{O_2} injure and restrict the pulmonary vascular bed by altering the structure and function of the pulmonary vascular wall. Injury to the normal lung by hyperoxia leads first to edema and then to the development of pulmonary hypertension (PH) as the walls of pulmonary blood vessels are restructured. After extended hyperoxia (28 days), return to lower tensions represents relative hypoxia, and pulmonary arteries constrict. In the normal lung, hypoxia causes vasoconstriction and pulmonary hypertension develops as the walls of pulmonary blood vessels restructure. After prolonged breathing of hypoxia (14 days), return to air represents relative hyperoxia and causes edema. (Reproduced from Jones and Reid [28].)

ventitial fibroblast each show a peak. The increased labeling of the fibroblast is the greatest of any of the vascular cells.

Since hyperoxia produces necrosis, a broad range of mitogens released from disintegrating or migrating cells can be invoked; and yet the smooth muscle cell, the cell type most often suggested to respond to PDGF in systemic arteries, shows no increase until after some weeks of hyperoxia. The pericyte does divide, but much less than in hypoxia. Division of the endothelial cell and interstitial fibroblast is less than for the alveolar epithelial cell. Interleukin-1, a mediator derived from endothelial and/or mononuclear cells, could be responsible for division of the fibroblast and the smooth muscle cell. TGF-β, another product of the mononuclear cell, promotes collagen synthesis and could suppress pericyte division: its production by the fibroblast can be induced by the action of TNF released from the mononuclear cell (46).

After the relative hypoxia of weaning, no increased mitotic activity is seen in the endothelial cell, pericyte, or fibroblast population, yet the smooth muscle cells maintain a raised level of division. PDGF is not sufficiently selective to explain this. The endothelial cells increase their mitotic rate. It is now that fibrosis, particularly in the interstitium, becomes obvious. This could represent activity by the fibroblasts that have developed during the stage of hyperoxia; or it could be a response by fibroblasts changed by hyperoxic injury to the TGF-β released from the relatively hypoxic mononuclear cells.

After a lag period of 2 weeks in air, there is a burst of activity in all cells except those that still have the features of precursor cells. The alveolar epithelial cell that gives a greater mitotic response to hyperoxia than the endothelial cell, on return to air, responds less than the endothelial cell.

A clear conclusion from comparing hypoxia with hyperoxia is that as a tissue adapts to a new environment, the phenotype of its constituent cells changes and that this persists. These cells do not rapidly revert to normal. The cells of the artery adapted to hyperoxia respond to relative hypoxia differently from cells of the normal artery. We have shown a relatively simple example of this in vitro. In culture, pericytes and smooth muscle cells obtained from chronically hypoxic rats grow more slowly than those from control rats, even in a mitogen-rich culture medium and in ambient air. Pericyte growth is slowed by heparin only in the first few days, smooth muscle cell growth only after 7 days. This pattern is preserved in hypoxic cells (Davies, personal communication: 6). It is clear how far we are from identifying the growth factors that are responsible for proliferation of the vascular wall cells in situ. To be able to show an in vitro effect is not enough. It is important that we be able to explain the selectivity of the cell response and also time relationships.

Sepsis and Endotoxemia: Recurrent and Continuous

In the four models produced by combinations of the two types of injury and two patterns of delivery, remodeling of the pulmonary circulation has been produced, but only one of them has been associated with the development of pulmonary hypertension (27,31,32). Continuous endotoxemia produces a biphasic pulmonary hypertension—an early short-lived constrictor response followed later by a mild hypertension that persists at rest (31). The importance of this group of models is that the structural changes represent severe vascular injury, but there is not necessarily a pulmonary hypertension present at rest. This does not mean that pulmonary hypertension does not develop more quickly on challenge.

The injury produced by these agents is associated with focal dilatation and thinning of the alveolar wall. The mediators responsible for this structural adaptation could be important in "neutralizing" the effect of injury that elsewhere in the vascular bed is associated with restriction.

In the isolated perfused lung system, the response of the vascular bed in each of these four models is different. In this preparation it is possible, using a pressure driven system, to partition the contribution to resistance to three levels, upstream, and downstream from the capillary bed, and to the capillary level (17).

For a given level of increased resistance which can be detected in the isolated perfused lung, the distribution of resistance is different. The response of the vascular bed to several constrictors showed a pattern characteristic of the injury. It is also of clinical interest that the response to the metabolites of oxygen is different; for example, challenge with these metabolites produced virtually a vasospasm on the venous side that persisted for the whole of the hour studied. In no other model of injury was there a response of this order. In all models when there was a response, the response was worse on the venous than on the arterial side. Thus, changed sensitivity to a variety of injurious stimuli is a feature of the structural remodeling considered here.

Primary Pulmonary Hypertension (Idiopathic, Essential, Cryptogenic): Arterial or Venous

In primary pulmonary artery hypertension as in the previously discussed disorders, the disease seems to cause injury and remodeling in the pulmonary microcirculation (1,2,34). Although the reason for the remodeling is not known, it seems to be the essential feature. There is no evidence pointing just to constriction as the primary cause of disease. It is not certain that constriction is even present in all patients since certainly not all patients respond to vasodilators.

In long-standing cases of primary pulmonary artery hypertension or in any type of heart failure, thromboembolism occurs that makes the pulmonary changes appear similar, regardless of the onset (28). To sort out the differences between so-called primary pulmonary hypertension and the thromboembolic varieties, we chose to look at the earliest cases available for examination, those dying soon after development of symptoms (2). In such cases, the disease is at a stage at which obliteration is occurring in the peripheral arteries, particularly those less than 40 μ in diameter (Fig. 9). These are the precapillary alveolar units in which the structure, by light microscopy, is nonmuscular and in which the normal contractile cell is the pericyte (Fig. 10). In certain early cases, the diffusion coefficient is extremely low in keeping with obliteration of peripheral arteries (34). If the patient survives, however, the residual patent bed undergoes dilatation and adaptation, and the diffusion coefficient returns to more normal levels.

The early obliteration of the small arteries suggested an endothelial abnormality as an early, perhaps primary change. Ultrastructurally fenestrated capillary walls have been shown as well as an increase in the connective tissue in the nonmuscular wall (34). Recently, we have demonstrated that von Willebrand ris-

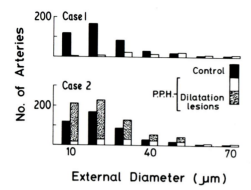

External Diameter (μm)

Figure 9: Reduction in the number of nonmuscular arteries less than 40 μm in diameter in primary pulmonary hypertension (PPH). Case 1: the patient with the shortest clinical history had no dilatation lesions. Case 2: a patient with a longer clinical history did have dilatation lesions. (Reproduced from Anderson et al. [2].)

tocetin cofactor activity is abnormally high in these patients (15): whereas the concentration of the antigen protein is normal, its activity is considerably increased to give an abnormally high ratio of activity to concentration. This is in contrast to the findings in nonspecific injury, such as in acute respiratory failure of the adult, in which a high concentration of antigen is present, but this is associated with appropriate activity so that the ratio is within the normal range of one (3). In a larger series of a patients, including those with the familial form as well as the sporadic variety, a similar pattern of abnormality is also present.

There is an idiopathic form of pulmonary hypertension in which the lesion is primarily in the veins (9). The designation "idiopathic" focuses attention on some intrinsic abnormality of the vessels, although the brunt of the changes can be either at the arterial or the venous end. This is one more example of the significant differences between parts of the pulmonary vascular loop.

In both the arterial and venous types of idiopathic pulmonary hypertension, the effect upstream from the obstruction is to increase pressure and shift blood flow. The arteries, and in the case of the venous obstruction also the capillaries, show hypertrophy and hyperplasia of all coats.

High Flow Injury: Pulmonary Vascular Obstructive Disease

In several cases of thromboembolism that were studied soon after the initial lesion, the patent, or normal, part of the vascular bed showed diffuse dilatation (2). The high velocity and high flow conditions of the residual bed lead rapidly to characteristic changes which, in their extreme forms, have been described as pulmonary vascular obstructive disease (7,28).

The blood vessels adapt in a somewhat similar way to reduced, as well as to high, flow. The pulmonary arteries supplying a scar show marked crenation of the internal elastic lamina suggesting constriction and additional, but usually partial, occlusion of the lumen by a nonspecific hyaline deposit. After bone marrow trans-

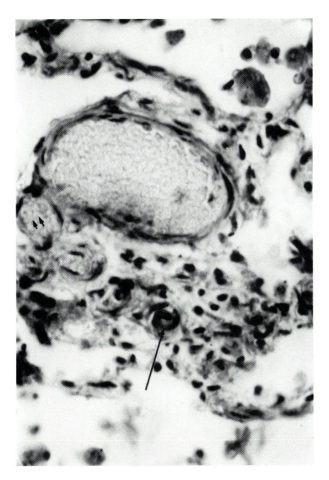

Figure 10: Small arteries from a patient with idiopathic primary pulmonary arterial hypertension who died within 6 months of the first symptom. Arteriogram showed fine peripheral pruning. A small patent muscular artery and its side branch (arrowheads) is filled with injectate: artery at arrow is replaced by concentric arrangement of fibrils and nuclei (4-μm section; Verhoeff's elastic van Gieson; original magnification X500). (Reproduced from Anderson et al. [2].)

plant, the material causing a hepatic venoocclusive lesion includes fibrinogen and factor VIII-related antigen but is not positive for the platelet-membrane molecule tested (glycoprotein 1B) (49). In contrast to the endothelium (33), the platelet does not seem to be the essential criminal in such changes.

After removal of thrombi or emboli from large arteries a "reflow injury" develops—another example of adaptation by the vascular bed to a new set of conditions. Angiomatoid and plexiform lesions develop in response to block downstream: shear injury is probably the critical factor. Narrowing or occlusion of a medium- or small-sized pulmonary artery leads to the opening up of collateral channels so that small vessels dilate and conduct blood to regions distal to an obstruction. This is one of several ways in which so-called plexiform lesions form (47).

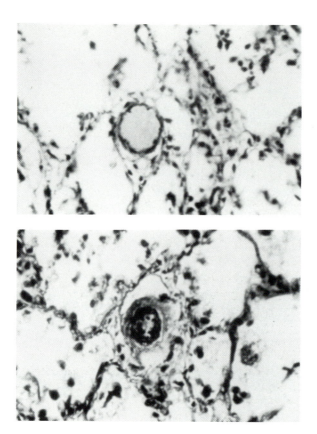

Figure 11: A normal intraacinar pulmonary artery (above), and one from an infant with persistent pulmonary hypertension of the newborn (below), showing a well-developed medial muscle layer and dense collagen sheath including a lymphatic vessel. (Reproduced from Murphy et al. [40].)

Persistent Pulmonary Hypertension of the Newborn

Pulmonary hypertension is the normal state of the pulmonary vascular bed before birth. In the first minutes and hours after birth, pressure and resistance normally fall rapidly in the pulmonary vascular bed. This normal adaptation has a functional as well as a structural component. Arteries dilate and the smallest resistance arteries show an increased distensibility (28). Although the tempting first assumption is that the reason for persistent pulmonary hypertension of the newborn (first described as "persistent fetal circulation") is a failure of these adaptations, in fatal cases the structure of the lung's microcirculation is abnormal (Fig. 11) (19,40,41). In the normal newborn, light microscopy reveals that all arteries within the respiratory region (i.e., within the acinus) are free of muscle (Fig. 12). In fatal cases, there is a thick muscular coat with a well-formed internal and external elastic lamina as well as a dense collagen sheath—all of these associated with a narrowing of the lumen and also of the external diameter (Fig. 11). The density of these arteries is normal and the veins are not affected. These structural

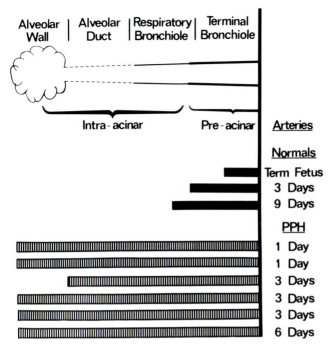

Figure 12: Diagrammatic representation of location of muscle in the walls of the intraacinar arteries of normal infants and those with idiopathic persistent pulmonary hypertension of the newborn. Muscle (as in Fig. 10) was apparent in the small intraacinar arteries. (Reproduced from Murphy et al. [40].)

changes point to an abnormal restructuring of the microcirculation before birth. In some cases, the increase in distensibility that normally occurs in the upstream resistance arteries also occurs in the intra-acinar arteries.

We expected that fatal cases of meconium aspiration might reflect a failure of adaptation: although all infants who died after meconium aspiration had "persistent fetal circulation" (11), neither pulmonary hypertension nor clinical outcome had correlated with the severity of the aspiration as assessed by radiographic changes, or with blood gases. Therefore, it seemed unlikely that the meconium aspiration had caused the hypertension or the death of the infant. In a morphologic study of the pulmonary vascular structure, we found that in all but one of eleven fatal cases of "meconium aspiration," the abnormal muscle was similar to that described above for persistent pulmonary hypertension of the newborn. We concluded that the passage of meconium in these infants is perhaps a marker of the same abnormality that caused the abnormalities in pulmonary arterial muscle.

The possibility of intrauterine hypoxia or of premature or partial closure of the ductus have both been advanced as possible causes of persistent pulmonary hypertension of the newborn. However, experimental studies using hypoxia or indomethacin have failed to produce these changes (14,39). We need to identify the hormones or growth factors that control intrauterine growth and differentiation; the explanation probably lies in their malfunction.

COMMENT

In all types of pulmonary hypertension considered above, the fundamental change is restriction of the pulmonary vascular bed starting in, and affecting particularly, the microcirculation. For example, in hypoxia and in high flow pulmonary hypertension, the restriction is due to structural remodeling that affects all coats of the precapillary arterial segment and the resistance arteries. By contrast, in high oxygen injury, there is vascular cell necrosis, obliteration of many microvessels, and a simultaneous remodeling of the patent microcirculation. In hyperoxia, arteries and veins in the alveolar wall are affected. The precursor smooth muscle cells in the lesion caused by high flow or hypoxia show obvious phenotypic change as they develop into smooth muscle cells: their pattern of matrix production also changes to one that is similar but still different from that of normal smooth muscle cells. Endothelial cells and fibroblasts multiply and adapt to the new metabolic environment.

Upstream from the level of restriction, the cell of each vascular layer also reacts. Although in the upstream arteries hypertrophy of the muscle or medial cell layer has long held center stage, multiplication of the adventitial fibroblast and endothelial cell is, in fact, greater: the fibroblast, for example, seems to lead the endothelial reaction, and the endothelial cell, at least ultrastructurally, shows striking if not necessarily fatal injury. Although all vascular coats of the upstream vessels show hypertrophy in all types of pulmonary hypertension, the reactivity of these vessels—with respect to both the site of response and the degree—is modified by the original cause of the hypertension. The biological response in these larger pre-acinar vessels is influenced by the cause or nature of the original injury as well as by the degree of pulmonary hypertension. This altered reactivity has important implications for the pharmacotherapy of the various forms of hypertension (4,6,17,49).

The catalogue of mediators capable of stimulating vascular cells to multiply in vitro grows apace. These have largely been investigated for systemic cells and in culture. Even for systemic cells, evidence is rare that what happens in vitro is what is happening in vivo. Therefore, to apply systemic results to the pulmonary circulation is doubly unjustified. The systemic studies are largely driven by an interest in atheroma, a condition of large arteries. In pulmonary hypertension, it is remodeling of the small vessels that must be the focus. The response to a given injury is so orchestrated, with point and counterpoint by each cell type, that there is characteristic timing and response for each injury. The challenge is to identify the instruments effecting this orchestration.

REFERENCES

1. Anderson G, Reid L, Simon G: The radiographic appearances in primary and in thrombo-embolic pulmonary hypertension. Clin Radiol 24 : 113–120, 1973.

2. Anderson EG, Simon G, Reid L: Primary and thrombo-embolic pulmonary hypertension: A quantitative pathological study. J Pathol 110:273–293, 1973.

3. Carvalho AC, Bellman SM, Saullo VJ, Quinn D, Zapol WM: Altered factor VIII in acute respiratory failure. N Engl J Med 307:1113–1119, 1982.

4. Coflesky JT, Jones RC, Reid LM, Evans JN: Mechanical properties and structure of isolated pulmonary arteries remodelled by chronic hyperoxia. Am Rev Respir Dis 136:388–394, 1987.

5. Davies P, Burke G, Reid L: The structure of the wall of the rat intraacinar pulmonary artery: an electron microscopic study of microdissected preparations. Microvasc Res 32:50–63, 1986.

6. Davies P, Hu L-M, Reid L: Effects of heparin on the growth of lung pericytes and smooth muscle cells in vitro. Fed Proc 46:663a, 1987.

7. Davies P, Jones R, Schloo B, Reid L: Endothelium of the pulmonary vasculature in health and disease, in Ryan US (ed), *Pulmonary Endothelium in Health and Disease*, in Lenfant C (exec ed), *Lung Biology in Health and Disease, Vol 32*. New York, Marcel Dekker, 1987, pp 375–445.

8. Davies P, Maddalo F, Reid L: Effects of chronic hypoxia on structure and reactivity of rat lung microvessels. J Appl Physiol 58:795–801, 1985.

9. Davies P, Reid L: Pulmonary veno-occlusive disease in siblings: case reports and morphometric study. Hum Pathol 13:911–915, 1982.

10. Davies P, Smith BT, Maddalo FB, Langleben D, Tobias D, Fujiwara K, Reid L: Characteristics of lung pericytes in culture including their growth inhibition by endothelial substrate. Microvasc Res 33:300–314, 1987.

11. Fox WW, Gewitz MH, Dinwiddie R, Drummond WH, Peckham GJ: Pulmonary hypertension in the perinatal aspiration syndromes. Pediatrics 59:205–211, 1977.

12. Fried R, Falkovsky G, Newburger J, Gorchakova AI, Rabinovitch M, Gordonova MI, Fyler D, Reid L, Burakovsky V: Pulmonary arterial changes in patients with ventricular septal defects and severe pulmonary hypertension. Pediatr Cardiol 7:147–154, 1986.

13. Fried R, Reid L: Early recovery from hypoxic pulmonary hypertension: a structural and functional study. J Appl Physiol 57:1247–1253, 1984.

14. Geggel RL, Aronovitz MJ, Reid LM: Effects of chronic in utero hypoxemia on rat neonatal pulmonary arterial structure. J Pediatr 108:756–759, 1986.

15. Geggel RL, Carvalho AC, Hoyer LW, Reid LM: von Willebrand factor abnormalities in primary pulmonary hypertension. Am Rev Respir Dis 135:294–299, 1987.

16. Goldstein JD, Reid L: Pulmonary hypoplasia resulting from phrenic nerve agenesis and diaphragmatic amyoplasia. J Pediatr 97:282–287, 1980.

17. Gore RG, Jones R: Pulmonary vascular reactivity in hyperoxic pulmonary hypertension in the rat. J Appl Physiol 65:2617–2623, 1988.

18. Groves BM, Reeves JT, Sutton JR, Wagner PD, Cymerman A, Malconian MK, Rock PB, Young PM, Houston CS: Operation Everest II: elevated high-altitude pulmonary resistance unresponsive to oxygen. J Appl Physiol 63:521–530, 1987.

19. Haworth SG, Reid L: Persistent fetal circulation: Newly recognized structural features. J Pediatr 88:614–620, 1976.

20. Hislap A, Reid L: Arterial changes in *Crotalaria spectabilis*-induced pulmonary hypertension in rats. Br J Exp Pathol 55:153–163, 1974.

21. Hislop A, Reid L: New findings in pulmonary arteries of rats with hypoxia-induced pulmonary hypertension. Br J Exp Pathol 57:542–554, 1976.

22. Hislop A, Reid L: Changes in the pulmonary arteries of the rat during recovery from hypoxia-induced pulmonary hypertension. Br J Exp Pathol 58:653–662, 1977.

23. Hu L-M, Geggel R, Davies P, Reid L: The effect of heparin on the haemodynamic and structural response in the rat to acute and chronic hypoxia. Br J Exp Pathol. In Press.

24. Hu L-M, Jones R: Injury and remodeling of pulmonary veins by high oxygen. A morphometric study. Am J Pathol 134:253–262, 1989.

25. Jones R, Adler C, Farber F: Lung vascular cell proliferation in hyperoxic pulmonary hypertension and on return to air: [³H]Thymidine pulse-labeling of intimal, medial and adventitial cells in distal vessels and at the hilum. Am Rev Respir Dis. Submitted.

26. Jones R, Farber F, Adler C: ³H-thymidine labelling of rat pulmonary microcirculation in hyperoxic pulmonary hypertension. Fed Proc 46:3946, 1987.

27. Jones R, Kirton OC, Zapol WM, Reid L: Rat pulmonary artery wall injury by chronic intermittent infusions of *Escherichia coli* endotoxin. Obliterative vasculitis and vascular occlusion. Lab Invest 54:282–294, 1986.

28. Jones RC, Reid LM: Structural basis of pulmonary hypertension, in Simmons D (ed), *Current Pulmonology*, Vol 8. Chicago, Year Book Medical Publishers, 1987, pp 175–210.

29. Jones R, Zapol WM, Reid L: Pulmonary artery remodeling and pulmonary hypertension after exposure to hyperoxia for 7 days. A morphometric and hemodynamic study. Am J Pathol 117:273–285, 1984.

30. Jones R, Zapol WM, Reid L: Oxygen toxicity and restructuring of pulmonary arteries—a morphometric study. The response to 4 weeks' exposure to hyperoxia and return to breathing air. Am J Pathol 121:212–223, 1985.

31. Kirton OC, Jones R: Rat pulmonary artery restructuring and pulmonary hypertension induced by continuous *Escherichia coli* endotoxin infusion. Lab Invest 56:198–210, 1987.

32. Kirton OC, Jones R, Zapol WM, Reid L: The development of a model of subacute lung injury after intra-abdominal infection. Surgery 96:384–394, 1984.

33. Langille BL, O'Donnell F: Reductions in arterial

diameter produced by chronic decreases in blood flow are endotheliumdependent. Science 231:405–407, 1986.

34. Meyrick B, Clarke SW, Symons C, Woodgate DJ, Reid L: Primary pulmonary hypertension: a case report including electron microscopic study. Br J Dis Chest 68:11–20, 1974.

35. Meyrick B, Reid L: The effect of continued hypoxia on rat pulmonary arterial circulation. An ultrastructural study. Lab Invest 38:188–200, 1978.

36. Meyrick B, Reid L: Hypoxia and incorporation of 3H-thymidine by cells of the rat pulmonary arteries and alveolar wall. Am J Pathol 96:51–70, 1979.

37. Meyrick B, Reid L: Endothelial and subintimal changes in rat hilar pulmonary artery during recovery from hypoxia. A quantitative ultrastructural study. Lab Invest 42:603–615, 1980.

38. Meyrick BO, Reid LM: Crotalaria-induced pulmonary hypertension. Uptake of 3H-thymidine by the cells of the pulmonary circulation and alveolar walls. Am J Pathol 106:84–94, 1982.

39. Murphy JD, Aronovitz MJ, Reid LM: Effects of chronic in utero hypoxia on the pulmonary vasculature of the newborn guinea pig. Pediatr Res 20:292–295, 1986.

40. Murphy JD, Rabinovitch M, Goldstein JD, Reid LM: The structural basis of persistent pulmonary hypertension of the newborn infant. J Pediatr 98:962–967, 1981.

41. Murphy JD, Vawter GF, Reid LM: Pulmonary vascular disease in fatal meconium aspiration. J Pediatr 104:758–762, 1984.

42. Rabinovitch M, Gamble W, Nadas AS, Miettinen OS, Reid L: Rat pulmonary circulation after chronic hypoxia: hemodynamic and structural features. Am J Physiol 236:H818–H827, 1979.

43. Rabinovitch M, Haworth S, Castaneda AR, Nadas SA, Reid LM: Lung biopsy in congenital heart disease: A morphometric approach to pulmonary vascular disease. Circulation 58:1107–1122, 1978.

44. Reid L: The pulmonary circulation: remodeling in growth and disease. The 1978 J. Burns Amberson Lecture. Am Rev Respir Dis 119:531–546, 1979.

45. Reid L: Structure and function in pulmonary hypertension. New perceptions. 7th Simon Rodbard Memorial Lecture. Chest 89:279–288, 1986.

46. Reid L, Davies P: The control of cell proliferation in pulmonary hypertension, in Weir EK, Reeves JT (eds), *Pulmonary Vascular Physiology and Pathophysiology*. New York, Marcel Dekker, in press.

47. Rendas A, Brown ER, Avery ME, Reid LM: Prematurity, hypoplasia of the pulmonary vascular bed and hypertension: fatal outcome in a ten-month old infant. Am Rev Respir Dis 121:873–880, 1980.

48. Rendas A, Lennox S, Reid L: Aorta-pulmonary shunts in growing pigs. Functional and structural assessment of the changes in the pulmonary circulation. J Thorac Cardiovasc Surg 77:109–118, 1979.

49. Shulman HM, Gown AM, Nugent DJ: Hepatic veno-occlusive disease after bone marrow transplantation. Immunohistochemical identification of the material within occluded central venules. Am J Pathol 127:549–558, 1987.

50. Vender RL, Clemmons DR, Kwock L, Friedman M: Reduced oxygen tension induces pulmonary endothelium to release a pulmonary smooth muscle cell mitogen(s). Am Rev Respir Dis 135:622–627, 1987.

Robert F. Grover, M.D., Ph.D.

20

Chronic Hypoxic Pulmonary Hypertension

Chronic hypoxic pulmonary hypertension is a term closely associated with cor pulmonale which, in turn, generally evokes a picture of recurrent heart failure in the patient with chronic obstructive airways disease. But, millions of normal, healthy people also have chronic hypoxic pulmonary hypertension as a consequence of living in an atmosphere of relative hypoxia at moderate altitudes. Although these individuals have pulmonary arterial pressures comparable to those of patients with chronic lung disease, they live normal, active lives and are free of any signs of heart failure.

The condition of chronic hypoxic pulmonary hypertension is one in which pulmonary arterial pressure is sustained at abnormally high levels as a consequence of persistent airway hypoxia. An analysis of 106 published values indicates that in resting, supine individuals near sea level, the pulmonary arterial pressure averages 14 ± 3 (SD) mmHg (31). Accordingly, pulmonary hypertension is defined as a mean pressure greater than 18 mmHg.

In 1947, Motley et al. (24) reported that in five normal men, lowering alveolar oxygen tension (PA_{O_2}) increased pulmonary arterial pressure. Subsequent observations have shown that the dose-response curve approximates a hyperbola (Fig. 1), the pulmonary arterial pressure increasing at a progressively more rapid rate below arterial P_{O_2} values of about 75 mmHg (31). The mechanism underlying pulmonary hypertension in response to chronic hypoxia is generally considered to be an extrapolation of the acute response, i.e., vasoconstriction, although it may be augmented by morphological and hematological changes. Consequently, chronic pulmonary hypertension would be expected to occur when PA_{O_2} remains less than about 75 mmHg. This degree of hypoxia corresponds to an altitude of about 2100 m.

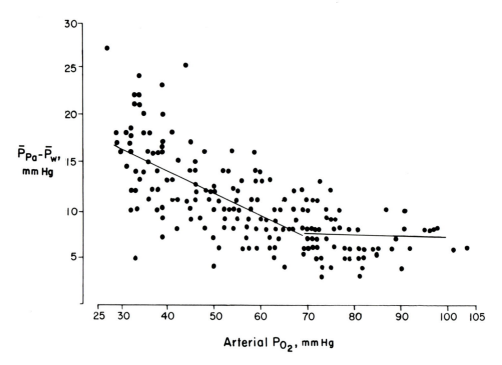

Figure 1: Pulmonary pressor response to acute hypoxia in 50 patients with normal pulmonary arterial pressures living near sea level. Mean pulmonary arterial (PPA) and pulmonary wedge (PW) pressures, and systemic arterial oxygen tension (Pa$_{O_2}$) were measured while each patient breathed ambient air and three hypoxic gas mixtures. Below a Pa$_{O_2}$ of approximately 70 mmHg, the pulmonary vascular pressure gradient (PPA − PW) increases progressively. Although the original figure indicated this threshold by the intersection of two straight lines (as shown), the overall pattern of response appears to be hyperbolic. (Modified after Reeves et al. [31].)

PULMONARY HYPERTENSION AT HIGH ALTITUDE

Geographical Distribution

Pulmonary arterial pressures at high altitude have been determined in different parts of the world (Table 1).

NORTH AMERICA

Extensive data have been gathered in Denver, Colorado (1600 m), where the pulmonary arterial pressures in 56 normal adults averaged 15 ± 3 mmHg, not different from 14 ± 3 mmHg at sea level (30). Among observations at a higher altitude (Leadville, Colorado, 3100 m), the corresponding average in 50 individuals was 24 ± 7 mmHg, i.e., the residents there do have pulmonary hypertension. At intermediate altitudes, the pulmonary arterial pressure falls between these limits: in Flagstaff, Arizona (2100 m), the average pulmonary arterial mean pressure in seven normal adults was 19 ± 6 mmHg (28). These observations on individuals

TABLE 1 RESTING PULMONARY ARTERIAL PRESSURES AT VARIOUS ALTITUDES

Altitude (meters)	Site	PA pressure (mmHg)	Site	PA pressure (mmHg)
<1000	Sea level[31]	14 ± 3 (106)	Lima, Peru[27]	12 ± 2 (25)
	Hangzhou, China[45]	18 ± 3 (16)		
	Lexington, Kentucky[30]	16 ± 3 (35)		
	Bern, Switzerland[11]	14 ± 3 (45)		
1000–2000	Denver, Colorado[30]	15 ± 3 (56)		
2000–2500	Flagstaff, Arizona[28]	19 ± 6 (7)	Mexico City, Mexico[6]	15 ± 2 (21)
	Xining, Qinghai, China[45]	22 ± 4 (31)		
2500–3000			Bogota, Colombia[25]	13 ± 3 (18)
3000–3500	Leadville, Colorado[30]	24 ± 7 (50)		
3500–4000	Chengduo, Qinghai, China[45]	28 ± 8 (22)	Leh, Ladakh, India[33]	20 ± 4 (7)
			La Paz, Bolivia[18]	20 ± 3 (10)
			La Paz, Bolivia[34]	23 ± 4 (11)
			La Paz, Bolivia[23]	23 ± 3 (18)
			La Oroya, Peru[14]	22 ± 4 (24)
4000–4600			Cerro de Pasco, Peru[23]	19 ± 4 (9)
			Cerro de Pasco, Peru[14]	22 ± 4 (9)
			Morococha, Peru[27]	28 ± 10 (38)

Pressures expressed as mean ± SD. Values in parentheses indicate number of subjects.

who are chronically hypoxic are consistent with the proposition above that chronic pulmonary hypertension does not develop until PA_{O_2} remains below 75 mmHg; this occurs at altitudes higher than 2100 m.

MEXICO AND SOUTH AMERICA

In contrast to the residents of the Rocky Mountains on whom the observations cited above were made, the Quechua and Aymara Indians of the Andes of Peru and Bolivia have lived at altitude for perhaps hundreds of generations rather than for only a few generations. In these individuals residing at 2240 to 2640 m, pulmonary arterial hypertension was not present: sea level values for mean pulmonary arterial pressure in 25 individuals averaged 12 ± 2 mmHg whereas the corresponding pressures at altitude were 15 ± 2 mmHg at 2240 m (n = 21) and 13 ± 3 mmHg at 2640 m (n = 18) (6,25). However, at higher altitudes, pulmonary hypertension did become evident: at 3700 to 4370 m, the pressures averaged 19 ± 4 to 23 ± 4 mmHg (14,18,23,34); and at 4540 m, the pulmonary hypertension was even more marked, averaging 28 ± 10 mmHg (27). Therefore, in these populations, the hypoxic pulmonary pressor response curve seems to be displaced, i.e., they do develop pulmonary hypertension at high altitude, but only at altitudes above 3500 m. This suggests that one manifestation of very long-term adaptation to chronic hypoxia is a decreased sensitivity of the pulmonary vasculature to hypoxia as a vasoconstrictive stimulus. However, another reasonable alternative is that the blunted vasoconstrictor response, like the low ventilatory sensitivity to acute hypoxia reported among Peruvians living at sea level, is genetically determined (3).

AFRICA AND ASIA

On the continent of Africa, much of Ethiopia lies above 2000 m, and cities such as Addis Ababa and Ankaber have large populations living up to 2600 m. The high plateau of the Pamirs in central Asia has populations living above 3600 m. Unfortunately, data from these areas are not available. However, in seven natives of Leh (3600 m), in northwest India on the southern slopes of the Himalayas, pulmonary arterial pressures averaged 20 ± 4 mmHg (33).

In 31 natives of Qinghai Province on the Tibetan Plateau (45), mean pulmonary arterial pressures of 22 ± 4 mmHg were found at 2260 m as compared to an average pressure of 28 ± 8 mmHg in 22 individuals at 3950 m. These data indicate a greater degree of pulmonary hypertension on the Tibetan Plateau than in the Andes, and comparable to that in the Rocky Mountains. They also bear on the idea that prehistoric man migrated to North and South America from Asia. Human occupation of the Pacific coast of South America dates back to 8500 B.C., with evidence of man living in the Andes above 4000 m for the past 9500 years.

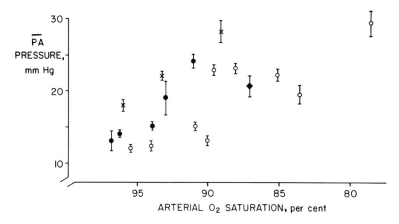

Figure 2: Resting pulmonary arterial (PA) pressures (group mean ± SEM) in populations living at the various altitudes indicated in Table 1. At each altitude, the level of arterial O_2 saturation provides an index of the hypoxic stimulus. Note that at each level of arterial hypoxemia, the pulmonary hypertensive response is greater in residents of the United States (closed circles) and China (Xs) than in populations living in Latin America (open circles) and India (closed diamond). See Table 1 for references.

TABLE 2 EXERCISE PULMONARY ARTERIAL PRESSURES AT VARIOUS ALTITUDES

Altitude (meters)	Site	PA pressure mean ± SD (range) (mmHg)
<100	Sea level[31]	21 ± 4 (12–33) (n = 46)
150	Lima, Peru[2]	18 ± 3 (15–22) (n = 22)
550	Bern, Switzerland[11]	19 ± 5 (4–33) (n = 45)
1600	Denver, Colorado[37]	24
2100	Flagstaff, Arizona[28]	32 ± 10 (21–50) (n = 7)
3100	Leadville, Colorado[37]	54 ± 19 (23–109) (n = 28)
3600	Leh, Ladakh, India[33]	26 ± 5 (n = 7)
3750	La Paz, Bolivia[18]	32 ± 8 (19–60) (n = 10)
4540	Morococha, Peru[2]	60 ± 17 (32–115) (n = 35)

In most studies, oxygen uptake during exercise, 1000–1200 ml/min.

Although presumably Tibet was populated even earlier, the natives of the Tibetan Plateau have more severe pulmonary hypertension than the Andean natives. These observations do not lend support to the hypothesis that the lesser degree of pulmonary hypertension in the Andes is the result of long-term adaptation to chronic hypoxia. Indeed, they strengthen the concept that genetic (racial) factors are more important.

Racial Differences

Although values for alveolar P_{O_2} at altitude are not consistently reported, values for arterial oxygen saturation can be used as a reasonable approximation of the hypoxic stimulus. In Figure 2, pulmonary arterial pressure is examined relative to arterial saturation. In accord with the observations above, at each level of arterial hypoxemia, pulmonary arterial pressure is higher among Caucasians than among Latin Americans. Also, the level of pulmonary hypertension is higher in natives of the Tibetan Plateau than in Latin Americans, and very similar to that of Caucasians. The lesser degree of pulmonary hypertension in the Ladakhis of northwest India may reflect their racial distinction from the population studied on the Tibetan Plateau. Overall, instead of the greater pulmonary hypertension among Caucasians and Chinese reflecting a more severe hypoxic stimulus, it seems to represent a greater pulmonary vascular response to comparable stimuli.

Although examination of pulmonary arterial pressures at rest does provide evidence of pulmonary hypertension at high altitude, the increments in pressure are fairly modest. However, during exercise, the findings are more impressive. As a rule, the intensity of exercise at altitude has sufficed to increase oxygen uptake to 1000 to 1200 ml/min, thereby approximately doubling the cardiac out-

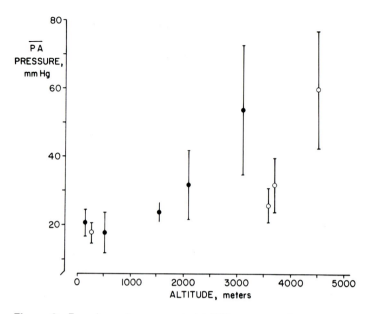

Figure 3: Exercise pulmonary arterial (PA) pressures (group mean ± SD) at the various altitudes listed in Table 2. As in Figure 2, the severity of pulmonary hypertension at each altitude is greater in Caucasians (closed circles) than in Latin Americans (open circles), suggesting a racial difference in the pulmonary vascular response to hypoxia. Note the increase in interindividual variability with increasing altitude. See Table 2 for references.

put at rest. This level of exercise at, or near, sea level increases mean pulmonary arterial pressure to 18 to 21 mmHg (2,11,29); rarely do individual values exceed 25 mmHg (Table 2). At higher altitudes in the United States, pulmonary arterial pressures during exercise are higher: in Flagstaff (2100 m), pressures were 32 ± 10 (SD) mmHg (28); in Leadville (3100 m), pressures were 54 ± 19 mmHg (37). In the Andes, exercise pressures were 32 ± 8 mmHg at 3700 m, and 60 ± 17 mmHg at 4540 m. Variability appears to increase at the higher altitudes, with some individuals developing mean pressures greater than 100 mmHg. As at rest, the increase in pulmonary arterial pressure during exercise at progressively higher altitudes appears to be greater among residents of North America than in natives of the Andes or northern India (Fig. 3).

Effect of Pulmonary Hypertension on Gas Exchange

Question has been raised about whether the pulmonary hypertension of high altitude facilitates, in some way, adaptation to life in chronic hypoxia. Indeed, it has been proposed that, at high altitude, an increase in pulmonary arterial pressure would tend to offset the influence of gravity and render lung perfusion more uniform (4). The problem with this argument is that at rest, when the metabolic demands for oxygen are relatively low, inefficient gas exchange would pose little problem. It is during exercise, when oxygen demands increase, that efficient gas exchange is most desirable. Even at sea level, the onset of mild exercise is associated with increased blood flow to the apices of the lungs so that pulmonary blood flow overall becomes quite uniform (13). Consequently, there is no need to invoke pulmonary hypertension to accomplish this end. Moreover, minimizing the topographical lung perfusion gradient at high altitude does not necessarily render the distribution of localized ventilation/perfusion more uniform throughout the lung. Rather, pulmonary gas exchange at high altitude is rendered more efficient because of an increase in diffusing capacity (5). It seems reasonable to conclude that, at sea level, the phenomenon of hypoxic pulmonary vasoconstriction serves primarily to match local perfusion to local airway hypoxia; at high altitude, where this phenomenon applies to the entire lung, it ceases to serve this function.

Components of Increased Pulmonary Vascular Resistance

MEDIAL HYPERTROPHY AND HYPERPLASIA

Even though the muscular media of the small muscular pulmonary arteries is thin, they are capable of constricting sufficiently to double the pulmonary arterial pressure when stimulated by acute airway hypoxia or other appropriate agonists. In most species, including humans exposed to chronic hypoxia, the normally thin media undergoes hypertrophy. In addition, smooth muscle appears more distally in the pulmonary arterial tree. This "work hypertrophy" is taken as evidence of sustained vasoconstriction (38). The presence of this medial hypertrophy/hyperplasia, per se, probably reduces the lumen of these small vessels. In addition, the more muscular small arteries are probably capable of more powerful vasoconstriction. Together, the anatomical and functional aspects of this medial hypertrophy probably account for most of the increased resistance to blood flow through the lungs in chronic hypoxia.

Recently, an additional feature of the pulmonary vascular smooth muscle in chronic hypoxia has been described. The muscle cells take on a secretory function and produce a substance that is a powerful stimulant for the growth of connective tissue (21), thereby altering further the structure of the small pulmonary arteries and probably rendering them less distensible.

POLYCYTHEMIA, BLOOD VISCOSITY

Polycythemia is a well-recognized feature of adaptation to chronic hypoxia. At high altitude, the increase in red cell mass combined with a reduction in plasma volume results in a rise in hematocrit. Although the relationship between hematocrit and blood viscosity is complex, hematocrits above 50 percent do increase significantly the resistance to blood flow in the lungs as well as in other organs. In the dog lung (with left atrial pressure held constant), pulmonary vascular resistance increases exponentially as the hematocrit increases. Furthermore, the effects of acute hypoxia on pulmonary vascular resistance are greatly augmented by increasing hematocrit. In the Andes at 4540 m, pulmonary hypertension averaging 28 ± 10 mmHg was associated with an average hematocrit of 59 ± 7 percent.

VASOCONSTRICTION

Reversibility of Vasoconstriction. Administration of 100% O_2 to high altitude natives at 3700 m lowered resting pulmonary arterial pressures from 23 to 16 mmHg

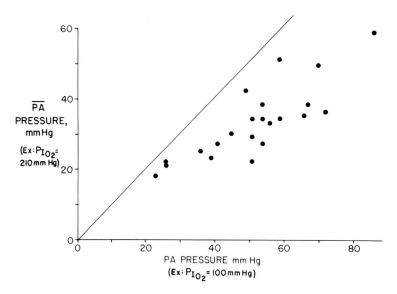

Figure 4: Exercise pulmonary arterial (PA) pressure in 23 individuals living at 3100 m (Leadville, Colorado). Each person exercised first breathing ambient air with an inspired oxygen tension (P_{IO_2}) of 100 mmHg (abscissa). Then P_{IO_2} was increased to 210 mmHg (ordinate) and the same intensity of exercise was again performed. Acute relief of the chronic atmospheric hypoxia lowered PA pressure by one third; all points fell below the line of identity. (Data from Vogel et al. [37].)

(n = 11) (34), and from 23 to 17 mmHg (n = 21) (15); however, 30% O_2 had no effect (17). In these studies, the resting pressures were only modestly elevated, so that there was relatively little potential for pressure reduction.

During exercise at high altitude, pulmonary arterial pressure rises markedly, thereby amplifying the potential for vasodilation in response to breathing oxygen. In Leadville residents (Fig. 4), relief of hypoxia in 23 individuals consistently lowered exercise pulmonary arterial pressures by one third. The higher the pressures before oxygen, the greater the reduction during oxygen breathing. Also, in five individuals breathing ambient air, pulmonary arterial pressures during exercise were reduced 40 percent by the pulmonary vasodilator tolazoline; adding 44% O_2 in two of these produced even greater reductions in pressure (37). These observations provide strong evidence that readily reversible pulmonary vasoconstriction is a major contributor to the pulmonary hypertension in these native residents at high altitude.

The effect of sustained relief of chronic hypoxia was examined in 11 men native to 4540 m in the Andes. Pulmonary arterial pressure at high altitude was 24 ± 5 mmHg at rest and increased to 54 ± 12 mmHg with exercise. After 2 years at sea level, their pressures were 12 ± 2 mmHg at rest and 25 ± 4 mmHg during comparable exercise, i.e., pulmonary vascular resistance at rest underwent a 68 percent reduction and the pulmonary hypertension of high altitude resolved completely. Unusually severe pulmonary hypertension at altitude could also be relieved in this way (10). Similar results were obtained in India: the resting pulmonary arterial pressures in seven permanent residents of Ladakh at 3600 m were 20 ± 4 mmHg; five weeks after descent to sea level, their pressures had decreased to 14 ± 2 mmHg.

TABLE 3 PULMONARY HEMODYNAMICS IN HIGH ALTITUDE NATIVES

Altitude	Condition	Cardiac output (1/min)	Pulmonary artery pressure (mmHg)	Wedge pressure (mmHg)	Pulmonary vascular resistance (units)
3750m [18]	Rest	7.0 ± 1.5	20 ± 3	7 ± 4	1.9 ± 0.6
(n = 10)	Exercise	11.9 ± 1.8	32 ± 8	7 ± 3	2.1 ± 0.5
4540m [2]	Rest	6.2 ± 1.1	29 ± 11	5 ± 2	4.2 ± 2.3
(n = 35)	Exercise	11.9 ± 2.0	60 ± 17	6 ± 4	4.6 ± 1.8

Values expressed as mean ± SD.

Vasoconstriction During Exercise. In the normal individual resting supine at sea level, pulmonary vascular resistance is low and remains essentially constant in the face of rising intravascular pressures as cardiac output increases during exercise (29). Two reports, one from La Paz, Bolivia (3750 m) (17), and the other from Morococha, Peru (4540 m) (2), yielded identical results: with mild exercise (less than twice the resting cardiac output), pulmonary vascular resistance failed to decrease even though pulmonary arterial pressure increased remarkably at the higher altitude (Table 3). However, the same exercise performed while breathing oxygen evoked less of an increase in pulmonary arterial pressure (Fig. 4), implying a decrease in resistance, i.e., vasodilation. These observations are consistent with the idea that the pressor influence of a decrease in alveolar P_{O_2} is enhanced by lowering the P_{O_2} of mixed venous blood (12). Indeed, it has been proposed that during exercise at high altitude, when mixed venous P_{O_2} falls, the intravascular hypoxemia augments the extravascular airway hypoxia, thereby increasing the hypoxic stimulus to the intervening vascular wall. Accordingly, oxygen breathing would be expected to lessen pulmonary vasoconstriction during exercise by not only removing the stimulus of airway hypoxia but also by raising the mixed venous P_{O_2} (Fig. 4).

Pulmonary Vascular Reactivity

In sea level residents, the hypoxic response curve is relatively flat, and the overall increase in resistance with hypoxia is only 1.3 units (Fig. 5). With the greater muscularity of the small pulmonary arteries in high altitude residents comes an exaggerated pressor response to acute hypoxia; the overall increase in pulmonary vascular resistance is more than twice as great as at sea level. The pressor effect of acute hypoxia is much greater than the depressor effect that occurs when the stimulus of ambient hypoxia is removed (Fig. 5). This pattern of response at 3100 m in the Rocky Mountains is supported by observations in men native to 3700 m in the Andes: acute hypoxia that lowered arterial oxygen saturation from 89 percent to 59 percent increased pulmonary vascular resistance by 3.0 units, whereas oxygen breathing lowered resistance only by 0.5 units (15). Enhanced pulmonary vascular reactivity has also been reported in dogs living at high altitude (8,40).

This enhanced reactivity would seem to indicate that after chronic hypoxic pulmonary hypertension has become established, the individual may be more vul-

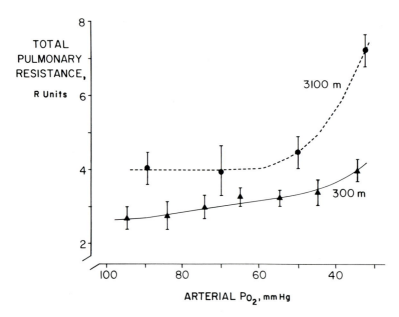

Figure 5: Progressive acute hypoxia, indicated by decreasing arterial P_{O_2}, increases "total pulmonary resistance" (calculated as the mean PA pressure/cardiac output). The upper curve (broken line) is based on 43 measurements in 24 residents at high altitude. The lower curve (solid line) is based on 129 measurements in 37 subjects. The data are shown as mean ± SEM. Pulmonary vascular reactivity to hypoxia is greater in high altitude residents at 3100 m than in persons living near sea level at 300 m. Note that in the high altitude residents, when the ambient hypoxia (Pa_{O_2} 50 mmHg) is enhanced, the increase in resistance is much greater than the decrease following acute relief of the ambient hypoxia. (R. F. Grover, unpublished observations.)

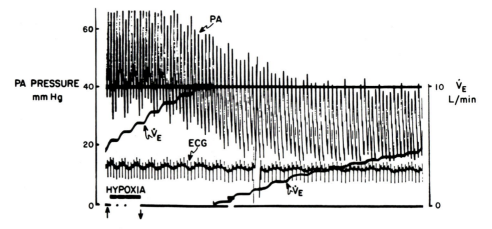

Figure 6: Pulmonary vascular reactivity in a normal woman living at 3100 m since birth. Acute hypoxia for 5 min increased her pulmonary arterial (PA) pressure to 65/37 mmHg associated with an increase in heart rate (ECG) and ventilation ($\dot{V}E$). Removal of the increased hypoxic stimulus, i.e., return to the lesser ambient hypoxia of room air (down arrow at left edge of figure), produced a prompt fall in PA pressure to 40/18 mmHg, together with a decrease in both heart rate and ventilation. This illustrates the increased reactivity of high altitude natives indicated in Figure 5.

nerable to the pulmonary pressor effects of added hypoxia (Fig. 6), e.g., as occurs during hypoventilation while asleep. However, in 11 male residents of Leadville (3100 m) studied by right heart catheterization, while awake and during sleep, in whom arterial P_{O_2} fell from 55 ± 3 to 50 ± 6 mmHg (and arterial P_{CO_2} rose from 34 ± 3 to 39 ± 9 mmHg), the pulmonary arterial mean pressure for the group did not change significantly on average (28 ± 6 versus 30 ± 9 mmHg) even though the pressure did increase significantly in two individuals (by 13 and 18 mmHg, respectively).

Variability in response to a given stimulus is characteristic of all biological systems and the pulmonary hypertensive response to hypoxia is no exception. In fact, when dealing with the hypoxia of high altitude, variability occurs not only in the pulmonary vascular pressor response, but also in the stimulus itself, alveolar hypoxia.

VARIABILITY IN STIMULUS

The stimulus to pulmonary vasoconstriction is primarily the oxygen tension in the distal airways, PA_{O_2}. This is determined by a number of factors including not only the inspired (ambient) P_{O_2} but also the alveolar ventilation. Lowering of arterial P_{O_2} is a powerful stimulus to ventilation so that hyperventilation is a normal aspect of adaptation to the chronic hypoxia of high altitude. But individuals vary markedly in their ventilatory responses to acute isocapnic hypoxia (7), a factor that, in turn, influences the level of ventilation attained following adaptation to high altitude. This inherent ventilatory sensitivity may determine the individual's tolerance to hypoxia, i.e., a low ventilatory sensitivity *permits* hypoxia to persist or intensify.

An additional aspect of ventilatory sensitivity to hypoxia is that after years of hypoxia, sensitivity diminishes progressively. Among populations at high altitude, children with relatively few years of exposure have normal ventilatory sensitivities, whereas adults with more cumulative years of hypoxia lose this sensitivity (16). Hence, it is not surprising that when normal individuals are studied at the same high altitude, we find considerable variability in their level of arterial hypoxia. For example, in 38 normal men living at 4540 m, the range of arterial oxygen saturation at rest was 66 to 88 percent ($78 \pm 5SD$) (27).

VARIABILITY IN RESPONSE

The magnitude of the pulmonary hypertension that results from comparable degrees of hypoxia shows marked variability among individuals. Apparently, this variability in pulmonary vascular reactivity was inherent in the lungs prior to any stimulus. This conclusion is based on extensive evidence mainly from cattle, a species that develops remarkable pulmonary hypertension when exposed to hypoxia. Investigation of this phenomenon began about 30 years ago (43). It was soon realized that in a group of normal Hereford steers exposed to 3000 m for several months, some developed severe pulmonary hypertension (90 ± 25 mmHg) whereas others developed more moderate pulmonary hypertension (45 ± 4 mmHg) (43). Subsequently, in cattle exposed to 3850 m (43), it was found that after 8 weeks of exposure, the range of pulmonary arterial pressures was 50 to 102 mmHg.

Those steers with lower pressures were categorized as relatively "resistant" to hypoxia (hyporesponders) whereas those with more severe pulmonary hypertension were considered "susceptible" (hyperresponders). A breeding program succeeded in transmitting the traits of hypo- and hyperresponsiveness, thereby establishing that pulmonary vascular reactivity is a genetic trait (43). Recently, hypo- and hyperreactivity of the airways of mice was shown to be determined by a single autosomal recessive gene (17). Perhaps the gene responsible for hypo- and hyperreactivity of the pulmonary arteries will also be identified soon.

The basis for the greater reactivity in the "susceptible" individuals proved to be greater muscularization of the small pulmonary arteries that rendered them more sensitive not only to hypoxia but also to other stimuli, e.g., prostaglandin $F_{2\alpha}$ (41). Not only is this true among individuals of the same species, but it appears to explain interspecies variability as well. Subsequent investigations established a positive correlation between the amount of lung vascular smooth muscle in a variety of species prior to exposure to hypoxia and the magnitude of the pulmonary hypertension that these species developed upon exposure to high altitude (36).

At low altitude, "resistant" calves exposed to acute hypoxia manifested less of an increase in pulmonary arterial pressure than that which occurred in the "susceptible" calves. These differences correlated highly with the responses to chronic hypoxia in these same individuals (44), lending further support to the concept that the pulmonary hypertensive response to chronic hypoxia is a direct extension of the pressor response to acute hypoxia, i.e., predominantly vasoconstriction.

Thus, we have evidence that the marked individual variability in the severity of pulmonary hypertension among individuals at high altitude reflects both variability in alveolar ventilation (the stimulus) as well as variability in pulmonary vascular reactivity (the response), and that both are inherited traits.

GENDER

Among residents of Leadville at 3100 m, women (n = 12) had higher levels of arterial P_{O_2} (60.9 versus 57.2 mmHg) and lower levels of arterial P_{CO_2} (26.9 versus 33.3 mmHg) than men (n = 39) (39; LG Moore, unpublished observations). These results are attributable to sustained higher levels of ventilation prompted by female sex hormones, particularly progesterone.

Gender differences also exist in the pulmonary vascular response to acute airway hypoxia. In lungs of sheep perfused in situ, the hypoxic pressor response proved to be significantly less in females than in males (42). The blunted pulmonary vascular reactivity in the females was attributed to estradiol.

Gender also influences erythropoiesis. Following puberty, testosterone stimulates erythropoiesis at all altitudes, resulting in higher hematocrit and hemoglobin concentrations in men than in women. Chronic hypoxia, specifically arterial desaturation, also stimulates red cell production and increases total red cell mass (39). As a result, hematocrit and hemoglobin concentration are increased in men, women, and children who live at high altitude. However, the combined effects of testosterone and hypoxemia result in hematocrits above 50 percent in men at altitude, whereas hematocrits are usually less than 50 percent in women at altitude (8). In this crucial range, hematocrits increase significantly the resistance to blood flow through the lung. The net result could be higher pulmonary artery pressures in men than in women at high altitude.

However, gender is apparently without influence on the severity of pulmonary hypertension at high altitude (20). After 4 weeks of exposure of male and female swine to rather extreme hypoxia (simulating 5490 m), females were less hypoxic, had higher levels of Pa_{O_2} and lower levels of Pa_{CO_2}, and developed slightly less right ventricular hypertrophy. However, pulmonary hypertension was equally severe in both males and females, with mean pulmonary arterial pressures of 78 ± 4 and 74 ± 2 mmHg, respectively. Moreover, in 10 female adolescents of Leadville, Colorado (3100 m), resting pressures averaged 25 ± 3 (SEM) mmHg whereas they averaged 24 ± 2 mmHg in 18 young men (37). During exercise, mean pressures were 48 ± 8 mmHg in the females and 58 ± 4 mmHg in the males; the higher cardiac outputs achieved by the males accounted for this difference.

HYPOVENTILATION WITH PULMONARY HYPERTENSION

Alveolar Hypoventilation at Sea Level

With respect to the cardiovascular response, the most significant difference between the chronic hypoxia of altitude and that associated with chronic obstructive airways disease at sea level is the coexistence of hypoxia, hyperventilation, and hypocapnia at altitude and of hypoxia, hypoventilation, and CO_2 retention in chronic obstructive airways disease.

CARDIAC OUTPUT, MYOCARDIAL FUNCTION

Soon after ascent to high altitude, hematocrit increases, reflecting a decrease in plasma volume associated with the hypocapnia that results from hyperventilation. As plasma volume falls, there is a parallel decrease in cardiac stroke volume without a compensatory increase in heart rate. Consequently, cardiac output is subnormal at high altitude, even in long-term residents, while myocardial function remains normal. In contrast, the patient with alveolar hypoventilation has CO_2 retention, a normal or increased plasma and blood volume, and a normal cardiac output (9).

More importantly, myocardial function is apparently impaired by hypercapnia (32). In contrast to the normal heart which responds to an increase in right ventricular afterload by increasing the stroke work of the right ventricle with little increase in its end-diastolic pressure, the heart in chronic hypercapnic acidosis has a serious impairment in its ability to increase right ventricular stroke work and right ventricular end-diastolic pressure increases. This difference may explain why chronic hypoxic pulmonary hypertension is well tolerated by the normal individual at high altitude but often poorly tolerated by the hypoxemic, hypercapnic patient with chronic obstructive airways disease.

COR PULMONALE

Some patients with chronic obstructive airways disease develop pulmonary hypertension and cor pulmonale whereas others do not. The discrepancy may be due to inherited differences in the ventilatory sensitivity to hypoxia and CO_2, and in pulmonary vascular reactivity. Those patients in whom pulmonary hypertension complicates chronic obstructive airways disease are hypoxemic and hypercapnic, i.e., they are hypoventilators. The hypercapnic patients also have a low ventilatory sensitivity to CO_2, and perhaps to hypoxia. One reasonable conclusion is that the patient with chronic obstructive airways disease who is born with a normal ventilatory sensitivity to CO_2 and hypoxia will make the added respiratory effort to overcome the obstruction and maintain relatively normal blood gases. However, the comparable patient with an inherently low ventilatory sensitivity to CO_2 and hypoxia will tolerate hypoxemia and CO_2 retention, i.e., he will lack the "drive" to overcome the airways obstruction; the resulting hypoventilation and alveolar hypoxia will stimulate pulmonary vasoconstriction that will be enhanced by hypercapnic acidosis. If, in addition, the patient with low ventilatory sensitivity to the respiratory gases also inherited a pulmonary vascular bed that is highly sensitive to hypoxia, he will be even more "susceptible" to hypoxic pulmonary hypertension. In addition, other influences that decrease alveolar ventilation, such as obesity, sleep, or lower respiratory infection, will intensify the hypoxic stimulus and the resulting pulmonary vasoconstriction. The same factors that lower arterial oxygen saturation promote polycythemia and operate synergistically to increase the severity of his pulmonary hypertension. Therefore, the patient who is prone to develop pulmonary heart disease is one who has inherited a double handicap (7). Just as the pulmonary hypertension of high altitude is largely reversible by removal of the hypoxic stimulus, so is the vasoconstrictive component of the pulmonary hypertension reversible in patients with chronic obstructive airways disease.

Hypoventilation at High Altitude

CHRONIC MOUNTAIN SICKNESS

Residents at high altitude who were previously well adapted may develop alveolar hypoventilation from any one of a number of causes. In this situation, the effects of atmospheric hypoxia and of hypoventilation are additive, and the individual becomes more hypoxic than normal individuals at the same altitude. In response to this greater hypoxic stimulus, pulmonary hypertension increases because of vasoconstriction and is exaggerated by excessive polycythemia, resulting in the syndrome of chronic mountain sickness (CMS).

In a group of men with CMS living in Colorado at 3100 m, some were found to have mild obstructive airways disease whereas others breathed shallowly so that the dead space/tidal volume ratio was increased, and in some the central control of breathing appeared to be depressed by the hypoxia. Moreover, many experienced a marked fall in arterial oxygen saturation during sleep. However, regardless of the initiating mechanism, loss of the ventilatory response to hypoxia in these individuals enabled the hypoxemia to persist (16).

Patients with CMS have severe pulmonary hypertension. In 10 patients with CMS living in Peru at 4300 m, arterial saturations were 69 ± 5 percent (normal 81 ± 5 percent), hematocrits were 79 ± 4 percent (normal 59 ± 5 percent), and resting mean pulmonary arterial pressures of 47 ± 18 mmHg compared with 23 ± 5 mmHg in normal residents at that altitude (26). That this pulmonary hypertension is the result of hypoxic pulmonary vasoconstriction augmented by polycythemia was demonstrated by the rapid decrease in pulmonary arterial pressure that occurred in these individuals within days of descent to sea level.

CHRONIC OBSTRUCTIVE AIRWAYS DISEASE

For patients with chronic obstructive airways disease, residence at high altitude would seem to invoke the risk of increasing the degree of hypoxemia, of aggravating polycythemia, of augmenting pulmonary hypertension, and of increasing mortality. Contrary to this expectation, 28 patients with stable chronic obstructive airways disease who lived in Mexico City at 2240 m had less pulmonary hypertension than did comparable patients at sea level (19). Furthermore, in patients in whom arterial oxygen saturations were lower than 76 percent, pulmonary arterial pressures were also somewhat lower in Mexico City (37 ± 12 mmHg) than at sea level (44 ± 14 mmHg). These seemingly paradoxical findings may reflect the same phenomenon observed in healthy individuals (Table 1), i.e., that Latin American populations apparently develop less pulmonary hypertension at high altitude (hypoxemia) than do Caucasians.

Nevertheless, altitude does seem to have an adverse effect on patients with chronic obstructive airways disease. Mortality from emphysema is greater in Colorado than at lower altitudes, supporting similar findings from New Mexico and Utah (22).

SUMMARY AND CONCLUSIONS

Among human populations, pulmonary hypertension appears above 2000 m in the United States and China, but only above 3500 m in Mexico, South America, and India, implying racial differences in response. Humans rarely live permanently above 4500 m, and at this altitude, where PA_{O_2} is approximately 50 mmHg, the average pulmonary arterial pressure at rest is about 28 mmHg, or roughly twice as high as at sea level. This rather modest pulmonary hypertension at rest becomes much more impressive during exercise when mean pressures often reach 50 to 60 mmHg and may even exceed 100 mmHg in some individuals. Nonetheless, pulmonary hypertension in normal people appears to present no handicap to life or physical performance at high altitude.

Marked individual variability is characteristic of the severity of pulmonary hypertension at high altitude. This reflects variability in the intensity of the hypoxic *stimulus* due to differences in ventilation, as well as differences in the pulmonary vasoconstrictive *response* reflecting inherited differences in pulmonary vascular reactivity. Another variable is the degree of secondary polycythemia, since increased hematocrit and blood viscosity also contribute to the increased resistance to blood flow through the lung. Although absolute levels of hematocrit are higher in men than in women (at all altitudes), and men are more prone to hypoventilate and hence be more hypoxic, particularly during sleep, limited data indicate no influence of gender on the severity of hypoxic pulmonary hypertension.

Many lessons learned from normal people exposed to the atmospheric hypoxia of high altitude apply to patients at low altitude with hypoxia due to alveolar hypoventilation, as in chronic obstructive airways disease or to the obesity-hypoventilation syndrome. Inherited differences in ventilatory sensitivity to CO_2 and hypoxia, and in pulmonary vascular reactivity, help to explain the variable clinical picture of chronic obstructive airways disease. Those individuals who inherit the double handicap of a low ventilatory response to hypoxia and CO_2 combined with a high pulmonary vascular reactivity appear to be most prone to develop pulmonary heart disease if they develop chronic obstructive airways disease. In contrast to the normal individual at high altitude, in patients with chronic obstructive airways disease, pulmonary hypertension is poorly tolerated. This difference probably relates to the basic fact that hyperventilation at high altitude causes CO_2 to fall, whereas in chronic obstructive airways disease accompanied by hypoventilation, CO_2 retention occurs. The resulting hypercapnic acidosis impairs the ability of the right ventricle to work against an increased afterload, predisposing to congestive heart failure.

REFERENCES

1. Banchero N, Cruz JC: Hemodynamic changes in the Andean native after two years at sea level. Aerospace Med 41 : 849–853, 1970.

2. Banchero N, Sime F, Penaloza D, Cruz J, Gamboa R, Marticorena E: Pulmonary pressure, cardiac output, and arterial oxygen saturation during exercise at high altitude and at sea level. Circulation 33 : 249–262, 1966.

3. Cruz JC, Zeballos R: Influencia racial sobre la respuesta ventilatoria a la hipoxia e hipercapnia. Acta Physiol Lat Am 25 : 23–32, 1975.

4. Dawson A, Grover RF: Regional lung function in natives and long-term residents at 3,100 m altitude. J Appl Physiol 36 : 294–298, 1974.

5. DeGraff AC Jr, Grover RF, Johnson RL Jr, Hammond JW Jr, Miller JM: Diffusing capacity of the lung in Caucasians native to 3,100 m. J Appl Physiol 29 : 71–76, 1970.

6. De Micheli A, Villacis E, Guzzy de la Mora P, Rubio Alvarez V: Observaciones sobre los valores hemodinamicos y respiratorios obtenidos en sujetos normales. Arch Inst Cardiol Mexico 30 : 507–520, 1960.

7. Grover RF: New concepts in pulmonary heart disease. Med Times 110 : 32–37, 1982.

8. Grover RF, Johnson RL Jr, McCullough RG, McCullough RE, Hofmeister SE, Campbell WB, Reynolds RC: Pulmonary hypertension and pulmonary vascular reactivity in beagles at high altitude. J Appl Physiol 65 : 2632–2640, 1988.

9. Grover RF, Reeves JT: Oxygen transport in man during hypoxia: High altitude compared with chronic lung disease. Bull Europ Physiopath Respir 15 : 121–128, 1979.

10. Grover RF, Vogel JHK, Voigt GC, Blount SG: Reversal of high altitude pulmonary hypertension. Am J Cardiol 18 : 928–932, 1966.

11. Gurtner HP, Walser P, Fässler B: Normal values for pulmonary hemodynamics at rest and during exercise in man. Prog Respir Res 9 : 295–315, 1975.

12. Hales CA: The site and mechanism of oxygen

sensing for the pulmonary vessels. Chest 88 : 235S–240S, 1985.

13. Harf A, Pratt T, Hughes JHM: Regional distribution of $\dot{V}_A/\dot{Q}$ in man at rest and with exercise measured with krypton-81m. J Appl Physiol 44 : 115–123, 1978.

14. Hultgren HN, Kelly J, Miller H: Pulmonary circulation in acclimatized man at high altitude. J Appl Physiol 20 : 233–238, 1965.

15. Hultgren HN, Kelly J, Miller H: Effect of oxygen upon pulmonary circulation in acclimatized man at high altitude. J Appl Physiol 20 : 239–243, 1965.

16. Kryger MH, Grover RF: Chronic mountain sickness. Sem Respir Med 5 : 164–168, 1983.

17. Levitt RC, Mitzner W: Expression of airway hyperreactivity to acetylcholine as a simple autosomal recessive trait in mice. FASEB J 2 : 2605–2608, 1988.

18. Lockhart A, Zelter M, Mensch-Dechene J, Antezana G, Paz-Zamora M, Vargas E, Coudert J: Pressure-flow-volume relationships in pulmonary circulation in normal highlanders. J Appl Physiol 41 : 449–456, 1976.

19. Lupi HE, Sandoval J, Seoane M, Bialostozky D: Behavior of the pulmonary circulation in chronic obstructive pulmonary disease. Am Rev Respir Dis 126 : 509–514, 1982.

20. McMurtry IF, Frith CH, Will DH: Cardiopulmonary responses of male and female swine to simulated high altitude. J Appl Physiol 35 : 459–462, 1973.

21. Mecham RP, Whitehouse LA, Wrenn DS, Parks WC, Griffin GL, Senior RM, Crouch EC, Stenmark KR, Voelkel NF: Smooth muscle-mediated connective tissue remodeling in pulmonary hypertension. Science 237 : 423–426, 1987.

22. Moore LG, Rohr AL, Maisenbach JK, Reeves JT: Emphysema mortality is increased in Colorado residents at high altitude. Am Rev Respir Dis 126 : 225–228, 1982.

23. Moret P, Covarrubias E, Coudert J, Duchosal F:

Cardiocirculatory adaptation to chronic hypoxia. III. Comparative study of cardiac output, pulmonary and systemic circulation between sea level and high altitude residents. Acta Cardiol 27: 596–619, 1972.

24. Motley HL, Cournand A, Werko L, Himmelstein A, Dresdale D: The influence of short periods of induced acute anoxia upon pulmonary artery pressures in man. Am J Physiol 150: 315–320, 1947.

25. Ordonez JH: Physiological observations in residents of Bogota, Columbia, altitude 8700 feet. Rocky Mtn Med J 66: 33–36, 1969.

26. Penaloza D, Sime F: Chronic cor pulmonale due to loss of altitude acclimatization (chronic mountain sickness). Am J Med 50: 728–743, 1971.

27. Penaloza D, Sime F, Banchero N, Gamboa R, Cruz J, Marticorena E: Pulmonary hypertension in healthy men born and living at high altitudes. Am J Cardiol 11: 150–157, 1963.

28. Rappoport WJ, Robinson JC: Research in high altitude pulmonary hypertension. Arizona Pub Health News 58: 2–8, 1964.

29. Reeves JT, Dempsey JA, Grover RF: Pulmonary circulation during exercise, in Weir EK, Reeves JT (eds), *Pulmonary Vascular Physiology and Pathophysiology*. Lenfant C (exec ed), *Lung Biology in Health and Disease*. New York, Marcel Dekker (in press).

30. Reeves JT, Grover RF: High-altitude pulmonary hypertension and pulmonary edema, in Yu PN, Goodwin JF (eds), *Progress in Cardiology, Vol 4*. Philadelphia, Lea & Febiger, 1975, pp 99–118.

31. Reeves JT, Groves BM: Approach to the patient with pulmonary hypertension, in Weir EK, Reeves JT (eds), *Pulmonary Hypertension*. Mount Kisco, NY, Futura, 1984, pp 1–44.

32. Rose CE Jr, VanBenthuysen K, Jackson JT, Tucker CE, Kaiser DL, Grover RF, Weil JV: Right ventricular performance during increased afterload impaired by hypercapnic acidosis in conscious dogs. Circ Res 52: 76–84, 1983.

33. Roy SB: *Circulatory and Ventilatory Effects of High Altitude Acclimatization and Deacclimatization of Indian Soldiers*. Delhi, General Printing Co., 1972, pp 32–44.

34. Spievogel H, Otero-Calderon L, Calderon G, Hartmann R, Cudkowicz L: The effects of high altitude on pulmonary hypertension of cardiopathies, at La Paz, Bolivia. Respiration 26: 369–386, 1969.

35. Spracklen FH, Overy HR, Muller B, Grover RF: Hemodynamic and blood gas changes during sleep at high altitude (Abstract). Circulation 38: VI–186, 1968.

36. Tucker A, McMurtry IF, Reeves JT, Alexander AF, Will DH, Grover RF: Lung vascular smooth muscle as a determinant of pulmonary hypertension at high altitude. Am J Physiol 228: 762–767, 1975.

37. Vogel JHK, Weaver WF, Rose RL, Blount SG Jr, Grover RF: Pulmonary hypertension on exertion in normal man living at 10,150 feet (Leadville, Colorado) in Grover RF (ed), *Normal and Abnormal Pulmonary Circulation*. Basel/New York, S. Karger, 1963, pp 269–285.

38. Wagenvoort CA, Wagenvoort N: *Pathology of Pulmonary Hypertension*. New York, J Wiley & Sons, 1977.

39. Weil JV, Jamieson G, Brown DW, Grover RF: The red cell mass-arterial oxygen relationship in normal man. J Clin Invest 47: 1627–1639, 1968.

40. Weir EK, Tucker A, Reeves JT, Grover RF: Increased pulmonary vascular pressor response to hypoxia in highland dogs. Proc Soc Exp Biol Med 154: 112–115, 1977.

41. Weir EK, Will DH, Alexander AF, McMurty IF, Looga R, Reeves JT, Grover RF: Vascular hypertrophy in cattle susceptible to hypoxic pulmonary hypertension. J Appl Physiol 46: 517–521, 1979.

42. Wetzel RC, Sylvester JT: Gender differences in hypoxic vascular response of isolated sheep lungs. J Appl Physiol 55: 100–104, 1983.

43. Will DH, Hicks JL, Card CS, Alexander AF: Inherited susceptibility of cattle to high-altitude pulmonary hypertension. J Appl Physiol 38: 491–494, 1975.

44. Will DH, Hicks JL, Card CS, Reeves JT, Alexander AF: Correlation of acute with chronic hypoxic pulmonary hypertension in cattle. J Appl Physiol 38: 495–498, 1985.

45. Yang Z, He ZQ, Liu XL: Pulmonary hypertension related to high altitude: An analysis of 83 cases with microcatheterization. Chinese J Cardiol 13: 32–34, 1985.

John H. Newman, M.D.
James E. Loyd, M.D.

21

Familial Pulmonary Hypertension

Several heritable diseases result in clinically important pulmonary hypertension. The two primary diseases of the pulmonary circulation are familial primary pulmonary hypertension (FPPH) and familial pulmonary veno-occlusive disease. Heritable disorders that cause secondary pulmonary hypertension are those associated with procoagulation, hypoventilation, interstitial lung disease, alveolar hypoxia, lung proteolysis, and perhaps exaggerated hypoxic vasoconstriction (Table 1). Familial primary pulmonary hypertension will be the main focus of this review, but other diseases will also be mentioned.

TABLE 1 HERITABLE DISEASES CAUSING PULMONARY HYPERTENSION

Heritable Diseases Causing Pulmonary Hypertension
Familial primary pulmonary hypertension
Alpha $_1$-antiproteinase deficiency
Cystic fibrosis
Antithrombin III deficiency
Protein C deficiency
Fibrinolytic defect
Familial veno-occlusive disease
Familial idiopathic pulmonary fibrosis
Heritable Influences on Pulmonary Arterial Pressure
Strength of hypoxic vasoconstriction
Blunted ventilatory drives to hypoxia or hypercarbia
Susceptibility to chronic bronchitis and emphysema?
Copper metabolism?

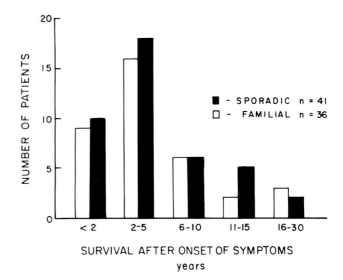

Figure 1: The distribution of survival after onset of symptoms for sporadic disease compared with 36 familial cases in which history of symptoms was available (20). Graph of sporadic cases was constructed by Voelkel and Reeves (25). (Reproduced from Loyd et al. [20].)

FAMILIAL PRIMARY PULMONARY HYPERTENSION

Familial primary pulmonary hypertension is a rare disease. Only 14 families in North America have been reported to have this disease (20,22). In addition, 12 families were entered in the NIH Registry for Primary Pulmonary Hypertension (23) and 15 others have been seen in our clinic during the last 6 years. The true incidence of familial primary pulmonary hypertension is unknown. The NIH Registry entered approximately 200 cases of primary pulmonary hypertension between 1981 and 1985, but because entry of previously diagnosed cases was permitted at the start of the Registry, these 200 cases reflect both prevalence and incidence (23). With this reservation, the 12 patients with familial disease entered in the Registry over these 4 years represent about 6 percent of the total group.

Familial primary pulmonary hypertension has the same clinical features as primary pulmonary hypertension in general. We have found a 2:1 female/male ratio, similar to the 1.7:1 female/male ratio found in sporadic primary pulmonary hypertension (23,25). The range and distribution of ages at the time of diagnosis are similar for familial and nonfamilial primary pulmonary hypertension: patients with familial disease have been diagnosed as young as one year of age and as old as age 65. Whether racial predilection exists in familial primary pulmonary hypertension is unknown; one of the 28 families in our records is black, the others are Caucasian. Survival from the onset of symptoms is similar among patients with familial and nonfamilial primary pulmonary hypertension (Fig. 1) (20,23,25). As is the case in nonfamilial primary pulmonary hypertension, in most patients with familial disease, the disease progresses rapidly and the patients die within 2 to 5 years; but some do survive for prolonged periods, even for 20 years or more.

Much of the information about the families of patients with familial primary pulmonary hypertension is historical, i.e., based on family history, review of old charts, and autopsy data. Primary pulmonary hypertension (PPH) was not rec-

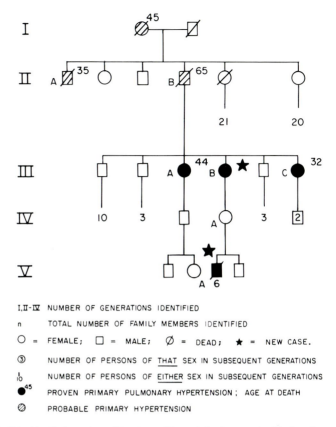

Figure 2: Pedigree of Family 5 in North American literature. The original cases in this family were III-A and III-C. In 1982, we discovered that a 6-year-old boy (V-A) had died of primary pulmonary hypertension, making his mother and grandmother obligatory carriers of the genetic susceptibility. In May of 1985, the grandmother III-B was discovered to have primary pulmonary hypertension at age 65. (Reproduced from Loyd et al. [20].)

ognized clinically until the Dresdale study of 1951 (7), and many instances have probably been missed or undiagnosed in the last 30 years. The advent of successful heart/lung transplantation for PPH and of successful therapy for diseases which mimic primary pulmonary hypertension, e.g., unresolved large pulmonary embolism, has improved the detection of such illnesses. Probably as a result of these developments, families with PPH are being recognized more often than previously. Little information is available in familial primary pulmonary hypertension about hemodynamics or drug responsiveness because many of these patients were treated in the 1960s and 1970s, i.e., before such measurements became routine.

We have found Raynaud's phenomenon in some families, and we suspect that there is a higher incidence of congenital heart defects, such as atrial septal defect, than would be expected as random events. We have not encountered any instance of either cirrhosis of the liver or collagen vascular disease in these families. The 12 patients with familial PPH reported to the Registry were not different with regard to physical findings, laboratory, or hemodynamic data from those with the sporadic form of the disease (23).

Inheritance

Familial primary pulmonary hypertension is an autosomal dominant disease. Autosomal disease was presumed for years because of the finding of disease in both sexes, but we were able to demonstrate male-to-male transmission in three families, effectively excluding X-linked disease (20,22). The involvement of most members of a sibship in several families provides reasonable evidence that the gene is dominant. On the other hand, the frequency of expression (penetrance) of this disease within families is highly variable. We have found transmission of the disease through five generations in one family but have been able to document only six cases in the 71 persons in this family.

One disturbing aspect of this disease is its ability to skip generations (Fig. 2: Family 5). Two sisters in this family died of primary pulmonary hypertension (20). A review of this family 15 years after the original report disclosed that a 6-year-old grandson of an asymptomatic sister of the two original cases had died of primary pulmonary hypertension. Recently, we discovered that the unaffected sister (patient IIIB) had been diagnosed as having the disease at age 65. Thus, her asymptomatic daughter (patient IVA), who appears clinically normal, also has either latent disease or the genetic predisposition to it. This pattern of clinical expression raises many important questions, including what controls the rate and progression of disease, what is the inciting mechanism, and why does disease occur at different ages?

Other Genetic Features

Apparently, familial primary pulmonary hypertension tends to occur at earlier ages in successive generations (16). In 10 families in which the disease occurred in two or more generations, we found that the mean age at death decreased from

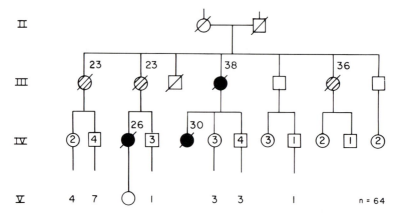

Figure 3: Family in which six women died of PPH over two generations. This family resides in Middle Tennessee, yet there was no insight that a family disease existed because of inaccurate diagnoses, poor, inadequate history taking, and lack of communication among separated family groups. (Reproduced from Loyd et al. [20].)

45.7 $\pm$ 3.5 SEM in the first recognized generation (n = 10), to 31.4 $\pm$ 4 (n = 14), and 14.2 $\pm$ 5.9 (n = 7) in the last generation.

The observation of accelerated disease in successive generations (genetic anticipation) has been criticized as potentially artifactual because of possible bias of ascertainment, i.e., that the finding of death from PPH at an earlier age in recent generations is simply due to heightened recognition of illness by the observer. However, this bias would be present only if members of earlier generations with disease are missed. We have complete pedigrees in several families over several generations, including up to 103 members in one family, so such bias should be minimal, if present at all. We have no explanation for the apparent acceleration of disease in subsequent generations.

The genetic basis of familial primary pulmonary hypertension is entirely unknown (24). Identification of the genetic basis of disease requires either that the gene be known, that there be a genetic probe available to hybridize to the segment of DNA being studied, that there be a known mutation at a known base pair substitution, or that restriction fragment length polymorphisms exist within a family. There are over 100,000 genes on the human genome; unless the gene responsible for familial primary pulmonary hypertension can be linked with some other known gene, a search for the FPPH gene would be a formidable problem. The families dealt with to date offer few clues to the genetic basis of familial primary pulmonary hypertension. For example, one family has a fibrinolytic defect (15); in two other families, both phenylketonuria and PPH have occurred. In addition, the incidence of cardiac anomalies in families with this disease seems to be higher than in the population at large. Our current approach to the genetic basis is to immortalize DNA from lymphocytes taken from members of families with this disease and to freeze red cells and plasma for linkage studies.

Families with Primary Pulmonary Hypertension (PPH)

Some instances of sporadic primary pulmonary hypertension may actually be familial. Failure to recognize the familial nature of the disease may be due to a low prevalence in a family because of a low frequency of genetic expression, poor intra-family communication, or failure of the physician to take a comprehensive family history. The basis for this belief stems from our experience with the first family that we encountered (Fig. 3) (20). The propositus was a 30-year-old woman whom we saw in 1980 and who reported no known family diseases. However, her extended family had several unusual deaths in young members during the prior two decades. Tracking down these family deaths, we found that a cousin had died in 1970 at Vanderbilt Hospital with the diagnosis of primary pulmonary hypertension. Our patient's mother had died in 1968 at age 38 at a local Nashville hospital with a history of dyspnea and peripheral edema. She experienced cardiovascular collapse during a contrast venogram performed in the attempt to diagnose the cause of ascites and leg edema; she died that evening. Rereview of her postmortem lung specimen 15 years later revealed lesions diagnostic of primary pulmonary hypertension. One maternal aunt with chronic dyspnea, edema, and cyanosis had died of hemoptysis, and two other aunts died suddenly after apparently normal childbirths without obstetric complication. Thus, there were six women in two generations with proven (n = 3) or probable (n = 3) familial pulmo-

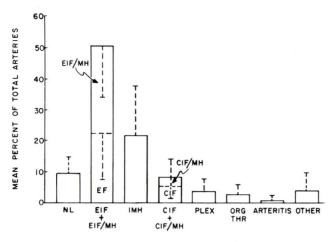

Figure 4: The individual types of pulmonary arterial lesions in all 23 patients shown as mean ± SD. NL = normal vessel; EIF = eccentric intimal fibrosis; EIF/MH = vessel with both eccentric intimal fibrosis and medial hypertrophy; IMH = isolated medial hypertrophy; CIF = concentric intimal fibrosis; CIF/MH = vessel with both concentric intimal fibrosis and medial hypertrophy; Plex = plexiform lesion; Org Thr = organized thrombus; Other = all other lesion types (see Table 4). (Reproduced from Lloyd et al. [18].)

nary hypertension. Nonetheless, familial disease was not initially suspected despite the fact that the entire extended family lived in Middle Tennessee and that two patients had died at local Nashville hospitals. Each of these cases was either misdiagnosed or was labeled "sporadic" primary pulmonary hypertension (PPH) until the sixth patient developed disease.

To test this hypothesis, we undertook to search for co-ancestry in apparently unrelated known PPH families residing in Tennessee (22). For this purpose, we employed a genealogical search company, Lineages Inc. of Salt Lake City, Utah. Lineages has access to the world's largest genealogic library, operated by the Mormon church. We have found eight PPH families in Tennessee, a relatively high concentration of the total of the 30 known families in the United States. Lineages focused on five families. The search, which took 1.5 years, revealed the surname "Hill" in three families. One family was traced to the Hatfield and McCoy families, both of which married into the Hills. The search involved 57 surnames and three of the lines were traced to the original immigrant—dates 1790, 1763, and 1744. Unfortunately, attempts to link the three Hill families in a genetic relationship were frustrated by poor record sources, typical of the early southern colonies. Further exhaustive study of our families would cost approximately $20,000 per family, a prohibitive cost. Thus, we were unable to document co-ancestry, and the hypothesis remains untested. An extremely interesting, albeit expensive, study would be a genealogic survey of all patients with primary pulmonary hypertension in the NIH Registry. Documentation of co-ancestry in some of these 187 patients might prove, or effectively negate, the idea that many cases of apparently nonfamilial PPH are, in fact, inherited.

Early Detection of Pulmonary Hypertension

Familial primary pulmonary hypertension offers a unique opportunity to detect disease before it is clinically evident. If disease could be detected before most of the vascular bed were obliterated, then therapeutic trials might have greater scientific merit, and tests directed at mechanisms of disease might be more meaningful. Because of this possibility, we have studied clinically unaffected members of two families in the middle Tennessee area with familial primary pulmonary hypertension (2). We are currently evaluating a variety of approaches to the early detection of pulmonary hypertension: echo-Doppler, the alveolar-arterial difference in P_{O_2} at maximal exercise, and the diffusing capacity for carbon monoxide under natural conditions and during the cold pressor test. As yet, each of these approaches must be regarded as investigational.

We have not performed right heart catheterization as a screening test in subjects from families with primary pulmonary hypertension because we believed invasive procedures could not be used for regular screening and might discourage prolonged follow-up. However, unaffected members of a family with primary pulmonary hypertension in Colorado have been catheterized (Dr. B. Groves, personal communication). In at least one patient, Groves found a mean pulmonary artery pressure that was borderline for pulmonary hypertension.

Pathological Lesions in Familial Primary Pulmonary Hypertension

Different opinions exist about the nature of the pathologic lesions in primary pulmonary hypertension, especially about whether different lesions represent different pathogenic mechanisms. Probably the two most controversial subsets in primary pulmonary hypertension are "thromboembolic" and "plexogenic" (3,13, 26–28). According to the consensus statement issued by the World Health Organization, *thromboembolic primary pulmonary hypertension* is characterized by eccentric intimal hyperplasia/fibrosis (EIF) of small arteries and lesions showing organized thrombosis. *Plexogenic arteriopathy* is characterized by the so-called plexiform lesion, which looks very much like a renal glomerulus, often associated with laminar concentric intimal fibroelastosis (CIF) of small pulmonary arteries (12).

We examined histologically lung sections from autopsies of 23 affected members of 13 families with PPH using elastic tissue stains as well as hematoxylin-eosin (18,19). The pathologists were unaware of the family history of the patients. Every artery and every abnormal vein on each section was categorized and each abnormal vessel was classified as showing either isolated medial hypertrophy, eccentric intimal fibrosis, concentric laminar intimal fibroelastosis, organized thrombus, arteritis, or plexiform lesions. Vessels that had more than one type of lesion, e.g., medial hypertrophy and eccentric intimal fibrosis (EIF), were recorded as having a "mixed" lesion rather than being tallied twice.

Figure 4 shows the distribution of lesion types in all 23 patients. Only 10 percent of all arteries found in the lung specimens were normal. Mixed lesions were the most common, occurring in about 32 percent of the vessels. Most of these mixed lesions had eccentric intimal fibrosis and medial hypertrophy (28 percent). CIF with medial hypertrophy occurred in only 3 percent and isolated medial hypertrophy in 22 percent.

Plexiform lesions were found in 18 patients and accounted for 3.4 percent of all arteries. Organized thrombi were found in 2.7 percent of arteries. Organized thrombi were found in 18 patients from 12 families, and plexiform lesions were

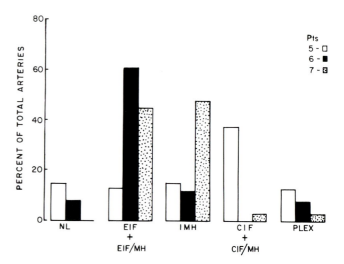

Figure 5: Distribution of types of pulmonary arterial lesions in each member of Family 12 (patients 5,6,7). NL = normal vessel; EIF = eccentric intimal fibrosis; EIF/MH = vessel with both eccentric intimal fibrosis and medial hypertrophy; IMH = isolated medial hypertrophy; CIF = concentric intimal fibrosis; CIF/MH = vessel with both concentric intimal fibrosis and medial hypertrophy; Plex = plexiform lesion. (Reproduced from Loyd et al. [18].)

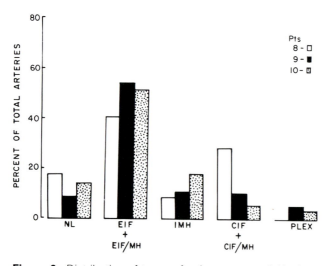

Figure 6: Distribution of types of pulmonary arterial lesions in each member of Family 13 (patients 8,9,10). NL = normal vessel; EIF = eccentric intimal fibrosis; EIF/MH = vessel with both eccentric intimal fibrosis and medial hypertrophy; IMH = isolated medial hypertrophy; CIF = concentric intimal fibrosis; CIF/MH = vessel with both concentric intimal fibrosis and medial hypertrophy; Plex = plexiform lesion. (Reproduced from Loyd et al. [18].)

found in 18 patients from 12 families. Organized thrombi and plexiform lesions coexisted in 14 patients and were found exclusive of each other in four patients each. Thus, organized thrombi and plexiform lesions were found together in the majority of patients but were found exclusive of each other in 8 of 23 (35 percent) patients. Arteritis and venous lesions were found in very few vessels, less than 0.5 percent of the total.

The distribution of lesions within two families is shown in Figure 5 and Figure 6. A wide spectrum of lesions was found in Family 12 (Fig. 5), yet the predominant lesion was different in each patient. Patient 5 had predominantly concentric intimal fibrosis, patient 6 had predominantly eccentric intimal fibrosis, and patient 7 had predominantly isolated medial hypertrophy. Despite these differences, each patient had plexiform lesions and, thus, would traditionally be classified as having plexogenic arteriopathy even though EIF lesions predominated in one patient. Similar heterogeneity is shown in Family 13 (Fig. 6). Ten plexiform lesions were found in patient 9, the most of any of the 23 patients in this study, and yet in patient 8 none were found. EIF, the lesion assumed to be most compatible with "thromboembolic" primary pulmonary hypertension, was the predominant lesion in every member of this family, yet all of these patients also had CIF lesions, purported to indicate a plexogenic arteriopathy.

This experience reaffirms that marked heterogeneity of lesions exists in familial primary pulmonary hypertension, both within families and among families. Thrombotic and plexiform lesions coexist, and marked differences in the predominant lesion type exist within families. We can only conclude that thrombotic lesions and eccentric intimal fibrosis may not necessarily represent a distinct pathogenesis in primary pulmonary hypertension. Moreover, it would appear that all different types of pathologic lesions in primary pulmonary hypertension represent different manifestations of a similar underlying pathogenesis.

These findings do not indicate or support any specific pathogenesis for the disease and do not imply that coagulation and thrombosis do not occur in primary pulmonary hypertension. It seems likely that activation of the coagulation cascade at the endothelial surface is a contributory mechanism in primary pulmonary hypertension. It also seems likely that some patients with primary pulmonary hypertension develop superimposed large vessel thromboembolic disease related to systemic venous stasis from low cardiac output. However, the nature of the pathologic lesions in primary pulmonary hypertension does not support the idea that microembolism occurs as a distinct pathogenetic mechanism. Nor do our data imply criticism of clinical studies in which anticoagulation is used to treat primary pulmonary hypertension (9): coagulation at the endothelial surface may be a mechanism of vascular disease and secondary thromboembolism can be a complication of abnormal endothelium regardless of the initiating lesion. Parenthetically, none of the lesions that we observed related to the syndrome of unresolved large vessel pulmonary embolism, a syndrome easily diagnosed by lung scan and arteriography and curable by surgery (21).

HERITABLE INFLUENCES ON PULMONARY ARTERIAL PRESSURE

Hypoxic vasoconstriction is a major determinant of pulmonary hypertension in a variety of diseases (8–11), including chronic bronchitis and emphysema, cystic fibrosis, alpha₁-antiproteinase deficiency, and probably idiopathic pulmonary fibrosis. The pulmonary vascular response to hypoxia also probably partly determines the susceptibility of persons to high altitude pulmonary edema, chronic mountain sickness, and sleep apnea syndromes. Marked differences exist in response to alveolar hypoxia among species and in individuals within species (see Chapter 9). The genetic basis of the strength of hypoxic pulmonary hypertension is not defined and the mechanism of hypoxic vasoconstriction remains unknown. Several characteristics may influence hypoxic vasoconstriction, including the extent of native muscularization of pulmonary arteries, the extent of collateral ventilation, and strength of ventilatory drive (8–11). The most investigated genetic susceptibility to pulmonary hypertension is in cattle, where "brisket" disease can be shown to be inherited. Brisket disease is right heart failure, manifested by edema of the dependent soft tissues of the neck (brisket) in cattle. This susceptibility appears to be transmitted by an autosomal dominant gene (14).

Individual variability in the strength of hypoxic vasoconstriction occurs in humans. Grover et al. studied 28 healthy high school students living at high altitude in Leadville, Colorado (elev. 10,200 ft) (10). Right heart catheterization was performed during vigorous supine exercise breathing the ambient air (Fig. 7). Twenty-five of the 28 students developed significant pulmonary hypertension during supine exercise, defined as mean pulmonary arterial pressure greater than 35 mmHg. The highest pulmonary arterial pressure, 165/95 mmHg (mean 118),

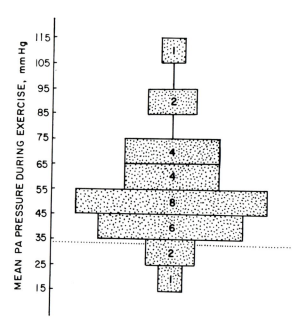

Figure 7: Twenty-eight normal high school students residing at high altitude (10,200 ft) were studied by right heart catheterization. During supine exercise, all but three developed significant pulmonary hypertension. The dotted line designates the upper limit of normal at sea level. (Reproduced from Grover [10].)

was achieved by a girl who was the local champion skier. The mechanisms responsible for the marked variability in pulmonary arterial pressure found in these 28 students are unknown, but probably represent multiple genetic and environmental influences.

There may also be racial differences in the susceptibility to pulmonary hypertension. The high pulmonary artery pressures of the Leadville natives, relative newcomers to altitude, contrasts sharply with the mild pulmonary hypertension of the Quechua Indians of the Peruvian Andes who have lived for 35,000 years at 15,000 feet, the highest altitude compatible with prolonged survival. It is likely that persons with genetic susceptibility to pulmonary hypertension were self-eliminated over time as this tribe continued to live at altitude. We are not aware of any reports of right heart catheterization of Tibetans, a race that has lived at high altitude for thousands of years. It is of interest that Tibetans have almost no incidence of chronic mountain sickness, a problem which does occur in the Quechua Indians. Clearly, racial differences exist in response to high altitude hypoxia.

OTHER HERITABLE DISEASES CAUSING PULMONARY HYPERTENSION

Table 1 lists a number of heritable diseases and disorders associated with pulmonary hypertension (17). Pulmonary hypertension results from a variety of mechanisms. Alpha$_1$-antiproteinase deficiency leads to obliterative pulmonary hypertension, subsequent to the unopposed proteinase digestion of the alveolar wall. It is likely that hypoxic pulmonary hypertension contributes in the later stages of this illness. Cystic fibrosis is a well-defined autosomal recessive illness causing secretion of abnormal mucus into the airways, which causes obstruction and chronic infection. Pulmonary hypertension in cystic fibrosis is probably predominantly due to widespread pulmonary vasoconstriction in underventilated portions of the lungs. There may be an element of obliterative pulmonary hypertension due to chronic infection and destruction of alveolar-capillary surface area.

Disorders of the clotting mechanism can also cause pulmonary hypertension. For example, antithrombin III deficiency is a rare but serious illness associated with pulmonary thromboembolism and perhaps even thrombosis in situ (5). Inappropriate coagulation is also seen in other disorders such as fibrinolytic defects and hereditary deficiencies of protein C (4). Protein C is a vitamin K-dependent lytic enzyme. Use of warfarin in patients with protein C deficiency can lead to paradoxical thrombus formation because of the inhibition of this lytic cofactor.

Idiopathic pulmonary fibrosis has been reported in a number of families. Abnormalities of copper metabolism have been reported in association with primary pulmonary hypertension (1). Pulmonary veno-occlusive disease has been reported in siblings (6), but we are unaware of parent-to-child transmission. A common exposure, i.e., viral infection rather than heritable disease, may be the inciting event for veno-occlusive disease. Clearly, the hereditary bases for pulmonary hypertension are not yet well understood.

ACKNOWLEDGMENTS

The study of pathological lesions reported in this chapter was a collaboration between the authors and Drs. James B. Atkinson, Department of Pathology, Vanderbilt; Dr. Renu Virmani, Armed Forces Institute of Pathology; and Dr. Giuseppe G. Pietra, Department of Pathology and Laboratory Medicine, University of Pennsylvania.

Support for this research was provided by NIH NHLBI 19153 SCOR in Pulmonary Vascular Disease, Clinical Research Center General Grant #M01 RR00095 and the Elsa S. Hanigan Fund of the Saint Thomas Foundation.

REFERENCES

1. Ahmed T, Sackner MA: Increased serum copper in primary pulmonary hypertension: A possible pathogenic link? Respiration 47 : 243–246, 1985.

2. Beard JT, Newman J, Loyd J, Byrd BF: Doppler estimation of changes in pulmonary artery pressure during hypoxia. Clin Research, In Press.

3. Bjornsson J, Edwards WD: Primary pulmonary hypertension: A histopathologic study of 80 cases. Mayo Clin Proc 60 : 16–25, 1985.

4. Broekman AW, Veltkamp JJ, Bertina RM: Congenital protein C deficiency and venous thromboembolism: A study of three Dutch families. N Engl J Med 309 : 340–344, 1983.

5. Cosgriff TM, Bishop DT, Hershgold EJ, Skolnick MH, Martin BA, Baty BJ, Carlson KS: Familial antithrombin III deficiency: Its natural history, genetics, diagnosis and treatment. Medicine (Baltimore) 62 : 209–220, 1983.

6. Davies P, Reid L: Pulmonary veno-occlusive disease in siblings: Case reports and morphometric study. Hum Pathol 13 : 911–915, 1982.

7. Dresdale DT, Schultz M, Michtom RJ: Primary pulmonary hypertension. I. Clinical and hemodynamic study. Am J Med 11 : 686–705, 1951.

8. Fishman AP: Pulmonary circulation, in Fishman AP, Fisher AB (eds), *Handbook of Physiology, Sect 3: The Respiratory System, Vol I: Circulation and Nonrespiratory Functions.* Bethesda, American Physiological Society, 1985, pp 93–165.

9. Fuster V, Steele PM, Edwards WD, Gersh BJ, McGoon MD, Frye RL: Primary pulmonary hypertension: Natural history and the importance of thrombosis. Circulation 70 : 580–587, 1984.

10. Grover RF: Pulmonary circulation in animals and man at high altitude. Ann NY Acad Sci 127 : 632–639, 1965.

11. Grover RF, Wagner WW, McMurtry IF, Reeves JT: Pulmonary circulation, in Shepherd JT, Abboud FM (eds), *Handbook of Physiology, Sect 2: The Cardiovascular System, Vol III: Peripheral Circulation and Organ Blood Flow, Part 2.* Bethesda, American Physiological Society, 1983, pp 103–136.

12. Hatano S, Strasser T (eds): *Primary Pulmonary Hypertension: Report on a WHO Meeting.* Geneva, World Health Organization, 1975, pp 7–45.

13. Heath D, Edwards JE: The pathology of hypertensive pulmonary vascular disease. Circulation 18 : 533–547, 1958.

14. Heath D, Williams DR: Pulmonary hypertension, in *Man at High Altitudes.* New York, Churchill Livingstone, 1981, pp 103–118.

15. Inglesby TV, Singer JW, Gordon DS: Abnormal fibrinolysis in familial pulmonary hypertension. Am J Med 55 : 5–14, 1973.

16. Kingdon HS, Cohen LS, Roberts WC, Braunwald E: Familial occurrence of primary pulmonary hypertension. Arch Intern Med 118 : 422–426, 1966.

17. Litwin SD (ed): *Genetic Determinants of Pulmonary Disease, Vol II,* in Lenfant C (ed), *Lung Biology in Health and Disease.* New York, Marcel Dekker, 1978.

18. Loyd JE, Atkinson JB, Pietra GG, Virmani R, Newman JH: Heterogeneity of pathological lesions in familial primary pulmonary hypertension. Am Rev Respir Dis 138 : 952–957, 1988.

19. Loyd JE, Atkinson JB, Virmani R, Pietra GG, Newman JH: Concentric and eccentric intimal fibrosis occur together in families with primary pulmonary hypertension. Am Rev Respir Dis 135 : A350, 1987.

20. Loyd JE, Primm RK, Newman JH: Familial primary pulmonary hypertension: Clinical patterns. Am Rev Respir Dis 129 : 194–197, 1984.

21. Moser KM, Daily PO, Peterson K, Dembitsky W, Vapnek JM, Shure D, Utley J, Archibald C: Thromboendarterectomy for chronic, major-vessel thromboembolic pulmonary hypertension. Ann Intern Med 107 : 560–565, 1987.

22. Newman JH, Loyd JE: Genetic basis of pulmonary hypertension. Sem Respir Med 7 : 343–352, 1986.

23. Rich S, Dantzker DR, Ayres SM, Bergofsky EH, Brundage BH, Detre KM, Fishman AP, Goldring RM, Groves BM, Koerner SK, Levy PC, Reid LM, Vreim CE, Williams GW: Primary pulmonary hypertension. A national prospective study. Ann Intern Med 107: 216–223, 1987.

24. Shapiro LJ, Comings DE, Jones OW, Rimoin DL: New frontiers in genetic medicine. Ann Intern Med 104: 527–539, 1986.

25. Voelkel NF, Reeves JT: Primary pulmonary hypertension, in Moser KM (ed), *Pulmonary Vascular Diseases.* New York, Marcel Dekker, 1979, pp 573–649.

26. Wagenvoort CA: Lung biopsy specimens in the evaluation of pulmonary vascular disease. Chest 77: 614–625, 1980.

27. Wagenvoort CA: Lung biopsy findings in secondary pulmonary hypertension. Heart Lung 15: 429–450, 1986.

28. Wagenvoort CA, Wagenvoort N: Primary pulmonary hypertension: A pathologic study of the lung vessels in 156 clinically diagnosed cases. Circulation 42: 1163–1182, 1970.

John T. Reeves, M.D.
Andrew J. Peacock, M.D.
Kurt R. Stenmark, M.D.

22

Animal Models of Chronic Pulmonary Hypertension

Animals develop chronic pulmonary hypertension in response to chronic hypoxia, chemical agents, inflammation, large pulmonary blood flow, high pulmonary venous pressure, and emboli. During the past decade, the use of animal models to gain insight into chronic pulmonary hypertension has increased considerably (11,49). This chapter provides an update of the subject.

NEONATAL PULMONARY HYPERTENSION

In the fetus, pulmonary arterial pressures are as high as, or higher than, pressures in the aorta. As a result, blood flows from the pulmonary artery to the aorta via the ductus arteriosus (4). Should pulmonary vascular resistance fail to decrease normally at birth, the fetal pulmonary hypertension would be expected to persist. Similarly, if a stimulus to pulmonary vasoconstriction were to occur early in postnatal life, pulmonary hypertension might easily recur. Indeed, pulmonary hypertension is a severe and rather frequent problem in the human newborn (14); it is associated with high mortality and debilitating complications in survivors.

Postnatal Hypoxia: The Newborn Calf at High Altitude

Newborn calves placed at high altitude (4300 m) develop severe pulmonary hypertension within a few days (53,55). Initially, pulmonary vasoconstriction pre-

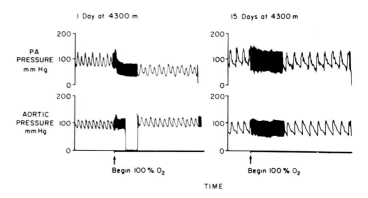

Figure 1: Pulmonary arterial and aortic pressures in a newborn calf at high altitude. When the calf, aged 2 days, had lived at 4300 m for 1 day, oxygen breathing (arrow) decreased pulmonary arterial pressure (left panel). After 15 days at 4300 m, oxygen breathing caused little change in pressure (right panel). (Reproduced from Stenmark et al. [53].)

dominates as the cause of the pulmonary hypertension since the high pulmonary vascular resistance is readily reversed by oxygen breathing or removal to a lower altitude. However, by 2 weeks, the pulmonary hypertension becomes more fixed and is not reversed by the acute administration of oxygen (Fig. 1).

The calf model of the hypertension is particularly remarkable because pressures in the pulmonary artery are higher than systemic arterial blood pressures. Before this devastating syndrome was produced in the calf, it had been shown that placing newborn calves at high altitude caused perpetuation of the fetal-type pulmonary circulation. But pulmonary arterial pressures had not exceeded systemic arterial pressures (50). The inordinate pulmonary hypertensive response to chronic hypoxia in the newborn calf stemmed from the coincidence of several influences operative at 4300 m: a susceptible species, exposure at an early age, and a severe hypoxic stimulus.

Many of the features in the calves resemble those of human infants with severe life-threatening neonatal pulmonary hypertension: low pulmonary blood flows, pulmonary arterial pressures in excess of systemic arterial pressures, right atrial hypertension (indicating the presence of right heart failure), and right-to-left shunts through the foramen ovale and the ductus arteriosus; the latter contributes to severe and progressive hypoxemia.

The altitude-exposed calves also resemble the human disease in that there are marked morphologic changes in the small pulmonary arteries and arterioles: endothelial swelling and proliferation of the media and adventitia (53,54) of a degree probably sufficient to compress the lumen (Fig. 2). Intrapulmonary pulmonary arteries are surrounded by a sleeve of pulmonary parenchyma. The space within the sleeve surrounding the pulmonary arteries is limited by the compliance of the alveolar septae. Should the perivascular space surrounding the pulmonary arterioles become filled with adventitial tissue, compression of the lumen would be likely to occur. High pulmonary vascular resistance would then result from vasoconstriction, endothelial swelling, increased hypertrophy of the medial layer, plus restriction imposed by the adventitia. The latter factor, in particular, has not been sufficiently examined.

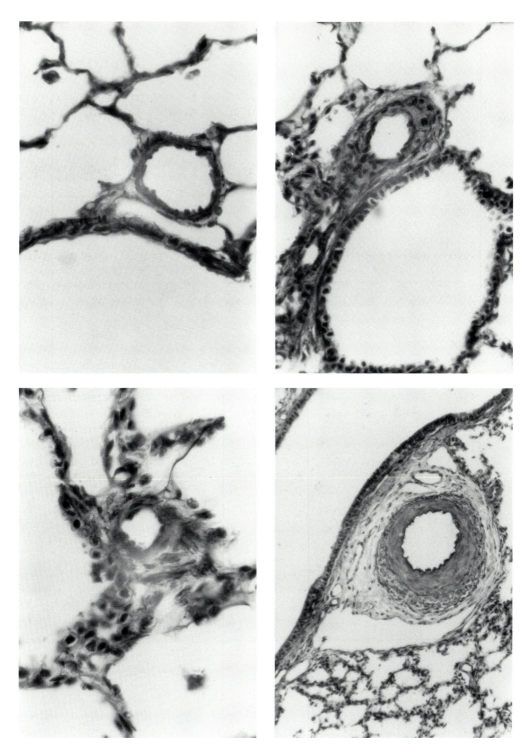

Figure 2: Photomicrographs of pulmonary arteries from 2-week-old calves. *Top left:* Arteriole from a control calf living at 1600 m. *Top right:* Arteriole from a calf at 4300 m. Proliferative cells and protein matrix fill the perivascular space. *Bottom left:* Muscularization of arteriole at alveolar duct level from a calf at 4300 m. Black strands of elastin can be seen. *Bottom right:* Muscular pulmonary artery from a calf to 4300 m. There is increased smooth muscle and marked adventitial thickening. Both collagen and elastin are increased. Pentochrome stain.

The pulmonary hypertensive calf presents advantages for study of the mechanisms underlying the hypertension as well as the vascular changes: the calf is convenient in size for hemodynamic measurements; bovine vascular cells are often cultured for experimental purposes; and the synthesis of the matrix proteins, elastin and collagen, can be explored (33). With respect to hemodynamic measurements in calves with suprasystemic pulmonary arterial pressures, acetylcholine proved to be particularly effective in decreasing the pulmonary vascular resistance as compared to oxygen inhalation or prostacyclin infusion (Fig. 3) (42). The more effective vasodilation with acetylcholine implies both that acute relief of chronic hypoxia by oxygen inhalation does not relieve completely the vasoconstrictive component and that endothelial-dependent vasodilator activity has probably been evoked in the pulmonary circulation. In contrast to these in vivo observations, endothelial-dependent relaxing activity is not seen in vitro in large pulmonary arteries obtained from hypertensive calves. This discrepancy suggests either that the large pulmonary arteries do not reflect behavior of the pulmonary microcirculation or that the in vitro environment does not reproduce that in vivo.

A second example of the value of animal models is the synthesis of the matrix proteins, elastin and collagen, which seems to be a key factor for the development of chronic pulmonary hypertension. In the rat, rendered pulmonary hypertensive by chronic exposure to hypoxia, synthesis of these matrix proteins increases and may play a role in the pathogenesis of the hypertensive process (25,26). In the high altitude calf, increases in collagen and in elastin are major factors contributing to the increased thickness of the adventitial layer (33,53,55). This response has been attributed to a "smooth muscle elastogenic factor" (SMEF) liberated by smooth muscle cells of the media, which stimulates the adventitial fibroblast to increase synthesis of the matrix proteins (33,53,55). Thus, the calf may be useful in the study of cellular and extracellular mechanisms of chronic pulmonary hypertension.

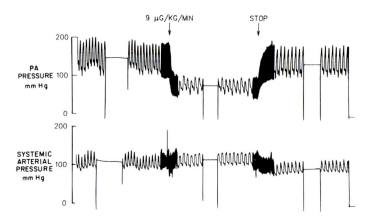

Figure 3: Pulmonary vasodilator effect of acetylcholine in a young calf at high altitude. Prior to acetylcholine infusion, the pulmonary arterial pressure exceeded systemic pressure; during the infusions of acetylcholine, the considerable drop in pulmonary arterial pressures and the increase in systemic arterial pressures reversed the relationship.

Prenatal Influences

An abnormal prenatal environment is possibly a cause of severe, and often persistent, pulmonary hypertension in the newborn infant. For example, it is conceivable that hypoxia in utero may cause an increased amount of pulmonary arterial smooth muscle in the newborn, possibly setting the stage for persistence of pulmonary hypertension even after alveolar P_{O_2} becomes normal (8). However, this hypothetical sequence has not withstood experimental scrutiny since prenatal hypoxia does not induce hypertrophy and hyperplasia in the pulmonary arterioles in newborn rats (7) and guinea pigs (40).

Whereas the effects of hypoxia on the fetal pulmonary circulation have been equivocal, the effects of increased pressure have not. Increase in pulmonary arterial pressure in the fetus—by unilateral renal artery constriction, constriction of the umbilical cord, or mechanical constriction of the ductus arteriosus—increases the amount of vascular smooth muscle in the fetal lung (28,29). Because inhibitors of the cyclooxygenase pathway oppose mechanisms that act to maintain patency of the ductus arteriosus (41), administration of indomethacin to the pregnant ewe would be expected to narrow the ductus arteriosus in utero. Indeed, chronic administration of indomethacin to the ewe does cause increased hypertrophy of the fetal pulmonary arterioles (29). Moreover, the right ventricle shows evidence of damage probably caused by elevated pressure. Although the fetuses in this study survived for a maximum of only 4 days, the authors postulate that application of less severe stimuli to ductal constriction in utero might enable the fetus to survive to birth and lead to persistent fetal hypertension. Preliminary observations on an animal model designed to test this hypothesis suggest that chronic (3 to 12 days) compression of the ductus arteriosus is associated with increased fetal pulmonary vascular resistance and a loss of normal vasodilator responses to oxygen (1). In addition, after birth, pulmonary arterial pressures remain high.

PULMONARY HYPERTENSION IN THE ADULT

The rat has proved particularly useful in developing animal models of pulmonary hypertension. A variety of stategies has been used in the species.

Hypoxic Pulmonary Hypertension in the Rat

The study of chronic hypoxic pulmonary hypertension in the rat has several advantages over that in the calf. Most important is that the rat is less expensive to procure and maintain and more readily exposed to hypoxia or altitude. With experience, pulmonary pressure and flow can be measured, even in the awake rat (10). Pulmonary arterial pressor responsiveness to hypoxia decreases with advancing age in the rat (60,61,62), probably as part of a generalized hyporeactivity of pulmonary and systemic vasculature with advancing age. Exposure of neonatal rats even to a modest altitude of 3000 m causes extreme right ventricular hypertrophy and, after 30 days, a marked increase in vascular reactivity to hypoxia

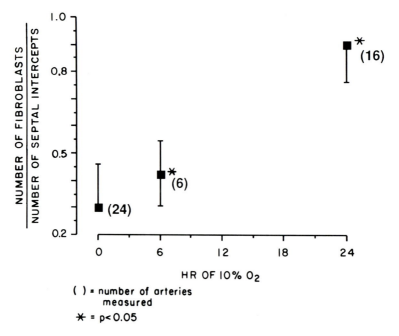

Figure 4: Increase in the number of fibroblasts around pulmonary arterioles during hypoxia in the rat. The arterioles were about 20 μ in diameter. Data presented as mean $\pm$ S.D. Time 0 = normoxia followed by data at 6 and 24 hr of breathing 10% O_2. The ordinate indicates the number of fibroblasts per number of alveolar septa intersecting or abutting the arteriole. After 24 hr, fibroblasts were considered to be in transition to smooth muscle cells. (Drawn from data in Table 2 of Sobin et al. [52].)

(61). The disadvantages of the rat are that the hypoxic pressor response is not quite as strong as in the calf, and the neonate is probably too small for hemodynamic measurements.

In both the rat and the calf, chronic hypoxic pulmonary hypertension is accompanied by increased protein synthesis and cell proliferation. But quite remarkable is the speed with which these changes begin to occur. For example, protein synthesis in the vessel wall increases within a few hours or days of initiating hypoxic exposure (31,39,63). The increase is not restricted to the small pulmonary arteries: collagen synthesis in the main pulmonary artery of the rat increases by more than 10-fold within 3 days (31). Within 24 hr, the number of fibroblasts within the arteriolar wall increases 3-fold (Fig. 4) (52). Whether the fibroblast (52) or the pericyte (38) ultimately becomes transformed into smooth muscle is uncertain, but it seems settled that cells move into the media. Previous observations suggesting that hypoxia causes loss of vessels (17) have not been substantiated (23). In chronic hypoxic pulmonary hypertension—in the calf, rat, or other species—a large part of the increased vascular resistance is a consequence of the increased thickness of the vascular wall. Hypoxic pulmonary hypertension does reverse on return to chronic normoxia (11), but thinning of vascular walls may be slow.

Attempts are being made to block the protein synthesis and the cellular proliferation that cause the increased thickness. Inhibitors of collagen production, beta-aminopropionitrile (26) and a proline analogue, cis-4-hydroxy-L-proline (25), have decreased the right ventricular hypertrophy, the pulmonary hypertension, and the collagen content of the vessel wall, implying that collagen synthesis is an important component of the chronic pulmonary hypertensive process. Heparin, which inhibits certain growth factors such as platelet-derived growth factor, has also successfully blunted the effects of hypoxic pulmonary hypertension in mice (9), implying that growth factors, possibly from platelets (24), also participate in the genesis of chronic pulmonary hypertension. Thus, the use of chronically hypoxic rats and mice provides clues to the mechanisms of hypoxic pulmonary hypertension and also suggests future directions of treatment in pulmonary hypertension.

Inhibition of angiotensin converting enzyme has relatively little effect on chronic hypoxic pulmonary hypertension in the rat (3,30), possibly because of the low level of converting enzyme activity in the pulmonary vessels of this species (3,22). However, chemical inhibition of the converting enzyme does decrease protein synthesis in the main pulmonary artery trunk (30).

The role of the autonomic nervous system in the development of chronic pulmonary hypertension continues to be of extreme interest. The pulmonary arterioles are richly supplied with adrenergic nerves in some species but not in others. McLean et al. (32) found that the small pulmonary arteries of the rat are devoid of adrenergic nerves and that the rat develops severe pulmonary hypertension during chronic hypoxia. They also noted that other animals, such as the calf and pig, which manifest large pressor responses to chronic hypoxia, lack adrenergic innervation of the arterioles. In contrast, less susceptible species, such as the dog and guinea pig, have rich adrenergic innervation. These authors suggest that the adrenergic nerves of the lung protect against pulmonary hypertension. Whether the proposed protection would stem from alpha or beta agonists is not clear. These observations have to be reconciled with others, e.g., that the presumed inhibition of alpha-adrenergic tone protects against pulmonary hypertension from embolism (13). Moreover, the idea that locally released adrenaline is protective against pulmonary hypertension stands in contrast to the adverse effect of systemically administered beta-adrenergic agonists (6,64). It seems that further investigation into the role of the adrenergic nerves in chronic pulmonary hypertension is warranted.

Monocrotaline in the Rat

Since the discovery by Lalich that monocrotaline induces inflammation in pulmonary vessels and that the process leads to pulmonary hypertension in the rat (21), the monocrotaline-treated rat has been used extensively as an animal model of pulmonary hypertension. Although it is not entirely clear which human disease is being mimicked, investigators consider that the mechanisms involved in the pathogenesis of pulmonary hypertension after monocrotaline administration may provide insights into factors that may cause chronic pulmonary hypertension in general.

After administration of monocrotaline, endothelial cell damage accompanied by vascular leak may be present at 24 hr and is clearly manifest by 2 to 3 days (56). Then follows a complex series of events involving inflammatory cells, chemical mediators of inflammation, and vasoactive substances (51), the net result of which is severe pulmonary hypertension that leads to death in 3 to 4 weeks. In the immediate postnatal period, the inflammatory process seems to be directed at alveoli leading to fatal retardation of alveolar development (59). After 4 weeks

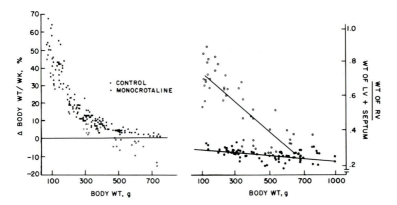

Figure 5: Effects of monocrotaline on growth. *Left:* Rate of decreases with age in control and monocrotaline-treated rats. *Right:* Hypertrophy of the right ventricle following mono-crotaline is more severe in young, rapidly growing rats, than in older, slower growing rats. (Modified after Sugita et al. [45].)

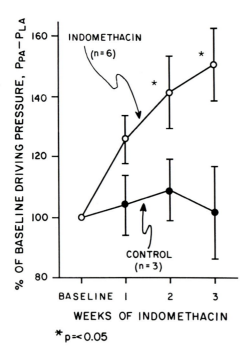

Figure 6: Effect of indomethacin on driving pressure. Repeated injections of indomethacin increase driving pressure ($P_{PA} - P_{LA}$) for pulmonary blood flow. Data presented as mean $\pm$ S.D. (Modified after Meyrick et al. [37].)

of age, monocrotaline causes pulmonary hypertension, the severity of which decreases as the rats grow older. Indeed, young rats which are rapidly growing develop severe pulmonary hypertension, whereas very old and slow growing rats may develop no pulmonary hypertension at all (Fig. 5) (57).

Although it has been proposed that inflammatory cells and/or their products of the inflammatory process are involved in the pathogenesis of monocrotaline pulmonary hypertension, this idea has not yet been substantiated (54). In favor of this hypothesis is an inhibitory effect of methylprednisolone (27) or dexamethasone (16), and blunting of the process by platelet depletion (51); the latter deserves further study, because neither inhibition of thromboxane release (51) nor of platelet-derived growth factor by heparin (5) seems to inhibit the monocrotaline effects.

The role of the neutrophil is not clear either: neutropenia induced by whole body radiation seems to enhance, rather than to blunt, the effects of monocrotaline (57); however, monocytes which are not depleted by radiation could play a role in the pathogenesis of the pulmonary hypertension (57). Chronic thoracic radiation has been used to cause mild pulmonary hypertension. This effect is presumably mediated by way of the release of oxygen radicals that damage the vessels (47). A pathogenetic sequence has been proposed to account for the pulmonary vascular changes in the monocrotaline rat model; this sequence entails leakage of pulmonary vessels, inflammation, and thickening of the media (36).

Other Inflammatory Agents

Although other methods of inducing chronic inflammation have been used to induce pulmonary hypertension, none have elicited pressures as high as those in the monocrotaline rat model. Repeated administration of carrageenan to the rat (12) or endotoxin to the sheep (34,35) induces mild chronic pulmonary hypertension. In the rat, endotoxin produces alveolar and vascular injury without pulmonary hypertension (19). Oddly enough, repeated administration of indomethacin to sheep causes pulmonary arterial pressure and resistance to increase; inflammation appears to have a causal role in this process (Fig. 6) (37).

The results using monocrotaline in rats and using other inflammatory agents in other animals indicate that chronic pulmonary inflammation can cause pulmonary hypertension. Inflammation is associated with severe pulmonary hypertension in human cystic fibrosis and in bronchopulmonary dysplasia, and with less severe pulmonary hypertension in interstitial lung disease. Future work must settle whether information gained from the animal models of pulmonary inflammation can be applied to human disease.

Pulmonary Hypertension from Increased Hematocrit

Hematocrit is directly related to pulmonary arterial pressure and relatively independent of hypoxia (2). The polycythemia that develops spontaneously at high altitude in the Hilltop strain of rats (45) is inordinate as compared to that developed by the Madison strain (43). In both strains, exposure to hypoxia evokes polycythemia, pulmonary arterial hypertension, and right ventricular hypertrophy; the level of polycythemia, within and between strains, is directly related to the level of pulmonary hypertension and the degree of right ventricular hypertrophy. Therefore, the Hilltop strain develops inordinate levels not only of polycythemia but also of pulmonary arterial pressure. The mechanisms responsible for the excessive polycythemia and severe pulmonary hypertension in the Hilltop strain are unclear (15,44).

Pulmonary Hypertension Associated with Increased Growth Rate

Although vasoconstriction is an important element in the pathogenesis of chronic pulmonary hypertension, proliferation of cells and synthesis of matrix protein in vessel walls ultimately cause death. If so, animal models that shed light on the proliferative process may provide insight into a central problem of chronic pulmonary hypertension. For example, the sparing of older animals from the ravages of monocrotaline-induced (57) or altitude-induced (62) pulmonary hypertension may result from the low potential of older animals for proliferation. By the same token, marked sensitivity of newborn animals to hypoxic (50,53,55, 60,61) or monocrotaline-induced (57) pulmonary hypertension may result from a heightened potential for excessive growth.

Particularly interesting is the possible impact of excessive growth rate on induction of pulmonary hypertension in the avian species. Ascites, right heart hypertrophy, and failure have been described in fast growing chickens bred for meat production (20). Chickens may be among the most rapidly growing vertebrates on earth. For example, a chick weighing 37 g at hatch, may at 6 weeks exceed 3 kg in weight (46), an increase of almost 100-fold over initial weight. In broiler chickens, a syndrome of ascites that causes mortality at the moderate altitude of about 6,000 ft on the Transvaal in the Union of South Africa (18) also occurs in fast growers at sea level (20). Ascites was associated with hypertrophy of the right ventricle, raising the possibility that right heart failure is the cause of the accumulation of the abdominal fluid.

The question is, then, what is the cause of the right ventricular hypertrophy? Certain evidence suggests that hypoxemia may be responsible (46): hypoxemia is maximal at the time that mortality from the syndrome is maximal; the high hematocrit indicates that the hypoxemia is chronic; both the hypoxemia and the high hematocrit are associated with right ventricular hypertrophy. Moreover, the hypoxemia is associated with high values of arterial P_{CO_2}, suggesting that hypoventilation is at least partially responsible for the hypoxemia. Morphometric analysis of the lung microvasculature in rapidly growing turkeys raised the additional prospect that deficient diffusing surface area for oxygen might contribute to the hypoxemia (58). Thus, arterial hypoxemia in this model may be due to both poor ventilatory control and a low diffusing capacity of the lung.

The poor ventilatory control and the low capacity for diffusion may reflect impairment of postnatal development. In keeping with this concept, surviving individuals show improvement in gas exchange as growth rate is slowed by reducing the amount of feed available (46). Associated with the improvement in gas exchange is an associated decrease in mortality from the right ventricular failure. Accordingly, in some individuals, rapid growth may induce arterial hypoxemia which, in turn, acts as a stimulus for pulmonary hypertension. At the same time, the potential for proliferation provides the milieu for an enhanced response to the hypoxic stimulus. As a corollary, the chicken and the turkey provide models for studying the relation of growth factors to the development of chronic pulmonary hypertension. What is particularly remarkable about these models is that apparently fatal hypoxic pulmonary hypertension develops spontaneously at sea level—a unique feature among animal models of pulmonary hypertension.

CONCLUSION

Progress in understanding the mechanisms of chronic pulmonary hypertension depends on integration of whole animal studies with those at the organ, cellular, and subcellular levels (48). Although studies in intact man and animals provide relevant questions, studies at the more fundamental levels afford the prospect of insight into certain mechanisms that cannot be explored in animals or humans. Among these are stimuli that act, either directly or via intercellular communication, to prompt lung vascular cells to change from a resting to a proliferative mode. The number, versatility, and relevance of animal models of pulmonary hypertension have increased dramatically in the last few years. Our understanding of the pulmonary hypertensive process has improved correspondingly.

REFERENCES

1. Abman SH, Shanley PF, Accurso FJ: Chronic intrauterine pulmonary hypertension alters perinatal pulmonary vasoreactivity and structure. Pediatr Res. In Press.

2. Barer GR, Bee D, Wach RA: Contribution of polycythaemia to pulmonary hypertension in simulated high altitude rats. J Physiol 336 : 27–38, 1983.

3. Caldwell RW, Blatteis CM: Effect of chronic hypoxia on angiotensin-induced pulmonary vasoconstriction and converting enzyme activity in the rat. Proc Soc Exp Biol Med 172 : 346–350, 1983.

4. Dawes GS: *Foetal and Neonatal Physiology.* Chicago, Year Book Publishers, 1968.

5. Fasules JW, Stenmark KR, Henson PM, Voelkel NF, Reeves JT: Neither anticoagulant nor nonanticoagulant heparin affects monocrotaline lung injury. J Appl Physiol 62 : 816–820, 1987.

6. Fried R, Reid LM: The effect of isoproterenol on the development and recovery of hypoxic pulmonary hypertension. Am J Pathol 121 : 102–111, 1985.

7. Geggel RL, Aronovitz MJ, Reid LM: Effects of chronic in utero hypoxemia on rat neonatal pulmonary arterial structure. J Pediatr 108 : 756–759, 1986.

8. Goldberg SJ, Levy RA, Siassi B, Betten J: Effects of maternal hypoxia and hyperoxia upon the neonatal pulmonary vasculature. Pediatrics 48 : 528–533, 1971.

9. Hales CA, Kradin RL, Brandstetter RD, Zhu YJ: Impairment of hypoxic pulmonary artery remodeling by heparin in mice. Am Rev Respir Dis 128 : 747–751, 1983.

10. Herget J, Palecek F: Pulmonary arterial blood pressure in closed chest rats. Changes after catecholamines, histamine, and serotonin. Arch Int Pharmacodyn Ther 198 : 107–117, 1972.

11. Herget J, Palecek F: Experimental chronic pulmonary hypertension. Int Rev Exp Pathol 18 : 347–406, 1978.

12. Herget J, Palecek F, Preclik P, Cermakova M, Vizek M, Petrovicka M: Pulmonary hypertension induced by repeated pulmonary inflammation in the rat. J Appl Physiol 51 : 755–761, 1981.

13. Herget J, Suggett AJ, Palecek F, Slavik Z: Effect of alpha-methyldopa on lung microembolism in the rat. Bull Eur Physiopathol Respir 18 : 687–692, 1982.

14. Heymann MA, Hoffman JIC: Persistent pulmonary hypertension syndromes in the newborn, in Weir EK, Reeves JT (eds), *Pulmonary Hypertension.* Mount Kisco, NY, Futura, 1984.

15. Hill NS, Ou LC: The role of pulmonary vascular responses to chronic hypoxia in the development of chronic mountain sickness in rats. Respir Physiol 58 : 171–185, 1984.

16. Hilliker KS, Roth RA: Alteration of monocrotaline pyrrole-induced cardiopulmonary effects in rats by hydralazine, dexamethasone, and sulphinpyrazone. Br J Pharmacol 82 : 375–380, 1984.

17. Hislop A, Reid L: New findings in pulmonary arteries of rats with hypoxia-induced pulmonary hypertension. Br J Exp Pathol 57 : 542–554, 1976.

18. Huchzermeyer FW, DeRuyck AM: Pulmonary hypertension syndrome associated with ascites in broilers. Vet Rec 119 : 94, 1986.

19. Jones R, Kirton OC, Zapol WM, Reid L: Rat pulmonary artery wall injury by chronic intermittent infusions of *Escherichia coli* endotoxin. Lab Invest 54 : 282–294, 1986.

20. Julian RJ, Friars GW, French H, Quinton M: The relationship of right ventricular hypertrophy, right ventricular failure, and ascites to weight gain in broiler and roaster chickens. Avian Dis 31 : 130–135, 1987.

21. Kay JM, Heath D: *Crotalaria spectabilis. The pulmonary hypertension plant.* Springfield, IL, Thomas, 1968.

22. Kay JM, Keane PM, Suyama KL, Gauthier D: Lung angiotensin converting enzyme activity in chronically hypoxic rats. Thorax 40:587–591, 1985.

23. Kay JM, Suyama KL, Keane PM: Failure to show decrease in small pulmonary blood vessels in rats with experimental hypertension. Thorax 37:927–930, 1982.

24. Kentera D, Zdravkovic M, Rolovic Z, Susic D: Platelets in rats with chronic normobaric hypoxic pulmonary hypertension. Respiration 48:159–163, 1985.

25. Kerr JS, Riley DJ, Frank MM, Trelstad RL, Frankel HM: Reduction of chronic hypoxic pulmonary hypertension in the rat by β-aminopropionitrile. J Appl Physiol 57:1760–1766, 1984.

26. Kerr JS, Ruppert CL, Tozzi CA, Neubauer JA, Frankel HM, Yu SY, Riley DJ: Reduction of chronic hypoxic pulmonary hypertension in the rat by an inhibitor of collagen production. Am Rev Respir Dis 135:300–306, 1987.

27. Langleben D, Reid LM: Effect of methylprednisolone on monocrotaline-induced pulmonary vascular disease and right ventricular hypertrophy. Lab Invest 52:298–303, 1985.

28. Levin DL, Hyman AI, Heymann MA, Rudolph AM: Fetal hypertension and the development of increased pulmonary vascular smooth muscle: A possible mechanism for persistent pulmonary hypertension of the newborn infant. J Pediatr 92:265–269, 1978.

29. Levin DL, Mills LJ, Weinberg AG: Hemodynamic, pulmonary vascular, and myocardial abnormalities secondary to pharmacologic constriction of the fetal ductus arteriosus. A possible mechanism for persistent pulmonary hypertension and transient tricuspid insufficiency in the newborn infant. Circulation 60:360–364, 1979.

30. McKenzie JC, Hung KS, Mattioli L, Klein RM: Reduction in hypertension-induced protein synthesis in the rat pulmonary trunk after treatment with Teprotide (SQ 20881). Proc Soc Exp Biol Med 177:377–382, 1984.

31. McKenzie JC, Klein RM: Protein synthesis in the rat pulmonary trunk during the early development of hypoxia-induced pulmonary hypertension. Blood Vessels 20:283–294, 1983.

32. McLean JR, Twarog BM, Bergofsky EH: The adrenergic innervation of pulmonary vasculature in the normal and pulmonary hypertensive rat. J Auton Nerv Syst 14:111–123, 1985.

33. Mecham RP, Whitehouse LA, Wrenn DS, Parks WC, Griffin GL, Senior RW, Crouch EC, Stenmark KR, Voelkel NF: Smooth muscle-mediated connective tissue remodeling in pulmonary hypertension. Science 237:423–426, 1987.

34. Meyrick B, Brigham KL: Vasoconstriction and remodeling in pulmonary hypertension. Chest 88:268S–270S, 1985.

35. Meyrick B, Brigham KL: Repeated *Escherichia coli* endotoxin-induced pulmonary inflammation causes chronic pulmonary hypertension in sheep. Structural and functional changes. Lab Invest 55:164–176, 1986.

36. Meyrick B, Gamble W, Reid L: Development of *Crotalaria* pulmonary hypertension: hemodynamic and structural study. Am J Physiol 239:H692–H702, 1980.

37. Meyrick B, Niedermeyer ME, Ogletree ML, Brigham KL: Pulmonary hypertension and increased vasoreactivity caused by repeated indomethacin in sheep. J Appl Physiol 59:443–452, 1985.

38. Meyrick B, Reid L: The effect of continued hypoxia on rat pulmonary arterial circulation. An ultrastructural study. Lab Invest 38:188–200, 1978.

39. Meyrick B, Reid L: Hypoxia and incorporation of ^{3}H-thymidine by cells of the rat pulmonary arteries and alveolar wall. Am J Pathol 96:51–70, 1979.

40. Murphy JD, Aronovitz MJ, Reid LM: Effects of chronic in utero hypoxia on the pulmonary vasculature of the newborn guinea pig. Pediatr Res 20:292–295, 1986.

41. Olley PM, Bodach E, Heaton J, Coceani F: Further evidence implicating E-type prostaglandins in the patency of the lamb ductus arteriosus. Eur J Pharmacol 34:247–250, 1975.

42. Orton EC, Reeves JT, Stenmark KR: Pulmonary vasodilation in calves with severe pulmonary hypertension: In vivo and in vitro comparison. J Appl Physiol. In Press.

43. Ou LC, Cai YN, Tenney SM: Responses of blood volume and red cell mass in two strains of rats acclimatized to high altitude. Respir Physiol 62:85–94, 1985.

44. Ou LC, Hill NS, Tenney SM: Ventilatory responses and blood gases in susceptible and resistant rats to high altitude. Respir Physiol 58:161–170, 1984.

45. Ou LC, Smith RP: Probable strain differences in rats in susceptibilities and cardiopulmonary responses to chronic hypoxia. Respir Physiol 53:367–377, 1983.

46. Peacock AJ, Pickett C, Morris K, Reeves JT: Spontaneous pulmonary hypertension in fast growing broiler chickens reared at sea level. Submitted to J Appl Physiol.

47. Perkett EA, Brigham KL, Meyrick B: Increased vasoreactivity and chronic pulmonary hypertension following thoracic irradiation in sheep. J Appl Physiol 61:1875–1881, 1986.

48. Pulmonary Circulation and Pulmonary Hypertension: 30th Annual Aspen Lung Conference. Voelkel NF (ed). Chest 93:79S–188S, 1987.

49. Reeves JT, Herget J: Experimental models of pulmonary hypertension, in Weir EK, Reeves JT (eds), *Pulmonary Hypertension.* Mount Kisco, NY, Futura, 1984.

50. Reeves JT, Leathers JE: Postnatal development of pulmonary and bronchial arterial circulations in the calf and the effects of chronic hypoxia. Anat Rec 157: 641–656, 1967.

51. Roth RA, Ganey PE: Arachidonic acid metabolites and the mechanisms of monocrotaline pneumotoxicity. Am Rev Respir Dis 136: 762–765, 1987.

52. Sobin SS, Tremer HM, Hardy JD, Chiodi HP: Changes in arteriole in acute and chronic hypoxic pulmonary hypertension and recovery in rat. J Appl Physiol 55: 1445–1455, 1983.

53. Stenmark KR, Fasules J, Hyde DM, Voelkel NF, Henson J, Tucker A, Wilson H, Reeves JT: Severe pulmonary hypertension and arterial adventitial changes in newborn calves at 4300 m. J Appl Physiol 62: 821–830, 1987.

54. Stenmark KR, Morganroth ML, Remigio LK, Voelkel NF, Murphy RC, Henson PM, Mathias MM, Reeves JT: Alveolar inflammation and arachidonate metabolism in monocrotaline-induced pulmonary hypertension. Am J Physiol 248: H859–H866, 1985.

55. Stenmark KR, Orton EC, Reeves JT, Voelkel NF, Crouch EC, Parks WC, Mecham RP: Vascular remodeling in neonatal pulmonary hypertension: Role of the smooth muscle cell. Chest 93: 127S–132S, 1988.

56. Sugita T, Hyers TM, Dauber IM, Wagner WW, McMurtry IF, Reeves JT: Lung vessel leak precedes right ventricular hypertrophy in monocrotaline treated rats. J Appl Physiol 54: 371–374, 1983.

57. Sugita T, Stenmark KR, Wagner WW, Henson PM, Henson JE, Hyers TM, Reeves JT: Abnormal alveolar cells in monocrotaline-induced pulmonary hypertension. Exp Lung Res 5: 201–215, 1983.

58. Timmwood KI, Hyde DM, Plopper CG: Lung growth of the turkey, *Meleagris gallopavo:* II. Comparison of two genetic lines. Am J Anat 178: 158–169, 1987.

59. Todd L, Mullen M, Olley PM, Rabinovitch M: Pulmonary toxicity of monocrotaline differs at critical periods of lung development. Pediatr Res 19: 731–737, 1985.

60. Tucker A, Alberts MK, Wilke WL: Vascular reactivity in lungs isolated from rats exposed from birth to moderate altitude and/or lead. Fed Proc 46: 1091, 1987.

61. Tucker A, Anderson KK, Babyak SD, White WL: Pulmonary hypertension and increased pulmonary vascular reactivity in rats exposed at 10,000 ft since birth. Chest 93: 185S, 1988.

62. Tucker A, Greenlees KJ, Wright ML, Migally N: Altered vascular responsiveness in isolated perfused lungs from aging rats. Exp Lung Res 3: 29–35, 1982.

63. Voelkel NF, Wiegers U, Sill V, Trautman J: Kinetic study on the lung DNA-synthesis stimulated by chronic high altitude hypoxia. Thorax 32: 578, 1978.

64. Winter R, Collins C, Ruddock PE, Rudd RM: The effect of systemic beta-2-adrenergic agonist therapy on the pulmonary hypertensive response to chronic hypoxia in rats. Am Rev Respir Dis 134: 763–767, 1986.

William D. Edwards, M.D.

23 _____

The Pathology of Secondary Pulmonary Hypertension

Chronic secondary pulmonary hypertension encompasses a spectrum of disorders, and its morphology is as varied as its causes. Vascular alterations are widespread and include medial hypertrophy, a variety of obstructive intimal lesions, and luminal thrombosis. Some lesions are common to all forms of pulmonary hypertension, and others are limited only to specific forms. Certain combinations of lesions tend to occur together, however, and form characteristic microscopic patterns that correspond to specific underlying causes.

GENERAL FEATURES

Pulmonary Manifestations

Medial hypertrophy of muscular pulmonary arteries is a constant feature of all forms of chronic pulmonary hypertension (2) (Fig. 1). It is thought to represent the morphological counterpart of chronic vasoconstriction and tends to be most severe in venous and plexogenic forms of pulmonary hypertension and least severe in embolic and hypoxic forms. Medial hypertrophy also occurs in the elastic pulmonary arteries but may be masked by arterial dilatation (Fig. 1). Muscularization of arterioles is frequently observed but tends to correlate better with increased pulmonary blood flow than with pressure.

Obstructive intimal lesions, also a feature of many forms of pulmonary hypertension, are related to proliferations of smooth muscle cells and by myofibroblasts

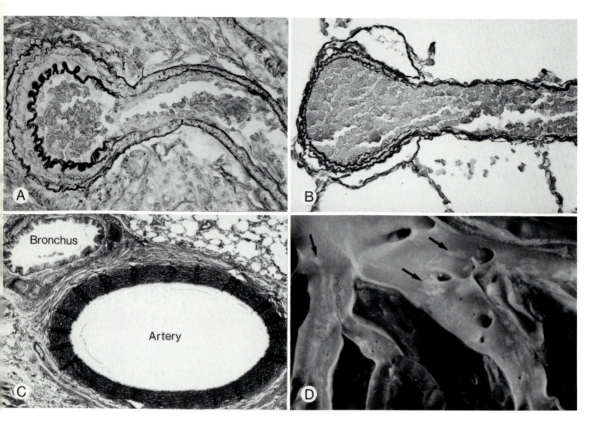

Figure 1: Pulmonary manifestations of chronic pulmonary hypertension.
A. Medial hypertrophy of muscular pulmonary artery and muscularization of arteriole.
B. Normal muscular pulmonary artery and arteriolar branch, for comparison with (A).
C. Dilatation and medial hypertrophy of elastic pulmonary artery. Normally, diameters of artery and adjacent bronchus should be similar.
D. Shallow atheromas (arrows) of large elastic pulmonary arteries.
(A to C, Elastic-van Gieson; A and B, X360; C, X36.) (A, C, and D, from Fuster V, McGoon MD, Dines DE, Edwards WD: Pulmonary hypertension [with specific reference to primary pulmonary hypertension], in Brandenburg RO, Fuster V, Guiliani ER, McGoon DC [eds], *Cardiology: Fundamentals and Practice.* Chicago, Year Book Medical Publishers, 1987, pp 1811–1829.) (B, from Edwards [2].)

that presumably are derived from the media. Several different forms of intimal proliferation are recognized and serve as distinguishing features among the various histopathologic types of pulmonary hypertension.

Chronic dilatation of hypertensive arteries may result in compression of the left main and right intermediate bronchi and thereby lead to recurrent obstructive pneumonias, especially in children with compliant bronchi. In mitral stenosis with chronic pulmonary venous hypertension, entrapment of the left bronchus between the distended left atrium, below, and the dilated left pulmonary artery, above, produces a so-called hemodynamic vise that not only elevates the bronchus but also compresses it. Rightward displacement of the aortic arch by the dilated pulmonary artery may also lead to compression of the left recurrent laryngeal

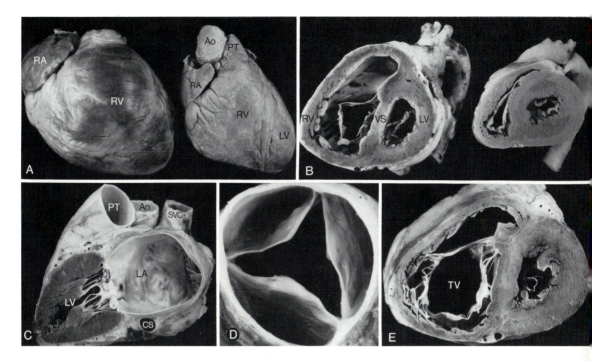

Figure 2: Cardiac manifestations of chronic pulmonary hypertension.

a. Right ventricular (RV) hypertrophy and dilatation and right atrial (RA) dilatation. Normal heart at right is for comparison. Ao = aorta; LV = left ventricle; PT = pulmonary trunk.

B. Marked right ventricular hypertrophy and dilatation with straightening of ventricular septum (VS) and resulting D-shaped ventricular chambers. Normal heart at right is for comparison. Perfusion-fixed specimens are dissected tomographically to simulate echocardiographic short-axis view.

C. Dilatation of pulmonary trunk and coronary sinus (CS). Left-sided two-chamber view of heart from patient with rheumatic mitral stenosis, left atrial (LA) dilatation, and chronic pulmonary venous hypertension. SVC = superior vena cava.

D. Pulmonary insufficiency due to dilatation of pulmonary trunk and valve annulus.

E. Tricuspid regurgitation due to dilatation of right ventricle and valve annulus. TV = tricuspid valve.

(A, from Edwards [2].) (B to D, from Edwards WD: Applied anatomy of the heart, in Brandenburg RO, Fuster V, Giuliani ER, McGoon DC [eds], *Cardiology: Fundamentals and Practice*. Chicago, Year Book Medical Publishers, 1987, pp 47–112.)

nerve, between the aorta and the trachea, and thereby produce hoarseness in some patients.

As in the systemic circulation, chronic hypertension in the pulmonary vascular bed is also attended by the development of atherosclerosis (Fig. 1). Only the elastic pulmonary arteries are involved, and the intimal plaques are characteristically shallow and nonobstructive.

Cardiac Manifestations

Right ventricular hypertrophy is a constant feature of chronic pulmonary hypertension (2) (Fig. 2). With time, dilatation of the right ventricular chamber occurs,

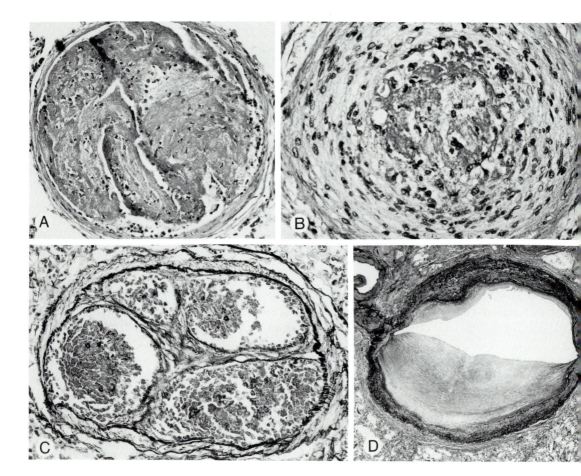

Figure 3: Microscopic features of thromboembolic pulmonary hypertension.
A. Recent occlusive thrombus.
B. Organizing occlusive thrombus.
C. Old organized and recanalized thrombus with luminal fibrous webs.
D. Old organized thrombus with resulting eccentric intimal fibrosis.
(A and B, Hematoxylin-eosin; C and D, Elastic-van Gieson; A, X180; B, X360; C, X240; D, X18.) (C and D, from Edwards [2].)

particularly along the outflow tract, and results in obliteration of the retrosternal space. Abnormal motion and geometric straightening of the ventricular septum also tend to occur as the right ventricle dilates (Fig. 2). The resulting changes in ventricular shapes coupled with hypoxemia may explain, in part, the *left* ventricular dysfunction that occurs in some patients with chronic pulmonary hypertension.

Microscopically, myocytes are hypertrophied and exhibit increased cell diameters and enlarged hyperchromatic nuclei. In dilated hearts, attenuation (stretching) of myocytes also occurs. Interstitial fibrosis of various degrees of severity is commonly observed and, in conjunction with myocyte hypertrophy, forms the morphologic substrate for decreased right ventricular compliance.

In chronic pulmonary hypertension, the pulmonary valve cusps become thickened, and dilatation of the pulmonary trunk may lead to valvular incompetence (Fig. 2). Similarly, right ventricular dilatation is commonly associated with dilatation of the tricuspid valve annulus and the production of tricuspid regurgitation (Fig. 2).

Dilatation of the right atrium may be associated with aneurysmal leftward bowing of the valve of the fossa ovalis or with left-to-right shunting across a patent foramen ovale. Dilatation of the venae cavae and their tributaries is associated with jugular venous distention and congestive hepatosplenomegaly. The coronary sinus is also dilated.

PRECAPILLARY OBSTRUCTION

Embolic Pulmonary Arteriopathy

Elevated pulmonary vascular resistance may develop because of arterial obstruction by embolic material. Recurrent thromboemboli from the leg veins or pelvic venous plexus account for most of the cases. Rarely, however, emboli arise from thrombi within the right atrium or along ventriculoarterial shunt catheters (for hydrocephalus) or from nonthrombotic sources (2).

RECURRENT THROMBOEMBOLI

Some patients experience typical episodes of pulmonary embolism, with acute dyspnea and chest pain, with or without hemorrhagic pulmonary infarction. Emboli are relatively large and, therefore, readily detected by ventilation-perfusion scan or by pulmonary angiography. In contrast, patients who experience only recurrent small thromboemboli and progressive dyspnea may be given the clinical diagnosis of primary pulmonary hypertension (1,16). Moreover, mediastinal fibrosis of adenopathy can cause appreciable compression of adjacent pulmonary arteries and veins and, thereby, mimic thromboembolic disease (2) (see Chapter 30).

Grossly, elastic pulmonary arteries may be focally obstructed by recent thromboemboli and by old fibrous or fibrocalcific lesions. Fibrous webs or bands created by organized and partially lysed thromboemboli are also commonly observed (Fig. 3). Microscopically, elastic and muscular pulmonary arteries harbor thromboemboli of various ages and stages of organization (Fig. 3). Luminal obstruction is responsible for increased pulmonary arterial resistance, and medial hypertrophy occurs as a secondary response. Plexiform lesions are not observed, and pulmonary veins and capillaries are not appreciably altered.

NONTHROMBOTIC EMBOLI

Rarely, neoplastic emboli, most commonly from the breast or lung, obstruct sufficient portions of the pulmonary arterial bed to cause elevated vascular resistance. Other rare forms of emboli that may produce pulmonary hypertension are ova in pulmonary schistosomiasis, talc in intravenous drug abuse, and hydatid cysts in echinococcosis (2).

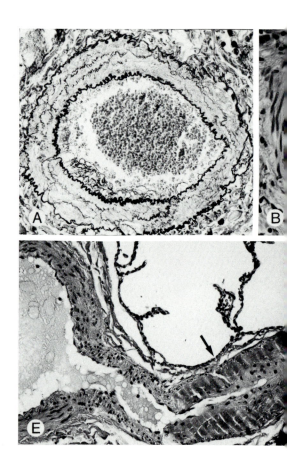

Plexogenic Pulmonary Arteriopathy

Plexogenic pulmonary arteriopathy is a form of pulmonary hypertension that may exist as a primary disorder or may be secondary to congenital cardiac shunts, portal hypertension, or the drug aminorex fumarate. Microscopically, it is characterized by a variety of pulmonary arterial lesions, one of which is the plexiform lesion. Because of the diversity of the observed lesions, some investigators consider the term "plexogenic arteriopathy" to be too confining and potentially misleading.

CONGENITAL CARDIAC SHUNTS

Plexogenic pulmonary arteriopathy occurs in patients with a ventricular septal defect (without pulmonary stenosis), a patent ductus arteriosus, or rarely, an atrial septal defect. In patients with complete transposition of the great arteries or truncus arteriosus, hypertensive pulmonary vascular disease tends to develop earlier than in those with an isolated ventricular septal defect (2). Among patients with a complete atrioventricular canal defect, pulmonary vascular disease may develop earlier in those with Down's syndrome, although some investigators disagree.

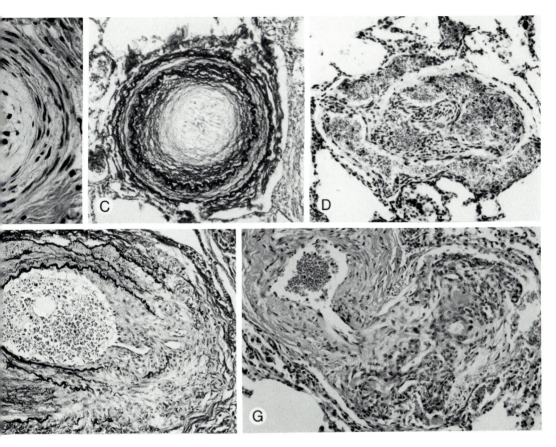

Figure 4: Microscopic features of plexogenic pulmonary arteriopathy.
A. Medial hypertrophy of muscular pulmonary artery.
B. Concentric intimal proliferation.
C. Concentric laminar intimal fibroelastosis.
D. Dilatation lesion.
E. Fibrinoid degeneration (arrow).
F. Healing arteritis (right lower quadrant of artery).
G. Plexiform lesion (compare with [E] and [F], precursors of plexiform lesions).
(A, C, and F, Elastic-van Gieson; B, D, E, and G, Hematoxylin-eosin; A, C to G, X180; B, X360.) (B, C, and G, from Fuster V, McGoon MD, Dines DE, Edwards WD: Pulmonary hypertension [with specific reference to primary pulmonary hypertension], in Brandenburg RO, Fuster V, Giuliani ER, McGoon DC [eds], *Cardiology: Fundamentals and Practice.* Chicago, Year Book Publishers, 1987, pp 1811–1829.) (E, from Edwards [2].) (F, from Bjornsson, Edwards [1].)

The various histopathological lesions tend to develop in a typical order, as described by Heath and Edwards (4) and later modified by Wagenvoort (13). Accordingly, the spectrum of observed lesions may have prognostic importance in lung biopsy specimens. Medial hypertrophy and muscularization of arterioles is the initial abnormality (grade 1) and is thought to reflect a state of chronic vasoconstriction (Fig. 4).

More recently, investigators have divided the grade 1 lesions into three types:

peripheral extension of smooth muscle (grade A), medial hypertrophy (grade B), and loss of distal arteries and arterioles (grade C) (6,11). Other investigators, however, have proposed that grade C lesions may represent an artifact of perfusion-fixation (9,10).

Additional pulmonary arterial lesions (Fig. 4), listed in order of development, are concentric intimal proliferation (grade 2), concentric laminar intimal fibrosis (grade 3), fibrinoid degeneration and necrotizing arteritis (grade 6), plexiform lesions (grade 4), and dilatation lesions (grade 5). Thrombosis and eccentric fibrosis are also commonly observed and may contribute to arterial obstruction.

Plexiform lesions generally involve small muscular pulmonary arteries near their origins from larger parent vessels. They are characterized by a proliferative tuft of intimal cells and capillary channels within a dilated arterial segment that is involved by focal medial disruption. The intimal proliferation represents smooth muscle cells, myofibroblasts, and fibrillary cells (vasoformative reserve cells). Platelet-fibrin thrombi are commonly observed within plexiform lesions and may be phagocytosed by the fibrillary cells.

The distinction between plexiform lesions and organized thrombi may be difficult in some cases (2). Organized thrombi, however, tend to involve arteries of various sizes and to be unassociated with medial disruption or aneurysmal dilatation. Moreover, plexiform lesions are generally more cellular than organized thrombi, although older lesions may become less cellular and even fibrotic.

The diversity of vascular lesions in plexogenic arteriopathy suggests the need for a semiquantitative descriptive diagnosis rather than the use of a single grade. In general, however, grades 1 and 2 lesions are potentially reversible, and grade 3 lesions are borderline. Grades 4 through 6 lesions, in contrast, indicate an extensively and irreversibly obstructed pulmonary arterial bed with a high fixed pulmonary vascular resistance. It is emphasized that the *numerical* Heath-Edwards grades are reserved *only* for the evaluation of hypertensive pulmonary vascular disease associated with congenital cardiac shunts.

PORTAL HYPERTENSION

Among patients with portal hypertension due to either cirrhosis or portal vein thrombosis, there is a group in whom pulmonary hypertension coexists. Their muscular pulmonary arteries are characterized by various combinations of plexogenic, thrombotic, and fibrotic lesions (3) (see Chapter 26).

AMINOREX FUMARATE

Between 1967 and 1972, an epidemic of pulmonary hypertension associated with the use of the appetite suppressant aminorex fumarate was reported in Switzerland, West Germany, and Austria. Although aminorex resulted in plexogenic pulmonary arteriopathy in humans, it has not produced similar hypertensive lesions in experimental animals (8) (see Chapter 29).

Hypoxic Pulmonary Vasculopathy

In humans, chronic alveolar hypoxia is a potent pulmonary vasoconstrictor and has numerous causes, the most common of which is chronic bronchitis. Secondary polycythemia, as well as acidosis, may contribute to the elevated pulmonary vascular resistance. In destructive disorders such as emphysema, the loss of regional capillary beds may also contribute to the hypertensive state (see Chapter 20).

As a result of chronic vasoconstriction, medial hypertrophy is characteristically observed in the muscular pulmonary arteries and small veins (12,17). Moreover, longitudinal muscle bundles may develop in the media, intima, and adventitia of pulmonary arteries and in the media of veins. Eccentric intimal fibrosis of arteries and muscularization of arterioles may also be encountered microscopically. Plexiform lesions are not observed. Bronchial arteries and veins commonly become dilated and tortuous, and arterial bronchopulmonary anastomoses are prominent, particularly in patients with bronchiectasis.

Fibrosing Pulmonary Vasculopathy

Pulmonary hypertension may develop in patients with various chronic fibrosing disorders of the lung, including interstitial pulmonary fibrosis and collagen vascular diseases. In most cases, vascular lesions are considered to be the result of parenchymal fibrosis and chronic alveolar hypoxia, and in situ thrombosis commonly occurs as a secondary process. Moreover, in scleroderma, for example, obstructive vascular lesions may develop even in patients without appreciable pulmonary fibrosis (20) (see Chapter 25).

Microscopically, the small pulmonary arteries and veins are the site of medial hypertrophy, eccentric intimal proliferation and fibrosis, focal organized and recanalized thrombi, and occlusive fibrotic plugs. In areas of dense parenchymal fibrosis, capillary beds may be obliterated. However, plexiform lesions do not develop. Bronchial vessels and arterial bronchopulmonary anastomoses are commonly dilated.

Dietary Pulmonary Vasculopathy

Ingested substances, either in native form or as metabolites, may affect the pulmonary circulation adversely. However, there is considerable interspecies and intraspecies variability in the responsiveness to vasoactive agents. Accordingly, substances that produce pulmonary hypertension in some subjects may not do so in others or in experimental animals.

TOXIC OIL SYNDROME

In Spain during 1981 and 1982, the illegal use of denatured rapeseed oil as a cooking substitute for olive oil resulted in the toxic oil syndrome. Pulmonary hypertension was a late manifestation in some subjects. By light microscopy, muscular pulmonary arteries were involved by medial hypertrophy, focal medial degeneration or destruction, eccentric intimal proliferation that was often highly obstructive, and adventitial lymphoplasmacytic cuffing (7). However, plexiform lesions were not observed. Arterioles were muscularized, and veins were the site of eccentric intimal proliferation and fibrosis (see Chapter 28).

PYRROLIZIDINE ALKALOIDS

Monocrotaline and fulvine cause pulmonary hypertension in various laboratory animals but not in humans (5). Jamaican bush-tea, which contains pyrrolizidine alkaloids, may produce *hepatic* veno-occlusive disease and cirrhosis in humans but has not been associated with *pulmonary* hypertension (see Chapter 22).

POSTCAPILLARY OBSTRUCTION

Thrombotic Pulmonary Venopathy

Pulmonary veno-occlusive disease is a rare disorder of unknown cause. It is characterized by progressive dyspnea and may be diagnosed as primary pulmonary hypertension (1,16). However, it is *not* related to *hepatic* veno-occlusive disease (see Chapter 24).

Organized and recanalized thrombi in the pulmonary venules and veins constitute the histopathologic hallmark of pulmonary veno-occlusive disease (18) (Fig. 5). Eccentric intimal fibrosis is also interpreted as organized mural thrombus. In addition, pulmonary veins are the site of medial hypertrophy and so-called arterialization (acquisition of a distinct external elastic lamina). Fresh thrombus and venous inflammation are rarely encountered.

A variety of microcirculatory lesions develop as a result of postcapillary obstruction. They include capillary congestion, interstitial and pleural edema, dilatation of interstitial and pleural lymphatics, and alveolar clusters of siderophages. These lesions are also observed in chronic pulmonary venous hypertension (Fig. 6). Pulmonary arteries are involved by medial hypertrophy, and small arteries may also exhibit eccentric intimal fibrosis and organized thrombi, similar to those observed in the pulmonary veins (19). Plexiform lesions, however, are not observed.

Congestive Pulmonary Vasculopathy

Obstruction distal to the pulmonary veins is the most common cause of pulmonary hypertension and may result from mitral or aortic valve disease, left ventricular hypertrophy or dysfunction, or other causes (2). Chronic pulmonary venous hypertension is associated with engorgement of the entire pulmonary circulation, which may affect pulmonary function, and produces secondary changes throughout the pulmonary vascular bed (14). Although the hypertensive lesions are reversible once the cause of obstruction is eliminated, their regression may take months to years.

Microscopically, veins and venules are the site of medial hypertrophy, arterialization, dilatation, and eccentric intimal fibrosis (Fig. 6). The pulmonary microcirculation is involved by capillary congestion, edema of interlobular septa and pleurae, dilatation of interstitial and pleural lymphatics, and alveolar hemosiderosis. Medial hypertrophy of muscular pulmonary arteries may be quite striking, and muscularization of arterioles is commonly observed. Intimal fibrosis is also a frequent finding and is thought to represent organized in situ stasis thrombosis

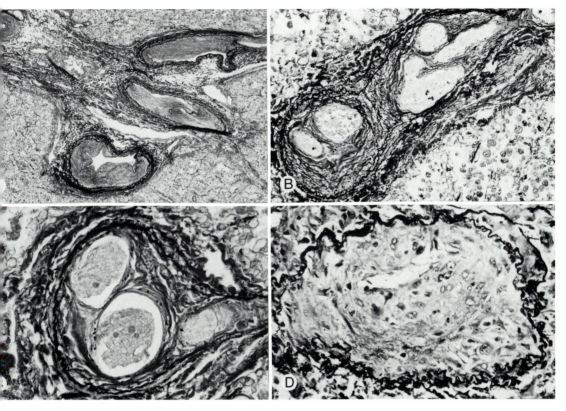

Figure 5: Microscopic features of pulmonary veno-occlusive disease.
 A. Obstructive eccentric intimal fibrosis of pulmonary veins.
B and C. Old organized and recanalized thrombi of pulmonary veins.
 D. Severely obstructive intimal proliferation with early recanalization channels in small pulmonary vein.
(A, Elastic-van Gieson, X45; B, X180; C and D, X360.) (A, B, and D, from Edwards [2].) (C, rom Edwards WD, Edwards JE: Recent advances in the pathology of the pulmonary vasculature. Monogr Pathol 19:235–261, 1978.)

within arterial segments. Plexiform lesions, however, are not a feature of chronic pulmonary venous hypertension, regardless of its duration or severity. Dilatation of muscular and elastic arteries may be prominent.

COEXISTENT FORMS

In certain instances, two different forms of pulmonary hypertension may coexist in the same patient. A subject with chronic heart failure and chronic bronchitis, for example, may have lesions of both the venous and the hypoxic forms of pulmonary hypertension. Moreover, a patient with mitral stenosis and chronic pulmonary venous hypertension may, because of limited activity and sluggish blood

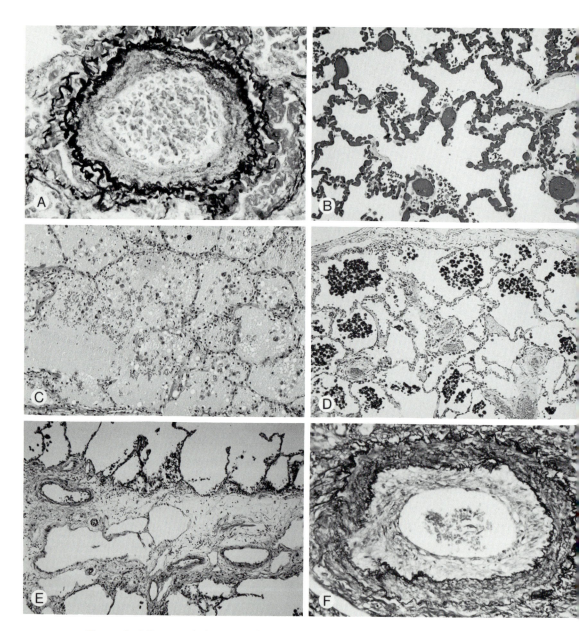

Figure 6: Microscopic features of chronic pulmonary venous hypertension.
A. Eccentric intimal fibrosis of pulmonary vein.
B. Dilatation and engorgement of alveolar capillaries.
C. Hemorrhagic alveolar edema.
D. Alveolar clusters of hemosiderin-laden macrophages.
E. Edema of interlobular septum and dilatation of septal lymphatics.
F. Medial hypertrophy and intimal fibrosis of pulmonary artery.
(A and F, Elastic-van Gieson; B to E, Hematoxylin-eosin; A, X360; B and F, X180; C to E, X90.) (A to C, E, from Edwards [2].) (D, from Fuster V, McGoon MD, Dines DE, Edwards WD: Pulmonary hypertension [with specific reference to primary pulmonary hypertension], in Brandenburg RO, Fuster V, Giuliani ER, McGoon DC [eds], *Cardiology: Fundamentals and Practice.* Chicago, Year Book Publishers, 1987, pp 1811–1829.)

flow, develop systemic venous thrombosis and thromboembolic pulmonary hypertension. As another example, if chronic heart failure develops in a patient with a ventricular septal defect, the lesions of chronic pulmonary venous hypertension may coexist with those of plexogenic pulmonary arteriopathy.

OPEN LUNG BIOPSY

The evaluation of hypertensive pulmonary vascular disease by open lung biopsy is usually performed in two abnormal states: congenital heart disease and primary pulmonary hypertension (15). If the disease process is not uniformly distributed, biopsies of both lungs or of upper and lower lobes may be necessary. After formalin fixation in a distended state, the biopsy tissue is sectioned so that the arteries and their adjacent bronchi are cut in cross section. Slides are prepared from several levels in the paraffin block and are stained with both hematoxylin-eosin and elastic-van Gieson.

For patients with congenital cardiac shunts, the various lesions of plexogenic arteriopathy should be described both qualitatively and semiquantitatively. Moreover, if left-sided valvular disease or heart failure is present, the lesions of pulmonary venous hypertension may also be observed. The Heath-Edwards grading system is appropriate for the evaluation of plexogenic disease but *not* for venous hypertensive lesions.

Patients with only a single functional ventricle (e.g., tricuspid atresia or double-inlet left ventricle) may undergo the Fontan operation, in which the right atrium is anastomosed directly to the pulmonary arteries. Postoperatively, pulmonary blood flow is maintained primarily by the respiratory bellows-action of the thoracic cage and, to a lesser degree, by right atrial contractions. Accordingly, even only moderate degrees of medial hypertrophy or intimal fibrosis may be associated with pulmonary resistances high enough to produce life-threatening obstruction to pulmonary blood flow. Moreover, right atrial mural thrombus may be a source of recurrent pulmonary embolization.

REFERENCES

1. Bjornsson J, Edwards WD: Primary pulmonary hypertension: a histopathologic study of 80 cases. Mayo Clin Proc 60 : 16–25, 1985.

2. Edwards WD: Pathology of pulmonary hypertension. Cardiovasc Clin 18 : 321–359, 1988.

3. Edwards BS, Weir EK, Edwards WD, Ludwig J, Dykowski RK, Edwards JE: Coexistent pulmonary and portal hypertension: Morphologic and clinical features. J Am Coll Cardiol 10 : 1233–1238, 1987.

4. Heath D, Edwards JE: The pathology of hypertensive pulmonary vascular disease: a description of six grades of structural changes in the pulmonary arteries with special reference to congenital cardiac septal defects. Circulation 18 : 533–547, 1958.

5. Heath D, Kay JM: Diet, drugs, and pulmonary hypertension. Prog Cardiol 7 : 125–140, 1978.

6. Hislop A, Haworth SG, Shinebourne EA, Reid L: Quantitative structural analysis of pulmonary vessels in isolated ventricular septal defect in infancy. Br Heart J 37 : 1014–1021, 1975.

7. Kay JM, Heath D: Pathologic study of unexplained pulmonary hypertension. Semin Respir Med 7 : 180–192, 1985.

8. Kay JM, Smith P, Heath D: Aminorex and the pulmonary circulation. Thorax 26 : 262–270, 1971.

9. Kay JM, Suyama KL, Keane PM: Failure to show decrease in small pulmonary blood vessels in rats with experimental pulmonary hypertension. Thorax 37 : 927–930 1982.

10. Mooi W, Wagenvoort CA: Decreased numbers of pulmonary blood vessels: reality or artifact? J Pathol 141 : 441–447, 1983.

11. Rabinovitch M, Reid LM: Quantitative structural analysis of the pulmonary vascular bed in congenital heart defects. Cardiovasc Clin 11 : 149–169, 1980.

12. Shelton DM, Keal E, Reid L: The pulmonary circulation in chronic bronchitis and emphysema. Chest 71 : 303–306, 1977.

13. Wagenvoort CA: Hypertensive pulmonary vascular disease complicating congenital heart disease: a review. Cardiovasc Clin 5 : 43–60, 1973.

14. Wagenvoort CA: Pathology of congestive pulmonary hypertension. Prog Respir Res 9 : 195–202, 1975.

15. Wagenvoort CA: Open lung biopsies in congenital heart disease for evaluation of pulmonary vascular disease: predictive value with regard to corrective operability. Histopathology 9 : 417–436, 1985.

16. Wagenvoort CA, Wagenvoort N: Primary pulmonary hypertension: a pathologic study of the lung vessels in 156 clinically diagnosed cases. Circulation 42 : 1163–1184, 1970.

17. Wagenvoort CA, Wagenvoort N: Hypoxic pulmonary vascular lesions in man at high altitude and in patients with chronic respiratory disease. Pathol Microbiol (Basel) 39 : 276–282, 1973.

18. Wagenvoort CA, Wagenvoort N: The pathology of pulmonary veno-occlusive disease. Virchows Arch [A] 364 : 69–79, 1974.

19. Wagenvoort CA, Wagenvoort N, Takahashi T: Pulmonary veno-occlusive disease: involvement of pulmonary arteries and review of the literature. Hum Pathol 16 : 1033–1041, 1985.

20. Young RH, Mark GJ: Pulmonary vascular changes in scleroderma. Am J Med 64 : 998–1004, 1978.

C.A. Wagenvoort, M.D.

24

Pulmonary Veno-Occlusive Disease

Pulmonary veno-occlusive disease is an uncommon condition of unknown etiology that is likely to cause considerable diagnostic problems for the clinician and, occasionally, for the pathologist. The clinical signs and symptoms are those associated with pulmonary hypertension; the most striking and characteristic morphological alteration is obstruction of pulmonary veins by intimal fibrosis. Pulmonary veno-occlusive disease was originally described by Höra in 1934 (13) but remained exceedingly rare until the last 15 years when it was afforded more attention and was recognized with increasing frequency.

TERMINOLOGY

The term pulmonary veno-occlusive disease was first used by Heath et al. by analogy with veno-occlusive disease of the liver (12). Although it has become clear that the pulmonary arteries are often affected, suggesting that *vaso-occlusive* disease might be more appropriate (18), the designation is so well established that most investigators, pathologists, and clinicians prefer to retain it.

INCIDENCE, AGE, AND SEX

In 1972, only 11 cases could be traced in the literature (26); by 1985, the number had risen to 67, including some unpublished cases (30). Since then, the number has continued to increase. Although the major account for this increase is undoubtedly a greater awareness of the condition, not only by the clinician but also by the pathologist, an absolute increase in incidence cannot be discounted. There are no apparent geographic distinctions in the occurrence of the disease: pulmonary veno-occlusive disease has been reported from all parts of the world. The younger age groups are primarily affected, and the disease is rare in patients more than 50 years old. The oldest patient on record is 67 years (30). Occasionally, the disease occurs in infants, e.g., as young as 8 weeks (28) or even 9 days (16). In children, the ratio of boys to girls is equal whereas in adults, males are approximately twice as often affected as females (30).

CLINICAL DIAGNOSIS AND TREATMENT

In 1975, a committee of the World Health Organization listed pulmonary veno-occlusive disease as one of the three conditions usually responsible for unexplained pulmonary hypertension, the other two being silent recurrent thromboembolism and primary plexogenic arteriopathy (11). Pulmonary hypertension is a constant feature of veno-occlusive disease; clinical distinction between the pulmonary veno-occlusive disease and the other two categories of unexplained pulmonary hypertension may be exceedingly difficult.

The symptomatology includes progressive dyspnea on exertion, fatigue, cyanosis, hemoptysis, and syncope. In these respects, the symptoms do not differ from those in several other forms of severe pulmonary hypertension. The chest radiograph may reveal a diffuse reticular nodular pattern and the presence of Kerley B lines indicating interstitial edema; however, the left atrium is not dilated. Sometimes a pleural effusion is present. In several cases, the radiographic findings did enable the clinical diagnosis to be made or suspected (1,7,22). More often, the diagnosis is established by open lung biopsy.

Cardiac catheterization invariably reveals pulmonary arterial hypertension. However, the pulmonary wedge pressure can vary greatly: although it may be high, more often it is normal so that it is not a reliable indicator for the diagnosis.

Pulmonary veno-occlusive disease pursues an insidious course and usually the outcome is fatal. The duration of the disease, from first symptoms until death, usually ranges from 6 months to one year but is occasionally longer, i.e., for several years. Sudden death occurred in one infant (3).

Treatment is rarely successful. Anticoagulant therapy has been tried. However, since almost all vascular lesions are fibrotic, there is little chance that the process can be reversed; whether anticoagulation prevents further progression is unclear. Temporary improvement of the condition has been reported following treatment with hydralazine and azathioprine (5,21).

MORPHOLOGY

As the name implies, in pulmonary veno-occlusive disease the *pulmonary veins* are particularly affected. The most striking lesion is intimal fibrosis, involving medium-sized and large, but predominantly small, veins. On histological section, the number of veins involved in this process is often very high, in some instances constituting as much as 60 to 75 percent of all veins (25). The average degree of luminal obstruction of uninjected pulmonary veins varies greatly (30).

The intimal thickening usually consists of a loose, paucicellular connective tissue (Fig. 1) with few collagen fibers and without elastic fibers (29). The loose appearance of the intimal fibrosis is due to interstitial edema rather than to mucoid change since the alcian blue stain for mucopolysaccharides is usually negative. Sometimes the pulmonary venous intimal fibrosis is more compact and collagen-rich with occasional elastic fibers. In some patients, the latter type predominates; it is believed to represent an older stage of the disease.

Recanalization of the intimal fibrosis is a regular occurrence. It varies from small channels to large luminal spaces, which may become so wide that remnants of intimal fibrosis stand out between them as intravascular fibrous septa (Fig. 2). Occasionally, recanalization is excessive so that abundant channels, penetrating the vascular walls and the surrounding obstructed veins, mimic small angiomas (9) (Fig. 3). Recent thrombi are usually absent or scarce (30).

A regular finding in the pulmonary veins of patients with pulmonary veno-occlusive disease is arterialization of their walls (Fig. 4). This designation implies that the normally irregular elastic configuration of the venous wall is changed in such a way that distinct internal and external elastic laminae are formed, just as in a pulmonary artery. It is usually associated with hypertrophy of the venous media. Pulmonary phlebitis has been described but is rare.

Systemic veins are not affected in patients with pulmonary veno-occlusive disease. The only exception to this rule is the occasional involvement of small bronchial veins (29). However, involvement is due to extension of the process from the pulmonary veins by way of veno-venous anastomoses.

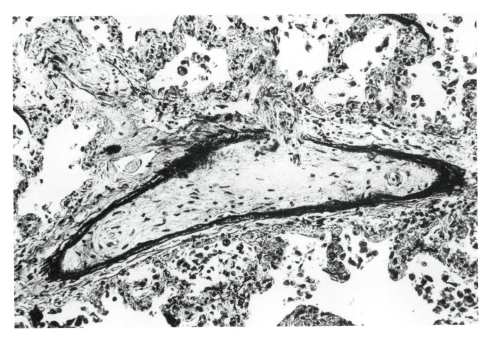

Figure 1: Pulmonary vein completely occluded by loose, paucicellular edematous intimal fibrosis. Elastic-van Gieson. X140.

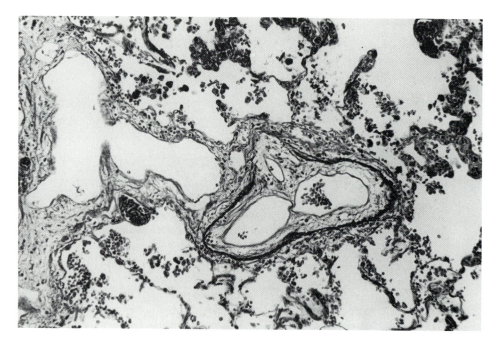

Figure 2: Pulmonary vein with intimal fibrosis. Recanalization channels are separated by intravascular septa. Elastic-van Gieson. X140.

The muscular *pulmonary arteries* in pulmonary veno-occlusive disease exhibit medial hypertrophy and intimal fibrosis to varying extent. Medial hypertrophy is particularly severe in infants and children. Intimal fibrosis of the arteries may be absent or mild; but, in approximately half of the cases, intimal fibrosis is prominent and similar in type to that affecting the pulmonary veins (Fig. 5). The often loose, paucicellular structure, the tendency to obliteration of the lumen, and the extensive recanalization of the intimal thickening are rather characteristic.

The intimal fibrosis in pulmonary veno-occlusive disease does not resemble that seen in patients with pulmonary venous hypertension caused by interference with pulmonary venous outflow: in mitral valve disease, for example, complete obstruction of the arterial lumen, as well as recanalization, are uncommon whereas in pulmonary veno-occlusive disease intravascular fibrous septa are often present. Sometimes pulmonary arteries, just like the pulmonary veins, undergo excessive recanalization resulting in angioma-like clusters of vessels outside of the arterial contour (30). One difference is that the arterial lesions occasionally suggest a more recent development than do those in the veins (25).

Recent thrombi, clearly recognizable as such despite early organization, are commonly observed in pulmonary arteries of patients with pulmonary veno-occlusive disease, even more often than in the veins (10,30). Arteritis or fibrinoid necrosis is rare; dilatation lesions or plexiform lesions have never been reported in this disease.

The *lung tissue* in pulmonary veno-occlusive disease often reveals characteristic changes, consisting of small foci of severe congestion and interstitial fibrosis

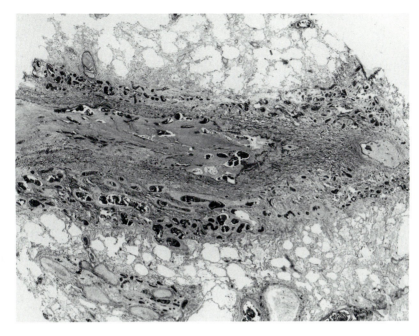

Figure 3: Large pulmonary vein, longitudinally cut and obstructed by intimal fibrosis. Multiple recanalization channels, within and outside the original venous wall, produce an angioma-like appearance. Hematoxylin-eosin. X7.

Figure 4: Small pulmonary vein with intimal fibrosis, medial hypertrophy, and arterialization, resembling a small artery. Elastic-van Gieson, X140.

Figure 5: Muscular pulmonary artery with prominent intimal fibrosis of a type similar to that in the veins. Elastic-van Gieson, X230.

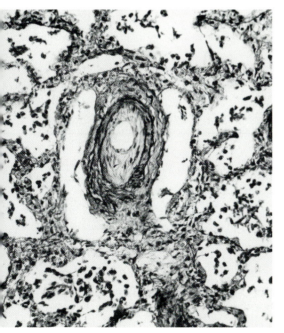

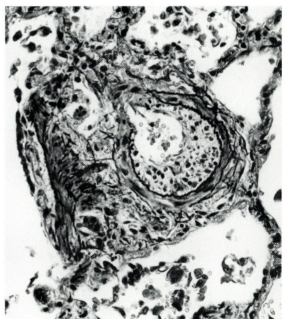

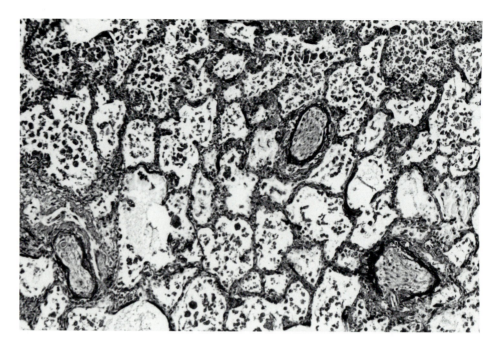

Figure 6: Lung tissue with congestion, interstitial fibrosis, and hemosiderosis, containing several occluded pulmonary veins. Elastic-van Gieson. X90.

(Fig. 6). Regularly, a number of small pulmonary veins in or around such areas are severely narrowed or obstructed. In some cases, the thickened alveolar walls contain some lymphocytes and plasma cells. Occasionally, these foci coalesce to form large areas of interstitial fibrosis.

Hemosiderosis is another characteristic alteration; it is rarely absent and sometimes very severe so that confusion with primary pulmonary hemosiderosis has occurred. Interstitial edema is a common feature, resulting in broad inter-lobular fibrous septa and a thickened pleura. The pulmonary lymphatics are markedly dilated. Hemorrhagic infarction of lung tissue has been reported but is not common. In some instances, hyperplasia of mucous glands within the bronchial walls respectively increased numbers of goblet cells within the epithelium of bronchi and bronchioli have been observed (29).

PATHOGENESIS

There is strong evidence that the process causing narrowing or occlusion of the lung vessels in pulmonary veno-occlusive disease is based on thrombosis; in keeping with this idea is the irregular and eccentric type of intimal thickening with its tendency to obliteration of the lumen and recanalization. Intravascular fibrous septa, very commonly found in pulmonary veins as well as in arteries of these patients, result from recanalization and are pathognomonic for a thrombotic origin.

It may be argued that recent thrombi are usually scarce or absent in the pulmonary veins. However, the transition by organization from fresh thrombi to fibrotic masses occurs within a few weeks. Thus, it is not surprising that thrombi are generally no longer recognizable as such by the time that lung tissue becomes available for study. Also, in patients with thromboembolic pulmonary hypertension, recent thrombi in pulmonary arteries are usually scarce or completely absent, although the thrombotic nature of the intimal plaques in these cases is not in doubt.

The loose, pale, paucicellular aspect of the intimal fibrosis has been interpreted as a myxoid change, unrelated to postthrombotic alterations (16). In our own experience, this appearance is not based upon a myxoid alteration, since the alcian-blue stain was consistently negative, but upon interstitial edema which is virtually always present throughout the lungs.

When pulmonary arteries are also affected in pulmonary veno-occlusive disease, they often contain recent thrombi. The other lesions also seem to have developed later than those in the veins. Moreover, it is possible that the endothelium of the pulmonary veins is more susceptible to noxious agents and thrombus formation than is that of the arteries. Therefore, it seems reasonable that the process starts in, and is often limited to, the pulmonary veins but that in some patients the pulmonary arteries may also become involved. Unfortunately, interest in examining the early lesions in vascular endothelium has been hampered by the unavailability of early stages for examination.

Although increased medial thickness of the muscular pulmonary arteries can be readily attributed to the increase in pulmonary arterial pressure, medial hypertrophy and arterialization of the pulmonary veins is more difficult to rationalize. It has been assumed that obstruction of larger veins evokes these alterations in the more proximal smaller veins. This possibility cannot be excluded because in some instances both large and small veins are involved. However, occasionally arterialization of the smaller pulmonary veins is prominent while the more distal larger veins are patent. In these instances, a primary injury to the venous wall may be involved (30).

The most common changes in the lung tissue, including interstitial edema, hemosiderosis, and various degrees of congestion and interstitial fibrosis, undoubtedly result from generalized pulmonary venous obstruction.

ETIOLOGY

The cause of pulmonary veno-occlusive disease is enigmatic. One reason for the failure to elucidate its etiology is that there is likely to be a variety of causes rather than a single one, so that it is a morphologic but not an etiological entity (27). In principle, any stimulus or agent that may elicit thrombosis within the lung vessels may be involved in its development. This, however, is more likely to be brought about by damage to the vascular wall, in particular to its endothelium, than by disturbances in the clotting mechanism which have never been conclusively demonstrated in these patients.

It has been suggested that respiratory infections, especially viral infections, are involved in the etiology of pulmonary veno-occlusive disease (6,15). Indeed, some patients with pulmonary veno-occlusive disease appear to have suffered attacks of acute respiratory disease in the early stages of the condition. It is, of course, uncertain that this implies a causal relationship, and it has even been suggested that the symptoms of the infection were the result rather than the cause of the vascular obliteration (3). However, the respiratory disorder almost always preceded the symptoms of pulmonary veno-occlusive disease by several weeks or months and subsided before the latter condition became evident. Moreover, the interstitial infiltration with lymphocytes and plasma cells and the hyperplasia of bronchial mucous glands and goblet cells in several cases, could well be consistent with a viral infection. The occasional association of pulmonary veno-occlusive disease with hyaline membranes in the lungs or with acute myocarditis (29), could also be interpreted in this way. Moreover, unilateral pulmonary veno-occlusive disease, an uncommon form of the disease, has also been suggested to be viral in origin (17,19).

Although the possibility of a viral factor in the etiology of the disease cannot be dismissed out of hand, it is unlikely that this is the only, or even the most common, cause. In most patients, neither the clinical history nor the morphological findings provide any indication for this supposition.

Several investigators have proposed that an immunological disorder is involved in the etiology of pulmonary veno-occlusive disease. The arguments have been based on the association with Raynaud's phenomenon (21,23), on its development following renal transplantation (4), and also on the demonstration of immune complexes in the lung tissues (8).

The possibility that hormonal factors play a part in pulmonary veno-occlusive disease must also be considered since the disease is twice as common in adult men as in adult women, whereas the sex ratio is the same in children. In contrast, in primary plexogenic arteriopathy, the sex ratio in adults is 3 or 4 to 1 in favor of women but again the same in children.

The occasional familial occurrence of pulmonary veno-occlusive disease may indicate a genetic influence. It has occurred in siblings in the absence of recognizable common environmental factors.

Toxic agents are sometimes implicated in the etiology of pulmonary veno-occlusive disease. An important reason to consider this possibility has been the analogy with veno-occlusive disease of the liver, in which a toxic etiology has been demonstrated (2). In hepatic veno-occlusive disease, the venous obstruction is caused by intimal fibrosis of a type similar to that in the pulmonary variety. Although a thrombotic origin of this tissue was originally denied, more recent studies of veno-occlusive disease of the liver have indicated that the venous alterations begin with endothelial injury, followed by gradual coagulation (24).

Hepatic veno-occlusive disease is known to be caused particularly by herbal toxins, including pyrrolizidine alkaloids that occur in species of *Crotolaria*, *Senecio*, and other genera, and by toxic agents from contaminated grain products. None of these have been demonstrated to produce such a disease in the lungs. Nor is any case on record in which liver and lungs were affected simultaneously. Although these data are of little help in elucidating the cause or one of the causes of pulmonary veno-occlusive disease, they reaffirm that a toxic etiology cannot be excluded. Sniffing of household cleanser could have played a part in one patient (14), and several patients developed the condition following chemotherapy for malignant disease which may have been accompanied by immunological disorders (20).

Therefore, although the etiology of pulmonary veno-occlusive disease remains unsolved, the available evidence suggests that there is no single cause (27); in all likelihood, a variety of agents may injure the endothelium of the pulmonary blood vessels. Apparently, the insult particularly affects endothelium of the pulmonary veins. But, in some instances, and probably at a later stage, the endothelium of the arteries may also be injured. This endothelial damage may then trigger co-agulation which, in turn, leads to vascular obstruction as a result of organization of the clot.

REFERENCES

1. Anderson JL, Durnin RE, Ledbetter MK, Angevine JM, Gilbert EF, Edwards JE: Clinical Pathologic Conference. Am Heart J 97: 233–240, 1979.

2. Bras G, Jelliffe DB, Stuart KL: Venoocclusive disease of the liver with non-portal type of cirrhosis occurring in Jamaica. Arch Pathol 57: 285–300, 1954.

3. Cagle P, Langston C: Pulmonary veno-occlusive disease as a cause of sudden infant death. Arch Pathol Lab Med 108: 338–340, 1984.

4. Canny GJ, Arbus GS, Wilson GJ, Newth CJ: Fatal pulmonary hypertension following renal transplantation. Br J Dis Chest 79: 191–195, 1985.

5. Capewell SJ, Wright AJ, Ellis DA: Pulmonary veno-occlusive disease in association with Hodgkin's disease. Thorax 39: 554–555, 1984.

6. Carrington CB, Liebow AA: Pulmonary veno-occlusive disease. Hum Pathol 1: 322–324, 1970.

7. Chawla SK, Kittle CF, Faber LP, Jensik RJ: Pulmonary venoocclusive disease. Ann Thorac Surg 22: 249–253, 1976.

8. Corrin B, Spencer H, Turner-Warwick M, Beales SJ, Hamblin JJ: Pulmonary veno-occlusion—an immune complex disease? Virchows Arch [Pathol Anat] 364: 81–91, 1974.

9. Daroca PJ, Mansfield RE, Ichinose H: Pulmonary veno-occlusive disease: Report of a case with pseudo angiomatous features. Am J Surg Pathol 1: 349–355, 1977.

10. Hasleton PS, Ironside JW, Whittaker JS, Kelly W, Ward C, Thompson GS: Pulmonary veno-occlusive disease. A report of four cases. Histopathology 10: 933–944, 1986.

11. Hatano S, Strasser T: *Primary Pulmonary Hypertension*. Report of WHO Committee. Geneva, World Health Organization, 1975, pp 1–46.

12. Heath D, Segel N, Bishop J: Pulmonary veno-occlusive disease. Circulation 34: 242–248, 1966.

13. Höra J: Zur Histologie der klinischen "primären Pulmonalsklerose." Frankfurt Z Pathol 47: 100–118, 1934.

14. Liu L, Sackler JP: A case of pulmonary veno-occlusive disease. Etiological and therapeutic appraisal. Angiology 23: 299–304, 1972.

15. McDonnell PJ, Summer WR, Hutchins GM: Pulmonary veno-occlusive disease. Morphological changes suggesting a viral cause. JAMA 246: 667–671, 1981.

16. Moragas A, Huguet P, Toran N, Rona V: Morphogenesis of pulmonary veno-occlusive disease in a newborn. Pathol Res Pract 176: 176–184, 1983.

17. Nasrallah AT, Mullins CE, Singer D, Harrison G, McNamara DG: Unilateral pulmonary vein atresia: Diagnosis and treatment. Am J Cardiol 36: 969–973, 1975.

18. Pääkkö P, Sutinen S, Remes M, Paavilainen T, Wagenvoort CA: A case of pulmonary vascular occlusive disease: comparison of post-mortem radiography and histology. Histopathology 9: 253–262, 1985.

19. Pajewski M, Reif R, Manor H, Starinsky R, Katzir D: Pulmonary veno-occlusive disease in a unilateral hypertransradiant lung. Thorax 36: 397–399, 1981.

20. Rose AG: Pulmonary veno-occlusive disease due to bleomycin therapy for lymphoma. S Afr Med J 64: 636–638, 1983.

21. Sanderson JE, Spiro SG, Hendry AT, Turner-Warwick M: A case of pulmonary veno-occlusive disease responding to treatment with azathioprine. Thorax 32: 140–148, 1977.

22. Scheibel RL, Dedeker KL, Gleason DF, Pliego M, Kieffer SA: Radiographic and angiographic characteristics of pulmonary veno-occlusive disease. Radiology 103: 47–51, 1972.

23. Scully RE, Mark EJ, McNeely BU: Case records of the Massachusetts General Hospital. N Engl J Med 308: 823–834, 1983.

24. Shulman HM, Gown AM, Nugent DJ: Hepatic veno-occlusive disease after bone marrow transplantation. Immunohistochemical identification of the material within occluded central venules. Am J Pathol 127: 549–558, 1987.

25. Thadani U, Burrow C, Whitaker W, Heath D: Pulmonary veno-occlusive disease. Q J Med 44: 133–159, 1975.

26. Wagenvoort CA: Vasoconstrictive primary pulmonary hypertension and pulmonary veno-occlusive disease. Cardiovasc Clin 4: 97–113, 1972.

27. Wagenvoort CA: Pulmonary veno-occlusive disease. Entity or syndrome? Chest 69:82–86, 1976.

28. Wagenvoort CA, Losekoot G, Mulder E: Pulmonary veno-occlusive disease of presumably intrauterine origin. Thorax 26:429–434, 1971.

29. Wagenvoort CA, Wagenvoort N: The pathology of pulmonary veno-occlusive disease. Virchows Arch [Pathol Anat] 364:6979, 1974.

30. Wagenvoort CA, Wagenvoort N, Takahashi T: Pulmonary veno-occlusive disease: involvement of pulmonary arteries and review of the literature. Hum Pathol 16:1033–1041, 1985.

Bruce H. Brundage, M.D.

25 ⸻⸻⸻⸻⸻⸻⸻⸻

Pulmonary Hypertension in Collagen Vascular Disease

Pulmonary hypertension is an uncommon but well recognized complication of some collagen vascular diseases. Pulmonary hypertension with cor pulmonale is quite common in patients with scleroderma in whom it is often a consequence of involvement of lung parenchyma. However, some patients with scleroderma and others with mixed connective tissue disease—systemic lupus erythematosus, polymyositis, dermatomyositis, rheumatoid arthritis, and juvenile rheumatoid arthritis—have pulmonary hypertension with little or no evidence of parenchymal lung disease (1–6,10–14). As in primary pulmonary hypertension, the cause of pulmonary hypertension in these patients is unknown. However, the pathologic changes in the lungs are often those of plexogenic arteriopathy, similar to those seen in primary pulmonary hypertension and Eisenmenger's complex.

METHODS

Because of the similarity between primary pulmonary hypertension and pulmonary hypertension without parenchymal lung disease in patients with collagen vascular disease, the NIH Registry on Primary Pulmonary Hypertension enrolled patients who had collagen vascular disease in association with pulmonary hypertension that was disproportionate to the extent and severity of the parenchymal lung disease.

All in all, the Registry enrolled 236 cases of unexplained pulmonary hypertension. Twenty-six cases were associated with cirrhosis or intravenous drug abuse (11 percent) and 18 were in patients with collagen vascular disease (8 percent).

TABLE 1 COMPARISON OF PATIENTS WITH COLLAGEN VASCULAR DISEASE ASSOCIATED WITH PULMONARY HYPERTENSION (CVPH) AND PATIENTS WITH PRIMARY PULMONARY HYPERTENSION (PPH): DEMOGRAPHY AND HEMODYNAMICS

	CVPH*	PPH**	p
Height, cm	161.2 ± 1.9	163.0 ± 1.1	
Weight, kg	59.0 ± 2.6	66.2 ± 1.4	
Age at symptom onset, yrs	43.2 ± 4.2	32.8 ± 1.1	<0.016
Age at baseline cath, yrs	45.3 ± 4.2	36.2 ± 1.1	<0.033
Heart rate, per min	82.4 ± 3.6	87.4 ± 1.4	
PAP (mean), mmHg	50.1 ± 3.1	61.1 ± 1.3	<0.012
PPCW, mmHg	6.9 ± 0.6	8.3 ± 0.3	
$\dot{Q}$ index	1.8 ± 0.1	2.30 ± 0.08	
PVR (indexed)	27.2 ± 3.7	26.4 ± 1.2	
Systemic arterial pressure (mean), mmHg	92.9 ± 3.5	91.4 ± 1.1	
PRA, mmHg	11.2 ± 1.4	9.61 ± 0.46	
SVR (indexed)	24.0 ± 3.1	26.2 ± 1.1	
PVR (indexed)/SVR (indexed)	1.1 ± 0.04	1.03 ± 0.01	=0.014
Systemic arterial pH	7.5 ± 0.01	7.4 ± 0.004	

All data presented as mean ± S.E.; p values shown for statistically significant differences.
* = based on 18 patients.
** = based on varying numbers of patients ranging from 157 to 192.

TABLE 2 COMPARISON OF PATIENTS WITH COLLAGEN VASCULAR DISEASE ASSOCIATED WITH PULMONARY HYPERTENSION (CVPH) AND PATIENTS WITH PRIMARY PULMONARY HYPERTENSION (PPH): HISTORICAL AND CLINICAL

	CVPH	PPH	p
Age			
20 years	2	22	
20–40 years	4	96	
40 years	12	74	
Sex			
Male	1	72	
Female	17	120	<0.05
Family History of PPH			
Absent	18	178	
Present	0	14	
Smoking History			
Never	12	104	
Ever	6	88	
Oral Contraceptive Use			
Never	13	54	
Ever	4	61	<0.05
High Altitude Residence			
No	16	162	
Yes	2	30	
Raynaud's Phenomenon			
Absent	3	176	
Present	15	16	<0.001
Antinuclear Antibodies			
Absent	1	96	
Present	17	96	<0.001

p values shown for statistically significant differences.

The remaining 192 cases were categorized as primary pulmonary hypertension. The patients with collagen vascular disease are the subject of this report.

RESULTS

A number of demographic and hemodynamic variables were compared between the patients with collagen vascular disease and pulmonary hypertension and those with primary pulmonary hypertension (Tables 1 and 2). Because of the small size of the group with collagen vascular disease, differences between mean values of all continuous variables for the two groups (collagen vascular pulmonary hypertension and primary pulmonary hypertension) were tested using nonparametric and parametric methods. The nonparametric test was the Wilcoxon Rank Sum; the parametric tests were Student's T-test and ANOVA. For the most part, comparison between parametric and nonparametric procedures revealed no differences in test results. Therefore, variables found significant ($p < .05$) remained significant.

The baseline descriptors of patients with primary pulmonary hypertension have been previously reported (8). The patients with pulmonary hypertension and collagen vascular disease were almost exclusively females, older, had lower pulmonary arterial pressures, a tendency to lower cardiac indices, and a much higher incidence of Raynaud's phenomenon and positive ANA titer than did patients with primary pulmonary hypertension. The incidence of dyspnea, fatigue, chest pain, syncope, palpitations, and peripheral edema did not differ significantly in the two groups; dyspnea and fatigue were by far the most common symptoms in both groups. Routine laboratory tests were similar in both groups. Azotemia and a lower hemoglobin concentration were slightly more common in the patients with collagen vascular disease ($p < .05$). Chest radiographic and electrocardiographic findings were similar; pulmonary arterial enlargement and right ventricular hypertrophy were present in 85 percent or more.

Pulmonary function tests were considerably more abnormal in patients with collagen vascular disease; the findings were consistent with restrictive lung disease (Table 3) even though patients were preselected for pulmonary hypertension that was out of proportion for the amount of parenchymal disease. Comparison

TABLE 3 COMPARISON OF PULMONARY FUNCTION TESTS AND BLOOD GAS VARIABLES IN THE TWO GROUPS OF PATIENTS

Variable	CVPH	PPH	p
DL_{CO}, ml/min/mmHg	11.9 ± 1.5	17.55 ± 0.6	<0.01
TLC, L	4.0 ± 0.2	5.01 ± 0.1	<0.01
FEV_1, L/sec	1.9 ± 0.1	2.62 ± 0.1	<0.001
FVC, L	2.4 ± 0.1	3.31 ± 0.1	<0.001
FEV_1/FVC, L	0.81 ± 0.0	0.81 ± 0.0	
Pa_{O_2}, mmHg	68.6 ± 7.8	68.0 ± 1.4	
Pa_{CO_2}, mmHg	30.0 ± 1.3	30.4 ± 0.4	
Systemic arterial O_2, ml/dl	16.2 ± 0.6	19.0 ± 0.3	<0.001
Pulmonary arterial O_2, ml/dl	8.7 ± 0.6	11.8 ± 0.5	<0.01
V_{O_2}, ml/min	177.7 ± 17.0	277.7 ± 36.6	<0.1

All values expressed as mean ± S.E.; p values shown for statistically significant differences. DL_{CO} = CO diffusing capacity; TLC = total lung capacity; FEV_1 = volume of air expired during the first second of the FVC; FVC = forced vital capacity.

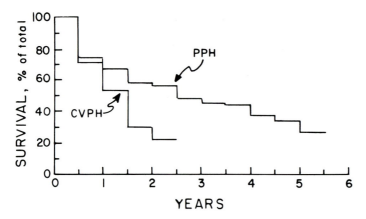

Figure 1: A Kaplan-Meir life table analysis comparing survival of patients with primary pulmonary hypertension (PPH) and collagen vascular disease with pulmonary hypertension (CVPH).

with patients who have primary pulmonary hypertension indicates that restrictive lung disease is often present in patients with pulmonary hypertension and collagen vascular disease even though the chest radiograph does not suggest it. These findings also suggest the possibility of a different mechanism for the development of pulmonary hypertension in the two groups.

Ventilation scans were more often abnormal in patients with collagen vascular disease (46 percent versus 20 percent, p = 0.166). Abnormal perfusion scans, albeit of low probability for pulmonary emboli, were common in both groups (56 percent versus 58 percent).

A Kaplan-Meir life table analysis depicted a mean survival of 471 days for patients with collagen vascular disease compared to 975 days for patients with primary pulmonary hypertension (Fig. 1). However, because of the small number of patients with collagen vascular disease, the differences were not significant.

DISCUSSION

The most interesting outcome of the comparison of patients who have collagen vascular disease and pulmonary hypertension with those who have primary pulmonary hypertension is the clear differences in pulmonary function testing: diffusing capacity, total lung capacity, forced expiratory volume at one second, forced vital capacity, and systemic arterial O_2 content were all significantly lower in the collagen vascular disease group indicating a much more severe restrictive lung abnormality than in the primary pulmonary hypertension group. The results suggest that despite criteria designed to exclude from the Registry patients with collagen vascular disease who had significant interstitial restrictive lung disease, a subtle form of the abnormality can escape detection. In progressive systemic sclerosis, it was originally believed that pulmonary fibrosis was the primary cause of pulmonary hypertension. However, attention has recently focused on obliterative vascular disease as the leading cause (11). Similarly, authors have tended to downplay the significance of interstitial lung disease in reported cases of pulmonary hypertension associated with other collagen vascular disease even though such pathology is often present, albeit mild to moderate in degree (1,6,10,11). Moreover, pulmonary function tests have often been abnormally compatible with a restrictive defect (1,10,12). Therefore, a continuum of restrictive lung abnormality appears to exist, at one end of which is primary pulmonary hypertension associated with a mild restrictive defect and at the other end of which is progressive systemic sclerosis associated with marked pulmonary fibrosis. Any collagen vascular disease, including progressive systemic sclerosis, can fall between these two extremes, with vascular disease predominating in some instances, fibrosis in others, or a combination of the two.

Although there are differences between patients who have pulmonary hypertension and collagen vascular disease and patients who have primary pulmonary hypertension, there are also similarities. The occurrence of positive ANA serologies in primary pulmonary hypertension has been known for years (7). However, recently the incidence of positive ANA tests was shown to be 40 percent higher than previously thought (9). This finding has been confirmed by the National Registry on Primary Pulmonary Hypertension in which the incidence of positive ANA tests in primary pulmonary hypertension patients was 50 percent (Table 2). This frequency of positive ANA tests places primary pulmonary hypertension between rheumatoid arthritis and systemic sclerosis, suggesting a link between primary pulmonary hypertension and the collagen vascular diseases (Fig. 2). The histologic lesion of the lung in collagen vascular disease patients with pulmonary hypertension has been reported to be a plexogenic arteriopathy similar to that seen in some patients with primary pulmonary hypertension (1,6,12).

Pulmonary hypertension in patients with collagen vascular disease sometimes appears to be out of proportion to the evidence of parenchymal lung disease. However, careful pulmonary function testing often indicates a more significant restrictive defect than in patients with primary pulmonary hypertension. These patients are almost always women whose symptoms and physical examinations

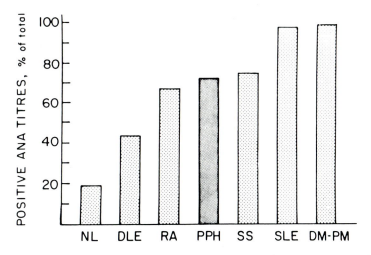

Figure 2: Relative frequency of positive (1–80) antinuclear antibody titers in various collagen vascular diseases. NL = normal; DLE = discoid lupus erythematosus; RA = rheumatoid arthritis; PPH = primary pulmonary hypertension; SS = systemic sclerosis; SLE = systemic lupus erythematosus; DM-PM = dermatomyositis-polymyositis. (Reproduced from Rich et al. [9].)

are virtually identical to those of patients with primary pulmonary hypertension. Their pulmonary artery pressures are markedly elevated but somewhat less so than in primary pulmonary hypertension. Once pulmonary hypertension is identified in patients with collagen vascular disease, life expectancy is very short (mean 471 days), even worse than that seen in primary pulmonary hypertension (975 days). Despite these differences, the high incidence of positive ANA tests in patients with primary pulmonary hypertension coupled with the frequent occurrence of the same lung pathology, plexogenic arteriopathy, raises the possibility of a similar etiology.

ACKNOWLEDGMENT

I wish to express my thanks and appreciation to Janet Kernis, M.P.H., for her invaluable assistance in the preparation of this manuscript.

REFERENCES

1. Bunch TW, Tancredi RG, Lie JT: Pulmonary hypertension in polymyositis. Chest 79:105–107, 1981.

2. Caldwell IW, Aitchison JD: Pulmonary hypertension in dermatomyositis. Br Heart J 18:273–276, 1956.

3. Fayemi AO: Pulmonary vascular disease in systemic lupus erythematosus. Am J Clin Pathol 65: 284–290, 1976.

4. Jordan JD, Snyder CH: Rheumatoid disease of the lung and cor pulmonale: Observations in a child. Am J Dis Child 108:174–180, 1964.

5. Kay JM, Banik S: Unexplained pulmonary hypertension with pulmonary arteritis in rheumatoid disease. Br J Dis Chest 71:53–59, 1977.

6. Kobayashi H, Sano T, Ii K, Hizawa K, Yamanoi A, Otsuka T: Mixed connective tissue disease with fatal pulmonary hypertension. Acta Pathol Jpn 32:1121–1129, 1982.

7. Rawson AJ, Woske HM: A study of etiologic factors in so-called primary pulmonary hypertension. Arch Intern Med 105:233–243, 1960.

8. Rich S, Dantzker DR, Ayres SM, Bergofsky EH, Brundage BH, Detre KM, Fishman AP, Goldring RM, Groves BM, Koerner SK, Levy PC, Reid LM, Vreim CE, Williams GW: Primary pulmonary hypertension: A national prospective study. Ann Intern Med 107: 216–223, 1987.

9. Rich S, Kieras K, Hart K, Groves BM, Stobo JD, Brundage BH: Antinuclear antibodies in primary pulmonary hypertension. J Am Coll Cardiol 8:1307–1311, 1986.

10. Rosenberg AM, Petty RE, Cumming GR, Koehler BE: Pulmonary hypertension in a child with mixed connective tissue disease. J Rheumatol 6:700–704, 1979.

11. Salerni R, Rodnan GP, Leon DF, Shaver JA: Pulmonary hypertension in the CREST syndrome variant of progressive systemic sclerosis (scleroderma). Ann Intern Med 86:394–399, 1977.

12. Schwartzberg M, Lieberman DH, Getzoff B, Ehrlich GE: Systemic lupus erythematosus and pulmonary vascular hypertension. Arch Intern Med 144: 605–607, 1984.

13. Trell E, Lindstrom C: Pulmonary hypertension in systemic sclerosis. Ann Rheum Dis 30:390–400, 1971.

14. Young RH, Mark GJ: Pulmonary vascular changes in scleroderma. Am J Med 64:998–1004, 1978.

Bertron M. Groves, M.D.
Bruce H. Brundage, M.D.
C. Gregory Elliott, M.D.
Spencer K. Koerner, M.D.
Jeffrey D. Fisher, M.D.
Robert H. Peter, M.D.
Stuart Rich, M.D.

Janet Kernis, M.P.H.
David R. Dantzker, M.D.
Alfred P. Fishman, M.D.
Kenneth M. Moser, M.D.
Daniel A. Pietro, M.D.
John T. Reeves, M.D.
Sharon I.S. Rounds, M.D.

26

Pulmonary Hypertension Associated with Hepatic Cirrhosis

Since 1951, several reports have stressed the coexistence of pulmonary hypertension and hepatic cirrhosis complicated by portal hypertension. This chapter deals with four aspects of this association: (1) the pulmonary abnormalities known to occur in association with hepatic cirrhosis are considered with respect to the likelihood that they might produce, or aggravate, pulmonary hypertension; (2) published reports that suggest that the rare coexistence of pulmonary hypertension and cirrhosis is more than a statistical coincidence are reviewed; and (3) hypotheses that attempt to explain the pathophysiological interrelationships between cirrhosis, portal hypertension, and pulmonary hypertension are presented; and (4) comparison is made between the clinical presentation, laboratory results, and hemodynamic findings of the 17 patients with combined cirrhosis and pulmonary hypertension in the NIH Registry on Primary Pulmonary Hypertension (PPH) and the 192 patients in the Registry considered to have "pure" PPH.

PULMONARY ABNORMALITIES ASSOCIATED WITH CIRRHOSIS

An excellent recent review by Krowka and Cortese summarized numerous pulmonary abnormalities which have been associated with hepatic cirrhosis (19). Approximately 15 to 45 percent of cirrhotic patients have one or more of the following: arterial hypoxemia ($Pa_{O_2} < 80$ mmHg) in conjunction with hemoglobin desaturation (2,5,34), clubbing, and hyperventilation. Pulmonary vascular abnormalities contributing to the hypoxemia include intrapulmonary shunting (1,36), portopulmonary shunting (4), pleural shunting (3), impaired hypoxic pulmonary vasoconstriction (9,13,27), ventilation-perfusion mismatching (14), and, more rarely, pulmonary hypertension (19). Intrapulmonary shunting may produce the unusual and debilitating symptoms of orthodeoxia and platypnea: orthodeoxia is defined as arterial desaturation made worse in the upright position and improved by reclining; platypnea is dyspnea aggravated by the erect posture and relieved by lying down (33). Both of these symptoms may be caused by the presence of vascular shunts in the lung bases. The effect of gravity in the sitting or standing posture is to increase the right-to-left intrapulmonary shunting by redistributing pulmonary blood flow to the bases, thus producing more severe hypoxemia. Pleural effusions which can contribute to the severity of hypoxemia are found in 5 to 10 percent of cirrhotic patients and may occur in the absence of ascites and intrinsic lung disease (23).

COEXISTENCE OF CIRRHOSIS AND PULMONARY HYPERTENSION

In 1951, Mantz and Craige reported the association of plexogenic pulmonary hypertension and portal vein stenosis in a 53-year-old woman with a history of recurrent hematemesis, who died from cor pulmonale. The autopsy findings were thought to be consistent with pulmonary hypertension secondary to pulmonary emboli from a spontaneously developed, cavernous, partially thrombosed portacaval shunt (24). Numerous subsequent reports have demonstrated the association of pulmonary hypertension and portal hypertension secondary to cirrhosis (6–8,29,30,39).

Whether the association of liver disease and pulmonary hypertension is causally related or coincidental is unknown. Lebrec found the prevalence of pulmonary hypertension to be 0.25 percent in 2,000 patients with portal hypertension (21). The observation that pulmonary hypertension occurred so rarely in patients with cirrhosis (0.26 percent or 2 of 765 hepatic cirrhotics over 20 years of age autopsied at the University of Zurich) caused Ruttner to conclude that the association may be coincidental (35). McDonnell reviewed 17,901 patients over the age of 1 year autopsied at Johns Hopkins Hospital from 1944 through 1981 and found that PPH occurred with a prevalence of 0.13 percent in all patients but with a prevalence of 0.73 percent in patients with cirrhosis ($p < 0.001$). In the same report, 2,459 patients with the clinical diagnosis of cirrhosis based upon hepatic biopsy findings had a clinical prevalence of PPH of 0.61 percent which was also significantly higher than the prevalence of PPH among all autopsied patients ($p < 0.001$). Thus, McDonnell concluded that the coexistence of hepatic cirrhosis and the development of the vascular lesions of pulmonary hypertension were not coincidental (25).

PATHOPHYSIOLOGY OF PULMONARY HYPERTENSION ASSOCIATED WITH CIRRHOSIS

To explain the development of pulmonary hypertension in patients with portal hypertension, most early reports emphasized the potential etiologic role of thromboemboli originating from the portal vein and gaining access to the pulmonary circulation by passing through portal-systemic venous shunts which develop spontaneously or are created surgically to control bleeding varices (20,21,37,40).

In 1974, Fishman hypothesized that pulmonary hypertension, in patients with cirrhosis and portal hypertension, might be caused by the inability of cirrhotic livers to detoxify vasoactive substances which are normally absorbed from the gastrointestinal tract and inactivated before entering the pulmonary circulation or by blocking a metabolic pathway that normally would exert an antihypertensive pulmonary arterial effect. Thus, he introduced the classification of "dietary" pulmonary hypertension (12). Since most patients with cirrhosis, with or without portal hypertension and a surgical portacaval shunt, do not develop pulmonary hypertension, a genetic predisposition to vascular endothelial injury from such toxins may be a prerequisite for the development of pulmonary hypertension. Some patients with primary and secondary pulmonary hypertension have been noted to have abnormalities of von Willebrand factor antigenic activity (16,31). This finding suggests the presence of significant endothelial cell injury which might predispose to thrombosis of the pulmonary microvasculature which has been observed in both PPH and pulmonary hypertension associated with cirrhosis (10,41). The clinical significance of these findings is uncertain since it is not known if abnormalities of von Willebrand factor production or degradation are etiologically important in the pathogenesis of pulmonary hypertension or serve as a secondary marker of damaged pulmonary endothelium.

Evidence suggesting that a substance taken by mouth could produce obliterative pulmonary vascular lesions and pulmonary hypertension in man was provided by a European epidemic of pulmonary hypertension which included many clinical and histologic features similar to PPH. Following the November 1965 release of an appetite suppressant, aminorex (5-amino-5-phenyloxazoline whose chemical structure resembles epinephrine and amphetamine), there was a 20-fold increase in the incidence of pulmonary hypertension in Switzerland, Austria, and Germany between 1966 and 1968 (18) (see chapter by Gurtner). The pulmonary arterial lesions in these patients were identical to the intimal and plexiform lesions considered typical of PPH. After aminorex was banned in 1968, the epidemic ended. Since researchers were unable to produce pulmonary hypertension by administering aminorex to animals, it was never proven to be the cause of the epidemic.

The potential occurrence of "dietary" pulmonary hypertension has also been suggested in humans who were (1) treated with phenformin (a biguanide) used to treat adult onset diabetes until it was removed from the market in 1977 because of the occasional complication of severe lactic acidosis (11), and (2) poisoned with toxic rapeseed cooking oil (which contained oleoanilide, a chemical by-product formed when industrial grade rapeseed oil reacts with aniline and acetanilide dyes used to mark the oil as unfit for human consumption) in a recent epidemic of pulmonary hypertension in Spain (15).

Abnormal pulmonary vascular reactivity in patients with cirrhosis uncompli-

TABLE 1 BASELINE CHARACTERISTICS OF CIRRHOTIC PATIENTS WITH PULMONARY HYPERTENSION

#	Patient	Center	Age	Sex	BSA	Etiology	PC-shunt	Var-ices	DOE	Ede-ma	Syn-cope	RVH
01	14013	U Penn	59	F	1.57	Chr Act Hep	+	+	+	−	−	−
02	15005	Harvard U	54	M	1.95	Alcoholic	+	+	+	+	−	+
03	15010	Harvard U	40	M	1.74	Alcoholic	−	−	+	−	+	+
04	19001	Cornell U	61	M	2.29	Postnecrotic	−	−	+	−	−	+
05	20002	Duke U	36	F	1.72	Micronodular	+	+	+	−	−	+
06	21001	Boston U	65	M	1.64	Alcoholic	+	+	+	+	−	+
07	21002	Boston U	58	F	1.36	Prim Bili	−	−	+	−	−	+
08	42005	U Mich	60	F	1.80	Alcoholic	+	−	+	+	−	+
09	49018	U Ill	59	F	1.41	Alcoholic	+	+	+	−	−	−
10	71009	UC San Fran	55	M	1.98	Postnecrotic	+	+	+	−	−	+
11	72005	U Utah	33	F	2.05	Alcoholic	+	+	+	−	−	+
12	73011	U Colo	47	F	1.71	Alcoholic	+	−	+	+	−	−
13	73015	U Colo	43	M	2.08	Alcoholic	+	+	+	−	+	−
14	73029	U Colo	30	F	1.78	Cong Hep Fib	+	+	+	+	−	+
15	73032	U Colo	60	F	1.53	Alcoholic	+	−	+	+	+	+
16	74007	Ced Sinai, LA	41	F	1.57	Alcoholic	−	+	+	+	−	+
17	76021	UC San Diego	58	F	1.25	Alcoholic	+	+	+	−	−	+
Mean			50.5		1.73							
Std			10.8		0.27							
n		12 Centers	17	11F	17		13+	11+	17+	7+	3+	13+

BSA = body surface area in square meters; PC-Shunt = portacaval shunt; DOE = dyspnea on exertion; RVH = right ventricular hypertrophy by ECG; Hgb = hemoglobin gm%; Hct = hematocrit %; Plt = platelet count × 1000; PT = prothrombin time in seconds; Bili = total bilirubin mg%; Alk = alkaline phosphatase units per ml; SGOT = serum glutamic oxalacetic transaminase units per ml; LDH = lactate dehydrogenase units per ml; ANA = abnormal anti nuclear antibody titer; Chr Act Hep = chronic active hepatitis; Prim Bili = primary biliary cirrhosis; Cong Hep Fib = congenital hepatic fibrosis; NA = not available; UNL = upper normal limit; Status = survival as of 7/1/88; A = alive; D = dead; Std = +/− one standard deviation from the mean.

cated by pulmonary hypertension was suggested by Daoud and Reeves in 1971 when they reported an impaired pulmonary vasoconstrictor response to severe inspiratory hypoxia (FI_{O_2} = .08 to .14) in 10 anemic (mean hematocrit = 36 percent), hyperkinetic (mean cardiac index = 5.6 L/min/M_2) patients with decompensated cirrhosis (9). Subsequent studies by Naeije in 24 patients with mildly to moderately decompensated cirrhosis revealed an average increase in pulmonary vascular resistance of 56 percent in response to breathing 12.5 percent O_2 for 10 min; on the average, this response was considered to be comparable to those reported for normal individuals subjected to a similar degree of hypoxia. However, taken individually, 7 of the 24 cirrhotic patients had a *blunted* hypoxic pulmonary vasoconstriction, i.e., an increase in pulmonary vascular resistance of less than 20 percent (27,28).

Observations on patients with the carcinoid syndrome may reflect the potential importance of normal hepatic function in protecting the pulmonary vasculature from vasoactive substances. Endothelial lesions in the right heart are seen in the carcinoid syndrome only when serotonin is produced by hepatic metastases and released directly into the hepatic veins. In contrast, the serotonin released by intestinal carcinoids into the splanchnic venous circulation is destroyed by normal hepatic metabolism and does not damage the endothelium of the right side of the heart (17). Even though the pulmonary and tricuspid valves may be signifi-

TABLE 1 *(continued)*

Hgb	Hct	Plt	ANA	PT	Bili	Alk	Alk/ UNL	SGOT	SGOT/ UNL	LDH	LDH/ UNL	Current status
14.1	42	152	+	10.3	0.8	231	1.2	44	1.8	379	1.1	A
13.0	37	87	−	15.0	1.9	138	1.2	106	2.7	288	1.3	D
15.6	46	199	+	13.0	0.7	180	1.6	50	1.3	183	0.8	D
16.2	47	79	−	10.1	1.4	55	1.1	38	0.5	346	1.4	A
14.3	40	89	+	13.0	2.4	532	4.8	106	3.0	294	1.2	D
14.8	45	147	NA	14.5	1.4	65	0.9	23	1.0	155	1.3	D
16.2	49	190	−	13.8	2.3	368	5.2	41	1.9	158	1.3	D
14.7	43	102	+	13.0	0.8	70	0.8	69	2.0	221	1.1	A
13.5	43	147	−	13.8	1.3	391	1.5	118	3.6	321	1.7	D
15.9	46	121	+	12.3	1.4	79	1.1	37	1.0	195	1.3	A
12.7	38	127	−	12.4	1.1	72	0.6	32	0.8	324	1.5	A
15.9	48	108	+	13.5	2.0	66	0.8	37	1.5	271	2.3	D
15.7	46	39	+	13.4	1.1	279	1.3	40	1.6	136	1.1	A
13.8	43	195	+	12.1	1.2	49	0.2	31	1.2	56	0.5	A
13.9	42	148	+	12.6	0.9	41	0.5	24	1.0	116	1.0	A
10.6	33	100	−	14.7	5.5	253	2.3	102	2.0	802	3.6	D
12.1	36	82	NA	14.8	5.2	123	0.9	42	0.9	384	1.9	D
14.3	43	124		13.1	1.8	176	0.9	55	1.2	272	1.0	
1.5	4	44		1.4	1.4	141	1.3	31	0.8	162	0.9	
17	17	17	9+	17	17	17	17	17	17	17	17	9D

cantly involved in the carcinoid syndrome, we are unaware of any patient who has had appreciable pulmonary hypertension secondary to the carcinoid syndrome. Why the pulmonary vasculature seems to be immune to toxic levels of serotonin and its metabolites is an unexplained medical curiosity.

Plexogenic lesions, the hallmark of PPH (41), are frequently found in patients with coexistent cirrhosis and pulmonary hypertension (10). However, scarring of the liver need not be in the form of cirrhosis for pulmonary hypertension to occur. For example, in a 25-year-old man with a history of neonatal omphalitis, hepatic vein sclerosis and portal hypertension was complicated by pulmonary hypertension. At autopsy, the architecture of the liver was preserved, but the liver was fibrotic—without regenerative nodules—and the portal veins were obliterated (10). Other instances have also been reported in which pulmonary hypertension and portal hypertension have been associated without cirrhosis (21,22,38). Therefore, portal hypertension, rather than cirrhosis, seems to be the prerequisite for the development of pulmonary hypertension. Moreover, histologic examination of the pulmonary vasculature cannot be used to distinguish PPH from pulmonary hypertension associated with portal hypertension with or without cirrhosis (10).

CLINICAL COMPARISON OF PATIENTS WITH PULMONARY HYPERTENSION ASSOCIATED WITH HEPATIC CIRRHOSIS AND PPH

Many clinical features of patients with primary pulmonary hypertension and pulmonary hypertension associated with hepatic cirrhosis are similar. Patients with cirrhosis are known to have anemia, increased cardiac output, decreased systemic vascular resistance, and mild hypoxemia (28). Studying the differences between patients with PPH and pulmonary hypertension associated with cirrhosis might provide useful insights regarding the pathophysiology and treatment of pulmonary hypertension from any etiology. In 1981, the NIH Registry on Primary Pulmonary Hypertension made provision for the recruitment of patients with pulmonary hypertension associated with cirrhosis so that a clinical comparison between the two disorders might be made. The following summarizes the findings in 17 patients from 12 participating centers who had combined pulmonary hypertension and hepatic cirrhosis and compares them with the findings in 192 patients with PPH from 32 centers, studied over the same interval, who did not have hepatic cirrhosis (32).

The baseline characteristics of the patients with combined pulmonary hypertension and cirrhosis are presented in Table 1. The mean age of the cirrhotic patients was 50.5 years (range from 30 to 65 years). There were 11 females and 6 males. The etiology of cirrhosis was alcohol abuse in 11, chronic active hepatitis in 1, micronodular cirrhosis in 1, primary biliary cirrhosis in 1, postnecrotic cirrhosis in 1, and congenital hepatic fibrosis in 1. Fourteen had a history of a surgical portacaval shunt. Eleven had experienced at least one episode of bleeding varices. All 17 complained of dyspnea on exertion. Edema had occurred in 7 and syncope in 3. Right ventricular hypertrophy was evident on the electrocardiogram in 13. The mean hemoglobin concentration was 14.3 gm per 100 ml, and the hematocrit averaged 43 percent. The mean platelet count was lowered to 124,000 per mm^3; in 5 patients, the platelet counts were less than 100,000. The ANA titer was increased in 9 of 15. Mean liver function test results were: prothrombin time, 13.1 seconds; total bilirubin, 1.8 mg percent; alkaline phosphatase, 0.9 times the upper limit of normal (range 0.2–5.2); SGOT, 1.2 times the upper limit of normal (range 0.5–3.6); and LDH, 1.0 times the upper limit of normal (range 0.5–3.6).

Comparisons of selected demographic, historical, laboratory and hemodynamic variables were made between the 17 patients with pulmonary hypertension associated with hepatic cirrhosis and the 192 patients with "pure" PPH. Statistical methods used included the Student's T-Test and Chi-square Test. Since the sample size of the cirrhotic group was small, all continuous variables were re-tested with the nonparametric method of the Wilcoxon Rank-Sum Test to confirm differences which were considered to be significant. Estimates of mean survival time were generated using the Kaplan-Meier product-limit method. The differences in mean survival time were tested by Logrank and Wilcoxon tests.

Several obvious differences were found in the distribution of selected demographic and medical history variables between the cirrhotic pulmonary hypertension and PPH patients (Table 2). The youngest cirrhotic patient with pulmonary hypertension was 30 years old whereas 34 percent of the PPH patients were less than 30 years of age. The mean age at onset of symptoms was 47 years for the cirrhotic patients versus 32.8 years for the PPH patients (p < .001). The mean age at baseline catheterization was 49.5 versus 36.2 years, respectively (p < .001). There was no significant difference in the sex distribution since 59 percent of the cirrhotic patients and 62 percent of the PPH patients were female. A positive family history was found in 7 percent of the PPH patients whereas none of the cirrhotic patients had a family history of pulmonary hypertension (p = NS). There was a history of smoking in 82 percent of the cirrhotic patients

TABLE 2 COMPARISON BETWEEN CIRRHOTIC PH AND PPH—DEMOGRAPHIC AND HISTORY VARIABLES

Variable	Cirrhotic PH (n=17)	PPH (n=192)	p value
Symptom onset to baseline catheterization (yrs)	2.5	3.5	NS
Age at symptom onset (yrs)	47.0	32.8	***
Age at baseline catheterization			
Mean age (yrs)	49.5	36.2	***
<20 Years (%)	0.0	11.5	**
20–40 Years (%)	17.6	50.0	**
>40 Years (%)	82.4	38.5	**
Sex—female (%)	58.8	62.5	NS
Family history of PH (%)	0.0	7.3	NS
Functional class			
I–II (%)	47.1	29.2	NS
III–IV (%)	52.9	70.8	NS
Raynaud's phenomenon (%)	0.0	16.0	NS
Smoking history (%)	82.4	45.8	**
Symptom—at any time (%)			
Dyspnea on exertion	100.0	97.4	NS
Fatigue	70.6	72.4	NS
Chest pain	35.3	46.9	NS
Near syncope	17.6	42.2	*
Syncope	17.6	37.0	NS
Edema	35.3	35.9	NS
Palpitations	35.3	32.3	NS

$* = p < .05; ** = p < .01; *** = p < .001;$ NS = not significant.

and only 46 percent of the PPH patients ($p < .01$). A history of Raynaud's phenomenon was reported in none of the cirrhotic patients and in 8 percent of the PPH patients (p = NS). There was a trend for fewer cirrhotic patients to be in functional classes III and IV compared to the PPH patients, 53 percent versus 71 percent (p = NS). Dyspnea on exertion was reported in 100 percent of the cirrhotic patients and 97 percent of the PPH patients. Fatigue occurred in 71 percent versus 72 percent, respectively. Chest pain was noted in 35 percent of the cirrhotic patients versus 47 percent of the patients with PPH (p = NS). The frequency of near syncope was 18 percent versus 42 percent (p = .048); for syncope, the frequency was 18 percent versus 37 percent, respectively (p = NS). A history of palpitations was recorded in 35 percent of the cirrhotic patients and in 32 percent of the PPH patients; edema was noted in 35 percent versus 36 percent.

The chest radiograph did not reveal any significant differences between the two groups when analyzed for increase in the size of the main or hilar pulmonary arteries, decrease in the size of peripheral vessels, or combined increase in the size of the main and hilar pulmonary arteries. Electrocardiography revealed no difference in the prevalence of right ventricular hypertrophy (86 percent of the cirrhotic patients versus 85 percent of the PPH patients). Although there was a difference in the frequency of abnormal ventilation scans (64 percent cirrhotic patients versus 28 percent PPH: $p < .05$), the presence of patchy diffuse abnormalities in the lung perfusion scans was the same (41 percent cirrhotic patients versus 40 percent PPH).

TABLE 3 COMPARISON BETWEEN CIRRHOTIC PH AND PPH—LABORATORY STUDIES

Variable	Cirrhotic PH (n=17)	PPH (n=192)	p value
Hemoglobin (gm%)	14.1	15.5	**
Hematocrit (%)	42.2	46.5	**
Prothrombin time (sec)	13.1	12.7	NS
Platelet count (× 1000)	124.1	225.7	***
BUN (mg%)	12.6	17.2	**
Creatinine (mg%)	1.0	1.3	NS
Bilirubin (mg%)	1.9	1.3	NS
Alkaline phosphatase (units)	181.9	124.2	NS
SGOT (units)	57.3	32.7	***
LDH (units)	273.4	235.4	NS
Arterial blood gases			
pH	7.5	7.4	NS
Pa_{CO_2} (mmHg)	29.7	30.4	NS
Pa_{O_2} (mmHg)	66.0	68.0	NS
Pulmonary function tests			
FEV_1 (liters)	2.46	2.62	NS
FVC (liters)	3.34	3.31	NS
FEV_1/FVC	0.74	0.81	**
TLC (liters)	5.1	5.0	NS
$D_{L_{CO}}$ (ml/min × mmHg)	16.8	17.6	NS

BUN = blood urea nitrogen; SGOT = serum glutamic oxalacetic transaminase; LDH = lactate dehydrogenase; Pa_{CO_2} = partial pressure carbon dioxide; Pa_{O_2} = partial pressure oxygen; Sa_{O_2} = saturation of hemoglobin with oxygen; FEV_1 = one second forced expired volume; FVC = forced vital capacity; TLC = total lung capacity; $D_{L_{CO}}$ = total lung carbon monoxide diffusing capacity; * = p < .05; ** = p < .01; *** = p < .001; NS = not significant.

The comparison of results from hematological and biochemical laboratory studies in the two groups is presented in Table 3. PPH patients had significantly higher hemoglobin and hematocrit values, perhaps due, in part, to the occurrence of variceal hemorrhage in the cirrhotic patients. The platelet count was lower in the cirrhotic patients, presumably secondary to hypersplenism. The blood urea nitrogen and serum creatinine concentrations tended to be higher in the PPH patients, perhaps reflecting their lower cardiac index. Although only the increase in SGOT was significantly higher in the cirrhotic patients, all their liver function tests, including the prothrombin time, total serum bilirubin, alkaline phosphatase, and LDH had a tendency to be higher than in the PPH patients. The pulmonary function tests were similar in the two groups since exclusion criteria eliminated enrollment of all patients with significant ventilatory abnormalities. Resting arterial blood gases demonstrated no difference in pH, P_{CO_2}, or P_{O_2}. Pulmonary function tests were similar in the two groups since exclusion criteria eliminated enrollment of all patients with significant ventilatory abnormalities.

Table 4 compares the hemodynamic variables derived from the baseline cardiac catheterizations in the cirrhotic pulmonary hypertensive patients with those who had PPH. The slightly higher heart rate and right atrial pressures in PPH were not statistically significant. The pulmonary arterial diastolic and mean pressures were significantly higher in the PPH patients. There was no difference in the pulmonary capillary wedge or systemic arterial pressures. The oxygen content of mixed venous pulmonary arterial blood was identical. However, the systemic arterial blood oxygen content in the cirrhotics was lower than in the PPH

TABLE 4 COMPARISON BETWEEN CIRRHOTIC PH AND PPH—BASELINE HEMODYNAMIC VARIABLES

Variable	Cirrhotic PH (n=17)	PPH (n=192)	p value
Heart rate (beats/min)	80.9	87.5	NS
Pressures (mmHg)			
Right atrium—mean	6.9	9.6	NS
Pulmonary artery			
Systolic	83.8	91.5	NS
Diastolic	35.2	44.4	**
Mean	51.4	61.1	*
Pulmonary capillary			
Wedge—mean	8.1	8.3	NS
Systemic artery			
Systolic	128.9	121.6	NS
Diastolic	73.2	75.6	NS
Mean	93.3	91.4	NS
Oxygen content (ml/dl)			
Systemic arterial	16.5	18.5	**
Pulmonary arterial	11.8	11.8	NS
Oxygen consumption (ml/min)	234.3	277.7	NS
Cardiac index (L/min/m²)	2.8	2.3	**
Stroke volume index (cc/beat/m²)	36.7	26.8	**
Resistances (Wood units/m²)			
Total pulmonary	12.2	19.5	**
Total systemic	22.6	28.4	*

* = p < .05; ** = p < .01; NS = not significant.

patients (16.5 versus 18.5 ml/dl; $p < 0.1$). Since the oxygen consumption for the two groups was comparable, the higher arteriovenous O_2 difference in the PPH patients reflected their lower cardiac index and stroke volume index. Therefore, the total and vascular pulmonary and systemic resistances were significantly higher in the PPH patients.

There was no significant difference in the mean survival time of the cirrhotic and PPH groups when tested by Logrank and Wilcoxon tests. However, the small size of the cirrhotic group and short duration of follow-up prior to March 1987 rendered this statistical analysis problematic.

SUMMARY

Comparison of the clinical presentation, laboratory results, and hemodynamic findings of 17 patients in whom pulmonary hypertension was associated with cirrhosis with those of 192 patients with "pure" primary pulmonary hypertension enrolled in the NIH Patient Registry on Primary Pulmonary Hypertension, indicated that patients with cirrhosis and pulmonary hypertension were older and less likely to have experienced syncope or Raynaud's phenomenon. They were more likely to have a history of smoking cigarettes. They had lower values for hemoglobin, hematocrit, platelet count, and arterial oxygen content, but higher values for SGOT. The pulmonary arterial diastolic and mean pressures were lower and the cardiac outputs were higher; thus, both the pulmonary and systemic resistances were lower. Even though the hemodynamic abnormalities of the cirrhotic pulmonary hypertensive patients were less severe, long-term survival did not differ from that of the patients with primary pulmonary hypertension.

ACKNOWLEDGMENTS

We wish to acknowledge the contribution of the participating investigators at the 32 centers who, by enrolling PPH patients in the Registry, provided the data base of "pure PPH" for the comparisons made in this chapter.

This research was supported by Contract 1-HR-14000 from the National Heart, Lung, and Blood Institute and Grant RR-00051 from the General Clinical Research Center Program of the Division of Research Resources, National Institutes of Health.

REFERENCES

1. Bank ER, Thrall JH, Dantzker DR: Radionuclide demonstration of intrapulmonary shunting in cirrhosis. AJR 140 : 967–969, 1983.

2. Bashour FA, Cochran P: Alveolar-arterial oxygen tension gradients in cirrhosis of the liver. Am Heart J 71 : 734–740, 1966.

3. Berthelot P, Walker JG, Sherlock S, Reid L: Arterial changes in the lungs in cirrhosis of the liver—lung spider nevi. N Engl J Med 274 : 291–298, 1966.

4. Calabresi P, Abelmann WH: Porto-caval and porto-pulmonary anastomoses in Laennec's cirrhosis and in heart failure. J Clin Invest 36 : 1257–1265, 1957.

5. Caldwell PRB, Fritts HW Jr, Cournand A: Oxyhemogloblin dissociation curve in liver disease. J Appl Physiol 20 : 316–320, 1965.

6. Cohen N, Mendelow H: Concurrent "active juvenile cirrhosis" and "primary pulmonary hypertension." Am J Med 39 : 127–133, 1965.

7. Chun PK, San Antonio RP, Davia JE: Laennec's cirrhosis and primary pulmonary hypertension. Am Heart J 99 : 779–782, 1980.

8. Cryer PE, Kissane J (eds): Clinicopathologic conference: Chronic active hepatitis and pulmonary hypertension. Am J Med 63 : 604–613, 1977.

9. Daoud FS, Reeves JT, Schaefer JW: Failure of hypoxic pulmonary vasoconstriction in patients with liver cirrhosis. J Clin Invest 51 : 1076–1080, 1972.

10. Edwards BS, Weir EK, Edwards WD, Ludwig J, Dykoski RK, Edwards JE: Coexistent pulmonary and portal hypertension: morphologic and clinical features. J Am Coll Cardiol 10 : 1233–1238, 1987.

11. Fahlen M, Bergman H, Helder G, Ryden L, Wallentin I, Zettergren L: Phenformin and pulmonary hypertension. Br Heart J 35 : 824–828, 1973.

12. Fishman AP: Dietary pulmonary hypertension. Circ Res 35 : 657–660, 1974.

13. Fishman AP, Fritts HW, Cournand A: Effects of acute hypoxia and exercise on the pulmonary circulation. Circulation 22 : 204–215, 1960.

14. Furukawa T, Hara N, Yasumoto K, Inokuchi K: Arterial hypoxemia in patients with hepatic cirrhosis. Am J Med Sci 287 : 10–13, 1984.

15. Garcia-Dorado D, Miller DD, Garcia EJ, Delcan J-L, Maroto E, Chaitman BR: An epidemic of pulmonary hypertension after toxic rapeseed oil ingestion in Spain. J Am Coll Cardiol 1 : 1216–1222, 1983.

16. Geggel RL, Carvalho AC, Hoyer LW, Reid LM: von Willebrand factor abnormalities in primary pulmonary hypertension. Am Rev Respir Dis 135 : 294–299, 1987.

17. Grahame-Smith DG: The carcinoid syndrome. Am J Cardiol 21 : 376–387, 1968.

18. Gurtner HP: Hypertensive pulmonary vascular disease: Some remarks on its incidence and aetiology, in Baker SB (ed), *Proceedings of the 12th Meeting of the European Study of Drug Toxicity, Uppsala, 1970.* Amsterdam, Excerpta Medica, 1971, pp 81–88.

19. Krowka MJ, Cortese DA: Pulmonary aspects of chronic liver disease and liver transplantation. Mayo Clin Proc 60 : 407–418, 1985.

20. Lal S, Fletcher E: Pulmonary hypertension and portal venous system thrombosis. Br Heart J 30 : 723–725, 1968.

21. Lebrec D, Capron JP, Dhumeaux D, Benhamou J-P: Pulmonary hypertension complicating portal hypertension. Am Rev Respir Dis 120:849–856, 1979.

22. Levine OR, Harris RC, Blanc WA, Mellins RB: Progressive pulmonary hypertension in children with portal hypertension. J Pediatr 83:964–972, 1973.

23. Lieberman FL, Hidemura R, Peters RL, Reynolds TB: Pathogenesis and treatment of hydrothorax complicating cirrhosis with ascites. Ann Intern Med 64:341–351, 1966.

24. Mantz FA, Craige E: Portal axis thrombosis with spontaneous portacaval shunt and resultant cor pulmonale. Arch Pathol 52:91–97, 1951.

25. McDonnell PJ, Toye PA, Hutchins GM: Primary pulmonary hypertension and cirrhosis: are they related? Am Rev Respir Dis 127:437–441, 1983.

26. Morrison EB, Gaffney FA, Eigenbrodt EH, Reynolds RC, Buja LM: Severe pulmonary hypertension associated with macronodular (postnecrotic) cirrhosis and autoimmune phenomena. Am J Med 69:513–519, 1980.

27. Naeije R, Hallemans R, Mols P, Melot C: Hypoxic pulmonary vasoconstriction in liver cirrhosis. Chest 80:570–574, 1981.

28. Naeije R, Melot C, Hallemans R, Mols P, Lejeune P: Pulmonary hemodynamics in liver cirrhosis. Am Rev Respir Dis 7:164–170, 1985.

29. Naeye RL: "Primary" pulmonary hypertension with coexisting portal hypertension. A retrospective study of six cases. Circulation 22:376–384, 1960.

30. Pare PD, Chan-Yan C, Wass H, Hooper R, Hogg JC: Portal and pulmonary hypertension with microangiopathic hemolytic anemia. Am J Med 74:1093–1096, 1983.

31. Rabinovitch M, Andrew M, Thom H, Trusler GA, Williams WG, Rowe RD, Olley PM: Abnormal endothelial factor VIII associated with pulmonary hypertension and congenital heart defects. Circulation 76:1043–1052, 1987.

32. Rich S, Dantzker DR, Ayres AM, Bergofsky EH, Brundage BH, Detre KM, Fishman AP, Goldring RM, Groves BM, Koerner SK, Levy PC, Reid LM, Vreim CE, Williams GW: Primary pulmonary hypertension: A national prospective study. Ann Intern Med 107:216–223, 1987.

33. Robin ED, Laman D, Horn BR, Theodore J: Platypnea related to orthodeoxia caused by true vascular lung shunts. N Engl J Med 294:941–943, 1976.

34. Rodman T, Sobel M, Close HP: Arterial oxygen unsaturation and the ventilation-perfusion defect of Laennec's cirrhosis. N Engl J Med 263:73–77, 1960.

35. Ruttner JR, Bartschi J-P, Niedermann R, Schneider J: Plexogenic pulmonary arteriopathy and liver cirrhosis. Thorax 35:133–136, 1980.

36. Rydell R, Hoffbauer FW: Multiple pulmonary arteriovenous fistulas in juvenile cirrhosis. Am J Med 21:450–460, 1956.

37. Sallam M, Watson WC: Pulmonary hypertension due to micro-thromboembolism from splenic and portal veins after portacaval anastomosis. Br Heart J 32:269–271, 1970.

38. Saunders JB, Constable TJ, Heath D, Smith P, Paton A: Pulmonary hypertension complicating portal vein thrombosis. Thorax 34:281–283, 1979.

39. Segel N, Kay JM, Bayley TJ, Paton A: Pulmonary hypertension with hepatic cirrhosis. Br Heart J 30:575–578, 1968.

40. Senior RM, Britton RC, Turino GM, Wood JA, Langer GA, Fishman AP: Pulmonary hypertension associated with cirrhosis of the liver and with portacaval shunts. Circulation 37:88–96, 1968.

41. Wagenvoort CA, Wagenvoort H: Primary pulmonary hypertension: Pathologic study of the lung vessels in 156 classically diagnosed cases. Circulation 42:1163–1184, 1970.

Michael A. Heymann, M.D.
Scott J. Soifer, M.D.

27 ————————————————————————————

Persistent Pulmonary Hypertension of the Newborn

The clinical syndrome of persistent pulmonary hypertension in the immediate newborn period (PPHN), sometimes called persistent fetal circulation syndrome, is characterized by failure of certain aspects of the circulation to undergo normal transition from the fetal to the postnatal state. The primary abnormality is maintenance of the high pulmonary vascular resistance found normally in the fetus, with consequent reduction of pulmonary blood flow; in addition, there is persistence of right-to-left shunting through the foramen ovale, or the ductus arteriosus, or both. Many factors are responsible for the physiological and physical control of pulmonary vascular resistance and for its normal fall after birth; therefore, the syndrome of persistent pulmonary hypertension of the newborn probably is caused by alterations in or failure of several mechanisms acting together rather than a single cause. The resultant syndrome, which generally occurs in otherwise normal full-term infants, leads to severe, often lethal, cardiorespiratory distress regardless of the etiology.

CLINICAL SYNDROME

The syndrome of persistent pulmonary hypertension of the newborn (PPHN) is characterized by early onset (generally within 4 to 8 hours after birth) of cyanosis and tachypnea, often with moderate or even severe respiratory distress. It occurs most commonly in full-term infants, occasionally in postmature infants, and very rarely in premature infants who are otherwise apparently normal (11,14). The clinical presentation may be indistinguishable from certain forms of congenital heart disease or primary pulmonary disease, such as group B beta-hemolytic streptococcal pneumonia. Structural cardiac disease must be excluded very early in the management of these infants; in the rare instance when clinical, electrocardiographic, radiographic, or two-dimensional echocardiographic and Doppler evaluation is not conclusive, cardiac catheterization may be warranted. Even without definite bacteriological evidence to the contrary, antibiotic treatment of streptococcal pneumonia is usually initiated until cultures prove to be sterile. A small group of infants with congenital malformations, such as diaphragmatic hernia or chest wall abnormalities, have hypoplastic lungs with a decreased pulmonary vascular bed; usually, they have pulmonary hypertension.

Infants with the true persistent pulmonary hypertension syndrome can be considered in two general groups: (1) those in whom pulmonary hypertension is associated with some type of aspiration; although usually it is meconium that is aspirated, aspiration of blood can also lead to the development of pulmonary hypertension; and (2) those in whom no intrinsic pulmonary disease is apparent. The incidence of PPHN is unknown but has been estimated to be about one in 1,500 live births (14). Although no accurate data are available, mortality is high: estimates vary from 20 to 50 percent, with the highest mortality in those infants who have aspiration syndromes.

The clinical features of both groups are similar. In addition to the signs noted above, there generally is a history of a difficult or abnormal labor and delivery or perinatal asphyxia. Apgar scores are often low; often, there is a history of meconium staining of amniotic fluid. Hypoglycemia, hypocalcemia, increased hematocrit, and acidemia are common. Low platelet counts occur in some infants, particularly after several days' illness; these infants, who usually are the most severely ill, probably have microthromboembolism of the small pulmonary arteries (28). In many infants, a systolic murmur can be heard; the murmur is attributed either to myocardial dysfunction or to increased afterload that results in dilatation of either or both ventricles and secondary tricuspid (more commonly) or mitral valve regurgitation, or both; bronchoconstriction with increased airway resistance is commonly associated with the cardiac dysfunction.

Right-to-left intrapulmonary or atrial shunting (usually across a patent foramen ovale) is evidenced either by subnormal oxygen saturation or tension in blood, either directly by sampling from an artery that arises from the ascending aorta (right radial) or indirectly by transcutaneous determination of P_{O_2} in the upper part of the body. Right-to-left atrial shunting is confirmed by Doppler evaluation or by contrast two-dimensional echocardiography; for this purpose, saline is injected into a vein and microcavitations are observed entering the left atrium across the interatrial septum. A right-to-left shunt through the ductus arteriosus is evidenced by Doppler evaluation, by a difference in arterial $P_{O_2} > 5$ mmHg between blood samples drawn simultaneously from an artery arising from the ascending aorta and from the descending aorta (usually via an indwelling umbilical arterial catheter), or by differences in transcutaneous measurements. These differences correlate roughly with the magnitude of right-to-left flow across the ductus arteriosus as well and, when the ductus arteriosus is open, with the degree of pulmonary hypertension; the difference in P_{O_2} is more easily demonstrated when pure O_2 is breathed.

The chest radiograph in infants without aspiration syndromes usually shows relatively clear lung fields; in those who have aspirated, parenchymal changes are seen. However, the radiographic appearance of the lungs is quite variable, so that severe hypoxemia is not reflected in the radiographic picture. Cardiomegaly is seen in perhaps half of the infants. Although the electrocardiogram is nonspecific, it may show increased right ventricular forces for age because the pulmonary hypertension does not allow normal postnatal regression of the free wall of the right ventricle.

THE NORMAL PULMONARY CIRCULATION

Morphological Development

In the fetus and immediate newborn, small pulmonary arteries of all sizes have a thicker muscular coat compared to the external diameter of the vessels than do similar arteries in the adult (see Chapter 19). This greater muscularity is generally held responsible, at least in part, for the vasoreactivity and for the high pulmonary vascular resistance found in the fetus, particularly as it draws close to term. In fetal lamb lungs fixed at perfusion pressures similar to those found normally in utero, the medial smooth muscle coat is most prominent in the smallest arteries (fifth and sixth generation arteries; external diameter 20–50 μm); during about the latter half of gestation, the medial smooth muscle thickness remains constant in relationship to external diameter of the artery (27). Similar observations utilizing slightly different techniques have been made in human lungs (19,37). After birth, particularly within the first several weeks, the medial smooth muscle involutes and the thickness of the media of the small pulmonary arteries decreases rapidly and progressively (20).

Toward the periphery of the lung, the completely encircling smooth muscle of the media gives way to a region of incomplete muscularization (37); in these partially muscularized arteries, the smooth muscle is arranged in a spiral or helix. More peripherally, the muscle disappears from arteries that are still larger than capillaries (nonmuscularized small pulmonary arteries). In these nonmuscular small pulmonary arteries, an incomplete pericyte layer is found within the endothelial basement membrane; in the nonmuscular portions of the partially muscular small pulmonary arteries, intermediate cells, i.e., cells intermediate in position and structure between pericytes and mature smooth muscle cells, are found (31). These cells are precursor smooth muscle cells; under certain conditions, such as hypoxia, they may rapidly differentiate into mature smooth muscle cells (31).

Small pulmonary arteries are conveniently identified by their relationship to airways. Preacinar pulmonary arteries lie proximal to or with terminal bronchioli; intra-acinar pulmonary arteries course with respiratory bronchioli, alveolar ductus, or within the alveolar walls. In the fetus during the last quarter of gestation, only about half of the pulmonary arteries associated with respiratory bronchioli (precapillary) are muscularized or partially muscularized, and the alveoli are free of muscular arteries (19). In the adult, complete circumferential muscularization extends peripherally along the intra-acinar arteries so that the majority of small pulmonary arteries in relationship to alveoli are completely muscularized. Between birth and teen age, the arteries undergo progressive peripheral muscularization; the adultlike pattern is reached at about the time of puberty.

During fetal growth in lambs, the number of small arteries increase greatly, not only in absolute terms but also per unit volume of lung (27). In the human, the main preacinar pulmonary arterial branches that accompany the larger airways are developed by 16 weeks (19). However, the development of the intra-acinar circulation relates more closely to the alveolar development that occurs late in gestation and perhaps even predominantly after birth (20): as the alveoli multiply, so do the arteries, a process that is generally complete by 10 years of age. In the early period of postnatal life (first 2 years in humans), pulmonary arterial growth is more rapid than alveolar growth (20).

Physiology

THE NORMAL FETAL CIRCULATION

In the fetus, normal gas exchange occurs in the placenta and pulmonary blood flow is low, supplying nutritional requirements for lung growth and perhaps serving metabolic or "para-endocrine" function (see Chapter 12). Pulmonary blood flow in near-term fetal lambs (term 145 days gestation) is about 100 ml/100 g wet lung weight, representing between 8 and 10 percent of total (combined left and atrial ventricular; 400–500 ml/kg/min) output of the heart (40,41). Pulmonary blood flow is low despite the dominance of the right ventricle, which in the fetus ejects about two-thirds of total cardiac output. Most of right ventricular output is diverted away from the lungs through the widely patent ductus arteriosus to the descending thoracic aorta, from which a large proportion reaches the placenta through the umbilical placental circulation for oxygenation. In young fetuses (about 0.5 of gestation), 3 to 4 percent of total cardiac output perfuses the lungs; this value increases to about 6 percent at about 0.8 gestation, corresponding temporally with the onset of the release of surface active material into lung fluid followed by another progressive slow rise to reach about 8 to 10 percent near term (41). Fetal pulmonary arterial blood pressure increases progressively during gestation; at term, mean pulmonary arterial blood pressure is about 50 mmHg (39), generally exceeding mean aortic blood pressure by about 1 to 2 mmHg. Pulmonary vascular resistance early in gestation is extremely high relative to that in the infant or adult, probably due to the low number of small arteries. Pulmonary vascular resistance falls progressively during the last half of gestation (39), new arteries develop, and cross-sectional area increases (27); however, baseline pulmonary vascular resistance is still much higher than after birth.

THE NORMAL TRANSITIONAL CIRCULATION

After birth and the start of pulmonary ventilation, pulmonary vascular resistance falls rapidly accompanied by an 8- to 10-fold increase in pulmonary blood flow. In normal full-term lambs, pulmonary arterial blood pressure falls to near adult levels within 1 to 2 hr. In the human this takes longer, so that by 24 hr of age mean pulmonary arterial blood pressure may be only half systemic (32). After the initial rapid fall in pulmonary vascular resistance and pulmonary arterial blood pressure, they continue to fall progressively, reaching adult levels 2 to 6 weeks after birth (39). With the large increase in pulmonary blood flow, pulmonary venous return into the left atrium increases, leading to a reversal of the pressure difference between the left and right atria. As a result, the valve of the foramen ovale closes, thereby preventing any significant right-to-left shunting of blood. In addition, the ductus arteriosus constricts and closes functionally within several hours, effectively separating the pulmonary and systemic circulations.

PHYSICS OF FLOW THROUGH THE PULMONARY VASCULAR BED

The physical factors that control flow through the pulmonary circulation can be estimated by applying the hydraulic equivalent of Ohm's law and the Poiseuille-Hagen relationship (38). The hydraulic equivalent of Ohm's law states that the resistance to flow between two points along a tube equals the pressure fall between the two points divided by flow. For the pulmonary vascular bed with resistance R and pulmonary blood flow $\dot{Q}$, the pressure fall occurs from the pulmonary artery (Ppa) to the pulmonary vein (Ppv). Thus:

$$R = (Ppa - Ppv)/\dot{Q} \tag{1}$$

Because we are interested in assessing changes in pulmonary arterial blood pressure, this can be rearranged to give:

$$Ppa = Ppv + R \cdot \dot{Q} \tag{2}$$

From Eq. (2), it can be seen that an elevation of pulmonary arterial blood pressure may occur with an increase of pulmonary venous pressure, pulmonary vascular resistance, or pulmonary blood flow. However, these factors are not necessarily independent. For example, pulmonary arterial blood pressure may remain constant in the face of increased pulmonary blood flow because the increased flow has caused pulmonary vascular resistance to fall by dilating, and perhaps recruiting, arteries; the product $R \cdot \dot{Q}$ does not change, and pulmonary arterial blood pressure does not increase.

Other factors that affect the relationship of pressure (P) and flow can be defined by a Poiseuille-Hagen relationship (38), which describes the relationship of P and $\dot{Q}$ of a Newtonian fluid flowing through a straight glass tube of round cross section:

$$Resistance = P_1 - P_2/\dot{Q} = (8/\pi)(l/r^4)(\eta), \tag{3}$$

where l is the length of the tube, r is its internal radius, and η is the viscosity of the perfusion fluid.

Before applying these formulae to the lung, differences between physical and biological systems should be considered. For example, although blood is not a Newtonian fluid, this is probably of little importance at normal hematocrits (2). Also, even though the walls of the small pulmonary arteries are not smooth, and the arteries branch, curve, and taper, and flow rates are low, the hemodynamic consequences of these factors are probably minimal (38). Because blood flow into the lungs is pulsatile, additional energy (and, therefore, higher pressure) is needed to accelerate the blood at each ejection; these inertial energy requirements are probably not large. Because of the relatively short distances between arterial branch points, laminar flow is unlikely in the lung, and viscous pressure losses would be greater than in the physical model. Since pulmonary vessels are distensible, changing transvascular pressure may alter their radii. Consequently, pressure-flow relations are not linear, as in a glass tube, even if Newtonian fluids are used as the perfusate (38). The lung compromises many blood vessels in parallel; these vessels are not all open all the time and may differ in radii in different lung zones.

Despite these differences from physical models, the general effects of changes in physical factors, such as viscosity or radius, do apply. Pulmonary vascular resistance is directly related to the viscosity of blood perfusing the lungs and inversely related to the cross-sectional area of the pulmonary vascular bed (radius[4]). Increasing viscosity or decreasing vessel radius, therefore, leads to an elevation of both Ppa and pulmonary vascular resistance. A change in luminal radius is the major factor responsible for maintaining a high pulmonary vascular resistance in the fetus. Consideration of these factors, particularly viscosity and cross-sectional area of the vascular bed, is important in evaluating the pathophysiology of persistent pulmonary hypertension syndrome in the newborn infant.

REGULATION OF PULMONARY VASCULAR RESISTANCE

In the fetal lung, pulmonary vascular resistance is initially high and, as previously discussed, falls throughout the final third of gestation. This high resistance is associated with the normally low blood oxygen tension (P_{O_2} in pulmonary arterial blood of 17 to 20 mmHg). Resistance is increased by hypoxemia (39) and decreased either by increasing oxygen tension (18) or by a vasodilator, such as acetylcholine (39), bradykinin (5), or the prostaglandins PGE_2 and PGI_2 (6,8,9); the latter are cyclooxygenase-mediated products of arachidonic acid metabolism that are present in the fetal circulation and are also produced by the fetal vasculature (52).

Pulmonary vascular resistance in the fetus is high despite the presence of these endogenous vasodilators, indicating an overwhelming vasoconstrictor influence. In addition to the hypoxic environment, strong candidates for the role of pulmonary vasoconstrictors in the fetus are the leukotrienes (LT) C_4 and D_4, which are also products of arachidonic acid metabolism, but through the lipoxygenase pathway. The leukotrienes are potent pulmonary vasoconstrictors. Although their role as mediators of hypoxic pulmonary vasoconstriction in adults has been challenged (3,45), a role for them has been proposed in newborn lambs (42), and the possibility remains that they may be tonically active in utero. In fetal lambs, end-organ antagonism (receptor blockade) or synthesis inhibition of leukotrienes (21,48) increases pulmonary blood flow about 8-fold, i.e., to levels corresponding to those that accompany normal ventilation after birth. These observations strongly suggest a physiologic role for leukotrienes in maintaining pulmonary vasoconstriction and, thereby, a low pulmonary blood flow in the fetus. In some systems, leukotriene effects may be mediated by inducing the production of thromboxane A_2. However, this does not seem to apply to the fetal lamb because inhibition of thromboxane synthesis does not affect pulmonary vascular resistance nor the response to leukotriene end-organ antagonism (10). Of the vasoactive leukotrienes, LTD_4 appears to be the active substance (44).

After birth, with the initiation of pulmonary ventilation, pulmonary vascular resistance falls and pulmonary blood flow increases markedly (39,51). Previously, these changes were thought to be mainly due to the increase in alveolar oxygen tension with some contribution from the physical expansion of the lung; the primary role of oxygen was supported by experiments indicating that pulmonary flow increased after exposure to hyperbaric oxygen without ventilation (18). However, part of the pulmonary vasodilation can be achieved by inflating the lungs with a low oxygen gas mixture that does not change arterial blood gas composition (22,51). Adding oxygen appears to complete the vasodilator process. Inflating the lung with a hypoxic gas mixture may lower pulmonary vascular resistance by either physical or chemical mechanisms: one mechanism may operate through alveolar surface tension; another is the release of cyclooxygenase-mediated products of arachidonic acid (16,22). Of the prostaglandin products, PGI_2 appears to have the most dominant physiological role at the start of ventilation.

The prostaglandins may also be involved in the initial postnatal pulmonary vasodilation. Exogenous PGE_2, and particularly PGI_2, decrease pulmonary vascular resistance in fetal goat or lamb lungs that are isolated and perfused either in situ or in intact fetuses (9,39). Moreover, indomethacin given before ventilation is begun attenuates the decrease in pulmonary vascular resistance that follows the initial rapid decrease in resistance, i.e., that occurs in the first 30 sec or so (23). However, PGE_2 and PGI_2 also produce systemic vasodilation in intact term fetal animals, whereas systemic vascular resistance normally increases soon after ventilation begins. Therefore, they probably are not the only prostaglandins involved in pulmonary vasodilation.

Among the other prostaglandins, PGD_2 has attracted particular interest. PGD_2 given to newborn animals produces greater pulmonary vasodilation than systemic vasodilation (7,49). This differential effect is lost by about 12 to 15 days of age, when PGD_2 produces pulmonary vasoconstriction; a similar pattern of response follows the administration of histamine which is a modest pulmonary vasodilator in the immediate perinatal period but subsequently becomes a pulmonary vasoconstrictor (13). Both PGD_2 and histamine are released from mast cells. In fetal rhesus monkeys, mast cell numbers increase in the lungs over the last portion of gestation; after birth, they decrease markedly (46). Therefore, the stimulus of lung expansion may cause mast cells to degranulate and release PGD_2 and histamine which contribute to the initial postnatal pulmonary vasodilation.

Bradykinin, another vasoactive agent, also has been shown to be a potent pulmonary vasodilator in the fetus (18). After ventilating the lungs of fetal lambs with oxygen or exposing the fetuses to hyperbaric oxygen, the concentration of kininogen, the bradykinin precursor, decreases and the concentration of bradykinin in blood increases (18). Accordingly, bradykinin may be one of the agents responsible for the component of the pulmonary vasodilator response that is unaffected by indomethacin, which blocks prostaglandin production. Bradykinin has been shown to stimulate PGI_2 production in intact fetal lungs and in pulmonary vascular endothelial cells in culture (30). Therefore, stimulation of local PGI_2 production by bradykinin may also contribute to the pulmonary vasodilation.

Another possible mechanism for PGI_2 production involves angiotensin II (AII), which increases in concentration at birth and has been shown to stimulate PGI_2 production by the lung (35). Moreover, stimulation of PGI_2 production by the neonatal lung is far more sensitive to AII than by the fetal or adult lung (35). If, as discussed above, mast cell degranulation does occur at birth, the resultant release of histamine could also stimulate production of PGI_2, as occurs in endothelial cells in culture (30). Another possible mechanism for PGI_2 release involves the physical effects of increased blood flow which, by producing an increase in shear forces, induces PGI_2 production by pulmonary vascular endothelial cells (53). If pulmonary blood flow is increased by any other cause, e.g., in response to O_2 or to bradykinin, a subsequent shear-induced PGI_2 production could enhance or sustain pulmonary vasodilation.

Not only PGI_2 but also a second lipid mediator, platelet-activating factor (PAF), could be involved in regulation of the postnatal pulmonary circulation. Small amounts of PAF produce pulmonary vasodilation in isolated rat lungs (54). Because PAF is not a circulating substance and probably acts only very close to the endothelial cell from which it is derived (30), the fact that pulmonary vasodilation was found with small, possibly physiologic, amounts of PAF whereas large, probably pharmacologic, amounts produced pulmonary vasoconstriction, supports the idea that PAF plays a role in pulmonary vascular regulation. PAF also seems to elicit pulmonary vasodilation in fetal sheep (1). Production of PAF by endothelial cells can be stimulated by the same agonists that produce PGI_2, i.e., bradykinin (B_2 receptor) and histamine (H_1 receptor) (30). Furthermore, AII apparently also stimulates PAF production in endothelial cell culture. Therefore, the possibility arises that both PGI_2 and PAF, independently or together with varying dominance, produce and/or maintain a dilated pulmonary circulation after birth. Production of each or both could be stimulated by bradykinin, AII, histamine, or some other mediator.

In conclusion, control of the perinatal pulmonary circulation probably reflects a balance between factors producing active pulmonary vasoconstriction (leukotrienes and hypoxia) and those leading to pulmonary vasodilation (several vasoactive substances and prostaglandins). The dramatic increase in pulmonary blood flow after birth most likely reflects a shift from active pulmonary vasoconstriction to active pulmonary vasodilation. It is possible that arachidonic acid metabolism shifts from lipoxygenase products in the fetus towards cyclooxygenase products due either to mechanical stimulation with lung expansion or to the higher oxygen environment after birth.

After the immediate postnatal period, the more important factors affecting pulmonary vascular resistance are O_2 concentration, pH, the effects of alveolar distention and perhaps certain vasoactive amines (histamine, 5-hydroxytryptamine), bradykinin, and metabolites of arachidonic acid by the cyclooxygenase (prostanoids and thromboxanes) and lipoxygenase (leukotrienes) pathways. The interaction of oxygenation and pH is particularly important. An increase in hydrogen ion concentration (decrease in pH) elicits pulmonary vasoconstriction; vasoconstriction occurs regardless of whether the decrease in pH is due to a metabolic acidosis or to a respiratory acidosis (43).

THE ABNORMAL PULMONARY CIRCULATION

Morphological Development

Pathological examination of the pulmonary vasculature of infants dying with the syndrome of persistent pulmonary hypertension of the newborn has defined fairly specific morphological changes associated with vascular remodeling (17,34, Chapter 19). The amount of circumferential medial smooth muscle in the walls of the small (resistance) pulmonary arteries increases, and a complete muscular coat replaces the partially muscularized coat in those arteries that normally do not have a complete layer; in addition, even the most peripheral (intra-acinar) arteries, which normally would have no muscle, are either completely or partially muscularized. Such extensive morphological changes point to more than an acute process that is confined to the immediate perinatal period. Indeed, they suggest a more prolonged period of stress in the fetus.

Although it was originally proposed that increased circumferential medial muscle occurs in rats exposed to chronic hypoxemia (15), this observation has not been confirmed in subsequent experiments (12). Nor does an increase in muscle mass occur in guinea pigs (33). However, these morphological changes do appear to occur in the lamb (47).

Administration of inhibitors of prostaglandin synthesis, such as aspirin or indomethacin, either to pregnant animals or to fetuses, produces constriction of the ductus arteriosus in utero (24,39). Because blood normally flows in the fetus from the main pulmonary artery to the descending aorta across the ductus arteriosus, constriction of the ductus arteriosus causes pulmonary hypertension and, in time, the development of increased pulmonary vascular medial smooth muscle (26). Although the use of these pharmacological agents during pregnancy has been linked to the development of the pulmonary hypertension syndrome (29,55), the association has not been proved.

Another possible cause of a reduction in the cross-sectional area of the pulmonary vascular bed is occlusion of the small pulmonary arteries either by emboli or thrombi. Microthromboembolism may play a significant part in the pathophysiology of persistent pulmonary hypertension of the newborn (28) and is apt to be associated with the severest and least responsive form of the disease (28).

In addition to changes in arterial muscularization, pathological changes have been observed both in endothelial cells and in the adventitia (4,34). Stenmark et al. have shown that functional maladaptation in the early postnatal period can lead to rapid and severe postnatal changes in structure (50): hypoxemia in newborn calves induced marked structural alterations, particularly of the adventitia, with thickening, cellular proliferation, and extracellular matrix deposition. In addition, therapeutic measures used in these infants (e.g., breathing of pure oxygen and rapid ventilation) could cause injury-related pathological changes.

Pathophysiology

The pathophysiological feature common to all infants with this syndrome is failure of the pulmonary vascular resistance to decrease normally with the start of ventilation. As a result, pulmonary blood flow is reduced, and pulmonary arterial pressure remains high at, or near, fetal levels. Associated with the pulmonary hypertension, right-to-left shunting may occur across the ductus arteriosus which remains patent in many of these infants. Right ventricular end-diastolic pressure is usually increased and, consequently, right atrial pressure also is increased; as a result, right-to-left shunting generally also occurs across the foramen ovale. The presence of tricuspid valve insufficiency, often associated with pulmonary hypertension and right ventricular dilatation, may accentuate this shunting. The ultimate pathophysiological effects are reduced pulmonary blood flow and reduced systemic oxygen delivery. As described above, the level of pulmonary vascular resistance is related to several factors, the most important in this clinical situation being pulmonary venous pressure, viscosity, and the cross-sectional area of the pulmonary vascular bed. Conditions that alter these factors adversely can lead to pulmonary hypertension in the newborn infant. Some causes are determinable. However, in many infants, no cause is found; these are the infants with the true idiopathic PPHN syndrome.

PULMONARY VENOUS PRESSURE EFFECTS

Associated with pulmonary venous hypertension of any etiology is an increase in mean capillary and pulmonary arterial blood pressures. Secondary to this may be increased fluid transduction into interstitial spaces, alveolar hypoxia, and further pulmonary vasoconstriction leading to pulmonary hypertension. In the immediate newborn period, fetal alveolar lung liquid passes into the interstitial spaces and is cleared from the lungs over a period of several hours. Pulmonary venous hypertension that interferes with this normal process may lead to pulmonary hypertension.

Congenital cardiac malformations that produce left ventricular failure also may cause pulmonary venous hypertension. Coarctation of the aorta or aortic stenosis are the most common causes in this group. Cor-triatriatum, congenital mitral stenosis, or variants thereof that obstruct blood flow into the left ventricle also may lead to pulmonary venous hypertension. In most instances, the clinical presentation, physical findings, electrocardiogram, chest radiograph, and 2-D echocardiographic/Doppler evaluation delineate the underlying cardiac anomaly as the cause of the pulmonary hypertension; rarely are such infants confused with those with persistent pulmonary hypertension syndrome. However, this need not be so in infants with total anomalous pulmonary venous connection and obstruction: infants with this disorder may have no specific clinical findings suggestive of cardiac disease. Usually, but not always, 2-D echocardiography with Doppler is helpful in separating these infants from those with the syndrome of persistent pulmonary hypertension of the newborn.

Intrinsic left ventricular myocardial dysfunction may lead to increased left ventricular end-diastolic pressure accompanied by left atrial and pulmonary venous hypertension. Myocardial dysfunction is associated with transient cardiomyopathy in infants of diabetic mothers or after asphyxia. Less commonly, primary cardiomyopathies of unknown etiology, myocardial tumors such as rhabdomyomas, and infectious viral myocarditis may produce myocardial dysfunction. Electrolyte imbalances, particularly hypocalcemia and hypoglycemia, may also depress myocardial performance. Although rare, anomalous origin of the left coronary artery may produce global left ventricular ischemia and dysfunction. Most of these disorders are clinically recognizable and generally are not confused with the syndrome of persistent pulmonary hypertension of the newborn. However, secondary left ventricular dysfunction, such as occurs with hypocalcemia, certainly may aggravate pulmonary hypertension in an infant with the syndrome of persistent pulmonary hypertension of the newborn.

INCREASED VISCOSITY

Blood viscosity is related to red cell number, fibrinogen concentration, and red cell deformability. An increased hematocrit increases viscosity, the amount depending on shear rate (2); an increased hematocrit may be found following twin-to-twin or maternal-to-fetal blood transfusion or delayed cord clamping. Pulmonary vascular resistance increases approximately logarithmically with the increase in hematocrit (2). Chronic intrauterine hypoxemia is associated with an increased hematocrit, as well as increased fibrinogen concentration (36), and infants born to diabetic mothers also may have an abnormally high hematocrit. A feature of newborn red cells is that they are less deformable than adult cells; acidemia accentuates the relative decrease in deformability.

REDUCED CROSS-SECTIONAL AREA

Infants with the syndrome of persistent pulmonary hypertension of the newborn fall into this category. Probably the most common cause for reduction in total pulmonary vascular cross-sectional area is failure of the fetal pulmonary circulation to undergo normal postnatal vasodilation. The mechanisms responsible for failure of the pulmonary vasculature to dilate are unknown. The most likely, but not proven, common denominator is perinatal hypoxemia or asphyxia. Why some infants exposed to this develop pulmonary hypertension whereas many others, who are equally stressed in the immediate perinatal period, do not, is unclear. As discussed above, medial smooth muscle is not only increased in the small pulmonary arteries, but the distribution of the smooth muscle along the length of the vessels is ontogenetically accelerated; the small distal pulmonary arteries, which in the normal newborn infant are only partially muscularized or not muscular at all, are completely muscularized, as in the adult. The possibility exists that these abnormally developed vessels exhibit an increased constrictor response to low oxygen or a vasoactive substance, either because of the increased muscle mass or because the developmental acceleration is not only structural but also functional. In fetal animal models, chronic intrauterine stress, such as chronic hypoxemia (15) or pulmonary hypertension (25), is known to produce an increased medial muscle mass in the small pulmonary arteries. In addition, chronic umbilical cord compression in the lamb delivered at term, which produces fetal hypoxemia, is associated with a pulmonary circulation that is overreactive to hypoxia (47). Infants exposed to similar intrauterine stresses may be at high risk for developing morphological and pathophysiological changes of the pulmonary vasculature followed by pulmonary hypertension.

A variety of other mechanisms can be postulated. Some relate to abnormal response or production of mediators and others to functional responses to morphological changes. However, convincing experimental support for such hypotheses remains to be adduced.

ACKNOWLEDGMENTS

The personal research referred to in this chapter was supported in part by U.S. Public Health Service Program Project Grant HL 24056, by grants HL 40473 and

HL 35518, and by BRSG Grant S07 RR05355 awarded by the Biomedical Research Support Program, Division of Research Resources, National Institutes of Health.

REFERENCES

1. Accurso F, Abman S, Wilkening RB, Worthen S, Henson PM: Exogenous PAF produces pulmonary vasodilation in the ovine fetus. Am Rev Respir Dis 133:11, 1986 (Abstract).

2. Agarwal JB, Paltoo R, Palmer WH: Relative viscosity of blood at varying hematocrits in pulmonary circulation. J Appl Physiol 29:866–871, 1970.

3. Ahmed T, Oliver W Jr: Does slow-reacting substance of anaphylaxis mediate hypoxic pulmonary vasoconstriction? Am Rev Respir Dis 127:566–571, 1983.

4. Allen K, Haworth SG: Impaired adaptation of intrapulmonary arteries to extrauterine life in the newborn pigs exposed to hypoxia: An ultrastructural study. J Pathol 150:205–212, 1986.

5. Campbell AGM, Dawes GS, Fishman AP, Hyman AI, Perks AM: The release of bradykinin-like pulmonary vasodilator substance in foetal and newborn lambs. J Physiol (Lond) 195:83–96, 1968.

6. Cassin S: Role of prostaglandins and thromboxanes in the control of the pulmonary circulation in the fetus and newborn. Semin Perinatol 4:101–107, 1980.

7. Cassin S, Tod M, Philips J, Frisinger J, Jordan J, Gibbs C: Effects of prostaglandin D_2 in perinatal circulation. Am J Physiol 240:H755–H760, 1981.

8. Cassin S, Tyler TL, Wallis R: The effects of prostaglandin E_1 on fetal pulmonary vascular resistance (38588). Proc Soc Exp Biol Med 148:584–587, 1975.

9. Cassin S, Winikor I, Tod M, Philips J, Frisinger S, Jordan J, Gibbs C: Effects of prostacyclin on the fetal pulmonary circulation. Pediatr Pharmacol 1:197–207, 1981.

10. Clozel M, Clyman RI, Soifer SJ, Heymann MA: Thromboxane is not responsible for the high pulmonary vascular resistance in fetal lambs. Pediatr Res 19:1254–1257, 1985.

11. Fox WW, Gewitz MH, Dinwiddie R, Drummond WH, Peckham GJ: Pulmonary hypertension in the perinatal aspiration syndromes. Pediatrics 59:205–211, 1977.

12. Geggel RL, Aronovitz BS, Reid LM: Effects of chronic in utero hypoxemia on rat neonatal pulmonary arterial structure. J Pediatr 108:756–759, 1986.

13. Goetzman BW, Milstein JM: Pulmonary vascular histamine receptors in newborn and young lambs. J Appl Physiol 49:380–385, 1980.

14. Goetzman BW, Riemenschneider TA: Persistence of the fetal circulation. Pediatr Rev 2:37–40, 1980.

15. Goldberg SJ, Levy RA, Siassi B, Betten J: The effects of maternal hypoxia and hyperoxia upon neonatal pulmonary vasculature. Pediatrics 48:528–533, 1971.

16. Gryglewski RJ, Korbut R, Ocetkiewicz A: Generation of prostacyclin by lungs in vivo and its release into the arterial circulation. Nature 273:765–767, 1978.

17. Haworth SG, Reid L: Persistent fetal circulation: Newly recognized structural features. J Pediatr 88:614–620, 1976.

18. Heymann MA, Rudolph AM, Nies AS, Melmon KL: Bradykinin production associated with oxygenation of the fetal lamb. Circ Res 25:521–534, 1969.

19. Hislop A, Reid LM: Intra-pulmonary arterial development during fetal life—branching pattern and structure. J Anat 113:35–48, 1972.

20. Hislop A, Reid LM: Pulmonary arterial development during childhood: Branching pattern and structure. Thorax 28:129–135, 1973.

21. Le Bidois J, Soifer SJ, Clyman RI, Heymann MA: Piriprost: A putative leukotriene synthesis inhibitor increases pulmonary blood flow in fetal lambs. Pediatr Res 22:350–354, 1987.

22. Leffler CW, Hessler JR, Green RS: The onset of breathing at birth stimulates pulmonary vascular prostacyclin synthesis. Pediatr Res 18:938–942, 1984.

23. Leffler CW, Tyler TL, Cassin S: Effect of indomethacin on pulmonary vascular response to ventilation of fetal goats. Am J Physiol 234:H346–H351, 1978.

24. Levin DL: Effects of inhibition of prostaglandin synthesis on fetal development, oxygenation and the fetal circulation. Semin Perinatol 4:35–44, 1980.

25. Levin DL, Hyman AI, Heymann MA, Rudolph AM: Fetal hypertension and the development of increased pulmonary vascular smooth muscle: A possible mechanism for persistent pulmonary hypertension of the newborn infant. J Pediatr 92:265–269, 1978.

26. Levin DL, Mills LJ, Weinberg AG: Hemodynamics, pulmonary vascular, and myocardial abnormalities secondary to pharmacologic constriction of the fetal ductus arteriosus. Circulation 60:360–364, 1979.

27. Levin DL, Rudolph AM, Heymann MA, Phibbs RH: Morphological development of the pulmonary vascular bed in fetal lambs. Circulation 53:144–151, 1976.

28. Levin DL, Weinberg AG, Perkin RM: Pulmonary microthrombi syndrome in newborn infants with unresponsive persistent pulmonary hypertension. J Pediatr 102:299–302, 1983.

29. Manchester D, Margolis HS, Sheldon RE: Possible association between maternal indomethacin therapy and primary pulmonary hypertension of the newborn. Am J Obstet Gynecol 126:467–469, 1976.

30. McIntyre TM, Zimmerman GA, Satoh K, Prescott SM: Cultured endothelial cells synthesize both platelet-activating factor and prostacyclin in response to histamine, bradykinin, and adenosine triphosphate. J Clin Invest 76:271–280, 1985.

31. Meyrick B, Reid L: The effect of continued hypoxia on rat pulmonary arterial circulation: An ultrastructural study. Lab Invest 38:188–200, 1978.

32. Moss AJ, Emmanouilides G, Duffie ER Jr: Closure of the ductus arteriosus in the newborn infant. Pediatrics 32:25–30, 1963.

33. Murphy JD, Aronovitz MJ, Reid LM: Effects of chronic in utero hypoxia on the pulmonary vasculature of the newborn guinea pig. Pediatr Res 20:292–295, 1986.

34. Murphy JD, Rabinovitch M, Goldstein JD, Reid LM: The structural basis of persistent pulmonary hypertension of the newborn infant. J Pediatr 98:962–967, 1981.

35. Omini C, Vigano T, Marini A, Pasargiklian R, Fano M, Maselli MA: Angiotensin II: A releaser of PGI_2 from fetal and newborn rabbit lungs. Prostaglandins 25:901–910, 1983.

36. Pickart LR, Creasy RK, Thaler MM: Polycythemia and hyperfibrinogenemia as factors in experimental intrauterine growth retardation. Am J Obstet Gynecol 124:268–271, 1976.

37. Reid LM: Structure and function in pulmonary hypertension. New perceptions. Chest 89:279–288, 1986.

38. Roos A: Poiseuille's law and its limitations in vascular systems. Med Thorac 19:224–238, 1962.

39. Rudolph AM: Fetal and neonatal pulmonary circulation. Ann Rev Physiol 41:383–395, 1979.

40. Rudolph AM, Heymann MA: The circulation of the fetus in utero. Methods for studying distribution of blood flow, cardiac output and organ blood flow. Circ Res 21:163–184, 1967.

41. Rudolph AM, Heymann MA: Circulatory changes during growth in the fetal lamb. Circ Res 26:289–299, 1970.

42. Schreiber MD, Heymann MA, Soifer SJ: Leukotriene inhibition prevents and reverses hypoxic pulmonary vasoconstriction in newborn lambs. Pediatr Res 19:437–441, 1985.

43. Schreiber MD, Heymann MA, Soifer SJ: Increased arterial pH, not decreased Pa_{CO_2}, attenuates hypoxia-induced pulmonary vasoconstriction in newborn lambs. Pediatr Res 20:113–117, 1986.

44. Schreiber MD, Heymann MA, Soifer SJ: The differential effects of leukotriene C_4 and D_4 on the pulmonary and systemic circulations in newborn lambs. Pediatr Res 21:176–182, 1987.

45. Schuster DP, Dennis DR: Leukotriene inhibitors do not block hypoxic pulmonary vasoconstriction in dogs. J Appl Physiol 65:1808-1813, 1987.

46. Schwartz LS, Osborn BI, Frick OL: An ontogenic study of histamine and mast cells in the fetal rhesus monkey. J Allergy Clin Immunol 56:381–386, 1974.

47. Soifer SJ, Kaslow D, Roman C, Heymann MA: Umbilical cord compression produces pulmonary hypertension in newborn lambs: A model to study the pathophysiology of persistent pulmonary hypertension in the newborn. J Devel Physiol 9:239–252, 1987.

48. Soifer SJ, Loitz RD, Roman C, Heymann MA: Leukotriene end organ antagonists increase pulmonary blood flow in fetal lambs. Am J Physiol 249:H570–H576, 1985.

49. Soifer SJ, Morin FC III, Kaslow DC, Heymann MA: The developmental effects of prostaglandin D_2 on the pulmonary and systemic circulations in the newborn lamb. J Devel Physiol 5:237–250, 1983.

50. Stenmark KR, Reeves JT, Voelkel NF, Crouch EP, Mecham RP: Altered pulmonary vascular elastin metabolism in severe hypoxic pulmonary hypertension. Fed Proc 46:517, 1987 (Abstract).

51. Teitel DF, Iwamoto HS, Rudolph AM: Effects of birth-related events on central blood flow patterns. Pediatr Res 22:557–566, 1987.

52. Terragno NA, Terragno A: Prostaglandin metabolism in the fetal and maternal vasculature. Fed Proc 38:75–77, 1979.

53. VanGrondelle A, Worthen S, Ellis D, Mathias MM, Murphy RC, Murphy RJ, Strife J, Reeves JT, Voelkel NF: Altering hydrodynamic variables influences PGI_2 production by isolated lungs and endothelial cells. J Appl Physiol 57:388–395, 1984.

54. Voelkel NF, Chang SW, Pfeffer KD, Worthen SG, McMurtry IF, Henson PM: PAF antagonists: Different effects on platelets, neutrophils, guinea pig ileum and PAF-induced vasodilation in isolated rat lung. Prostaglandins 32:359–372, 1986.

55. Wilkinson AR, Aynsley-Green A, Mitchell MD: Persistent pulmonary hypertension and abnormal PGE levels in preterm infants after maternal treatment with naproxen. Arch Dis Child 54:942–945, 1979.

Jose López-Sendón, M.D.
Miguel A. Gomez Sanchez, M.D.
María José Mestre de Juan, M.D.
Isabel Coma-Canella, M.D.

28

Pulmonary Hypertension in the Toxic Oil Syndrome

Dietary pulmonary hypertension has been categorized as a subset of primary pulmonary hypertension (6,26). It is caused by substances ingested as food, beverages, or medications. Among the etiologic agents that have been implicated to date are *Crotalaria* and other plants (13), the appetite-depressant, aminorex (12), and oral contraceptives (14). Less certain with respect to causal relationship is the coincidence of pulmonary hypertension and cirrhosis of the liver (2), but the association does underscore a relationship between the intestinal tract and pulmonary circulation.

Quite distinct from the etiologies above was an unusual epidemic of pulmonary hypertension that began in Spain in 1981. This outbreak has been designated the toxic oil syndrome (TOS) or toxic epidemic syndrome because of its occurrence after ingestion of toxic, denatured and re-refined rapeseed oil (1,3,8–11, 15–16,22,24,27–28).

THE TOXIC OIL SYNDROME

The Toxic Oil Syndrome is a multisystemic disease, the exact cause of which remains unproven, even though epidemiological evidence clearly implicates the consumption of an illegally marketed cooking oil (21,22). The first patient was seen in May 1, 1981. Since then, 20,486 cases have been reported and 671 individuals have died, most in the first months of illness; in 370 of these, the pathology at autopsy was attributable to the toxic oil syndrome. Moreover, 23 of the 370 deaths were directly related to pulmonary hypertension; in 9 other patients with the toxic oil syndrome who died, marked pulmonary hypertension was present although death was primarily due to severe neuromuscular involvement and its complications.

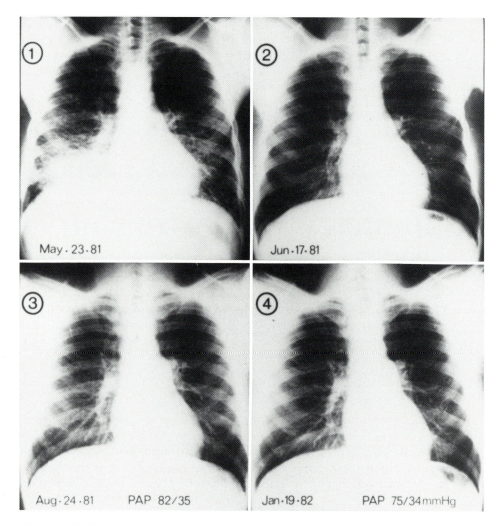

Figure 1: Typical radiographic evolution in a patient with the toxic oil syndrome.
1: Initial interstitial pulmonary edema characteristic of the acute phase.
2: Normal chest radiograph after several weeks of illness.
3: Development of pulmonary hypertension.
4: Persistence of radiographic signs of pulmonary hypertension 8 months after the onset of the disease. PAP = pulmonary arterial pressure, systolic and diastolic, mmHg.

General Clinical Picture of Toxic Oil Syndrome

Three stages can be differentiated in the course of the disease. In the first stage, from May to June 1981, the most striking feature was a toxic allergic pneumopathy with fever, myalgias, skin rash, respiratory distress (the main cause of death in this initial phase), and noncardiogenic pulmonary edema (Fig. 1). Blood eosinophilia was generally present: as a rule, the total eosinophilic count exceeded 500 cells/μl. The association of the toxic oil syndrome and the ingestion of denatured rapeseed oil was detected on June 10, 1981. Thereafter, as the oil was taken off the market and consumption ceased, the number of cases dropped sharply.

In July 1981, stage 2, the clinical picture started to change: 15 to 30 percent of the patients suffered a recrudescence of fever, myalgias, neurological symptoms, and heart failure. In this stage, the incidence of pulmonary hypertension assumed epidemic proportions. Meanwhile, the respiratory symptoms and chest radiographic findings disappeared (Fig. 1).

Stage 3 began in September 1981 when the toxic oil syndrome acquired another set of signs and symptoms, i.e., loss of weight, neuromuscular disorders, and scleroderma-like lesions that, in some instances, seemed to be part of the syndrome of progressive systemic sclerosis.

After January 1982, most patients remained free of major symptoms, but a few were left with neuromuscular disorders.

General Pathological Findings in Toxic Oil Syndrome

Despite the changing pattern of the clinical syndrome, all patients have shown vascular lesions which, taken together, differ from those of any other known disease. These lesions have been found in all organs in all phases of the syndrome. They have three outstanding features: (1) intimal lesions with swelling and cytoplasmic vacuolation of endothelial cells; (2) after July 1981, vascular wall infiltration by lymphocytes without fibrinoid necrosis, as well as intimal proliferation that partly obliterated vascular lumens; and (3) in advanced phases, obliterative fibrosis of the intima (18,21,22).

Etiology

There is a clear epidemiological relationship between the toxic oil syndrome and ingestion of an illegally marketed rapeseed cooking oil, fraudulently sold to the public as pure olive oil. Nearly all of the children and most adults with this syndrome had ingested an oil sold by door-to-door salesmen in 5l plastic bottles which bore no labels or evidence of sanitary controls (27).

RAPESEED OIL

Rapeseed oil, a second-class oil extracted from the rape or colza plant (*Brassica napus*), is used for cooking after being refined. Since it is illegal to import *edible* rapeseed oil into Spain, oil imported for industrial purposes is partially refined and, to indicate that the oil is not edible, aniline is added as an organic colorant. Those who substituted partially refined rapeseed oil for olive oil presumably tried to extract the aniline in order to restore the original color of the oil. In the process, they overlooked the formation of oleoanalides by the reaction of the aniline with the natural organic acids (mainly oleic and linoleic) in the oil as well as the possibility of other toxic substances (21).

THE NATURE OF THE TOXIC SUBSTANCE(S)

Despite the clear epidemiologic relationship between the syndrome and the sale and consumption of denatured and re-refined rapeseed oil, the etiologic agent(s) has not been identified. Moreover, the disease has not been completely reproduced in animals. Nonetheless, three toxic components are strongly linked with the disease: most important are the oleoanilides; other possibilities are peroxidants and free radicals derived from the oleoanilides (22). However, the likelihood is strong that the toxin will never be identified since it was unstable and could not be found in samples of the toxic oil.

TOXIC PROCESS

Several theories have been advanced to explain the toxic process. A direct action of the toxic material absorbed through the portal or lymphatic vessels or even inhaled during cooking has been postulated for the early stage of the disease. Later on, lipoperoxidation of cell membranes and activation of arachidonic acid resulting from damaged eosinophils may be a contributing mechanism (5,21,22). Lastly, an autoimmune process seems to be involved since autoantibodies have been found in some patients and many manifestations of the disease are the result of immunoallergic reactions (22,33). However, whether autoimmune reactions are the cause or effect of the clinical syndrome is unclear.

PULMONARY HYPERTENSION

Incidence

Pulmonary hypertension was first detected in June 1981 as one of the main manifestations of the toxic oil syndrome. From an initial incidence of 2.3 percent (27), the incidence of pulmonary hypertension increased rapidly thereafter so that between July and September 1981, estimates of incidence ranged from 9.3 percent (27) to 16 to 24 percent of patients with the toxic oil syndrome (1,3,8–11,15,21–22,24,28). After January 1982, the incidence of pulmonary hypertension decreased progressively. In December 1985, a randomized prospective study demonstrated an incidence of at least 1.5 percent in the population of patients who had suffered the disease. (H. Primero de Octubre and H. La Paz, unpublished observations). Recently, new cases of severe pulmonary hypertension have been detected, mainly in patients who had developed transient pulmonary hypertension in 1982.

Although risk factors for the development of pulmonary hypertension have not been found, a familial tendency has been found, with a higher prevalence in children 9 to 12 years old and in women (3:1) (1,8,9,15).

Course

In many patients, hemodynamic and clinical evidence of pulmonary hypertension, i.e., right ventricular hypertrophy and dilation of the pulmonary artery, faded within 6 months of onset. However, in 1 to 2 percent of the patients with the toxic oil syndrome, pulmonary hypertension persisted and became increasingly important after several years. Between 1986 and 1987, severe pulmonary hypertension was the leading cause of death among the sequelae of the toxic oil syndrome. Moreover, some patients who had experienced transient pulmonary hypertension in 1981, subsequently developed pulmonary hypertension after years of supposed return toward normotension.

Pathogenesis of Pulmonary Hypertension

The list of hypotheses to explain the development of pulmonary hypertension in the toxic oil syndrome includes pulmonary thromboembolism, hypoxic vasoconstriction, direct alpha-adrenergic stimulation by the toxic material, lactic acidosis, the release of endogenous catecholamines or vasoactive hormones, direct damage by toxic hepatic metabolites, and pulmonary endothelial swelling and proliferation. Of these, only the latter is based on well-documented data (18,22).

Our clinical and pathological experience permits the exclusion of some of these causes of pulmonary hypertension and favors certain pathogenic mechanisms. We performed right heart catheterization in 46 patients in whom pulmonary hypertension was suspected on clinical grounds. In those patients with moderate or severe pulmonary hypertension, pharmacological testing was done, including the administration of oxygen, tolazoline, isoproterenol, and other vasodilators. Angiograms were performed on seven patients, platelet function was studied in eight, and pulmonary biopsy specimens were obtained in two. This study was conducted in 1981; the postmortem studies that we reviewed from 32 patients covered the full span of the disease, including nine patients who died of severe pulmonary hypertension in the late stage.

Several possible pathogenetic factors were weighed in our studies: pulmonary fibrosis, obstruction of the pulmonary venous outflow, pulmonary thromboembolism, pulmonary vasoconstriction, platelet dysfunction, and pulmonary vascular lesions.

PULMONARY FIBROSIS

Pulmonary fibrosis seems to offer a ready explanation for pulmonary hypertension in patients who undergo an episode of diffuse and, in most cases, bilateral pneumonia that includes radiographic and anatomic evidence of diffuse interstitial exudation (21,22). Although all patients in our study did experience a bout of pneumonia, it was consistently followed by a period before the development of pulmonary hypertension during which the patient was free of pulmonary symptoms and radiographic signs of exudation or fibrosis (3,28). Moreover, no radiographic evidence of pulmonary fibrosis developed in the long-term follow-up of patients with toxic oil syndrome, regardless of pulmonary hypertension. Other reports based on radiographic (8,9,22) and anatomic studies (18,22) have also discounted the presence of pulmonary fibrosis.

OBSTRUCTION OF PULMONARY VENOUS OUTFLOW

Proliferative lesions in small pulmonary veins have been described in autopsy studies of patients with toxic oil syndrome (18). However, these lesions were found at random after toxic oil syndrome, without any relation to the occurrence of pulmonary hypertension; in general, the lesions were minor and localized. Moreover, if these lesions contributed to the pathogenesis of pulmonary hypertension, as in pulmonary veno-occlusive disease (25), the pulmonary capillary pressure would have been abnormally high. In our patients, as well as in all other patients who have undergone hemodynamic study for evaluation of pulmonary hypertension, pulmonary capillary pressure was consistently within normal limits (8,9,22) even when venous lesions were found in anatomic specimens.

PULMONARY THROMBOSIS AND EMBOLISM

Hematological disorders were manifested in patients with the toxic oil syndrome by moderate increases in prothrombin time and either thrombocytopenia or thrombocytosis (22). The incidence of these abnormalities increased in July 1981 when the epidemic of pulmonary hypertension began (22). Thromboembolic accidents, including pulmonary thrombosis and embolism, occur frequently in patients with the toxic oil syndrome (18,22). Indeed, pulmonary thromboembolism was once considered as a major factor in the development of pulmonary hypertension. However, in patients with documented pulmonary hypertension who came to autopsy, pulmonary thromboembolism was neither consistently present nor considered to be causally related (8,11). Radiographic manifestations of pulmonary embolism were not found in any of our patients. Nor could we demonstrate pulmonary vascular defects suggestive of embolism in eight patients subjected to pulmonary angiography (Fig. 2). For these reasons, it seems unlikely that pulmonary thromboembolism played an appreciable role in the pathogenesis of pulmonary hypertension associated with the toxic oil syndrome, at least in its first stages.

However, pulmonary thrombosis is a frequent postmortem finding in patients

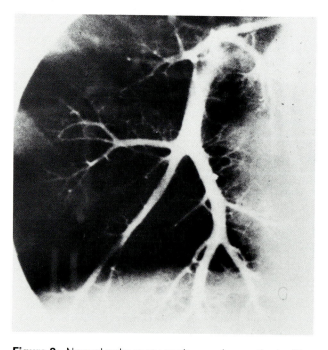

Figure 2: Normal pulmonary angiogram in a patient with severe pulmonary hypertension 4 months after initial symptoms of toxic oil syndrome. Pulmonary arterial pressure = 80/40 mmHg.

who died from pulmonary hypertension after 1985. The possible pathogenetic role of pulmonary vascular thrombosis is not clear, but pulmonary vascular thrombosis might be a contributing mechanism once the pulmonary hypertension is established.

PULMONARY VASOCONSTRICTION

Several lines of evidence suggest a major role for pulmonary vasoconstriction in the pathogenesis of the toxic oil syndrome. For example, calculated pulmonary vascular resistance was increased in all patients studied (Figs. 3 and 4) and was accompanied by a pressure gradient between the diastolic pulmonary and pulmonary wedge pressures. In addition, spontaneous or drug-induced swings in pulmonary arterial pressure and pulmonary vascular resistance were observed during the period of hemodynamic monitoring (Fig. 3). Finally, pulmonary hypertension proved to be reversible in many patients with the toxic oil syndrome (3,8,9) (Figs. 3 and 4), further supporting the presence of vasoconstriction in the early stages of the disease. Although the increase in pulmonary vascular resistance, the gradient between diastolic pulmonary and pulmonary wedge pressures and reversibility could reflect regression of pulmonary vascular lesions, it is difficult to explain the responses to pharmacological agents or the spontaneous fluctuations in pressure by other than changes in pulmonary vasomotor tone.

In addition to the spontaneous and drug-induced changes in pulmonary arterial pressure and vascular pulmonary resistances, up to 28 percent of patients with the toxic oil syndrome have manifested Raynaud's phenomenon (22). This observation is consistent with the idea of an increase in pulmonary arterial tone in those patients in whom Raynaud's phenomenon and pulmonary hypertension coexist (4,19,25).

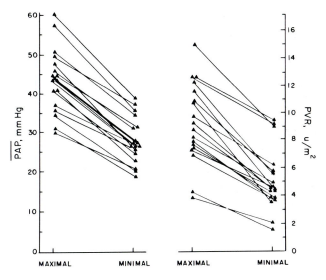

Figure 3: Spontaneous or drug-induced maximal and minimal values of mean pulmonary arterial pressure ($\bar{P}AP$) and pulmonary vascular resistance (PVR) during 3 days of hemodynamic monitoring (1981). U/m² = resistance units per square meter of body surface area.

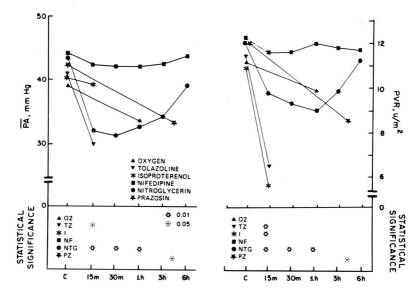

Figure 4: Mean values of pulmonary artery pressure and pulmonary vascular resistances before and after drug administration (1981). Tolazoline produced a marked reduction in both pulmonary arterial pressure and pulmonary vascular resistance; no significant changes occurred after oxygen administration; a varying, although significant, effect was observed after nitroglycerin, isoproterenol, and prazosin.

Other investigators using hydralazine, nifedipine, and diazoxide have failed to demonstrate that vasoactive drugs are effective in patients with the toxic oil syndrome (8,9). However, the number of patients in these acute studies was small. Verapamil studied in a larger group of 20 patients also proved ineffective (9). We used tolazoline, isoproterenol, nitroglycerin, and prazosin (Fig. 4), agents that were not used in the previous studies. Our results support the idea of pulmonary vasomotricity in the toxic oil syndrome. However, in a recent study involving nine patients with severe pulmonary hypertension (systolic pulmonary artery pressure > 80 mmHg) during 1986 and 1987, the oral and intravenous administration of different vasodilators failed to modify the values of pulmonary artery pressure or pulmonary vascular resistances (H. Primero de Octubre, unpublished observations). These divergent experiences with vasodilator agents in the toxic oil syndrome are difficult to reconcile but may reflect different stages in the evolution of pulmonary vascular lesions in the toxic oil syndrome.

Hypoxia, an important stimulus for pulmonary arterial vasoconstriction (4,19), was common early in the course of the toxic oil syndrome. However, in all patients whom we and others have studied, the acute illness and initial interstitial pneumonia subsided, arterial P_{O_2} values were greater than 70 mmHg when pulmonary hypertension was first detected (18). Moreover, oxygen administration failed to reduce pulmonary artery pressure or pulmonary vascular resistances (8,9) (Fig. 4). Later in the course, most patients with established pulmonary hypertension had low values for diffusing capacity alterations and for arterial P_{O_2}.

PLATELET DYSFUNCTION

It has been proposed that platelets are involved in the pathogenesis of pulmonary vasoconstriction and hypertension (4,17). Platelet factor 4 and/or beta thromboglobulin were abnormally increased in all the patients in our study, suggesting an abnormally increased platelet activation that might play an important role in evoking pulmonary vasoconstriction in the toxic oil syndrome. The values of these parameters were normal in a control group of 10 patients with the toxic oil syndrome studied hemodynamically who did not have pulmonary hypertension. Structural abnormalities in platelets have been demonstrated by electron microscopy.

Although platelet activation may be caused by direct action of the toxic material on platelets, it is more apt to be due to endothelial lesions in the pulmonary vessels. Platelet activation could play a major role in pulmonary vasoconstriction by releasing powerful vasoconstrictor substances, e.g., thromboxane A$_2$. Although the role of vasoactive substances released by platelets in the genesis of pulmonary hypertension remains speculative (17), it is possible that they contribute to the pulmonary vasoconstrictive component of pulmonary hypertension in the toxic oil syndrome (17,20).

VASCULAR LESIONS

Histological changes in the pulmonary vessels of patients with the toxic oil syndrome who develop pulmonary hypertension undergo a characteristic sequence (18,21,22). The initial lesions appear to be located in the pulmonary vascular endothelium and are characterized by cytoplasmic vacuolation and swelling. After July 1981, infiltration of the vascular lumen by lymphocytes (without fibrinoid necrosis) and cell proliferation and intimal fibrosis partially obliterated the vascular lumens of small arteries, arterioles, and capillaries. Later, progressively marked hypertrophy of the media in elastic and muscular pulmonary arteries was a constant finding. Plexiform lesions were first detected in postmortem specimens after 29 months and were found almost regularly in postmortem studies of patients who died of pulmonary hypertension after 1985 (eight of nine cases). Although these findings resemble those described in vasoconstrictive primary pulmonary hypertension (25), the general pathological picture of pulmonary hypertension after toxic oil syndrome is somewhat different. First, the initial lesion was located in the endothelium and muscular hypertrophy was a late finding. Additionally, in some cases, intimal fibrosis was eccentric and many patients presented with venous fibrosis and intravascular thrombi.

Although the observed vascular lesions may contribute to increased pulmonary vascular resistances, they do not discount the evidence for pulmonary vasomotricity. The mechanism responsible for the increase in pulmonary vascular tone is unclear. However, the possibility exists that damage to the pulmonary vascular endothelium may trigger the release of vasoactive materials, either directly by endothelial cells or by an interplay involving platelets and mast cells (4).

It is also noteworthy that even though pulmonary vascular lesions were found in many patients with the toxic oil syndrome (18), pulmonary hypertension developed in only about 20 percent of the affected population. The reported familial incidence, the prevalence of the disorder in women, and the occurrence of pulmonary hypertension in a fraction of those with the toxic oil syndrome suggest that individual susceptibility or hyperresponsiveness of the pulmonary arterial tree may be involved in the pathogenesis of pulmonary hypertension. Moreover, the demonstration of plexiform lesions in the late stages of the disease raises the prospect that some cases designated as primary pulmonary hypertension may

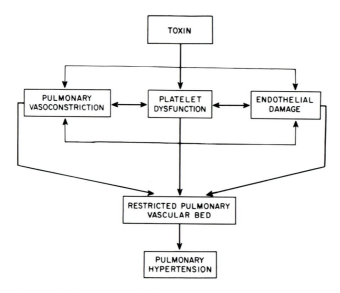

Figure 5: Hypothetical initiating mechanisms leading to pulmonary hypertension in the toxic oil syndrome.

have an exogenous, perhaps dietary, origin. Nevertheless, pulmonary hypertension in the toxic oil syndrome differs in many respects from other forms of dietary pulmonary hypertension.

In summary, it seems reasonable to exclude pulmonary fibrosis, pulmonary venous outflow obstruction, hypoxia, and pulmonary thromboembolism as major mechanisms of early pulmonary hypertension in the toxic oil syndrome. Instead, our experience favors pulmonary vasoconstriction, endothelial and platelet abnormalities, all factors that may be interrelated (7) (Fig. 5).

Unfortunately with respect to pathogenesis, many aspects of the pulmonary hypertension associated with the toxic oil syndrome remain difficult to assess: the ingredient of the toxin responsible for the syndrome has not been identified. Nor have studies of platelets and vasoactive materials been performed in comparable clinical settings. Nonetheless, there seems to be little doubt that the toxic oil syndrome is a distinct type of dietary pulmonary hypertension and that dietary pulmonary hypertension should be considered separately from the unexplained forms of pulmonary hypertension that are currently designated as "primary pulmonary hypertension."

REFERENCES

1. Bano-Rodrigo A, Herrainz I, Quero M, Hernandez M: Problemas cardiológicos en niños con síndrome tóxico. Simposium Nacional Síndrome Tóxico. Madrid, Ministerio de Sanidad y Consumo, 1982.

2. Chun PK, San Antonio PR, Davia JE: Laennec's cirrhosis and primary pulmonary hypertension. Am Heart J 99:779–782, 1980.

3. Coma-Canella I, López-Sendón J: Hemody-

namic effect of nifedipine, nitroglycerin and prazosin in pulmonary hypertension following ingestion of toxic oil. Eur Heart J 4:566–572, 1983.

4. Daoud FS, Reeves JT, Kelly DB: Isoproterenol as a potential pulmonary vasodilator in primary pulmonary hypertension. Am J Cardiol 42:817–822, 1978.

5. De la Morena E, Montero C: Low-serum L-carnitine concentrations in toxic oil syndrome. Lancet 1:904, 1982.

6. Fishman AP: Dietary pulmonary hypertension. Circ Res 35:657–660, 1974.

7. Fishman AP: Primary pulmonary hypertension, in Fishman AP (ed), *Pulmonary Diseases and Disorders*. New York, McGraw-Hill, 1980, pp 847–852.

8. García-Dorado D, Diller DD, García EJ, Delcán JL, Maroto E, Chaitman BR: An epidemic of pulmonary hypertension after toxic rapeseed oil ingestion in Spain. J Am Coll Cardiol 1:1216–1222, 1983.

9. Gomez Recio M, Martinez Elbal L, Rodrigo López JL, Salva Ariern J, Alcazar J, Zarco P: Hipertensión pulmonar en el síndrome tóxico. N Arch Fac Med 41:237–244, 1983.

10. Gomez Sanchez MA, Gomez Pajuelo C, Romanyk Cabrera JP, Dominguez Lozano MJ, Regato Pajares R: Hipertensión pulmonar en el síndrome tóxico. N Arch Fac Med 41:385–386, 1983.

11. Grupo del Hospital 1° de Octubre. Anatomía patológica del síndrome tóxico. Simposium Nacional Síndrome Tóxico. Madrid, Ministerio de Sanidad y Consumo, 1982.

12. Gurtner HP, Gertsch M, Salzmann C, Scherrer M, Stucki P, Wyss F: Haufen sich die primar vascularen formen des chronischen cor pulmonale? Schweiz Med Wochenschr 98:1579–1589, 1968.

13. Kay JM, Heath D: *Crotalaria Spectabilis. The Pulmonary Hypertension Plant*. Springfield, IL, Charles C. Thomas, 1969.

14. Kleiger RE, Boxer M, Ingham RE, Harrison DC: Pulmonary hypertension in patients using oral contraceptives. Chest 69:143–147, 1976.

15. López-Sendón J, Coma-Canella I: Patología cardiaca en el Síndrome Tóxico. Simposium Nacional Síndrome Tóxico. Madrid, Ministerio de Sanidad y Consumo, 1982.

16. López-Sendón J, Coma-Canella I: Pulmonary hypertension following ingestion of toxic cooking oil. Clin Respir Physiol 18:83, 1983.

17. Martin JF, Slater DN, Trowbridge EA: Abnormal intrapulmonary platelet production. A possible cause of vascular and lung disease. Lancet 1:793–796, 1983.

18. Martinez Tello FJ, Navas Palacios JJ, Ricoy JR, Gil Martin R, Conde Zurita JM, Colina Ruiz Delgado F, Tellez I, Cabello A, Madero García S: Pathology of a new toxic syndrome caused by ingestion of adulterated oil in Spain. Virchows Arch [Pathol Anat] 397:261–285, 1982.

19. Rounds S, Hill NS: Pulmonary hypertensive diseases. Chest 85:397–405, 1984.

20. Rubin LJ, Lazar JD: Influence of prostaglandin synthesis inhibitors on pulmonary vasodilatory effects of hydralazine in dogs with hypoxic pulmonary vasoconstriction. J Clin Invest 67:193–200, 1981.

21. Tabuenca JM: Toxic-allergic syndrome caused by ingestion of rapeseed oil denatured with aniline. Lancet 2:567–568, 1981.

22. Toxic epidemic syndrome, Spain, 1981. Toxic Epidemic Syndrome Study Group. Lancet 2:697–702, 1982.

23. Vicario JL, Serrano M, San Andres F, Arnaiz-Villena A: HLA-DR3, DR4 increase in chronic stage of Spanish oil disease. Lancet 1:276, 1982.

24. Villamor J, Rodriguez E, Pozo F: Descripción clínica de la enfermedad en adultos. Simposium Nacional Síndrome Tóxico. Madrid, Ministerio de Sanidad y Consumo, 1982.

25. Wagenvoort CA, Wagenvoort N: Primary pulmonary hypertension. Pathologic study of the lung vessels in 156 clinically diagnosed cases. Circulation 42:1163–1184, 1970.

26. Wagenvoort CA, Wagenvoort N: *Pathology of Pulmonary Hypertension*. New York, John Wiley & Sons, 1977.

27. Working group on denatured rapeseed toxic oil syndrome. El síndrome del aceite tóxico. Intoxicación alimentaria masiva en España. World Health Organization. Copenhagen. 1984, pp 1–87.

28. Yoldi M, López-Sendón J, Coma-Canella I, Sanz J, Martín Jadraque L: Hipertensión pulmonar en el síndrome tóxico. Correlacion clínico hemodinámica. Rev Esp Cardiol 35:I:59, 1982.

Hans Peter Gurtner, M.D.

29

Aminorex Pulmonary Hypertension

There has been an epidemic of chronic pulmonary hypertension in Austria, the Federal Republic of Germany (FRG), and Switzerland, which started in 1967, had its peak in 1968 and 1969, and disappeared after 1972. The mechanism leading to pulmonary hypertension was precapillary vascular obstruction due to plexogenic pulmonary arteriopathy. There was a close geographic as well as a temporal relationship between the epidemic and the marketing and the intake of the appetite-depressant drug, aminorex (MENOCIL*). The new disease followed a more rapid initial course; however, the long-term prognosis of aminorex associated pulmonary hypertension turned out to be less dismal than that of plexogenic primary and thromboembolic pulmonary hypertension and of pulmonary venoocclusive disease, respectively.

REVIEW OF THE EPIDEMIC OF AMINOREX ASSOCIATED PULMONARY HYPERTENSION

Initial Observations

In 1967 and even more so in the first half of 1968, we observed a sudden and marked increase in the incidence of chronic pulmonary hypertension of vascular

*This drug had not been approved by the Food and Drug Administration at the time of the epidemic's onset, nor has it been approved since.

origin (CPHVO) among the annual total of adult individuals investigated by means of cardiac catheterization. Within 12 months, the incidence had risen by a factor of 20 (10). Similar observations were made at the same time in Basel, Geneva, Lausanne, and Zurich and, somewhat later and less marked, in Austria and the Federal Republic of Germay (quoted in ref. 8).

For the sake of presentation, chronic pulmonary hypertension of vascular origin (CPHVO) is defined as a pathophysiological entity: precapillary pulmonary vascular resistance is abnormally high due to obstructive and/or obliterative lesions originating in the pulmonary arterioles and small muscular arteries. CPHVO is identified by excluding, by means of the appropriate hemodynamic and pulmonary function studies, the following: (1) precapillary vasoconstriction due to alveolar hypoxia, (2) restriction of the pulmonary vascular bed due to interstitial pulmonary parenchymal disease, (3) high flow pulmonary hypertension due to central left-to-right shunts, and (4) pulmonary venous congestion. CPHVO includes classical primary pulmonary hypertension, recurrent pulmonary thromboembolism, the rare condition of pulmonary hypertension in cirrhosis of the liver with portal hypertension, certain collagen diseases, schistosomiasis and congenital peripheral pulmonary stenosis, as well as aminorex-related pulmonary hypertension.

The patients with CPHVO whom we studied from 1967 to 1968 ("new" series) differed from those investigated prior to 1967 ("old" series) in several respects. A history of pulmonary embolism was rare (13 percent versus 62 percent). In the more recent population, the disease progressed rapidly; the interval between the onset of complaints and hospital admission lasted for only 10 months compared to more than 4 years in the old series. A lung biopsy taken in four patients gave no evidence of thromboembolic or inflammatory pulmonary vascular disease; instead, there was marked fibrosis and hyalinosis in the small pulmonary arteries and arterioles. Half of the patients studied since 1967 were more or less overweight in contrast to the one in eight in the old series. Seventeen out of the 23 new patients had tried to get rid of their effective (or imaginary) overweight by means of an appetite-depressant agent. They admitted ingesting the anorectic drug aminorex fumarate (MENOCIL) before the onset of first symptoms, i.e., dyspnea, syncope, and chest pain on exertion (10).

Aminorex

Aminorex (2-amino-5-phenyl-2-oxazoline) resembles adrenaline and ephedrine in its chemical structure. It acts as a potent anorexigen in most individuals and as a central stimulant in many. The drug was introduced on the Swiss market in November 1965 and withdrawn in October 1968.

Incidence of CPHVO, Bern, 1955–1986

In our institution, the average incidence of CPHVO (Fig. 1) was as low as 1.2 percent for the years 1955–1966. During the epidemic from 1967 to 1973, the average incidence increased to 8.0 percent, reaching a peak of 16.3 percent in 1968 and 16.0 percent in 1969. The rate of increase in incidence was similar to the

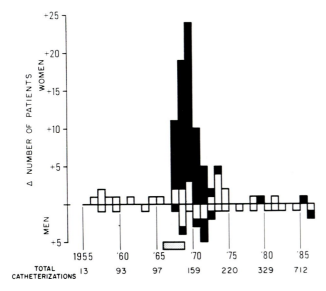

Figure 1: Frequency distribution of patients with chronic pulmonary hypertension of vascular origin (CPHVO) investigated in Bern, 1955–1986. The vertical columns represent the absolute number of individuals with CPHVO for each year: the female patients above the zero line; the male patients below the zero line. Individuals with a positive history of aminorex intake are indicated in black. The figure of catheterization procedures in adults is given at the bottom for each year. The average incidence of CPHVO in % of the catheterizations is indicated for various periods (plain type for all cases of CPHVO, bold type for aminorex-positive cases). The stippled horizontal bar refers to the duration of the aminorex marketing in Switzerland.

rate of decline. After 1973, the incidence of CPHVO in our patients dropped to lower than the pre-epidemic level (averaging 0.27 between 1974 and 1986); this low percentage is undoubtedly due to the increased number of catheterizations done in recent years in patients with ischemic heart disease.

During the epidemic, women were affected 4.5 times more frequently than men (f:m = 76:17). Almost six out of seven females (64/76) and slightly less than half of the males (7/17) had a history of aminorex intake prior to the onset of their symptoms. Thus, 76 percent of all 93 patients studied during the epidemic had a history of aminorex intake (9).

These observations correspond to those obtained by a German study group in Austria, the Federal Republic of Germany, and Switzerland (see section on Epidemiology).

CLINICAL AND FUNCTIONAL FINDINGS

CPHVO was identified in all patients by right heart catheterization, arterial blood gas analysis, plain chest radiographs, and pulmonary function studies. In this way, left-to-right shunts, alveolar hypoventilation, pulmonary parenchymal disease, and pulmonary venous congestion were ruled out as pathogenetic mechanisms. Pulmonary arteriography and perfusion scintigraphy, as well as the determination of the pulmonary diffusing capacity for oxygen (18), were carried out in a limited number of patients. So were the analyses of blood coagulation factors, the adhesivity and the life span of platelets. In addition, lung biopsies and autopsies were available by 1970.

A comparison of the patients with a positive history of aminorex intake (N = 71) and those without (N = 29) revealed that the two groups differed from each other only in that the aminorex-free group more often had of a history of pulmonary embolism (44 percent versus 12 percent) and no overweight (− 3 percent of the ideal weight versus + 15 percent) (8). Only the data of the aminorex-positive group are considered further below.

Symptoms and Signs

Dyspnea on exertion was the leading symptom (98 percent) followed by exertional chest pain (45 percent) and effort syncope (38 percent). A loud and often palpable second heart sound in the second left intercostal space was an important clue for the clinical diagnosis (94 percent). The same was true for the usually marked right axis deviation of the QRS-complex in the frontal plane of the electrocardiogram (+ 109 ± 44°). Central cyanosis (81 percent) and signs of right ventricular failure (67 percent) occurred frequently; pulmonary regurgitation was rare. Overweight was only moderate. Ninety percent of the patients were in the NYHA-classes III and IV and suffered from considerable exercise intolerance. Astonishingly, all patients were in regular sinus rhythm.

Lung Function, Arterial Blood Gases, and Hemodynamics

Arterial hypoxemia was slight (Sa_{O_2} 91 ± 4%) and arterial hypocapnia severe (Pa_{CO_2} 33 ± 3 mmHg), the latter reflecting alveolar hyperventilation. The residual volume, expressed as a percent of total lung capacity, was practically normal (31 ± 6%); so were the vital capacity and the forced expiratory volume, excluding chronic airways obstruction. Evidence of right ventricular failure was present in that both end-diastolic right ventricular (15 ± 7 mmHg) and mean right atrial (10 ± 5 mmHg) pressures were abnormally high. Marked pulmonary hypertension of the vaso-obstructive type was present (mean PA pressure of 50 ± 12 mmHg); the mean PA-wedge pressure did not exceed normal (9 ± 4 mmHg). The cardiac index averaged one third below normal (2.2 ± 0.7 L/min · m²). As a result, pulmonary vascular resistance was greatly increased, i.e., by more than 15 times (960 ± 392 dyn · sec/cm⁵).

Lung tissue from six biopsies and six autopsies demonstrated plexogenic pulmonary arteriopathy in all instances (14). Blood coagulation factors and the adhesivity and the life span of platelets were normal (10).

From the data presented in this section, it can be concluded that aminorex-associated pulmonary hypertension cannot be differentiated from classical primary pulmonary hypertension and from thromboembolic pulmonary hypertension by clinical and functional findings alone. Moreover, it shares with primary pulmonary hypertension the angiographic, scintigraphic and morphological findings. However, it differs from primary pulmonary hypertension in that its initial course and long-term prognosis are different (see section on Prognosis).

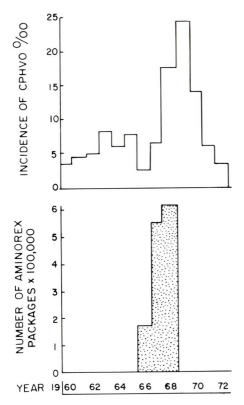

Figure 2: Incidence of patients with chronic pulmonary hypertension of vascular origin in % of catheterization procedures (upper ordinate). Data collected by a German study group and representing a total of 582 patients (1960–1972). The lower ordinates represent the number of aminorex packages sold (stippled columns). (Reproduced from Greiser [7] by permission of *Springer-Verlag*.)

RELATION BETWEEN EVENT AND FACTOR

In the following section the relationships between the epidemic of pulmonary hypertension and the etiological role of the anorexigen, aminorex, are analyzed in terms of epidemiology, pharmacology, and pharmacogenetics of drug hydroxylation.

Epidemiology

In a cooperative retrospective study, 23 centers from Austria, the Federal Republic of Germany, and Switzerland contributed to a collection of 582 cases with chronic pulmonary hypertension of vascular origin (CPHVO) that occurred during the period between 1960 and 1972 (7). As can be seen in Figure 2, pattern of distribution of incidence versus time is almost identical with that shown in Figure 1: starting to increase in 1967, peaking in 1968 and 1969, and reaching a maximum (3.1 percent) in 1969; subsequently, it drops to the pre-epidemic level (less than 0.6 percent). During the epidemic, 62 percent of affected patients gave a history of ingesting aminorex (alone or in combination with other anorectic drugs); a few patients had used anorexigens other than aminorex. These observations are epidemiologically noteworthy in four respects: (1) the epidemic was limited to those countries where aminorex had been sold; in countries that did not market the drug, the prevalence of CPHVO showed no more than random fluctuation from 1965 until 1972 (7); (2) in our institution, the onset of the typical symptoms of pulmonary hypertension generally followed the start of aminorex therapy by about 12 months; in addition, a corresponding lag in incidence occurred in West German hospitals (Fig. 2) (7); (3) the incidence of CPHVO during the epidemic did not increase above pre- and postepidemic levels by a mere 50 percent; instead, the peaks were as high as 13- and 60-fold, respectively; and (4) after the epidemic ended, the incidence of CPHVO returned to, and remained at, a low level in the Austrian, the West German, and the Swiss cardiology centers.

Even though the association between the epidemic and aminorex is strong with respect to time, geography, and frequency, it should be noted that the incidence of pulmonary hypertension in individuals who had no history of aminorex intake was also increased, especially during the early years of the epidemic (Fig. 1). However, this increase did not exceed the random changes in the prevalence of CPHVO that occurred during the same period in countries in which aminorex was not sold (7). In addition, some patients with CPHVO who originally denied the ingestion of aminorex, subsequently reversed themselves and admitted to ingesting the agent.

Anorexigens other than aminorex, such as chlorphentermine, phentermine, phenmetrazine, cloforex, pentorex, and amphetamine, were ingested by a minority of patients with CPHVO during the epidemic: in Switzerland, the fraction of such patients was minimal (29); in the cooperative study noted above, 33 percent of the patients gave no history of ingesting anorectic drugs, 48 percent had ingested aminorex alone, 13 percent had used aminorex in combination with other anorexigens, and 6 percent had consumed anorectic drugs other than aminorex. The German authors concluded that except for chlorphentermine and cloforex, there was no significant association between anorexigens other than aminorex and the development of CPHVO (7,16).

Pharmacology

Aminorex was synthesized by Poos in 1963 (20). Subsequently, Yelnosky et al., in open chest dogs anesthetized with phenobarbital, found that the drug increased transiently the contractile strength of the right heart, the systemic arterial pressure, and the heart rate; injection of a beta-blocking agent reduced the cardiac effect whereas an alpha-blocking drug diminished the effect on the systemic pressure. The effect on the pulmonary circulation was not studied (30). Borbely et al. studied 30 patients with acute aminorex intoxication. They called attention to tachycardia, an increase in systemic blood pressure, and hyperpnea; no fatal case was reported and late sequelae were not mentioned (2). The early clinical experience with aminorex, usually involving small numbers of patients, demonstrated marked weight-reducing and euphoric effects without severe side effects. After reviewing in 1970 the clinical tests done by various research groups at the request of the drug manufacturer of aminorex, Peters and Gourzis reported that in 4,400 subjects there occurred one instance of pulmonary hypertension; in addition, tachycardia, shortness of breath, edema, chest pain, fainting, and electrocardiographic changes were encountered in an appreciable number of patients (19).

After the initial clinical report suggesting the possibility of an association between the sudden increase in the incidence of CPHVO and the intake of aminorex, new and sophisticated pharmacological studies were undertaken in a variety of species: open and closed chest dogs, rats, monkeys, pigs, and calves, either in a single dose, in repeated doses, or chronically, i.e., up to 2 years' administration. The results of these experiments can be summarized as follows: (1) acute and subacute administration of aminorex leads to a marked, but transient, increase in pulmonary arterial pressure and in pulmonary vascular resistance in most of the species tested; and (2) however, it has not proved possible to induce chronic pulmonary hypertension or plexogenic pulmonary arteriopathy after chronic administration of the drug (see 8 and 9 for references).

How do these negative results using animals apply to the question whether aminorex played a conditioning or etiological role in the origin of the epidemic of pulmonary hypertension? In all likelihood, their implication for the human disorder is minimal: (1) too few animals were used for generalization since only 1 per 1,000 of those humans who took the drug developed pulmonary hypertension (7); (2) marked differences exist between animals and humans, among animals of different species, and even among different breeds of the same species, with respect to transport mechanisms and the metabolism of drugs. The varying response of different species to acute hypoxia is a case in point: the hypoxic pulmonary pressor response is marked in cattle, particularly in hyperreactive breeds, but it is small or even absent in the sheep, the cat, and the llama.

Dose-Response Relationship

A correlation between the total amount of aminorex ingested and the degree of pulmonary hypertension has not been demonstrated. However, it has been proposed that the risk of developing pulmonary hypertension does increase with the amount of aminorex consumed (7). In addition, the mortality was four times greater in patients who had taken a large total dose of aminorex (see section on Prognosis).

Pharmacogenetics of Drug Hydroxylation

It was noted above that the incidence of CPHVO among aminorex consumers was small. We undertook to find out if the responders are characterized by a pharmacogenetic predisposition, e.g., in the form of deficient drug hydroxylation.

There are three major ways by which a drug like aminorex can be eliminated: glomerular filtration, excretion via the liver into the bile, and metabolic transformation in the liver, e.g., hydroxylation, followed by renal elimination of the metabolites. It was known from previous studies that 80 percent of aminorex is metabolized and excreted in the urine; the remainder is eliminated in the feces. Since testing of aminorex in humans was felt to be unwarranted on ethical grounds, the hydroxylation of debrisoquine (D) and mephenytoin (M) was investigated in 17 patients who had aminorex-related pulmonary hypertension. Sixteen of the 17 proved to be efficient hydroxylators both with D and M (23). This result is comparable to the frequency distributions of efficient and inefficient hydroxylators in a healthy Swiss population. Therefore, the occurrence of pulmonary hypertension after the intake of aminorex cannot be attributed to a disturbance in the genetically controlled hydroxylation mechanism of D and M. However, this finding does not exclude the possibility of another defect of drug hydroxylation in these patients.

Morphology

It had been concluded as early as in 1968 that the morphological changes of the pulmonary vasculature in patients with aminorex-related pulmonary hypertension were not compatible with recurrent pulmonary thromboembolism. Two years later, based on a larger material, Laissue (14) and Widgren and Kapanci (28) concluded that the morphological changes in the small muscular pulmonary arteries were identical with those described by Heath and Edwards (13) in children with pulmonary hypertension and large congenital left-to-right shunts.

In 1977, Widgren published a report, based on material provided by eight Swiss pathological institutes, which detailed the morphological findings in 37 patients who had developed pulmonary hypertension after the intake of aminorex (26). The clinical and the autopsy findings can be summarized as follows: sex, 34 females and 3 males; age, 50 ± 2.3 years; duration of the aminorex treatment, 271 ± 40 days; total dose of aminorex consumed, 249 ± 33 tablets (14 mg per tablet); mean pulmonary artery pressure, 52 ± 2 mmHg (22 patients); pulmonary vascular resistance, 1258 ± 80 dyn $\cdot$ sec/cm^5 (20 patients); heart weight, 427 ± 15 g; and thickness of the right ventricular wall, 7.7 ± 0.6 mm (30 patients). Right ventricular failure was the cause of death in 26 out of 35 patients.

The lesions in the muscular pulmonary arteries that ranged in diameter between 100 and 1000 μ did not differ significantly from those of classical primary pulmonary hypertension or of high flow secondary pulmonary hypertension, i.e., from the pattern of lesions termed plexogenic pulmonary arteriopathy by a working group of the World Health Organization in 1973 (12). These lesions include (1) medial hypertrophy, (2) intimal hyperplasia, (3a) intimal fibrosis, (3b) diffuse dilatation lesions, (4) plexiform lesions, (5) angiomatoid lesions plus hemosiderosis, and (6) necrosis. Reports since then have confirmed that aminorex-related pulmonary hypertension shares a pattern of pulmonary vascular morphology with other forms of chronic pulmonary hypertension, e.g., primary pulmonary hypertension and congenital malformations of the heart with large left-to-right shunts. In addition, it occurs in some patients with cirrhosis of the liver and portal hypertension, and with schistosomiasis. The possibility then arises that plexogenic pulmonary arteriography represents a nonspecific pattern of pulmonary vascular reactivity.

LONG-TERM COURSE AND PROGNOSIS

Experience during the last 17 years has shown that the prognosis of aminorex-related pulmonary hypertension is better than that of both primary and thromboembolic pulmonary hypertension; in fact, partial remissions are common (1,3,6,22,24).

Between 1967 and 1973, 71 patients with aminorex-related pulmonary hypertension were investigated at our institution. They were characterized as follows:

sex, 64 females and 7 males; age, 49 years (28 to 68 years); aminorex consumption, 150 tablets (10 to more than 600); duration of aminorex intake, 2 weeks to more than 2 years; mean PA pressure, 50 mmHg (24 to 76 mmHg). From 1979 to 1980, we restudied a part of the original population. By October 1979, the beginning of the follow-up study, 34 patients had died; their average age was 53 years (37 to 71 years); the mean survival was 3.5 years (3 months to 10.5 years).

Aminorex-Positive Patients: Improvement Versus Deterioration

Of the 37 survivors, 20 patients were restudied (19 women and 1 man). This sample of 20 patients was representative of all survivors with respect to age, lean body mass, heart size, lung function, blood gases, pulmonary hemodynamics, and the amount of aminorex ingested at the time of the initial study. The interval between the original study and the reinvestigation was 10.5 years (7.7 to 12 years). The repeat study entailed a complete clinical investigation including a lung function study and right heart catheterization. Exercise testing during catheterization, either bicycle ergometry or handgrip, was limited to those patients in whom the restudy revealed a lower resting pulmonary arterial pressure than was found at the time of initial study. Treatment in the interval between the two studies was limited to digitalis and diuretics in those patients who were in right heart failure at the time of initial study or who developed right heart failure in the course of their disease. All patients but one was orally anticoagulated; anticoagulation was continued for at least 3 years in all patients and, in most, for the duration of the entire observation period (9,11).

The patients were divided into two subgroups depending on whether the mean PA pressure had fallen or risen during the observation period. In 12 patients, hemodynamics improved markedly; the cardiac index increased on the average by 50 percent, the mean PA pressure decreased by 24 mmHg or 50 percent, the pulmonary vascular resistance decreased by 67 percent, and the heart rate decreased by -20 percent. The right ventricular end-diastolic pressure decreased considerably, on the average by 8 mmHg, returning to normal in all who had initially been in frank right heart failure. In the subgroup with *worsened* hemodynamics (eight patients), the mean pulmonary arterial pressure increased by 23 percent and the pulmonary vascular resistance by 44 percent on the average; the cardiac index and the heart rate remained essentially unchanged. The right ventricular end-diastolic pressure normalized in half of the patients who had been in right heart failure when first studied.

The correlation between the change in hemodynamics and the change in complaints was disappointingly poor: although two-thirds of the *improved* group gave a history of an improved exercise tolerance together with the disappearance of effort angina and syncope, the same subjective improvement was reported by half of the worsened group.

In the *improved* group, the axis of QRS in the frontal plane shifted from a rightward deviation toward an intermediate position. Partial right bundle branch block disappeared in three out of six patients and a P pulmonale in seven out of eleven. In the worsened group, there was no significant change in the axis of QRS, and P pulmonale persisted in all patients who had this abnormality when first studied years before. Sinus rhythm was maintained in all patients of both groups, except in one patient who developed atrial fibrillation. In the *improved* group, the cardiothoracic ratio based on the chest radiograph diminished slightly and the arterial P_{CO_2} normalized, whereas in the *worsened* group, the heart size increased and hypocapnia became more marked.

Even though the workload during bicycle ergometry was small (47 watts during 4 min on the average) and the handgrip test was not tolerated for more than 5 min by most women, the pulmonary arterial pressure and the pulmonary vascular resistance increased in all 12 patients tested. The patients in whom resting pulmonary arterial pressure normalized during the observation period underwent the least marked hemodynamic changes during exercise. These findings suggest that pulmonary arteries and arterioles were still abnormal and unable to accommodate increased flow without sizable increments in pressure even in those individuals in whom resting vascular resistance had returned to normal levels. The only difference between the initial findings in the *improved* and *worsened* groups was that the patients who improved hemodynamically were 10 years younger on the average when they began to ingest aminorex.

Aminorex-Positive Patients: Survivors Versus Nonsurvivors

Looking back, there was no difference at the time of initial study, between survivors and nonsurvivors in age, in weight, and in the incidence of risk factors for pulmonary thromboembolism (Table 1). However, mean pulmonary arterial pressure and pulmonary vascular resistance were significantly higher, and right ventricular failure was more frequent initially in the deceased patients.

For the group of aminorex consumers as a whole, no correlation could be established between the total amount of aminorex ingested and mortality. Only if two extreme samples of patients are compared can such a correlation be suspected: in those in whom the total dose was small (less than 40 tablets, N = 9),

TABLE 1 PROGNOSIS OF CHRONIC PULMONARY HYPERTENSION OF VASCULAR ORIGIN (CPHVO): AMINOREX-POSITIVE PATIENTS

	Dead	Alive
Number of patients	34	37
Mean survival in years after diagnosis (cardiac catheterization)	3.5	
Time of first investigation; age, weight, risk factors for pulmonary thrombo-embolism	idem	
Mean pulmonary artery pressure (mmHg)	55 (+22%)	45[a]
Pulmonary arteriolar resistance (dyn · sec/cm[5])	1100 (+40%)	785[a]
Fraction of patients with rightsided cardiac failure	84%	58%[b]

Mortality versus total amount of aminorex ingested:
- whole group   (N = 71): no correlation
- subgroups: < 40 tabl.   (N = 9): mortality 22%
          >400 tabl.   (N = 5): mortality 80%

[a] p < .001
[b] p < .05
SOURCE: Data from Gurtner (9,11). Reproduced by permission.

**TABLE 2 PROGNOSIS OF CHRONIC PULMONARY HYPERTENSION OF VASCULAR ORIGIN (CPHVO):
AMINOREX-POSITIVE VERSUS AMINOREX-NEGATIVE PATIENTS**

	A-positive	A-negative
Number of patients	71	36
Median survival in years after diagnosis (cardiac cath.)	12	4.5
Probability of survival after 10 years	53%	34%[a]
Time of first investigation		
Age	idem	
Mean pulmonary artery pressure (mmHg)	50	52
Duration of symptoms prior to cardiac cath. (months)	14	40
Prevalence of risk factors for pulmonary embolism	idem	
Fraction of patients with long-term anticoagulation	87%	67%[b]
Subgroup with long-term anticoagulation and cardiac cath. 10 or more years ago: survival of 10 years	25/45	1/13[c]

[a]p < .05
[b]p < .025
[c]p < .01
SOURCE: Data from Gurtner (9,11). Reproduced by permission.

the mortality was 22 percent whereas in those with a high total dose (more than 400 tablets, N = 5), the mortality was very high, i.e., 80 percent. These two subgroups did not differ with respect to age and hemodynamics at their initial investigation (9,11).

Aminorex-Positive Versus Aminorex-Negative Patients

In Table 2, survival rates of the 71 aminorex-positive patients and 36 individuals with CPHVO who had no anorexigen exposure are compared. These patients were studied in our institution from 1955 to 1978. In the group without aminorex ingestion, the disease leading to pulmonary hypertension was usually considered, on clinical grounds, to be recurrent pulmonary thromboembolism or primary pulmonary hypertension. In some instances, pulmonary arteriography and autopsy were available. A comparison of survival rates of the two groups is shown in Figure 3. In the aminorex-positive patients, the median survival time was 12 years compared to 4.5 years in the aminorex-negative group. In the aminorex-positive group, the probability of survival is 67 percent after 5 years and 53 percent after 10 years; in the aminorex-negative group, the corresponding figures are 49 percent and 34 percent, respectively. At the time of initial study, the two groups did not differ with respect to age and the degree of pulmonary hypertension. However, the duration of symptoms prior to the hemodynamic investigation averaged 14 months in the aminorex-positive and 40 months in the anorexigen-free group.

It should be noted that long-term oral anticoagulation was instituted more often in the aminorex-positive group (87 percent versus 67 percent). In addition, there was a marked preponderance of females in the aminorex-positive group. Therefore, the two nonrandomized samples are not strictly comparable. However, if comparison of survival is confined to those patients in whom the initial diagnosis was made at least 10 years before, who had been on continuous oral

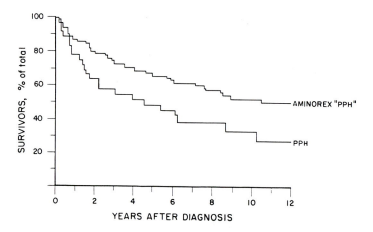

Figure 3: Survival of two groups of patients with chronic pulmonary hypertension of vascular origin: one that consisted of patients who had ingested aminorex (N = 71); the other had no exposure to aminorex. Cumulative monthly survival rates and the survival curves were calculated according to the method of Cutler and Ederer (4), and the two survival curves were compared by applying the log rank test.

anticoagulation, and in whom age (47 versus 49 years) and severity of pulmonary hypertension (mean PA pressure 50 versus 47 mmHg) were comparable, there is a remarkable difference of long-term survival: in the aminorex-positive group, 24 out of 45 patients survived for 10 years, whereas in the anorexigen-free group, only 1 of 13 survived for a corresponding period. Consistent with these results is a more recent experience with long-term use of anticoagulants in 154 pooled patients with primary pulmonary hypertension seen in Vienna and Bern. In the 91 who had taken aminorex and were chronically anticoagulated, aminorex survival was longer than in those who had not taken aminorex (8.48 versus 6.25 years). No statistically significant effect of anticoagulation on survival was found between the two groups who had not taken aminorex but had been anticoagulated even though those coagulated lived longer on the average than those who had not been anticoagulated (4.33 years for those who had taken aminorex and 3.65 years for those who had not) (Drs. Herbert Frank and Hans P. Gurtner, unpublished observations: Table 3). All told, these observations confirm the better prognosis of aminorex-related pulmonary hypertension and suggest a salutory effect of oral anticoagulation in PPH regardless of etiology.

TABLE 3 EFFECT OF CHRONIC ANTICOAGULATION ON SURVIVAL IN PRIMARY PULMONARY HYPERTENSION

	A-positive	A-negative
Number of patients	91	63
Survival, years		
Anticoagulated	8.48	4.33 p = 0.005
Not anticoagulated	6.25	3.65 p = 0.06
	p = 0.1	not significant

Data courtesy of Dr. Herbert Frank.

Therefore, the aminorex-related form of chronic pulmonary hypertension differs from primary and thromboembolic pulmonary hypertension both with respect to an accelerated initial course and a relatively favorable long-term prognosis. These conclusions are in agreement with those obtained from follow-up observations made in Austria (17) and the Federal Republic of Germany (25). A recent study from Geneva relating the histologic and morphometric findings in 10 women who had died between 9 and 18 years after their anorectic treatment points in the same direction (27).

CONCLUSIONS AND OUTLOOK

The tragedy with aminorex is one example, probably the first, of an epidemic of pulmonary hypertension. In the early 1980s, another epidemic took place in Spain, where a considerable fraction of the victims of the "toxic oil syndrome" developed severe pulmonary hypertension. In most instances, the pulmonary hypertension was only partially reversible. A generalized vasculitis, involving mainly the vessels of the mesentary and lungs, was held responsible (5).

The two epidemics are examples of "dietary" pulmonary hypertension in humans. They presented either in a pure form, i.e., without involvement of other organs (aminorex), or as a partial manifestation of a generalized intoxication (toxic oil syndrome). The uncomfortable prospect has to be faced that similar epidemics are apt to occur in the future because of new drugs or toxic ambient factors that are still unknown or unrecognized. In order to prepare for early recognition and intervention of a future epidemic, as well as to gain better understanding of the etiology, pathogenesis, natural history, and treatment of pulmonary hypertension of unknown cause, central registries for patients with primary pulmonary hypertension have been initiated by the National Institutes of Health (in 1981) and the International Society and Federation of Cardiology (in 1984).

The mechanism of aminorex-related plexogenic arteriopathy and pulmonary hypertension remains unsolved. There are numerous parallels between aminorex-associated and primary pulmonary hypertension, such as the identity of clinical, functional, and morphological findings as well as the preponderance of females. On the other hand, the two conditions differ with respect to their initial course, prognosis, and age distribution. In aminorex pulmonary hypertension, prognosis depends on the age of the patient at the time of the anorectic treatment, the initial severity of pulmonary hypertension and of right ventricular failure, and the amount of anorexigen ingested.

These observations are in agreement with the hypothesis that hypertensive plexogenic pulmonary arteriopathy, a morphological entity subscribed to by pathologists, can be caused or conditioned by more than one etiological factor. They lend support to the concept that plexogenic pulmonary arteriopathy is a nonspecific pattern of vascular reactivity and that the degree and extent of the lesions, the spontaneous reversibility of the pulmonary vascular obstruction and, therefore, the long-term prognosis may depend on the type of the etiologic agent, its dose, the duration of its activity, and the individual responsiveness. However, it is not known at present if the endothelial cell is the site of the initial changes caused by the noxious agent(s) followed by proliferation of subendothelial cells, vasoconstriction, hypertension, and medial hypertrophy (15). Nor has the role of platelet metabolites, particularly thromboxane B_2, which appears to be important in primary pulmonary hypertension (21), been studied in patients with aminorex disease. One possible remaining avenue of exploration might be studies done in vitro, to test the effects by aminorex in endothelial cell cultures and on the metabolism of blood platelets.

REFERENCES

1. Bass O, Gurtner HP: Verlauf der primär-vaskulären pulmonalen Hypertonie nach Einnahme von Aminorexfumarat (Menocil). Vorläufige Mitteilung, Schweiz med Wschr 103 : 1794, 1973.

2. Borbely F, Pasi A, Velvart J: Die akute perorale Vergiftung durch 2-amino-5-phenyl-oxazolinfumarat biem Menschen anhand von 30 Beobachtungsfällen. Arch Toxicol 26 : 117–124, 1970.

3. Corrodi P, Bühlmann AA: Zur Prognose des Cor pulmonale bei multipler Lungengefässobstruktion unter Dauerantikoagulation. Schweiz med Wschr 103 : 96–100, 1973.

4. Cutler MA, Ederer F: Maximum utilization of the life table method in analyzing survival. J Chron Dis 8 : 699–712, 1958.

5. Garcia-Dorado D, Miller DD, Garcia EJ, Delcan JL, Maroto E, Chaitman BR: An epidemic of pulmonary hypertension after toxic rapeseed oil ingestion in Spain. J Am Coll Cardiol 1 : 1216–1222, 1983.

6. Gertsch M, Stucki P: Weitgehend reversible primär vaskuläre pulmonale Hypertonie bei einem Patienten mit Menocil-Einnahme. Z Kreislauff 59 : 902–908, 1970.

7. Greiser E: Epidemiologische Untersuchungen zum Zusammenhang zwischen Appetitzüglereinnahme und primär vaskulärer pulmonaler Hypertonie. Internist 14 : 437–442, 1973.

8. Gurtner HP: Pulmonary hypertension, "plexogenic pulmonary arteriopathy" and the appetite depressant drug aminorex: post or propter? Bull Europ Physiopath Resp 15 : 897–923, 1979.

9. Gurtner HP: Chronische pulmonale Hypertonie vaskulären Ursprungs, plexogene pulmonale Arteriopathie und der Appetitzügler Aminorex: Nachlese zu einer Epidemie. Schweiz med Wschr 115 : 782–789, 818–827, 1985.

10. Gurtner HP, Gertsch M, Salzmann C, Scherrer M, Stucki P, Wyss F: Häufen sich die primär vaskulären Formen des chronischen Cor pulmonale? Schweiz med Wschr 98 : 1579–1589, 1695–1707, 1968.

11. Gurtner HP, Lépine JP, Mordasini RC: Long-term follow-up of pulmonary hypertension after the intake of the anorexigen aminorex, in Chazov EI,

Smirnov VN, Oganov RG (eds), *Cardiology, Proc. IX World Congress of Cardiology, Moscow 1982.* New York, Plenum Press, 1984, pp 1205–1215.

12. Hatano S, Strasser T: Primary pulmonary hypertension. Report on a WHO meeting. WHO, Geneva 1975.

13. Heath D, Edwards JE: The pathology of hypertensive pulmonary vascular disease. Circulation 18 : 533–547, 1958.

14. Laissue J: Ergebnisse pathologisch-anatomischer Untersuchungen bei Patienten mit primär vasculärer pulmonaler Hypertonie. Schweiz med Wschr 100 : 2152–2153, 1970.

15. Lockhart A: Actualité de l'artériopathie pulmonaire plexogénique de cause inconnue. Bull Europ Physiopath Resp 19 : 521–529, 1983.

16. Loogen F: Primäre pulmonale Hypertonie. Bericht der Kommission der Deutschen Gesellschaft für Kreislaufforschung. Verhandlg dt Ges Kreislaufforschg 38 : 134–141, 1972.

17. Mlczoch J, Probst P, Szeless S, Kaindl F: Primary pulmonary hypertension: Follow-up of patients with and without anorectic drug intake. Cor Vasa 22 : 251–257, 1980.

18. Obrecht HG, Scherrer M, Gurtner HP: Der Gasaustausch in der Lunge bei der primär vasculären Form des chronischen Cor pulmonale. Schweiz med Wschr 98 : 1999–2007, 1968.

19. Peters L, Gourzis JT: Pharmacological, toxicological and clinical observations with Aminorex in the United States, in Blankart R (ed), *Obesity, Circulation, Anorexigens.* Bern, Hans Huber, 1974, pp 61–77.

20. Poos GI, Carson JR, Rosenau JD, Roszkowski AP, Kelley NM, McGowin J: 2-amino-5-aryl-2-oxazolines. Potent new anorexigens. J Med Chem 6 : 266–272, 1963.

21. Rich S, Hart K, Kieras K, Brundage BH: Thromboxane synthetase inhibition in primary pulmonary hypertension. Chest 91 : 356–360, 1987.

22. Rivier JL, Jaeger M, Reymond CL, Desbaillets P: Hypertension artérielle pulmonaire primitive et anorexigène. Arch Mal Coeur 65 : 787–796, 1972.

23. Saner H, Gurtner HP, Preisig R, Küpfer A: Poly-

morphic debrisoquine and mephenytoin hydroxylation in patients with pulmonary hypertension of
vascular origin after aminorex fumarate. Eur J Clin
Pharmacol 31:437–442, 1986.

24. Turina J, Wirz P, Krayenbühl HP: Verlauf und
Prognose der primären pulmonalen Hypertonie.
Schweiz med Wschr 107:1825–1828, 1977.

25. Voss H, Feigel H, Bücking J: Langzeitverlauf
der primär vasculären pulmonalen Hypertonie mit
und ohne Einnahme von Appetitzüglern. Z Kardiol
72:215–221, 1983.

26. Widgren S: Pulmonary hypertension related to
Aminorex intake, in Grundmann E, Kirsten WH (eds),
Current Topics in Pathology. Berlin-Heidelberg-New
York, Springer, 64:1–64, 1977.

27. Widgren S: Survie prolongée en cas d'hypertension pulmonaire en relation avec la prise d'aminorex Schweiz med Wschr 116:918–924, 1986.

28. Widgren S, Kapanci Y: Menocilbedingte
pulmonale Hypertonie. Vorläufige morphologische
Ergebnisse über 8 pathologisch-anatomisch untersuchte Fälle. Z Kreislauff 59:924–930, 1970.

29. Wirz P, Arbenz U: Primär vasculäre pulmonale
Hypertension in der Schweiz 1965–1970. Schweiz
med Wschr 100:2147–2150, 1970.

30. Yelnosky J, Hewson RJ, Mundy J, Mitchell J:
The cardiovascular effects of Aminorex, a new anor-
exogenic agent. Arch Intl Pharmacodyn 164:412–
418, 1966.

Kenneth M. Moser, M.D.

30

Thromboembolic Pulmonary Hypertension

One factor that promotes increased recognition of hitherto neglected entities is the demonstration that they are potentially subject to treatment. Such a sequence appears to be occurring with respect to pulmonary hypertension secondary to chronic, major vessel thromboembolism.

This disorder has been known to exist for more than 30 years (1,3,20). Initial reports suggested that it was rare and of interest chiefly as an autopsy curiosity. Patients were described who complained of progressive dyspnea, fatigue, and right ventricular failure of obscure cause. At autopsy, they were found to have large, organized, endothelialized thromboemboli in the major (main, lobar, segmental) arteries and variable degrees of right ventricular hypertrophy/dilatation and right ventricular failure (1,3,20).

This "autopsy curiosity" remained as such for many years. However, advances in our understanding of cardiopulmonary pathophysiology, in diagnostic techniques, and in cardiac surgery combined to change its status. Among many such advances were the recognition that pulmonary infarction was an uncommon consequence of acute embolism, the wider application and improved safety of pulmonary angiography, and the development of cardiopulmonary bypass and hypothermia as adjuncts to complex cardiac surgical procedures. As these developments proceeded, reports began to appear of patients in whom the diagnosis was established antemortem, and successful correction by pulmonary thromboendarterectomy was achieved (21,23–25,36). These reports apparently kindled interest because, within the last several years, patients with pulmonary hypertension secondary to chronic major vessel thromboembolism are being recognized antemortem with increasing frequency.

Before reviewing the current status of this disorder, distinction should be drawn between this entity and certain other pulmonary hypertensive disorders, particularly those included under the rubric of "thromboembolic" pulmonary hypertension. In the past, this term has been applied to several different conditions. In one of these, obstruction involves the small (subsegmental and beyond) pulmonary arteries (41). The pathogenetic basis of these lesions is unknown. What is known is that a substantial number of such patients demonstrate histologic evidence of intravascular thrombosis in the small pulmonary arteries, i.e., organized, recanalized, endothelialized thrombotic residuals (41,42). Whether such thrombotic lesions imply a different pathogenesis than in other forms of 'primary' pulmonary hypertension is also unknown.

Unfortunately, it has become commonplace over the years to refer to patients with such widespread thrombotic lesions of the small pulmonary arteries as having thrombo*embolic* pulmonary hypertension (12). The implication of the designation *embolic* was that large numbers of small thrombi arising somewhere in the venous system had *embolized* to the pulmonary vascular bed and failed to resolve. There is, in fact, no evidence for such a sequence. Indeed, these patients consistently lack an embolic source in the periphery, they have no history suggestive of embolic episodes, and they mimic in all respects patients with primary pulmonary hypertension in whom such thrombotic lesions have not been identified (30). Thus, whether the entity of small vessel thrombo*embolic* pulmonary hypertension does exist is open to question. Instead, the lesions may represent thrombosis in situ, secondary to primary injury or dysfunction of the endothelial cells in small pulmonary arteries.

Because the literature on "thromboembolic pulmonary hypertension" often fails to distinguish between pulmonary hypertensive patients with small vessel thromboembolism and those with chronic emboli of major vessels, reports of "thromboembolic pulmonary hypertension" often deal with mixtures of such patients unless pulmonary angiography or autopsy has been done (6,10).

PATHOGENESIS

Patients with chronic pulmonary thromboembolism affecting major vessels constitute only a small fraction of the large population in which systemic venous thrombosis is complicated by pulmonary embolism. The patients with emboli affecting major pulmonary arteries are distinguished chiefly by extensive emboli that have *failed to resolve*. Instead, the emboli have undergone partial resolution, followed by organization, recanalization and endothelialization, resulting in chronic, obstructing lesions in major pulmonary arteries.

This is not the usual course of patients treated for acute pulmonary embolism (Fig. 1). In most of these patients, the emboli resolve rather completely and without residual pulmonary hypertension in days to weeks (5,26,39). Whether this sequence of resolution also applies to untreated patients is unknown since there is no corresponding series in which patients with known acute embolism have been followed without treatment.

No evidence has as yet been provided to indicate that patients who fail to resolve emboli have a recognized disorder of coagulation. In our series, fewer than 10 percent of patients have had either a deficiency in antithrombin III, pro-

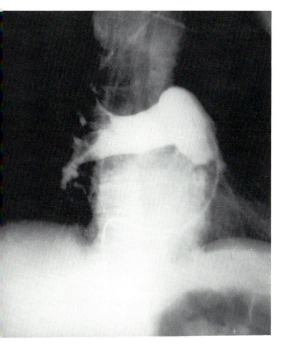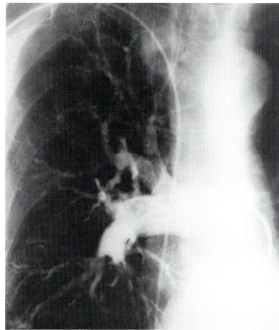

Figure 1: Massive, acute embolic occlusion.
A. Angiogram on admission.
B. Angiogram one week later while on heparin therapy. Substantial resolution is seen. Lung scan (not shown) normalized at 4 weeks.

tein C or protein S, or a lupus anticoagulant (23). In many of these patients, because the diagnosis of acute embolism had not been made, the disorder was untreated. Whether or to what degree failure to institute anticoagulant therapy contributes to the poor resolution is not known. However, lack of anticoagulant therapy for acute embolism cannot be the full explanation; the emboli failed to resolve in a significant proportion of our patients who did undergo anticoagulant therapy.

INCIDENCE

Major, chronic thromboembolic PH (C T-E PH) is not as uncommon as formerly believed. Between 1970 and 1983, we operated on 15 patients, or approximately one per year (25). Between 1983 and 1985, we operated on an additional 22 patients, or 9 per year (23). In 1986, 22 more patients underwent operation, and the pace accelerated further in 1987 and 1988. During this 18-year period, we have seen more than 80 other patients with C T-E PH who either did not meet our criteria for surgical intervention or are awaiting operation.

It is possible to venture a rough estimate of the frequency of this disorder in the United States. About 500,000 patients per year suffer a pulmonary embolic

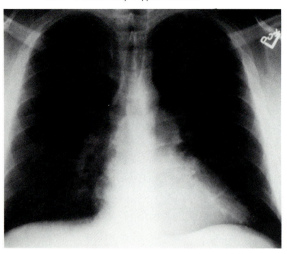 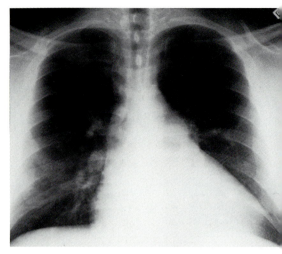

Figure 2: Chronic thromboembolic pulmonary hypertension in a 54-year-old man.
A. November 1985. On admission.
B. June 1986. Marked right ventricular and right atrial dilatation developed during the 7-month interval. Lung scans were unchanged. Successful thromboendarterectomy was performed.

event; 50,000 of these die (28). If we estimate that 0.1 percent of the remaining 450,000 patients have emboli that failed to resolve, an accumulation rate of 450 per year would occur.

NATURAL HISTORY

Although the natural history of this disorder is not yet fully defined, some insights have been gained (22,23). For example, *recurrent* embolic episodes have proved to be uncommon as a cause of clinical deterioration. Instead, clinical-scan-angiography-radiographic data indicate that most patients have experienced *one* major embolic event (often undiagnosed). After a 'honeymoon period' of months to years, manifestations of progressive deterioration of right ventricular function appear (Fig. 2). The deterioration seems to be attributable to three events: (1) the development of pulmonary hypertensive vascular changes in the nonoccluded vascular bed, (2) proximal extension of the thrombus in situ, and (3) progressive right ventricular hypertrophy and dilatation.

The development of hypertensive vascular changes in the nonoccluded pulmonary vascular bed has been documented by lung biopsy and autopsy. Not only are muscular hypertrophy and intimal thickening found in the small pulmonary arteries, but angiomatoid and plexiform lesions are also common. Such findings are not surprising because similar hypertensive changes occur in patients with congenital heart diseases in whom the pulmonary vascular bed is chronically subjected to high pressures and/or high flows (13,41); they also occur in severe mitral stenosis (29). These vascular changes lead to progressive increases in right ventricular afterload which, in turn, elicit right ventricular hypertrophy and dilatation and, in time, right ventricular failure.

The second postulated event, i.e., proximal extension of thrombus, has not been directly demonstrated. It is an inference drawn from the material removed at surgery: often, this material is "layered"; and, in some instances, the more proximal extensions consist of reddish granulation tissue whereas the more distal portions are densely fibrotic. Such proximal growth could, without altering the perfusion lung scan, further reduce the capacity of the pulmonary vascular bed and, thereby, increase the right ventricular afterload.

Although recurrent embolization seems to be the exception rather than the rule, some of these patients *have* had one or more embolic recurrences (documented either by scan or, less convincingly, by history). Recurrence could certainly contribute to deterioration. Another possibility is that obstruction of one major pulmonary artery can provide a nidus on which thrombi form, detach, and embolize other parts of the lungs.

One important question is, When can no further resolution be expected after an acute event? Resolution cannot be judged reliably on *clinical* grounds: many patients, in whom deficits on lung scans did not change, did improve *symptomatically* after a major embolic event. However, in time, right ventricular decompensation and clinical deterioration did occur. This period of improvement probably represents right ventricular compensation through hypertrophy and dilatation; when the limits of compensation are exceeded, frank right ventricular failure ensues. How quickly these limits are exceeded probably depends not only on the various events described above but also on other factors, such as coincident coronary arterial dysfunction, intrinsic lung disease, anemia, and the patient's life-style.

The reliable information about resolution of large emboli is based on serial scans in a small number of patients. These data indicate that resolution on the scans reaches its peak in 6 to 8 weeks; beyond then, no further resolution is to be anticipated. Accordingly, persistence of significant scan defects beyond 6 to 8 weeks should raise the prospect of chronic thromboembolic pulmonary hypertension (C T-E PH).

A second issue is the duration of survival in C T-E PH without surgical correction. Experience with 'untreated' C T-E PH is limited and, in view of the severe disability of most patients who have undergone surgery, a controlled series (operated versus nonoperated) does not appear to be ethical. However, we are aware of more than a dozen patients with C T-E PH who, after symptomatic periods of 6 months to 5 years, died between the time of referral and the time of scheduled arrival at our institution. The experience of Riedel et al. is similar (32). Finally, because of the many parallels between this condition and primary pulmonary hypertension, it seems reasonable to suggest that the survivorship periods are similar; i.e., an average of 2 to 3 years after the diagnosis is made (19). Moreover, as in primary pulmonary hypertension, a substantial portion of the survival period is spent in a state of marked disability.

PRESENTATION

The clinical manifestations of C T-E PH closely parallel those of primary pulmonary hypertension with respect to specifics and subtlety. As in primary pulmonary hypertension, the patients complain chiefly of dyspnea on effort and of easy fatigability (30). Other common complaints are effort near-syncope, substernal discomfort (due to right ventricular ischemia), right upper quadrant discomfort (due to hepatic congestion), and peripheral edema.

Perhaps surprisingly, a definite history of either deep vein thrombosis or pulmonary embolism can be elicited in less than one-half of the patients (23). However, this low incidence of *overt* venous thromboembolism is deceptive: a considerable number of patients with "no history" of venous thrombosis have had events compatible with that diagnosis, e.g., "calf strain" or "pulled muscle" or a brief period of leg swelling. Moreover, most patients can be shown by venography or impedance plethysmography to have objective evidence of prior deep venous thrombosis.

The same is true of a history of embolism: many patients with "no history" have had episodes of "pneumonia," "pleurisy," "hyperventilation," or "myocardial infarction" in the past, all without diagnostic confirmation.

Two historical features have been of particular interest to us. One is the presence of chronic, poorly productive cough. Often present for many months, this has occurred in about 15 percent of our patients. Its etiology is unclear. In these patients, fiberoptic bronchoscopy has disclosed a hyperemic, friable, boggy bronchial mucosa. The cough has subsided in all patients after surgery.

A second feature has been recurrent hemoptysis, rarely brisk. This may be related to the mucosal abnormalities noted above or to proliferation of bronchial arteries, i.e., collateral vessels; it does not appear to be related to pulmonary infarction. This recurrent hemoptysis has also resolved after surgery.

These historical features of C T-E PH are supplemented at presentation by physical and laboratory findings which are often subtle, because most depend, as in primary pulmonary hypertension, on the degree and duration of the pulmonary hypertension. Examination of the lungs is often unremarkable. Cardiac findings range from normal to overt manifestations of pulmonary hypertension: right ventricular lift, palpable P_2; right ventricular dilatation (tricuspid regurgitation); and right ventricular failure (S_3, fixed-split S_2, dilated and bounding neck veins, enlarged and pulsatile liver, ascites and peripheral edema).

One characteristic physical finding occurs in about 30 percent of patients: flow murmurs over the lung fields which mimic those of congenital pulmonary artery branch stenosis (9). These murmurs occur over main, lobar or segmental arteries which have been stenosed by organized thrombus. They are continuous, with systolic accentuation, and may be blowing or harsh. They may occur anywhere over the lung fields. Since physicians usually do not listen for murmurs over the lung fields, they are easily overlooked. Harsh murmurs may be attributed incorrectly to aortic stenosis or, when they radiate into the neck, to carotid artery narrowing.

In patients with C T-E PH who present with the complaint of dyspnea on exertion, findings of the usual laboratory studies depend on the stage of disease. For example, chest radiographs may appear normal, or the cardiac silhouette may be enlarged, sometimes to a remarkable degree. However, the size of the central pulmonary arteries in C T-E PH may suggest the diagnosis: in contrast to primary pulmonary hypertension, in which marked dilatation of the central vessels is the rule, in C T-E PH the central pulmonary arteries may either be quite normal in size (because of organized thrombus) or one side (which contains

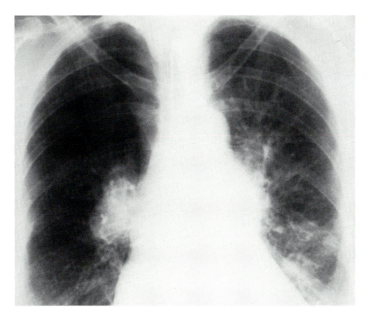

Figure 3: Chronic thromboembolic pulmonary hypertension. Right pulmonary artery is totally obstructed and lung appears hypoperfused. Left lung is hyperperfused.

organized thrombus) may seem small while the other side (which is free of proximal thrombus) may be markedly dilated. Similarly, the distribution of parenchymal blood flow may provide a clue: in primary pulmonary hypertension, blood flow is decreased, or normal, everywhere whereas in C T-E PH some areas of the lungs are hyperperfused and others are hypoperfused (Fig. 3). In some instances, the hyperperfusion has been misinterpreted as interstitial fibrosis.

The electrocardiogram and echocardiogram-Doppler of patients with C T-E PH mimic those of primary pulmonary hypertension and, again, reflect the severity and duration of pulmonary hypertension. However, in three of our patients, echocardiography has disclosed thrombus in the right atrium; in one other patient, "fluttering" thrombus in the right pulmonary artery was revealed.

Spirometry is usually normal but, as in primary pulmonary hypertension, some patients' lung volumes are smaller than predicted (15,34). Evidence of mild obstructive airways disease is found occasionally, particularly among those with a history of smoking cigarettes. Since the diffusing capacity for carbon monoxide (DL_{CO}) is often normal, a normal value cannot be used to rule out the diagnosis of C T-E PH (33,34). However, most patients show a mild to moderate decrease in the DL_{CO}.

Arterial blood gas analyses of blood drawn at rest usually show mild hypoxemia and hypocapnia. However, during exercise, more than 90 percent of our patients have shown a decrease in arterial P_{O_2} and/or oxygen saturation (34).

Among the noninvasive diagnostic procedures, the key tests for differential diagnosis are the lung perfusion and ventilation scans. In primary pulmonary hypertension, the lung scans either are consistently normal or demonstrate

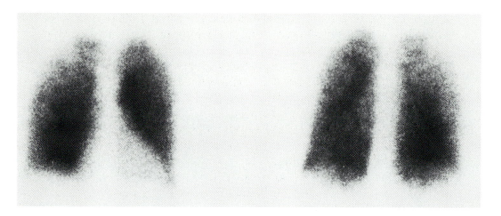

Figure 4: Perfusion lung scan in patient with severe primary pulmonary hypertension. Patchy subseqmental defects are present. Left: anterior; right: posterior.

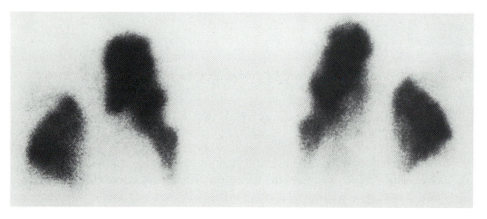

Figure 5: Perfusion lung scan in patient with chronic thromboembolic pulmonary hypertension. Multiple segmental defects are present on perfusion scan. Ventilation scan (not shown) was normal. Left: anterior; right: posterior.

patchy, subsegmental defects (8,31) (Fig. 4). In C T-E PH, all patients whom we have encountered have shown one or more segmental, or larger, perfusion defects that were "mismatched" with respect to a normal ventilation scan (8) (Fig. 5). However, the size of the defects on the perfusion scan has consistently, and sometimes strikingly, underestimated the severity of thrombotic obstruction (35). Thus, the presence of one or two segmental defects does not rule out severe obstruction of the major pulmonary arteries.

Clinical examination of the legs is not a reliable indicator of the presence of prior venous thrombosis: in most patients, examination of the lower extremities is normal. However, impedance plethysmography (IPG) is quite useful (16); in more than 60 percent of the patients who underwent surgery, IPG was positive (abnormal) either unilaterally or bilaterally. Although a very low cardiac output or a high right atrial pressure can cause IPG tests to become positive bilaterally, venous obstruction due to prior thrombi *is* the predominant cause as attested by a high incidence of abnormal venograms in many and the persistence of positive IPG tests after surgical correction has markedly improved cardiac output and reduced right atrial pressure.

In summary, the presenting features of patients with C T-E PH may be quite subtle, consisting of effort dyspnea and easy fatigability on effort with little evidence on either history, physical examination, or routine laboratory studies of either venous thrombosis or extensive pulmonary embolism. Therefore, it is not surprising that these patients often go undiagnosed or misdiagnosed for long periods of time: in our experience, the average duration of symptoms before definitive diagnosis is about 4 years.

In time, as evidence of right ventricular overload becomes manifest, the diagnosis becomes more evident. However, even at this juncture, alternative diagnoses, particularly primary pulmonary hypertension, are often entertained. The key to early recognition is awareness of the entity of C T-E PH and, in terms of diagnostic studies, the perfusion lung scan: a perfusion lung scan should be done in any patient who presents with dyspnea and easy fatigability of obscure cause on effort. If the scan shows one or more segmental defects, the aggressive diagnostic sequence described in the next section should be undertaken.

EVALUATION AND SELECTION OF CANDIDATES FOR SURGICAL CORRECTION

Not all patients with chronic embolic residua are candidates for surgical correction. Many have a modest occlusive residuum that does not pose the threat of right ventricular dysfunction or failure. Moreover, patients with other conditions that would *not* benefit from thromboendarterectomy must be excluded: cardiopulmonary bypass poses great risk to patients with severe pulmonary hypertension in whom the pulmonary hypertension is not relieved by surgery. Also, in patients who *are* to undergo correction for chronic T-E PH, definitive efforts to prevent future embolic recurrence should be made.

The following criteria for evaluation and selection of suitable candidates for thromboendarterectomy have evolved over the years in our center: (1) a value for pulmonary vascular resistance > 300 dynes $\cdot$ sec/cm^5; (2) demonstration that the chronic emboli *begin* in the main, lobar or segmental arteries; (3) absence of significant concurrent disease; and (4) the expressed desire of the patient to accept the risks of surgery (23). Some of the procedures for determining suitability are applied to all patients; others are confined to patients who have certain indications.

All patients undergo a detailed history and physical examination; an intense effort is made to obtain all outside records: review of the old records is not only essential in constructing a clear picture of the patient's history but may also avoid repetition of certain studies. In all patients, initial laboratory studies consist of a complete blood count, urinalysis, a routine panel of blood chemistries, determinations of blood levels of anti-thrombin III, Protein C, Protein S, Factor X and fibrinogen, and of the partial-thromboplastin time and the prothrombin time. In patients who are taking coumadin, the anticoagulant is stopped before invasive studies are begun; prophylaxis is maintained using subcutaneous heparin.

Other studies that are performed in all patients, unless they were done recently, include chest radiographs (posteroanterior and lateral), an electrocar-

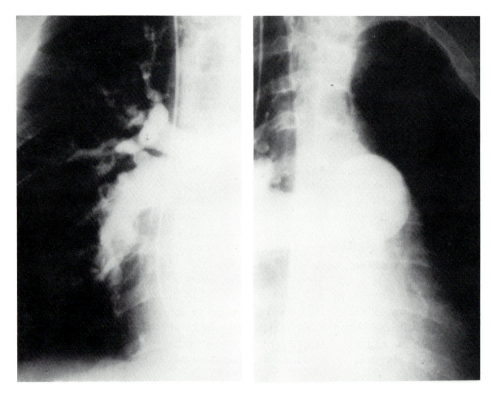

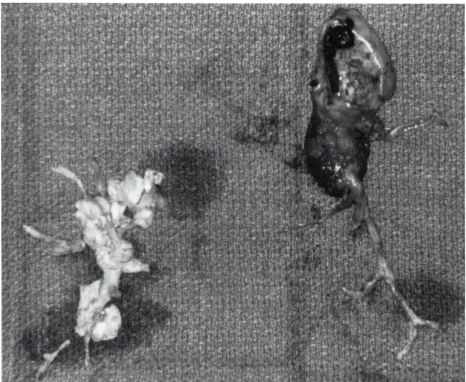

Figure 6: Chronic thromboembolic pulmonary hypertension.
A. Pulmonary angiogram previously interpreted as agenesis of pulmonary artery on the left and multiple branch stenoses on the right.
B. Chronic embolic material removed at surgery.

diogram, and an echocardiogram. The echocardiogram is analyzed for right ventricular and right atrial size and function, valvular function, left ventricular and left atrial size and function, and for the position and movement of the interventricular septum. All chambers are searched for evidence of mural or intramural thrombus. In addition, Doppler estimates are made of pulmonary artery pressure (14,44), and impedance plethysmography is performed. A psychiatric interview and detailed psychological testing also are carried out. In addition, interviews are held with the patient to assess his (or her) support structure, degree of physical limitation, and expectations.

Next, perfusion and ventilation lung scans are done and, whenever possible, compared with previous scans. Pulmonary spirometry is performed, including determination of the single breath diffusing capacity for carbon monoxide. Then, arterial blood gases are determined at rest and during exercise, according to a protocol designed to ensure patient safety.

If evaluation to this juncture has not disqualified the patient as a candidate for surgery, cardiac catheterization is done. The usual procedure consists of right heart catheterization that includes measurements of right atrial, right ventricular, pulmonary arterial and pulmonary wedge pressures, and determination of the cardiac output. Whenever feasible, these parameters are also assessed during exercise. Hypoxic patients breathe oxygen throughout the procedure.

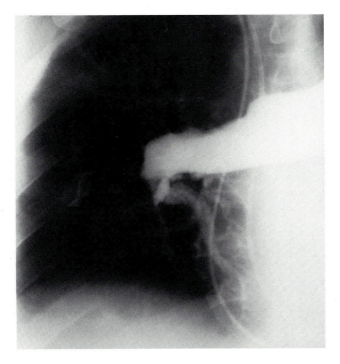

Figure 7: Chronic thromboembolic pulmonary hypertension. Unusual angiographic presentation of patient with chronic thrombus occluding the right main pulmonary artery and most branches.

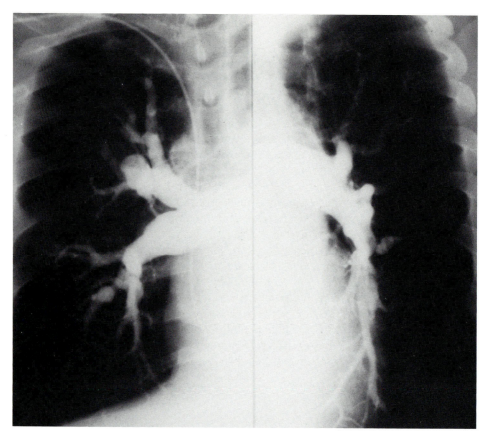

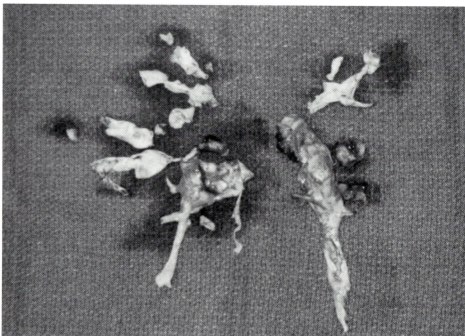

Figure 8: Chronic thromboembolic pulmonary hypertension.
A. Angiograms demonstrating obstructions, stenoses, and some vessels with poststenotic aneurysmal dilatations.
B. Chronic thrombus removed from pulmonary arteries. Same patient as Figure 2.

After the hemodynamic measurements, pulmonary angiography is done as described elsewhere (27). Of special importance with respect to angiography are its safety and its interpretation. Safety is particularly enhanced by restricting injections of contrast medium, whenever possible, to one injection per main pulmonary artery and by injecting small amounts of nonionic medium. The angiograms are interpreted immediately after unilateral injection before the catheter is moved. If the study is adequate, the other side is injected, and once again, the films are interpreted before the catheter is removed.

Unfortunately, the many patterns of central, chronic, organized thrombi found on pulmonary angiography cannot be described briefly. However, the findings do *not* resemble those characteristic of acute embolism. Moreover, without considerable experience in comparing the angiographic findings with those at thromboendarterectomy, misinterpretation can easily occur. Among the likely misinterpretations are branch stenosis and agenesis of the pulmonary artery (Figs. 6, 7, and 8).

In about one-third of our patients in whom excellent angiography has failed to reveal the proximal extent of thrombi in the pulmonary arterial tree, pulmonary angioscopy has proved extremely useful (37,38). It is critical for surgical success that the chronic emboli begin, at least as moderate intimal thickening, in the lobar branches or in the most proximal of the segmental branches (Fig. 9); if not, sur-

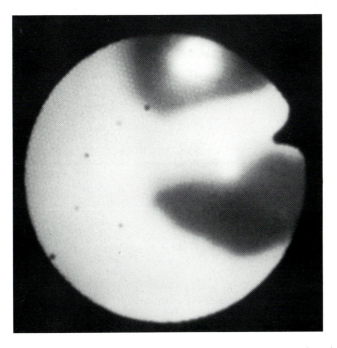

Figure 9: Chronic thromboembolic pulmonary hypertension. Angioscopic view of irregular, narrowed segmental arteries.

gical access is currently impossible. Pulmonary angioscopy has been extremely useful not only in defining the details of proximal extension but also, on occasion, in allowing the exclusion of competitive diagnoses such as fibrosing mediastinitis (2).

In all patients more than 35 years old, coronary angiography is also done routinely at the same time as right heart catheterization. This additional diagnostic study has been adopted because of postoperative episodes of myocardial infarction in some patients without antecedent history of angina or of findings suggestive of coronary arterial disease.

Finally, unless the inferior vena cava has previously been interrupted satisfactorily, or a source of emboli other than the legs has been identified, the inferior vena cava and the right or left iliac vein up to the entry of the common femoral vein are visualized using contrast medium. Ordinarily, the right heart catheterization, pulmonary angiography, coronary angiography, and inferior vena cava visualization are carried out as part of the same procedure. Pulmonary angioscopy is done as a separate procedure. If angiography identifies an alternative explanation for the patient's findings, then the other procedures are not done.

More recently, computed axial tomography (CAT scanning) of the chest has also been done routinely, for two reasons: (1) to rule out fibrosing mediastinitis (2), and (2) to identify pleural or parenchymal abnormalities that are questionable on routine chest radiographs.

It has been suggested that bronchial arteriography by "back perfusion" of the pulmonary arterial bed can be helpful in determining the distal extent of the pulmonary arterial thrombi (36). We have not found this procedure to be useful on several accounts: (1) "back perfusion" has *not* demonstrated, with any reliability, the distal extent of the chronic thrombotic process; (2) we have consistently found that chronic thrombi that begin in one order branch extend for only one or two further orders of branching beyond their origins; and (3) the procedure of bronchial angiography is not without morbidity. Since the procedure may mislead rather than guide, we do not do it.

Should this diagnostic work-up indicate that the patient is a suitable candidate for surgery, the patient's willingness to undergo thromboendarterectomy is determined. The final phase of preoperative preparation includes two measures directed at preventing future embolic recurrences: (1) a Greenfield filter is placed in all patients (11,17) (unless some obvious reason exists not to do so), and (2) anticoagulant therapy is continued.

SURGICAL CORRECTION

Pulmonary thromboendarterectomy is a formidable surgical procedure, even for the most experienced cardiothoracic surgeon. The techniques now used have evolved over the years with increasing experience (4,23,25).

Pulmonary thromboendarterectomy bears *no relationship* to acute pulmonary embolectomy. The chronic, fibrotic endothelialized structures which partially or completely obstruct pulmonary arteries in C T-E PH are incorporated into the arterial wall. To remove them safely and completely requires meticulous dissection and attention to detail. For surgical mortality and morbidity to be low and for optimal functional outcomes, surgeons undertaking to perform this procedure would be well advised to seek the collaboration of those who have already gained considerable experience with it.

The importance of experience is evident at the time that the involved pulmonary artery is opened. Because the neointima may be smooth or only slightly pitted, it is easy for the inexperienced surgeon to conclude that no thrombus is present. Indeed, there is no acute, red-fibrin thrombus. Recognition that the rather smooth intimal surface is really neointima, and that this is the chronic thrombus that must be removed, is the first critical step in achieving optimal surgical results.

Median sternotomy is the most effective approach to visualizing and manipulating the affected pulmonary arterial structures (4). Access to both the right and left pulmonary arteries is essential since endarterectomy must be done bilaterally if the severe pulmonary hypertension is to be relieved. Cardiopulmonary bypass is required for adequate bilateral endarterectomy. Moreover, hypothermia with periods of cardioplegia and circulatory arrest is essential to achieve the bloodless field required for proper visualization and dissection (4).

It also has become routine to search for a patent foramen ovale or atrial septal defect; if one is found, it is closed. Tricuspid insufficiency is no longer treated by annuloplasty since relief of the pulmonary hypertension by the endarterectomy is associated with spontaneous resolution of the tricuspid insufficiency as the right ventricular dilatation regresses (7).

Other procedures may be required at surgery. For example, lung biopsy may be indicated in some patients. In others, coronary artery bypass or correction of aortic stenosis may be required. Finally, if a Greenfield filter could not be placed preoperatively, it is placed under direct vision, at the time of the endarterectomy, through the right atrium.

Some patients have developed bilateral phrenic nerve paralysis, apparently due to a combination of deep hypothermia and local cooling in order to preserve myocardium. A special myocardial cooling blanket devised to alleviate the need for local cooling has resolved this problem (40).

POSTOPERATIVE COURSE

In addition to the usual problems encountered after cardiac surgery, such as bleeding, arrhythmias, pericarditis, and infection, bilateral thromboendarterectomy poses special challenges, including reperfusion lung edema, phrenic nerve injury, hemodynamic instability, venous thrombosis, and psychiatric disturbances.

Reperfusion lung injury (18) is of particular concern because it occurs in every patient and leads to arterial hypoxemia. The edema appears radiographically within 2 to 72 hours after surgery. On the radiograph, it is limited to regions of the lungs to which perfusion has been restored by endarterectomy (Fig. 10). Neither the onset nor duration bear any relationship to preoperative or postoperative hemodynamic values; in particular, the left atrial pressure is normal. Since the affected regions often comprise a high percentage of the pulmonary vascular bed, arterial hypoxemia can be quite severe. Perfusion lung scans indicate that flow continues to these edematous areas, thus creating zones of intrapulmonary shunt

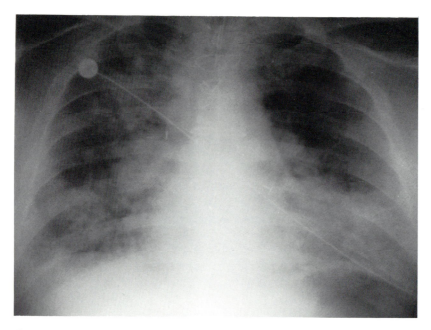

Figure 10: Chronic thromboembolic pulmonary hypertension. Reperfusion pulmonary edema following thromboendarterectomy. No obstructions were removed from right middle or left upper lobar arteries.

or low ventilation/perfusion ratio (18). Bronchoalveolar lavage samples are rich in protein as in the adult respiratory distress syndrome. Management requires high inspired concentrations of oxygen. Positive end-expiratory pressure may also be useful in some instances.

Bilateral phrenic nerve paresis is a severe complication requiring prolonged ventilatory assistance. It is easily detected in the early postoperative period by noting paradoxical motion of the diaphragm during spontaneous inspiratory efforts. Since late 1984 when the myocardial cooling blanket was introduced, bilateral and unilateral (right) paresis have each occurred only once. In all survivors of endarterectomy, normal diaphragmatic function has returned after 2 to 6 months.

A variety of psychiatric disturbances has occurred early in the postoperative course. They are transient but may pose management problems in the intensive care unit. The basis for these disturbances is not clear (43). They do not correlate well with preoperative psychological tests.

Four patients have manifested neurological sequelae involving sensory or motor function of one arm. In three, these sequelae appear to be poststernotomy brachial plexus injuries (40). In one, cerebral injury appears to have been involved, although brain CT scans were normal. All four patients have experienced gradual improvement.

Prevention of recurrent venous thrombosis is another important aspect of postoperative management. Most of these patients have chronic unilateral or bilateral obstruction in the deep venous system of the legs. Therefore, they are subject to recurrent venous thrombosis postoperatively. For prophylaxis, we place all patients on intermittent venous compressive devices during, and after, surgery. We also reinstitute low dose (5000–7500 u every 12 hr) subcutaneous heparin 48 to 72 hr after surgery and start coumadin 4 to 5 days after surgery.

Heparin is continued until the patient's prothrombin time has been in the desirable range (1.4 to 1.6 x control) for at least 3 days; the compressive devices are continued until the patient is fully ambulatory. Using this regimen, we have not encountered a single instance of postoperative recurrent venous thrombosis. Moreover, as noted above, virtually all patients have a Greenfield filter in place to prevent embolic recurrence (43).

POSTOPERATIVE OUTCOME

Review of the results of intervention can best be divided into short-term (in-hospital) and long-term (postdischarge) observations.

Short-Term

Following successful endarterectomy, the patients undergo substantial hemodynamic improvement (Table 1). Accompanying these hemodynamic changes are echocardiographic changes that demonstrate a decrease in right atrial and ventricular size, and return of the interventricular septum to, or toward, its normal position and a loss of paradoxical motion (7). If right axis was present preoperatively, the electrocardiogram shows reversion of the QRS axis toward normal. The perfusion lung scan demonstrates reperfusion of zones that were previously nonperfused.

The changes on physical examination depend on the preoperative findings. Pulmonary arterial valvular closure is less intense; fixed slitting of S_2 is replaced by normal inspiratory widening; tricuspid insufficiency moderates or disappears; dilated, pulsatile neck veins resolve; peripheral edema, if present, clears; the characteristic "stenosis" murmurs are absent.

Predischarge pulmonary function tests characteristically show a restrictive defect, and the diffusing capacity for carbon monoxide is subnormal. Arterial hypoxemia at rest that is exaggerated by exercise usually persists at the time of discharge.

TABLE 1 PRE- AND POSTOPERATIVE PULMONARY HEMODYNAMICS IN 64 PATIENTS WHO UNDERWENT THROMBOENDARTERECTOMY

Pulmonary artery mean (mmHg)		Pulmonary wedge (mmHg)		Cardiac output (L/min)		Pulmonary vascular resistance (dynes · sec/cm^5)	
Preop	Postop	Preop	Postop	Preop	Postop	Preop	Postop
49.6	28.4*	9.2	11.1	3.76	5.72**	904	272*
(±9.6)	(±7.9)	(±3)	(±3)	(±.86)	(±1.12)	(±348)	(+134)

The postoperative values are averages obtained during the period from return to the intensive care unit to discontinuation of monitoring (usually at 72 hr).
  * = significant (p < .001).
  ** = significant (p < .01).

TABLE 2 CAUSES OF DEATH IN 9 PATIENTS WHO DIED POSTOPERATIVELY

Case #	Age	NYHA classi-fication	Time postop (days)	Cause
4	65	4	19	Myocardial infarct (LV)
13	21	4	55	Adult Respiratory Distress Syndrome
17	56	4	<1	Myocardial infarct (RV)
19	70	4	126	Diaphragmatic paresis; multiple complications
21	67	4	45	Multiple complications
30	41	4	<1	No thrombus removed; progressive RV failure
36	37	4	4	Myocardial infarct (LV)
44	41	4	7	Gram-negative sepsis
50	72	4	47	Multiple complications

Nine of the 64 patients included in this analysis died (14 percent). All patients who died were in the New York Heart Association (NYHA) Class IV. The causes of death have been multiple (Table 2). In one instance, the thrombi could not be removed because they began at the segmental level. Severe Class IV status has not been a basis for denying surgical intervention if, despite awareness of high risk, the patient requested the operation. Mortality from the procedure has decreased slowly over the years, partly because of an increasing proportion of Class III patients and partly because of a decrease in mortality in Class IV patients; in 1986, mortality for Class IV patients was 15 percent (Table 3).

TABLE 3 NEW YORK HEART ASSOCIATION CLASSIFICATION OF PATIENTS WHO UNDERWENT SURGERY SINCE 1970

	Number of patients	NYHA class III	NYHA class IV	Number of deaths
1970–81	15	5	10	2
1982–84	12	2	10	3
1985	15	6	9	2
1986	22	9	13	2

**TABLE 4 PRE- AND POSTOPERATIVE CLASSIFICATION
OF SURVIVORS**

NYHA class	Preop	Postop
IV	33	0
III	22	1
II	0	12
I	0	42
Total	55	55

Long-Term

In 55 survivors, the period of follow-up has ranged from 10 months to 17 years, averaging 4.4 years. The most striking feature of the follow-up period in these patients has been a change in the NYHA category between the pre- and post-operative periods (Table 4). Functional improvement continues for up to 12 months after hospital discharge. Part of this improvement is undoubtedly due to recovery from the surgery itself, including resolution of postoperative anemia. However, in many patients, hemodynamic improvement also continues. As may be seen in Table 5, in the 24 patients who returned for recatheterization 6 to 14 months after surgery, improvement has been the rule. Although lung biopsy has not been repeated, this improvement probably reflects regression of pulmonary hypertensive changes in the pulmonary vascular bed. In keeping with the hemodynamic improvement is the progressive improvement in the perfusion lung scan at follow-up and the reversion of the preoperative echocardiographic and electrocardiographic findings.

Follow-up pulmonary angiograms have consistently documented extensive restoration of patency to pulmonary vessels (Fig. 11). The persistence of obstruction in some segmental or subsegmental vessels has corresponded well to decisions made at the time of surgery regarding obstructions beyond current access or not approached for reasons of safety.

TABLE 5 PULMONARY HEMODYNAMICS IN 24 PATIENTS STUDIED PRE- AND POSTOPERATIVELY

	Preoperative	Immediately postoperative**	4 to 14 months postoperative
Pulmonary arterial mean, (mmHg)	49.8 (±9.1)	29.2 (±8.4)	24.1 (±10.2)* +
Cardiac output, (L/min)	3.97 (±1.05)	5.71 (+1.12)*	5.70 (±0.75)*
Pulmonary capillary wedge (mmHg)	7.9 (±3.2)	9.3 (±1.6)	7.4 (±6.3)
Pulmonary vascular resistance (dynes · sec/cm^5)	978 (±431)	308 (±144)*	222 (+134)* +

* = significant (p < .05 versus preop).
+ = significant (p < .05 versus immediate postop).
** First 3 days after surgery.

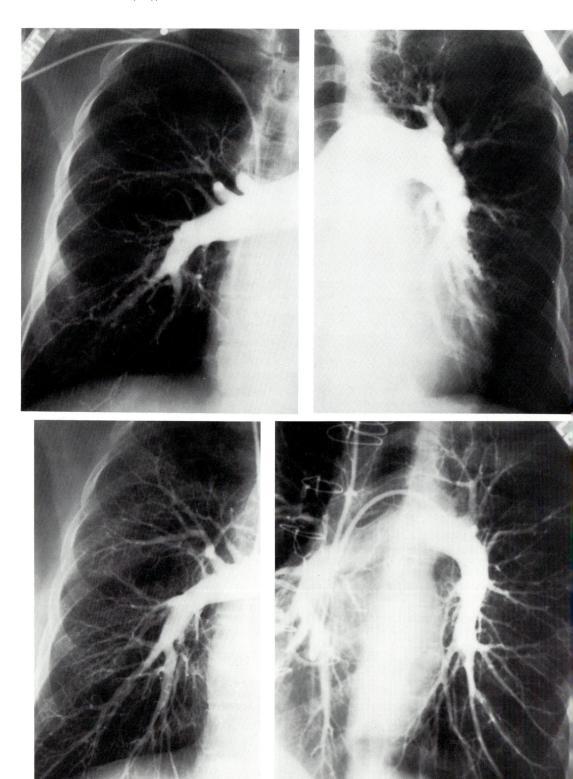

LEFT: **Figure 11:** Chronic thromboembolic pulmonary hypertension.
A. Preoperative right angiogram.
B. Preoperative left angiogram.
Extensive lobar and segmental obstructions are present. Extensive thrombus was removed. Pulmonary vascular resistance was 1266 dynes · sec/cm⁵.
C. Postoperative (6 months after surgery) right angiogram.
D. Postoperative left angiogram.
Marked restoration of vessel patency. Pulmonary vascular resistance had decreased to 214 dynes · sec/cm⁵.

REFERENCES

1. Ball KP, Goodman JF, Harrison CV: Massive thrombotic occlusion of the large pulmonary arteries. Circulation 14:766–783, 1956.

2. Berry DF, Buccigrossi D, Peabody J, Peterson KL, Moser KM: Pulmonary vascular occlusion and fibrosing mediastinitis. Chest 89:296–301, 1986.

3. Carroll D: Chronic obstruction of major pulmonary arteries. Am J Med 9:175–185, 1950.

4. Daily PO, Dembitsky WP, Peterson KL, Moser KM: Modifications of techniques and early results of pulmonary thromboendarterectomy for chronic pulmonary embolism. J Thorac Cardiovasc Surg 93:221–233, 1987.

5. Dalen JE, Banas JS, Brooks HL, Evans GL, Paraskos JA, Dexter L: Resolution rate of acute pulmonary embolism in man. N Engl J Med 280:1194–1199, 1969.

6. Dantzker DR, Bower JS: Mechanisms of gas exchange abnormality in patients with chronic obliterative pulmonary vascular disease. J Clin Invest 64:1050–1055, 1979.

7. Dittrich H, Nicod P, Moser KM: Early improvement of hemo-dynamic and echocardiographic abnormalities after pulmonary thromboendarterectomy. Circulation 74:II-445, 1986.

8. Fishman AJ, Moser KM, Fedullo PF: Perfusion lung scans versus pulmonary angiography in evaluation of suspected primary pulmonary hypertension. Chest 84:679–683, 1983.

9. Franch RH, Gay BB Jr: Congenital stenosis of the pulmonary artery branches. Am J Med 35:512–529, 1963.

10. Fuster V, Steele PM, Edwards WD, Gersh BJ, McGoon MD, Frye RL: Primary pulmonary hypertension: Natural history and the importance of thrombosis. Circulation 70:580–587, 1984.

11. Greenfield LJ, Peyton R, Crute S, Barnes R: Greenfield vena caval filter experience. Arch Surg 116:1451–1456, 1981.

12. Hatamo S, Strasser T (eds): Primary Pulmonary Hypertension. Report on a WHO meeting. Geneva, World Health Organization, 1975, pp 7–45.

13. Heath D, Edwards JE: The pathology of hypertensive pulmonary vascular disease. Circulation 18:533–547, 1958.

14. Horn M, Hoyt B, Watt C: Doppler-echocardiographic assessment of pulmonary hemodynamics in patients with lung disease. Chest 92:1065, 1987.

15. Horn M, Ries AL, Neveu C, Moser KM: Restrictive ventilatory pattern in precapillary pulmonary hypertension. Am Rev Respir Dis 128:163–165, 1983.

16. Hull R, Taylor DW, Hirsh J, Sackett DL, Powers P, Turpie AG, Walker I: Impedance plethysmography: The relationship between venous filling and sensitivity and specificity for proximal vein thrombosis. Circulation 58:898–902, 1978.

17. Kanter B, Moser KM: The Greenfield vena cava filter. Chest 93:170–175, 1988.

18. Levinson RM, Shure D, Moser KM: Reperfusion pulmonary edema after pulmonary artery thromboendarterectomy. Am Rev Respir Dis 134:1241–1245, 1986.

19. Levy PS, Rich S, Kerms J: Mortality follow-up of subjects in the Primary Pulmonary Hypertension Registry. Reported to International Conference on PPH. Philadelphia, PA, 1987.

20. Magidison O, Jacobson G: Thrombosis of the main pulmonary arteries. Br Med J 17:207–211, 1955.

21. Moser KM, Braunwald NS: Successful surgical intervention in severe chronic thromboembolic pulmonary hypertension. Chest 64:29–35, 1973.

22. Moser KM, Daily PO, Peterson KL: Management of chronic unresolved large vessel thromboembolism, in Weil JA, Dawson CA, Weir EK, Buckner CK (eds), *The Pulmonary Circulation in Health and Disease.* Orlando, FL, Academic Press, 1987.

23. Moser KM, Daily PO, Peterson K, Dembitsk W, Vapnek JM, Shure D, Utley J, Archibald C: Thromboendarterectomy for chronic, major vessel thromboembolic pulmonary hypertension. Immediate and long-term results in 42 patients. Ann Intern Med 107:560–564, 1987.

24. Moser KM, Houk VN, Jones RC, Hufnagel CC: Chronic massive thrombotic obstruction of the pulmonary arteries: Analysis of four operated cases. Circulation 32:377–385, 1965.

25. Moser KM, Spragg RG, Utley J, Daily PO: Chronic thrombotic obstruction of major pulmonary arteries: Results of thromboendarterectomy in 15 patients. Ann Intern Med 99:299–305, 1983.

26. Murphy ML, Bulloch RT: Factors influencing the restoration following pulmonary embolization of blood flow as determined by angiography and scanning. Circulation 38:1116–1126, 1968.

27. Nicod P, Peterson K, Levine M, Dittrich H, Buchbinder M, Chappuis F, Moser K: Pulmonary angiography in severe chronic pulmonary hypertension. Ann Intern Med 107:565–568, 1987.

28. NIH Consensus Conference: Prevention of venous thrombosis and pulmonary embolism. JAMA 256:744–749, 1986.

29. Ramirez A, Grimes ET, Abelmann WH: Regression of pulmonary vascular changes following mitral valvuloplasty: An anatomic and physiologic case study. Am J Med 45:975–982, 1968.

30. Rich S, Dantzker DR, Ayres SM, Bergofsky EH, Brundage BH, Detre KM, Fishman AP, Goldring RM, Groves BM, Koerner SK, Levy PS, Reid LM, Vreim CE, Williams GW: Primary pulmonary hypertension: A national prospective study. Ann Intern Med 107:216–223, 1987.

31. Rich S, Pietra GG, Kieras K, Hart K, Brundage BH: Primary pulmonary hypertension: Radiographic and scintigraphic patterns of histologic subtypes. Ann Intern Med 105:499–502, 1986.

32. Riedel M, Stanek V, Widimsky J, Prerovsky I: Longterm follow-up of patients with pulmonary thromboembolism. Chest 81:151–158, 1982.

33. Riedel M, Widimsky J, Stanek V: Steady-state pulmonary transfer factor in chronic thromboembolic disease. Bull Eur Physiopathol Respir 16:469–477, 1980.

34. Ryan KL, Fedullo PF, Clausen J, Moser KM: Pulmonary function in chronic thromboembolic pulmonary hypertension. Am Rev Respir Dis 133:A222, 1986.

35. Ryan KL, Fedullo PF, Davis GB, Vasquez TE, Moser KM: Perfusion scan findings understate the severity of angiographic and hemodynamic compromise in chronic thromboembolic pulmonary hypertension. Chest 93:1180–1185, 1988.

36. Sabiston DC, Wolfe WG, Oldham HN, Wechsler AS, Crawford FA, Jones KW, Jones RH: Surgical management of chronic pulmonary embolism. Ann Surg 185:699–712, 1977.

37. Shure D, Gregoratos G, Moser KM: Fiberoptic angioscopy: Role in the diagnosis of chronic pulmonary arterial obstruction. Ann Intern Med 103:844–850, 1985.

38. Shure D, Moser KM, Harrell JH, Hartman MT: Identification of pulmonary emboli in the dog: Comparison of angioscopy and perfusion scanning. Circulation 64:618–621, 1981.

39. Urokinase-Streptokinase Pulmonary Embolism Trial: A National Cooperative Study. JAMA 229:1606–1610, 1974.

40. Vander Salm TJ, Cereda JM, Cutler BS: Brachial plexus injury following median sternotomy. J Thorac Cardiovasc Surg 80:447–452, 1980.

41. Wagenvoort CA, Wagenvoort N: Primary pulmonary hypertension. A pathologic study of the lung vessels in 156 clinically diagnosed cases. Circulation 42:1163–1169, 1970.

42. Wagenvoort CA, Wagenvoort N: Pathology of pulmonary hypertension. New York, John Wiley & Sons, 1977.

43. Wragg RE, Dimsdale JE, Moser KM, Daily PO, Dembitsky WP, Archibald C: Operative predictors of delirium after pulmonary thromboendarterectomy. A model for postcardiotomy delirium? J Thorac Cardiovasc Surg 96:524–529, 1988.

44. Yock PG, Popp RL: Noninvasive estimation of right ventricular systolic pressure by Doppler ultrasound in patients with tricuspid regurgitation. Circulation 70:657–662, 1984.

PART FOUR

The Primary Pulmonary Hypertension Registry

Alfred P. Fishman, M.D.

31

Introduction to the National Registry on Primary Pulmonary Hypertension

The designation "primary pulmonary hypertension" is a synonym for unexplained or idiopathic pulmonary hypertension. By definition, it is a diagnosis of exclusion. Clinically the disorder was characterized by Dresdale almost 40 years ago (2). Since then, many clinical experiences with small groups of patients have been reported. Although reports of the histological features of primary pulmonary hypertension antedated the clinical reports (1), pathologists have remained unable to reach a comfortable consensus about the diagnostic microscopic features of this disorder.

The advent of powerful vasodilator agents in the late 1970s provided fresh impetus to attempts to treat this dread disease. However, testing the efficacy of the new agents in arresting or reversing the disorder was handicapped by the paucity of control data concerning its natural history: not only was the disease sporadic in incidence, but its etiologies were diverse. Indeed, except for medical centers in Europe that had dealt with the aminorex epidemic (4), no medical center could provide a homogeneous population that might serve as a control group for vasodilator therapy (3).

Recognizing this difficulty, the Division of Lung Diseases of the National Heart, Lung, and Blood Institute created a National Registry in 1981. The Registry was designed to pool data from different medical centers for the sake of sharing experiences and for assessing the effectiveness of pulmonary vasodilator therapy.

The Registry was based on two essential ingredients. At the core was a *computer-based facility* that was operated by epidemiologists and statisticians under the watchful eye of a steering committee, clinicians, clinical investigators,

TABLE 1 TYPES OF PULMONARY HYPERTENSION EXCLUDED FROM THE NATIONAL REGISTRY ON PRIMARY PULMONARY HYPERTENSION

Heart disease: congenital or acquired
Pulmonary thromboembolic disease
Obstructive airways disease
Interstitial lung disease
Hypoxic pulmonary hypertension
Overt collagen disease
Parasitic disease affecting the lungs
Pulmonary arterial stenoses: peripheral or central
Sickle cell disease with pulmonary arterial thromboses
Pulmonary venous hypertension
Pulmonary hypertension in the first year of life associated with congenital abnormalities of the lungs, diaphragm, and/or thorax

and pathologists; the task of this center was to collect, monitor, and analyze data gathered in a standardized way. Feeding into the core facility were medical centers which would provide data about individual patients diagnosed as having primary pulmonary hypertension (Table 1); special forms were used for reporting and by the end of 1988, 32 centers had delivered to the Registry almost 200 cases that had passed muster. A pathology center was also designated; the responsibility of this center was to provide uniform histological interpretations to the Registry based on lung tissue obtained by biopsy and at autopsy. Provision was also made to collect data about clues to the etiology of primary pulmonary hypertension (Table 2).

TABLE 2 SUBSETS OF PATIENTS IN WHOM PRIMARY PULMONARY HYPERTENSION IS ASSOCIATED WITH OTHER DISORDERS OR POSSIBLE CLUES TO ETIOLOGY

Hepatic cirrhosis (portal and pulmonary hypertension)
Collagen disease without overt symptoms or signs
Raynaud's phenomenon
Possible diet or drug etiologies
Familial history of pulmonary hypertension or unexplained cor pulmonale

The chapters that follow summarize the lessons learned from the Registry by the end of 1988. Although the Registry is now officially closed, analysis of the data goes on. To date, the Registry has been rewarding on several accounts. Not only has it provided fresh insights from analysis of the data, but its existence and its reports have heightened international interest in this disease and intensified efforts to develop effective pulmonary vasodilator agents. In addition, the Registry has promoted interchange between pathologists and clinicians leading to a more rational histological underpinning of the clinical disorder. Finally, the Registry has served to remind clinicians and pathologists that by the time they encounter a patient with primary pulmonary hypertension, the disease is approaching or has reached end-stage and that prospects for greater understanding and possibly for effective medical intervention rest heavily on earlier diagnosis and intervention.

REFERENCES

1. Brenner O: Pathology of the vessels of the pulmonary circulation. Arch Intern Med 56:976–1014, 1935.

2. Dresdale DT, Schultz M, Michtom RJ: Primary pulmonary hypertension: I. Clinical and hemodynamic study. Am J Med 11:686–694, 1951.

3. Fishman AP: Dietary pulmonary hypertension. Circ Res 35:657–660, 1974.

4. Gurtner HP: Pulmonary hypertension, "plexogenic pulmonary arteriopathy" and the appetite depressant drug aminorex: post or propter? Bull Eur Physiopathol Respir 15:897–923, 1979.

Edward H. Bergofsky, M.D.
Carol E. Vreim, Ph.D.

32

The Research and Clinical Dilemmas Encountered by the Primary Pulmonary Hypertension Registry

Patient registries are an effective mechanism that enables the prospective collection of data on a sufficient number of patients for analysis. The establishment of patient registries can be for a variety of far-reaching purposes. For example, among the registries supported by the National Heart, Lung, and Blood Institute, one acquired data on the natural history of sickle cell disease, while another acquired data on a new therapeutic tool, percutaneous transluminal coronary angioplasty. Yet another registry was a subcomponent of a randomized clinical trial on coronary artery surgery. The registry allowed data to be obtained on all patients referred to a clinical center for evaluation and treatment of coronary artery disease, including those not choosing to participate in the clinical trial.

A patient registry is not intended to test a scientific hypothesis, but rather to generate one. It does not establish the value of one therapy against another or one therapy against no therapy; that requires a clinical trial. It can, however, provide the necessary data upon which to design a clinical trial. In addition, a patient registry can contribute to the establishment of a scientific community where data is more rapidly communicated.

REGISTRY FOR PRIMARY PULMONARY HYPERTENSION

Although it had long been recognized that primary pulmonary hypertension (PPH) was a rare disease, there was an intense interest in the disease following an outbreak of unexplained pulmonary hypertension in Europe in 1967. This epidemic was eventually attributed to the appetite suppressant, aminorex. Because of the interest generated at the time in PPH, the World Health Organization convened a meeting in 1973 to review the limited scientific information that was available about the disease. As a result of this meeting, it was recommended that it would be helpful to establish a registry of these patients throughout the world (2). Although this has not been done, a number of countries and regions have established their own patient registries for PPH.

The Division of Lung Diseases of the National Heart, Lung, and Blood Institute convened a small working group in September 1978 to evaluate the Division's program in pulmonary hypertension. Recognizing the continued lack of progress in treating primary pulmonary hypertension and the relative rarity of the disorder, the working group recommended that the Division establish a national patient registry to collect data on PPH. The goal of the Registry was to obtain and analyze data on the natural history, etiology, pathogenesis, and treatment of PPH.

Because of the apparent differences in etiology and pathogenesis of PPH, as well as the rarity of the disorder, it had proven difficult to develop a consistent therapeutic approach for treating this disorder and, therefore, to decrease the high mortality associated with PPH. At that time, with the advent of powerful vasodilator drugs, new interest had been stimulated in attempting to relieve the vasoconstrictive component of the disease. It was felt that a registry would enable a much faster accumulation of data on these patients than could be obtained from an individual clinical center. The accumulated data might then serve the Registry or other investigators to provide new insights into the etiology and pathogenesis of PPH, to develop new strategies for earlier diagnosis, and to suggest beneficial therapeutic regimens. The Registry became operational in 1981 and consisted of five major components: participating clinical centers, the data and coordinating center, the pathology center, the steering committee, and the program office.

Thirty-two clinical centers from throughout the United States contributed data to the Registry. Criteria for inclusion as a clinical center included a minimum of three PPH patients per year, willingness to share information, availability of appropriate quality controlled hemodynamic and laboratory testing, and endorsement by the sponsoring department and institution. The clinical centers were to be reimbursed $150 for each patient enrolled and $25 for each follow-up form submitted. Follow-up forms were to be submitted every 6 months or more often if a major event occurred, such as rehospitalization or cardiac catheterization.

The responsibilities of the data and coordinating center included collecting the data from the clinical centers and monitoring its quality, analyzing it in accordance with the objectives of the Registry, and facilitating interaction among the participating clinical centers. They were also responsible for the preparation and distribution of periodic data reports to the program office and the participating clinical centers. In addition, they assisted in the coordination and management of steering committee meetings and of conferences held for the investigators.

The pathology center received, prepared, examined, and interpreted the tissue provided by the clinical centers.

A steering committee, under the direction of the Division of Lung Diseases, oversaw the general operation of the Registry. It was comprised of 13 members, representing several of the clinical centers, the data and coordinating center, the

TABLE 1 DILEMMAS OF A NATIONAL DISEASE REGISTRY

Effects of observation on natural history
Registry data requirements in excess of clinical indications
Preconceived definition of the disease
Communication among investigators
Compensation for record keeping
Geographic skewing

pathology center, and the program office. The steering committee established the patient entry criteria and developed and modified, as needed, standardized patient reporting forms used by all the clinical centers. It also reviewed the data at periodic intervals and was responsible for publication of the data. The program office provided guidance and coordination of the project in accordance with the policies of the NIH.

THE DILEMMAS OF THE REGISTRY

One of the goals of the Registry was to observe the natural history of primary pulmonary hypertension. To do so required the creation of an organization of considerable complexity which would include clinicians, investigators, pathologists, epidemiologists, and statisticians. They, in turn, would create a series of admission criteria and data requirements for the Registry which had the potential to change the makeup of the patient enrollment, as well as the diagnostic testing and therapeutic management offered to these patients. We sought to minimize the effects of these dilemmas on our goal of defining the natural history of PPH by carefully considering each one separately at the inception of the Registry and during its subsequent course by the use of the decision-making steering committee. The major dilemmas perceived at the outset are listed in Table 1 and discussed below, along with our efforts at their resolution.

The Effects of Observation

The Registry may create sufficient interest in the physician so that follow-up visits or interventions are more frequent than otherwise would be the case, even though not mandated by Registry requirements. This possibility could conceivably affect clinical outcome and natural history in both directions; more care resulting in prolonged survival or more intervention, such as additional cardiac catheterizations resulting in their attendant hazards. To obviate the observation effect, the Registry made few requirements for follow-up, except at 6-month intervals, so that clinically dictated follow-up visits would almost certainly intervene. No requirements for data derived from intervention, such as cardiac catheterization with or without drug treatment, were imposed by the Registry for follow-up. Whether additional invasive procedures or therapeutic measures were undertaken because of enthusiasm generated by the existence of the Registry and interinvestigator interaction (see below) is uncertain. However, a future analysis of the intervention (i.e., angiography, cardiac catheterization, changes in drug regimens, etc.) for individual clinical centers and investigators, with special emphasis on the intensity of communication with other centers, may shed some light on this phenomenon.

Data Requirements of the Registry

Entry requirements formulated by the Registry could in· lve procedures more hazardous than otherwise would be dictated by recommended clinical practice. From the diagnostic standpoint, two interventions required by the Registry would be classified as invasive. Invasive by definition would be associated with some clinical risk, even if very small, as opposed to a noninvasive diagnostic test, such as an echocardiogram, where virtually no risk is known. The first of these two interventions is the initial diagnostic cardiac catheterization. All patients required this for entry into the Registry. In some cases, this catheterization had been performed at a clinical center other than that which reported the case to the Registry.

The Registry regulations required (1) a cardiac catheterization performed in the clinical center or in a satellite center where the catheterization was known to the principal investigator to have been performed in an acceptable manner, (2) acceptable techniques to rule out intracardiac shunting indicative of congenital heart disease, and (3) acceptable measurements to rule out left heart disease. If any one of the three requirements were doubtful, entry into the Registry would require a repeat cardiac catheterization. As is apparent, fulfilling criteria #2 and #3 are merely consistent with good clinical practice and, even in the absence of the Registry, would have required recatheterization, unless a noninvasive technique offered a substitute approach acceptable to the patient's consulting physician. Thus, only criterion #1 would have elicited a second cardiac catheterization to comply with entry requirements to the Registry; this decision was of course taken only by the physician delivering primary care to the patient, whether or not he was also the principal investigator of the clinical center.

The actual ratio of previous to entry cardiac catheterizations is illustrated in Figure 1. The number varied from year to year reflecting total numbers of patients, but throughout the 5 years of the Registry, the ratio remained the same, i.e., about 70 percent of entered patients had had a previous cardiac catheterization. The performance of the cardiac catheterization which would be used for entry generally occurred after the patient's referral to a clinical center. The performance of this study was prompted by at least four possible incentives: (1) to rule out other diagnostic entities producing pulmonary hypertension, (2) to trace the progress of the disease, (3) to test pulmonary vasodilator drugs, and (4) to provide reliable data for the Registry. No data were collected by the Registry on the reasons for these repeat catheterizations. Many no doubt were for clinical reasons involving the first three possibilities listed above, especially the pharmacological trials. Where no clinical reason existed, appropriate institutional review and informed consent were a part of the initial criteria for participation in the Registry. Finally, though it was unclear how many cardiac catheterizations were solely for the purpose of entry into the Registry, no mortality and only

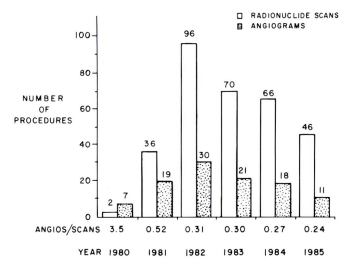

Figure 1: Ratio of previous to entry cardiac catheterization in patients entered in the Registry on Primary Pulmonary Hypertension, 1981–1985. Entry caths = all baseline cardiac catheterizations qualifying patients for entry, usually performed during the indicated year. Previous caths = a previous cardiac catheterization which could have been performed during the indicated year or, as usually occurred, during previous years. Entry caths = number of entered patients. As indicated, the ratio of previous to entry cardiac catheterizations was constant from year to year.

one minor morbidity incident were attributable to any of these diagnostic catheterizations.

The other example of entry requirement by the Registry was pulmonary angiography. However, this test was only required when pulmonary radionuclide perfusion scans in a given patient had been classified as high probability or indeterminant for pulmonary thromboembolism. In view of the fact that undiagnosed pulmonary hypertension was suspected in their patients, clinical prudence would already have indicated the need for pulmonary angiography in this group, without any such requirement by the Registry. Moreover, of the 163 perfusion scans analyzed, only five fell into the high probability to indeterminate category.

Thus, even though the Registry required for entry only five angiograms (and these would have been clinically indicated), the clinical centers together performed 106 angiograms (1980–1985). The incidence of these clinically dictated angiograms varied from center to center and appeared to reflect the clinical judgement of physicians and their suspicion of pulmonary thromboembolism. A bonus, of course, accrued to the Registry from an analysis of the results of these unsolicited angiograms: the incidence of adverse events during angiography was determined to be low, only one event (transient hypotension) in 106 angiograms, despite a large variation in degree of pulmonary hypertension. Figure 2 shows the ratio of angiograms to radionuclide perfusion scans in each year of the Registry. The indicated steady decline in the ratio from 1981 to 1985 suggests that greater familiarity with the disease may have decreased the clinical suspicion of thromboembolism.

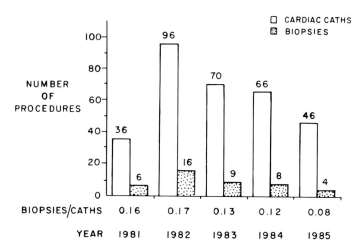

Figure 2: Ratio of pulmonary angiograms to radionuclide scans of patients entered in the Registry on Primary Pulmonary Hypertension, 1981–1985. The ratio appeared to decrease with time.

Definition of Disease

The preconceived description of the disease dictates the entry criteria to the Registry so that the classical notion of the disease becomes a self-fulfilling prophecy. There were several examples of this dilemma. They were most apparent in the exclusionary criteria for lung disease. Patients with lung volumes or expiratory flow rates in the abnormal range were excluded, but it is fully possible that some patients with PPH could have low lung volumes without having interstitial lung disease and some might have a combination of PPH and bronchial asthma. Thus, the description of PPH emerging from the Registry might be altered by this exclusion. The Steering Committee of the Registry elected, however, to risk this possibility in the interest of obtaining a group of patients with unquestioned PPH in order to fully describe the natural history of their disease.

Several other examples of exclusionary criteria were treated differently. For instance, patients with histories of intravenous drug abuse were considered to have either PPH or cotton-talc embolization of the pulmonary circulation. Without lung biopsy, these two categories could not be differentiated. All such patients, so long as they conformed in every other way to the Registry criteria, were entered, but segregated and analyzed separately (at least until new clinical data determined which category was appropriate). Neither open lung biopsy nor transbronchial biopsy were ever required for entry of any patient into the Registry. Where some doubt existed as to whether the pulmonary hypertension was primary, the patients were entered and considered for separate analysis at a later time. Such patients included not only the intravenous drug abusers, but also some with suspected scleroderma, collagen-vascular disease, and small thromboembolic disease, where the diagnosis was not yet definitive. These represented 19 percent of all patients entered.

Thus, the Registry developed two ways of dealing with exclusionary criteria. A finding (i.e., a physical or laboratory fact), such as a low lung volume, excluded patients altogether, whereas historical information, such as intravenous drug abuse, segregated the patients within the Registry. These differences in treatment of entry were, therefore, reasonably consistent. Although some patients who truly had PPH may have been excluded, the body of patients who were admitted to the Registry conformed to the present day conception of the clinical appearance of this disease and, thus, served as a suitable group in which to follow natural history of the disease.

Communication Among Investigators

The formation of the Registry would promote communication among a nationally distributed group of clinical investigators and, on this basis, produce more rapid evolution of treatment (good or bad) than would otherwise occur. Such an eventuality might very well change the natural history of the disease from that of previous generations. In fact, much has been made recently regarding the role of the observer in altering the phenomenon observed (3). However, PPH is not subatomic physics. It is possible for the physicist to alter observed events, but no alteration of all other examples of these events occurs in the universe. On the other hand, in PPH it is possible that natural history is changing now because the Registry indirectly caused more rapid dissemination of information about this disease; but, contrary to the situation in physics, the disseminated information will have forever changed the way patients are treated and, hence, bring about a definitive alteration for the moment of the natural history of PPH. When the Registry is concluded, it will be able to offer the clinician the present natural history of this disease, not what it was in 1891 (4) or 1951 (1) or probably even in 1981.

What kinds of clinical information which could influence management of PPH were subject to early dissemination by the Registry? Examples exist in three categories, of which the first is diagnosis. In this category, both pulmonary angiography and open lung biopsy occur. As indicated above, angiography was only required by the Registry for entry in case of an indeterminate or high probability radionuclide lung perfusion scan (there were five such patients). This entry criterion coincides with indicated clinical practice, in a patient with undiagnosed pulmonary hypertension. The additional 106 pulmonary angiograms were characterized by an unusual frequency with respect to time. At the beginning of the Registry in 1981, over one-half the entered patients (.52) had had pulmonary angiograms, whereas by 1985, the last year of the Registry, only 24 percent of the patients were having angiograms. Thus, angiography did not follow the usual pattern with accepted diagnostic procedures; its frequency of use decreased rather than increased. This usual pattern would be particularly expected since the Registry had already accumulated data showing virtually no adverse reactions to pulmonary angiography. The apparent decrease in use of this procedure may, therefore, be based on investigator interaction in which considerable experience was accumulated and exchanged even before reviewed publications were available. In this case, early doubts about the reliability of the normal radionuclide perfusion scan may have been dispelled by the Registry experience as disseminated by interinvestigator interaction.

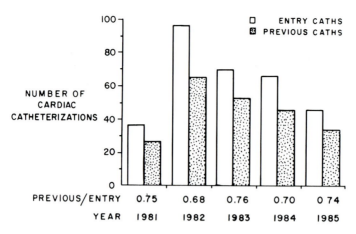

Figure 3: Ratio of open lung biopsies to total baseline cardiac catheterizations in patients entered in the Registry on Primary Pulmonary Hypertension, 1981–1985. The ratio appeared to decrease with time.

Open lung biopsy was not an entry criterion nor did the Steering Committee of the Registry make recommendations regarding its use. The time course of open lung biopsies from 1981 to 1985 is shown in Figure 3. The maximum ratio of biopsies to entered patients (reflected by cardiac catheterizations) was 0.17 in 1982 but decreased thereafter until, in the last year, the ratio was only 0.08. The high point of open lung biopsies, in 1981 and 1982, represented material referred from two sources: (1) an ongoing research study, independent of the Registry, of the role of lung biopsy in the management of these patients; and (2) random submissions apparently based on a differential diagnostic or other clinical indication. That all these submissions fell off over a 3-year period also suggests that early dissemination of information among the Registry participants may have played a role here.

The second category subject to the early communication effect is therapy. In this case, it is very possible that the dissemination of information and opinion among more than 30 clinical investigators could result in either more uniform approaches or changes in management earlier than would have been expected from publications in the medical literature. To the extent that the changes in therapy are rational, early dissemination of information within the Registry would be beneficial. There is, in fact, some evidence that a greater uniformity of therapy occurred: calcium channel blockers are now far more commonly used as vasodilators than they were at the inception of the Registry; it may be inferred that this was because of the existence of the Registry.

The third category subject to promotion by early dissemination of information is clinical research. This effort was, in fact, sought deliberately by the Registry as one of its desired by-products. An example of this category was the early dissemination of information regarding the incidence of antinuclear antibodies in PPH and the subsequent formation of groups outside the Registry to examine the association of this phenomenon to PPH.

Compensation for Clerical Work

Payment for completing long and tedious entry forms for each patient may act either to encourage entries into the Registry or to perform procedures not clinically indicated in order to facilitate acceptance. Did the $150 reimbursement for each accepted entry form act as a bounty? The Registry recognized that the principal investigators of the clinical centers would often be too busy to complete long forms. In the interest of facilitating entries, the payment of $150 was conceived for fellows or nurse clinicians who had the requisite expertise and time to perform this task. Thus, a separation of duties was largely achieved, with the principal investigator making the entry decision and with the associate receiving the stipend for the clerical work. Therefore, it would appear highly unlikely that the reimbursement fee affected clinical practice.

Geographic Skewing

Did the enthusiasm of a few investigators from cities at high altitude distort the geographic distribution of patients within the Registry or provide a patient subgroup whose natural history was influenced by the altitude? This was a carefully considered question at the outset of the Registry. As it developed, only two centers participating in the Registry were located at high altitude. They contributed 42 of the 238 patients accepted as of June, 1987, or 17.6 percent. The number appeared too small to affect materially the natural history of PPH; in addition, many patients at these two centers were referred from sea-level areas as well.

The above summary conveys the gist of the ethical and research dilemmas faced by the Registry Steering Committee.

One of the foremost of these dilemmas was the ability to satisfy entrance criteria by data which ordinary clinical indications would have accumulated. Every effort was made to restrict entrance criteria to clinically indicated testing. Thus, neither lung biopsy, vasodilator administration during cardiac catheterization nor pulmonary angiography (except when clinically indicated) was required for entrance. Cardiac catheterization occupied an intermediate position as an entry requirement. When the principal investigator could not vouch for the accuracy of a previous cardiac catheterization, Registry entry required recatheterization; however, clinical indications also necessitated recatheterization in order to (1) rule out shunts, left heart disease, and valvular stenosis; (2) perform pulmonary angiography; (3) determine rate of advancement of the disease; and (4) test vasodilator agents. Thus, there were always multiple factors dictating the need for repeat cardiac catheterization at the time of entry.

The other major dilemma we faced were the changes in the natural history of the disease brought about by alterations in clinical practice. Since we noted the development of uniformities of practice during the course of the Registry among its clinical centers and since these clinical centers managed the bulk of PPH patients in this country, the overall management of PPH may have changed more rapidly than during the natural course of dissemination of clinical information through journals and conferences. Until Registry data are further analyzed, it is uncertain whether changes in clinical practice altered the natural history of the disease.

ACKNOWLEDGMENTS

We are grateful to Paul Levy, Sc.D., and Janet Kernis, M.P.H., Director and Coordinator, respectively, of the PPH Data Coordinating Center, Chicago, Illinois, for supplying data used in this analysis.

REFERENCES

1. Dresdale DT, Schultz M, Michtom RJ: Primary pulmonary hypertension: I. Clinical and hemodynamic study. Am J Med II:686–694, 1951.

2. Hatano S, Strasser T (eds), *Primary Pulmonary Hypertension: Report on a WHO Meeting.* Geneva, World Health Organization, 1975.

3. Robin ED: Risk benefit analysis in chest medicine. The kingdom of the near dead. The shortened unnatural life history of primary pulmonary hypertension. Chest 92:330–334, 1987.

4. Romberg E: Veber Sklerose der Lungenarterien. Deutsche Arch Klinike 48:197–204, 1891.

Stuart Rich, M.D.

33 ⸺⸺⸺⸺⸺⸺⸺⸺⸺⸺

NIH Registry on Primary Pulmonary Hypertension: Baseline Characteristics of the Patients Enrolled

In 1981, the Division of Lung Diseases of the National Heart, Lung, and Blood Institute established a national registry for the characterization of patients with primary pulmonary hypertension (PPH). The goal of the registry was to collect prospectively data bearing on the natural history and treatment of PPH in the hope that fresh insights might be gained into the etiology and pathogenesis of the disease. A total of 191 patients who satisfied uniform criteria for entry were enrolled (17).

Primary pulmonary hypertension is, and is apt to remain, a diagnosis of exclusion. For that reason, the Registry enrolled patients only after certain secondary causes for pulmonary hypertension were excluded (Table 1).

TABLE 1 BASES FOR EXCLUSION FROM THE REGISTRY

Pulmonary hypertension within the first year of life, and congenital abnormalities of the lungs, thorax, and diaphragm

Congenital or acquired valvular or myocardial disease

Pulmonary thromboembolic disease evidenced either by a lung perfusion scan or positive pulmonary angiogram, a diagnosis of sickle cell anemia, or a history of intravenous drug abuse

Obstructive airways disease manifested by hypoxemia and reduced rates of airflow

Interstitial lung disease evidenced by a decrease in total lung capacity associated with pulmonary infiltrates on the chest radiograph

Arterial hypoxemia and hypercapnia

Collagen vascular disease

Parasitic disease affecting the lungs

Pulmonary arterial or valvular stenosis

Pulmonary venous hypertension manifested by pulmonary wedge pressures greater than 12 mmHg

FINDINGS OF THE REGISTRY

Demographics

The incidence of primary pulmonary hypertension in the general population has not been published, although the rate in patients undergoing right heart catheterization has been reported to be 1.1 percent (20). Although primary pulmonary hypertension occurs in the very young and elderly, its incidence is greatest between the ages of 20 and 45 years. The mean age of patients enrolled in the Registry was 36 years; it was similar for men and women. For women, the highest frequency was in the third decade; for men, it was in the fourth decade. Nine percent of the patients were more than 60 years old. The ratio of women to men was 1.7:1, regardless of decade. Symptoms at the time of presentation tended to be more severe in women than in men; 75 percent of the women were in functional class III or IV (New York Heart Association Classification) whereas 64 percent of the men fell into these categories (Fig. 1).

Several familial cases of PPH have now been reported in the American population (12). In the NIH Registry, the incidence was 7 percent. The familial type of disorder has been attributed to autosomal dominant inheritance with incomplete penetrance. Not infrequently, once the diagnosis of familial pulmonary hy-

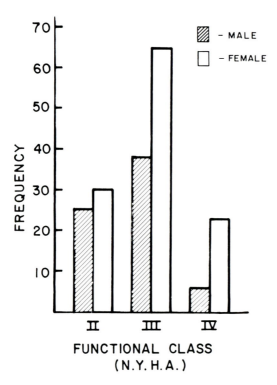

Figure 1: The distribution of patients entered in the NIH Registry on PPH is shown according to sex and functional class. Women tended to be more symptomatic at the time of diagnosis.

pertension is entertained for one or more individuals, retrospective analysis of family members who died without apparent cause has suggested that they too had died of primary pulmonary hypertension (12,22). Patients with a positive family history have the same clinical features as those with the nonfamilial disorder except for a shorter period from the onset of symptoms until diagnosis. The earlier diagnosis in the familial form has been attributed to a heightened awareness on the part of the patient or physician.

The Registry failed to identify a common etiology for primary pulmonary hypertension. Neither pregnancy (6,14) nor oral contraceptive use (11) could be implicated as an etiological factor.

Clinical Features

The clinical manifestations of patients who presented with primary pulmonary hypertension were diverse: dyspnea, fatigue, chest pain, palpitations, leg edema, near syncope, and syncope. Dyspnea was by far the most common initial symptom, occurring in 60 percent of the cases. However, virtually all patients admitted to dyspnea by the time the diagnosis was confirmed. Fatigue (19 percent), chest pain (7 percent), near syncope (5 percent), syncope (8 percent), leg edema (3 percent), and palpitations (5 percent) were less common initial symptoms. Twenty-nine percent of the patients had mild symptoms (functional class II) at the time of diagnosis; when compared to the more symptomatic patients (functional class III and IV), they were less likely to complain of fatigue and more apt to have peripheral edema.

The time between the onset of the first symptom and the diagnosis of primary pulmonary hypertension was 2.03 ± 4.9 years (median = 1.27 years); it was similar for men and women. Since dyspnea and fatigue are common in active people, it is understandable why patients failed to seek medical attention early, or why physicians may have delayed in pursuing the diagnosis.

The physical examination of a patient with PPH proved to be similar to that of patients with pulmonary hypertension due to a variety of causes. Right-sided third and fourth heart sounds were common; so were pulmonary ejection and regurgitant murmurs. Tricuspid regurgitation was extremely common, often the most notable auscultatory finding. The presence of a third heart sound and tricuspid regurgitation was associated with increased right atrial pressure and reduced cardiac output. Clubbing was not a manifestation of primary pulmonary hypertension.

The chest radiographic findings of patients with PPH typically showed enlargement of the main and hilar pulmonary arteries; pruning of the peripheral vasculature is common (1). As a rule, the lung fields were clear except for increased bronchovascular markings at the bases in patients with pulmonary veno-occlusive disease (3,23). Although upright posterior-anterior and lateral chest radiographs are important in helping to exclude lung disease as the underlying cause, clear lung fields on a chest radiograph did not exclude interstitial lung disease as a possible etiology (7).

In most patients, the electrocardiogram showed right axis deviation, right ventricular hypertrophy, and right ventricular strain; in all patients, the underlying rhythm was sinus in origin. Atrial fibrillation, which is common in cor pul-

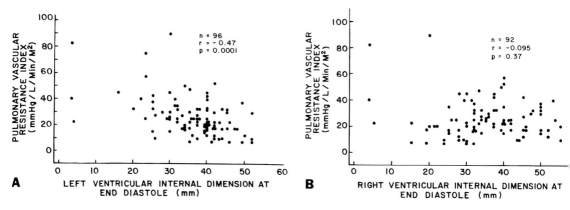

Figure 2: The relationship between pulmonary vascular resistance index and end-diastolic dimension of the left ventricle (A) and right ventricle (B) as measured on m-mode echocardiography is shown for patients entered in the PPH Registry. The inverse relationship with the left ventricle, although not very strong, was highly significant.

monale secondary to lung disease, was not seen. The reason for this discrepancy is speculative (13).

The echocardiogram (m-mode) showed a normal to small left ventricular end-diastolic internal dimension in all patients; in 75 percent, right ventricular enlargement was present. The calculated pulmonary vascular resistance index correlated inversely with left ventricular end-diastolic dimension ($r = 0.47$, $p < 0.001$) but not with right ventricular end-diastolic dimension (Fig. 2). Since, by definition, the filling pressure of the left ventricle is normal in primary pulmonary hypertension, this inverse relationship probably reflects decreased volume loading of the left heart as determined by the severity of the pulmonary vascular disease. Paradoxical septal motion was described in 59 percent and partial systolic closure of the pulmonic valve in 60 percent. In approximately 6 percent of patients, the chest radiograph, echocardiogram, and/or electrocardiogram were relatively normal despite significant pulmonary hypertension, thereby underscoring the lack of insensitivity of these tests in some patients.

Despite a 29 percent incidence of positive antinuclear antibodies in the blood, the frequency of Raynaud's syndrome—which occurred almost exclusively in the women—was only 11 percent, slightly greater than the 6 percent prevalence reported in normal controls (25). In keeping with previous studies, the female-to-male prevalence of positive antinuclear antibodies was 1.4 to 1 (16,18).

There were two predominant patterns of perfusion lung scans in these patients: 42 percent were interpreted as normal and 58 percent had diffuse patchy abnormalities. Previous studies describing these patterns of perfusion lung scans in patients with unexplained pulmonary hypertension have suggested that the normal pattern may be associated with plexogenic arteriopathy, whereas the patchy distribution may be indicative of microthrombi or veno-occlusive disease (19,24).

Measurements of pulmonary function revealed that patients with primary pulmonary hypertension generally have a mild restrictive defect without airways obstruction in association with arterial hypoxemia and respiratory alkalosis. However, no association was found between any parameter of airway flow or lung volume, and hemodynamics. A decrease in the diffusing capacity of the lungs was another common finding (8,10). Although obliteration of the small pulmonary arteries has been proferred as an explanation for this decrease (2), no significant correlation was found between the diffusing capacity and any index of the severity of the pulmonary hypertension. Because of the wide distribution of values which included normal lung volumes and/or diffusing capacities, pulmonary function tests proved to be insensitive markers of the disease.

Almost universal was the finding of mild to moderate arterial hypoxemia which is generally attributed to the combined effects of a low mixed venous Po_2 (resulting from a low cardiac output) and a mild degree of ventilation-perfusion inequality (5). In some instances, more severe degrees of hypoxemia may be attributable to right-to-left shunting via a patent foramen ovale. The chronic respiratory alkalosis is held to be due to an increase in ventilation caused by increased afferent stimulation originating either in intrapulmonary stretch receptors or intravascular baroreceptors (4,9,21).

Hemodynamic Features

As a rule, patients with PPH showed a characteristic constellation of hemodynamic features at the time of diagnosis: severe pulmonary hypertension with a three-fold increase in mean pulmonary artery pressure (60 $\pm$ 18 mmHg range 28–127 mmHg), mild-to-moderate increase in right atrial pressures (9 $\pm$ 6 mmHg, range 0–29 mmHg) with normal pulmonary wedge pressures, and mildly reduced cardiac indexes (2.27 $\pm$ 0.9 L/min/M^2, range 0.8–7.9 L/min/M^2). Patients with the more severe symptoms (functional class III and IV) had minimally higher mean pulmonary artery pressures than did their less symptomatic (functional class II) counterparts (62 versus 56 mmHg, p = 0.06). They also had higher right atrial pressures (11 versus 7 mmHg, p = 0.0001) and lower cardiac indexes (2.06 versus 2.73 L/min/M^2, p = 0.0003). In contrast, hemodynamic values for the two groups were indistinguishable with respect to duration of symptoms. Although young women have often been described as most severely afflicted by primary pulmonary hypertension, no significant differences in hemodynamics or functional class were found between women 15 to 34 years old and men and women 35 years old or older.

The hemodynamic findings suggest that the severity of symptoms can be related to increasing right atrial pressure and falling cardiac index, both of which are reflections of right ventricular function. The fact that the mean pulmonary artery pressures were similar in patients in whom the duration of symptoms was less than 1 year and in those who were symptomatic for more than 3 years suggests that the pulmonary artery pressure increases to high levels early in the course of the disease. Patients in whom dyspnea on effort was the sole complaint already had severe pulmonary hypertension. The onset of fatigue and edema, symptoms that reflect right ventricular failure, tended to appear later in the clinical course. Although physicians tend to relate the severity of the disease to the duration of symptoms, the hemodynamic comparisons did not support this practice. Indeed, the results raise the prospect that the severity of the disease process may not parallel the duration of the disease as reflected in symptoms; also, that progression of the disease may differ considerably from patient to patient.

Hazards of the Work-up

An important function of the Registry was to monitor the incidence of adverse experiences that might occur in the patients during diagnostic evaluation. There were no reported adverse consequences of perfusion lung scanning and only one mild adverse reaction (transient hypotension) in the 50 patients reported to have undergone pulmonary angiography. The low incidence of adverse reactions underscores the safety of using angiography to rule out chronic pulmonary thromboemboli in any patient who presents with unexplained pulmonary hypertension (15). Ten adverse experiences were reported to have occurred during diagnostic catheterization (exclusive of the drug evaluations); of these, six were probably related to the pulmonary hypertension itself. There were no deaths or sustained morbidity from any of the procedures.

CONCLUSION

Using uniform diagnostic criteria, the NIH Registry has characterized prospectively the demographic and clinical features of a large number of patients with primary pulmonary hypertension. The results indicate that the diagnosis is usually not made until advanced abnormalities exist in the physical examination, laboratory tests, and pulmonary hemodynamics. Although there is as yet no therapy that can cure primary pulmonary hypertension, the results emphasize a need to focus on strategies for making the diagnosis before pulmonary vascular abnormalities are severe and irreversible.

REFERENCES

1. Anderson G, Reid L, Simon G: The radiographic appearances in primary and thromboembolic pulmonary hypertension. Clin Radiol 24 : 113–120, 1973.

2. Anderson EG, Simon G, Reid L: Primary and thromboembolic pulmonary hypertension: A quantitative pathological study. J Pathol 110 : 273–293, 1973.

3. Dail DH, Liebow AA, Gmelich J, Carrington CB, Churg A: A study of 43 cases of pulmonary veno-occlusive disease. Lab Invest 38 : 340–350, 1978.

4. D'Alonzo GE, Gianotti LA, Pohil RL, Reagle RR, DuRee SL, Fuentes F, Dantzker DR: Comparison of progressive exercise performance of normal subjects and patients with primary pulmonary hypertension. Chest 91 : 57–62, 1987.

5. Dantzker DR, Bower JS: Mechanisms of gas exchange abnormality in patients with chronic obliterative pulmonary vascular disease. J Clin Invest 64 : 1050–1055, 1979.

6. Dawkins KD, Burke CM, Billingham ME, Jamieson SW: Primary pulmonary hypertension and pregnancy. Chest 89 : 383–388, 1986.

7. Epler GR, McLoud TC, Gaensler EA, Mikus JP, Carrington CB: Normal chest roentgenograms in chronic diffuse infiltrative lung disease. N Engl J Med 298 : 934–939, 1978.

8. Gazetopoulos N, Salonikides N, Davies H: Cardiopulmonary function in patients with pulmonary hypertension. Br Heart J 36 : 19–28, 1974.

9. Green JF, Sheldon MI: Ventilatory changes associated with changes in pulmonary blood flow in dogs. J Appl Physiol 54 : 997–1002, 1983.

10. Horn M, Ries A, Neveu C, Moser KM: Restrictive ventilatory pattern in precapillary pulmonary hypertension. Am Rev Respir Dis 128 : 163–165, 1983.

11. Kleiger RE, Boxer M, Ingham RE, Harrison DC: Pulmonary hypertension in patients using oral contraceptives. Chest 69 : 143–147, 1976.

12. Loyd JE, Primm RK, Newman JH: Familial primary pulmonary hypertension: Clinical patterns. Am Rev Respir Dis 129 : 194–197, 1984.

13. Louie EK, Rich S, Brundage BH: Doppler echocardiographic assessment of impaired left ventricular filling in patients with right ventricular pressure overload due to primary pulmonary hypertension. J Am Coll Cardiol 8 : 1298–1306, 1986.

14. McCaffrey RM, Dunn LJ: Primary pulmonary hypertension in pregnancy. Obstet Gynec Surv 19 : 567–591, 1964.

15. Moser KM, Spragg RG, Utley J, Daily PO: Chronic thrombotic obstruction of major pulmonary arteries: Results of thromboendarterectomy in 15 patients. Ann Intern Med 99 : 299–304, 1983.

16. Rawson AJ, Walke HM: A study of etiologic factors in so-called primary pulmonary hypertension. Arch Intern Med 105 : 233–243, 1960.

17. Rich S, Dantzker DR, Ayres SM, Bergofsky EH, Brundage BH, Detre KM, Fishman AP, Goldring RM, Groves BM, Koerner SK, Levy PC, Reid LM, Vreim CE, Williams GW: Primary pulmonary hypertension: A national prospective study. Ann Intern Med 107 : 216–223, 1987.

18. Rich S, Kieras K, Hart K, Groves BM, Stobo JD, Brundage BH: Antinuclear antibodies in primary pulmonary hypertension. J Am Coll Cardiol 8 : 1307–1311, 1986.

19. Rich R, Pietra GG, Kieras K, Hart K, Brundage BH: Primary pulmonary hypertension: Radiographic and scintigraphic patterns of histologic subtypes. Ann Intern Med 105 : 499–502, 1986.

20. Storstein O, Efskind L, Muller C, Rokseth R, Sanders S: Primary pulmonary hypertension with emphasis on its etiology and treatment. Acta Med Scand 79 : 197–212, 1966.

21. Theodore J, Robin ED, Morris AJR, Burke CM, Jamieson SW, Van Kessel A, Stinson EB, Shumway NE: Augmented ventilatory response to exercise in pulmonary hypertension. Chest 89 : 39–44, 1986.

22. Thompson P, McRae C: Familial pulmonary hypertension: Evidence of autosomal dominant inheritance. Br Heart J 32 : 758–760, 1970.

23. Wagenvoort CA, Wagenvoort N, Takahashi T: Pulmonary veno-occlusive disease: Involvement of pulmonary arteries and review of the literature. Hum Pathol 16 : 1033–1041, 1985.

24. Wilson AG, Harris CN, Lavender JP, Oakley CM: Perfusion lung scanning in obliterative pulmonary hypertension. Br Heart J 35 : 917–930, 1973.

25. Zahavi I, Chagnac A, Hering R, Davidovich S, Kuritzky A: Prevalence of Raynaud's phenomenon in patients with migraine. Arch Intern Med 144 : 742–744, 1984.

Giuseppe G. Pietra, M.D.

34

The Histopathology of Primary Pulmonary Hypertension

Pathologists have identified several patterns of pulmonary vascular lesions in patients diagnosed on clinical grounds as having primary pulmonary hypertension (1,3,7,17). In addition to the three pathological entities recognized by the World Health Organization (WHO) in 1973 (5), namely, plexogenic pulmonary arteriopathy, recurrent thromboembolism, and pulmonary veno-occlusive disease, two entities, pulmonary hemangioendotheliomatosis (9,14) and primary pulmonary arteritis (1), have recently been recently described as rare causes of primary pulmonary hypertension.

However, the histopathological classification of hypertensive pulmonary vascular disease proposed by the WHO has been criticized because it presumes well-defined pathogenetic mechanisms of pulmonary hypertension and does not take into consideration the complexities and severity of the pathological lesions seen in individual cases. Accordingly, the National Registry on Primary Pulmonary Hypertension has adopted a descriptive classification of hypertensive pulmonary vascular diseases which is based on the predominant type and location of pathological changes in the vascular wall. This classification will be used in this chapter and will be preceded by a description of the various pathological lesions that occur in adult patients with pulmonary hypertension.

HISTOPATHOLOGY OF THE HYPERTENSIVE PULMONARY VASCULATURE

The pulmonary blood vessels react to altered hemodynamics in a limited number of ways. On cross section, lesions may be confined to the media, to the intima, to the adventitia or may involve all components of the vascular wall, including the lumen. Along the length of the pulmonary vascular tree, the pathological changes may be limited to the pulmonary trunk and elastic arteries or extend to the muscular pulmonary artery and arterioles or even involve the entire length of the vascular tree. In primary pulmonary hypertension, the vascular lesions affect primarily the small pulmonary arteries, and changes in the elastic pulmonary arteries, such as intimal atheromas and fibrosis and medial hypertrophy, are considered to be secondary. In a few instances of primary pulmonary hypertension, both small arteries and veins are predominantly affected (1,11,15,17).

Muscular Pulmonary Arteries and Arterioles

In the muscular pulmonary arteries and arterioles, hypertensive pathological changes may affect the media, the intima, or the entire arterial wall.

Lesions of the Media

Medial hypertrophy is defined as an abnormal increase in smooth muscle mass and reduplication of elastic laminae in muscular arteries (Fig. 1), and as an extension of smooth muscle into partially muscularized or nonmuscularized intra-acinar arterioles (Fig. 2). It is present in each case of pulmonary hypertension but differs in severity from case to case and from vessel to vessel within the same lung.

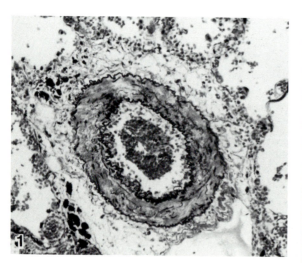
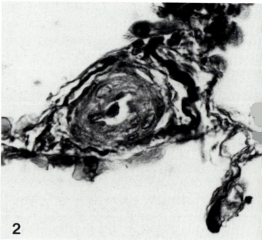

Figure 1: Moderate medial hypertrophy of a muscular pulmonary artery. The media is three times normal in thickness. Verhoeff-van Gieson stain. X200.

Figure 2: Muscularization of pulmonary arteriole. A thick muscle coat is present in the arteriole. Normally the muscle layer in this type of vessel is discontinuous. Verhoeff-van Gieson stain. X800.

Although medial hypertrophy sometimes occurs as an isolated lesion, more frequently it is associated with intimal lesions (as described below).

The hypertrophic smooth muscle of the media may undergo degeneration and be partially or totally replaced by fibrous tissue, presumably as a consequence of long-standing disease or high pressures. Since this process is a gradual one, medial hypertrophy and fibrosis may coexist in the same vessel. In time, atrophy and fibrosis of the medial muscle leads to dilatation of the vascular lumen and thinning of the media. Although the presence of medial fibrosis and smooth muscle atrophy in pulmonary muscular arteries has not been taken into account in recent attempts to correlate the extent of anatomical vascular lesions and abnormal hemodynamics (4,13), it was clearly described by Brenner (2) 30 years ago in his classic paper on the pathology of the vessels of the pulmonary circulation. There can be little doubt that vessels involved by medial fibrosis are apt to respond differently to vasodilator therapy than will vessels in which the media is hypertrophied. The degree and extent of medial fibrosis in the pulmonary vessels of patients with pulmonary hypertension warrants the attention of the pathologist.

Lesions of the Intima

Intimal lesions are found in association with mediae that are normal in thickness, hypertrophied, or atrophied. The intimal lesions are of two types: *eccentric intimal fibrosis* and *concentric laminar intimal fibrosis*.

Eccentric intimal fibrosis is characterized by intimal cushions that are composed of myofibroblasts, connective tissue fibers, and matrix (Fig. 3). In two recent large series of patients with primary pulmonary hypertension, eccentric

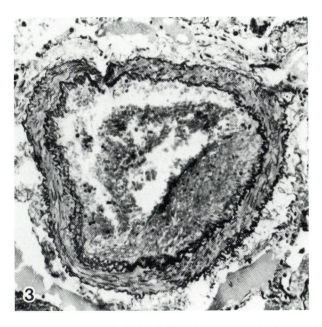

Figure 3: Eccentric intimal fibrosis characterized by patchy fibrous intimal thickening. Verhoeff-van Gieson stain. X200.

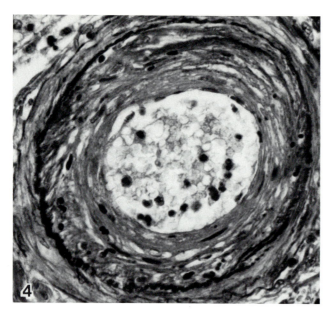

Figure 4: Concentric laminar intimal fibrosis. The arterial lumen is narrowed by concentric layers of myofibroblasts, connective tissue fibers, and matrix rich in proteoglycans. Verhoeff-van Gieson stain. X500.

intimal fibrosis was found to be the most common type of intimal lesion (1,11). Eccentric intimal fibrosis may be localized to a segment of the intima or involve the entire circumference of the intima; the involvement may be so extensive as to obliterate the arterial lumen completely (1). Eccentric intimal fibrosis may result from organization of either emboli or thrombi or from proliferation of intimal cells that can be triggered by a variety of insults to the vascular wall (10). Pathologists often assume that eccentric intimal fibrosis represents organization of a clot. Since, in the individual case, it is not possible on morphological grounds to determine which of the above mechanisms is responsible for the lesion, it seems preferable not to use the term *organized thromboemboli* as a synonym for *eccentric intimal fibrosis*.

Concentric laminar intimal fibrosis (Fig. 4) is a highly characteristic intimal lesion composed of concentric, onionskin-like layers of myofibroblasts and elastic fibers that are separated by an abundant acellular connective tissue matrix that is rich in proteoglycans. Concentric laminar intimal fibrosis is not unique for primary pulmonary hypertension although the WHO pathological classification did include it under the designation "plexogenic arteriopathy" (see below): identical lesions occur in the pulmonary hypertension that accompanies congenital heart disease with a shunt. It also occurs in the systemic and pulmonary muscular arteries of patients with progressive systemic sclerosis or chronic allograft rejection. In pulmonary hypertension, concentric laminar intimal fibrosis tends to be progressive, often accompanied by atrophy of the underlying media (1,17).

Lesions of the Adventitia

Isolated changes in the adventitia of muscular arteries are not observed in primary pulmonary hypertension. However, the adventitia is usually involved in lesions that affect the full thickness of the arterial wall.

Lesions of the Entire Arterial Wall

Three types of lesions can affect the full thickness of the arterial wall: arteritis, plexiform lesions, and dilatation lesions.

Arteritis is a primary inflammatory process that usually involves the intima and media and, less often, the adventitia. Arteritis may be necrotizing with fibrin insudation (*fibrinoid necrosis*) or entail infiltration of the arterial wall with polymorphonuclear leukocytes and lymphocytes. It may involve only one aspect of the arterial wall or its entire circumference. Healing of the arteritis can result in scarring of the vessel wall and deposition of calcium and iron on degenerated elastic fibers (ferruginization).

Plexiform lesions have generated a great deal of interest and controversy that seem to be inversely proportional to their functional significance and frequency. Plexiform lesions have been considered to be the hallmark of the arteriopathy seen in primary pulmonary hypertension. This view is reflected in the designation *plexogenic pulmonary arteriopathy* (5,17). Although distinctive, plexiform lesions may be difficult to distinguish from recanalized thromboemboli. The distinctive feature (Figs. 5 and 6) of a plexiform lesion is an aneurysmal dilatation of a muscular artery or arteriole near its origin from a larger parent vessel. The lumen of the aneurysm is filled with a complex network of thin-walled vessels, lined by plump endothelial cells (Fig. 6). The media is partially or totally destroyed and

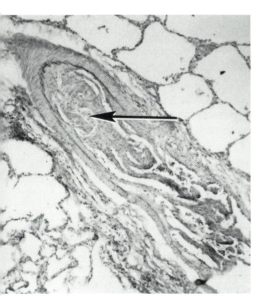
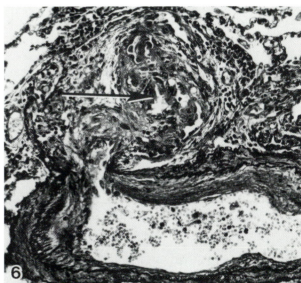

Figure 5: Recanalized thromboembolus (arrow). The arterial lumen is subdivided into multiple channels by fibrous septa and proliferated endothelial cells. Note that the arterial wall is not destroyed. Verhoeff-van Gieson stain. X180.

Figure 6: Plexiform lesion (arrow) arising at the origin of a pulmonary artery from parent vessels. The vessel wall has been destroyed locally, resulting in the formation of a microaneurysm that is filled with small blood channels and granulation tissue. Verhoeff-van Gieson stain. X200.

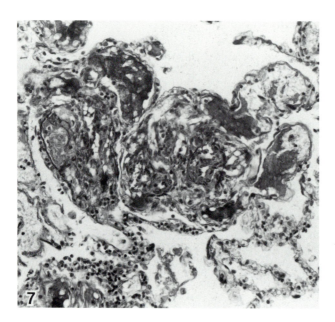

Figure 7: Dilatation lesion composed of a network of thin-walled dilated blood vessels. Verhoeff-van Gieson stain. X250.

the adventitia is replaced by granulation tissue. Proximally, the lumen of the parent artery is markedly narrowed and the intima undergoes fibrosis. Distally, the plexiform lesion feeds into a network of dilated thin-walled blood vessels. Plexiform lesions develop in vessels previously damaged by fibrinoid necrosis. Platelet or blood thrombi are often seen in their lumens.

Some authors have distinguished dilatation lesions from plexiform lesions (19). In their view, dilatation lesions consist of sinusoidal-like clusters of dilated thin-walled vessels (Fig. 7) that are not associated with plexiform lesions. However, whether dilatation lesions exist, per se, is questionable since it is often impossible to determine whether a dilatation lesion is only part of a plexiform lesion that is present at a different level of tissue section.

Lesions Involving the Arterial Lumen

The lumens of muscular pulmonary arteries and arterioles may be partially or totally occluded by thrombi or emboli in different stages of organization. Characteristically, organized thromboemboli cause eccentric patches of intimal fibrosis and fibrous septa that subdivide the vascular lumen into several endothelial-lined small channels (Fig. 5). As indicated above, recanalized thromboemboli may closely resemble plexiform lesions. Their true nature can be recognized by the absence of dilatation and medial destruction of the affected artery (Fig. 5), and by their random distribution in vessels of different size, without predilection for branching sites.

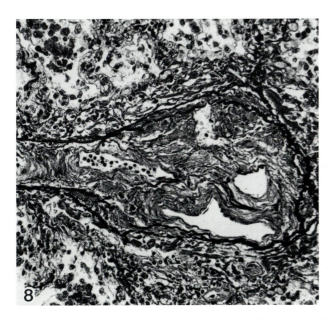

Figure 8: Pulmonary vaso-occlusive disease. The lumen of an intrapulmonary vein is sub-divided into small blood channels separated by broad fibrous septa. The adjacent pulmonary capillaries are markedly congested and the alveoli are filled with hemosiderin-laden macrophages. Verhoeff-van Gieson stain. X250.

Lesions of Pulmonary Venules and Veins

Hypertensive changes in pulmonary veins and venules are present in only a small percentage of patients having primary pulmonary hypertension. The hypertensive changes may involve the media, the intima, or the lumen. Medial hypertrophy and the formation of well-developed internal and external elastic laminae (arterialization) may be seen. The medial changes are associated with narrowing and obliteration of lumens by fibrous tissue, smooth muscle cells, and small vascular channels that resemble recanalized thrombi (Fig. 8); hence, the term *pulmonary veno-occlusive disease.*

THE WHO CLASSIFICATION OF THE PATHOLOGY OF PRIMARY PULMONARY HYPERTENSION

In 1973 the World Health Organization (WHO) held a conference on the pathology of primary pulmonary hypertension and codified criteria for the morphological diagnosis of this entity (5). The conference recognized that the clinical syndrome was associated with three distinct types of pulmonary vascular lesions. However, only one type, *plexogenic pulmonary arteriopathy,* was considered to be the characteristic lesion of vasoconstrictive pulmonary hypertension (17). With respect to the other two types of pulmonary vascular lesions, the pulmonary

TABLE 1 HISTOPATHOLOGICAL CLASSIFICATION OF PRIMARY PULMONARY HYPERTENSION

Present classification	WHO classification	Characteristic histopathological features*
Primary pulmonary arteriopathy with:		
Plexiform lesions, with or without thrombotic lesions	Plexogenic pulmonary arteriopathy (1,5,17)	*Plexiform lesions;* medial hypertrophy, eccentric or concentric-laminar intimal proliferation and fibrosis, fibrinoid degeneration-arteritis, dilatation lesions, and thrombotic lesions.
Thrombotic lesions	Thromboembolic pulmonary hypertension (1,15,17)	*Thrombi* (fresh, organizing, or organized, and recanalized—collander lesions), varying degrees of medial hypertrophy; *no* plexiform lesions.
Isolated medial hypertrophy	Plexogenic pulmonary arteriopathy (1,15,17)	*Medial hypertrophy; no* appreciable intimal or luminal obstructive lesions.
Intimal and medial hypertrophy	Plexogenic pulmonary arteriopathy (1,5,17)	*Eccentric or concentric-laminar proliferation and fibrosis;* varying degrees of medial hypertrophy; *no* thrombotic or plexiform lesions.
Isolated arteritis	Plexogenic pulmonary arteriopathy (1)	*Active or healed arteritis,* limited to pulmonary arteries; varying degrees of medial hypertrophy, intimal fibrosis, and thrombotic lesions; *no* plexiform lesions.
Pulmonary veno-occlusive disease	Pulmonary veno-occlusive disease (5,17)	*Intimal fibrosis and recanalized thrombi* (collander lesions) of pulmonary veins and venules; arterialized veins, capillary congestion, alveolar edema and siderophages, dilated lymphatics, pleural and septal edema and arterial medial hypertrophy, intimal fibrosis, and thrombotic lesions.
Pulmonary capillary hemangiomatosis (9,14)	—	*Infiltrating thin-walled blood vessels,* widespread throughout pulmonary parenchyma.

* Medial hypertrophy may be accompanied by muscularization of arterioles.

hypertension was considered to be the consequence either of recurrent silent pulmonary emboli (*thromboembolic pulmonary arteriopathy*) or of thrombosis of pulmonary veins (*pulmonary veno-occlusive disease*) (5,17,18).

Although the designation *plexogenic arteriopathy* derived its name from the plexogenic lesions, the term has been used somewhat indiscriminately in the past in categorizing the pathology findings in patients with the clinical manifestations of primary pulmonary hypertension. Indeed, it has even been applied to instances of isolated medial hypertrophy or of a combination of medial hypertrophy and concentric laminar intimal fibrosis in which plexogenic lesions could not be found. Additional ambiguity stems from the fact noted above that plexogenic arteriopathy is not unique to primary pulmonary hypertension, i.e., it occurs in pulmonary hypertension caused by congenital heart defects (6), schistosomiasis (8), and appetite suppressants (21). Reservations about usage of the term plexogenic pulmonary arteriopathy have prompted the National Registry to advocate reexamination of its diagnostic value.

A REVISED CLASSIFICATION OF THE HISTOPATHOLOGY
OF PRIMARY PULMONARY HYPERTENSION

The WHO Committee on the Pathology of Primary Pulmonary Hypertension deserves credit for having recognized that clinical primary pulmonary hypertension is associated with different patterns of vascular pathology, suggesting multiple etiologies and pathogenetic mechanisms. However, it has become apparent that there are several inconsistencies in the WHO classification: thromboembolic lesions are probably thrombotic, rather than embolic, in origin (1); plexiform lesions are absent in 30 percent of cases of "plexogenic arteriopathy" (17), "plexogenic" and "thromboembolic" lesions often coexist in the same patient (1,11), and medial hypertrophy is sometimes the only anatomic change present in some instances of so-called plexogenic pulmonary arteriopathy (1,7,17).

The WHO classification assumed not only that concentric laminar intimal fibrosis was pathognomonic for vasoconstrictive hypertension, but also that eccentric intimal fibrosis was pathognomonic for organized thrombi or emboli (17). However, neither in one large recent clinical-pathological study (1) nor in the Registry (Pietra, Edwards, Kay: personal observations) could evidence be adduced to support the idea of an embolic origin for the eccentric intimal lesions. Instead of the expected findings of pulmonary embolism, i.e., clinical and pathological evidence of emboli lodging in large elastic pulmonary arteries, both bodies of data indicated that in patients dying of primary pulmonary hypertension, eccentric intimal fibrosis was generally confined to the pulmonary muscular arteries and arterioles. Moreover, quantitative assessment of material submitted to the Registry failed to find any statistically significant difference between the degrees of medial hypertrophy in the plexogenic and thromboembolic pulmonary arteriopathies (11). Finally, in several instances, concentric and eccentric intimal fibrosis were found to coexist (11). Therefore, eccentric intimal fibrosis may be a secondary rather than a primary vascular hypertensive lesion.

With respect to *pulmonary veno-occlusive disease*, its association with widespread medial hypertrophy and with eccentric and concentric intimal fibrosis of muscular pulmonary arteries and arterioles has raised the possibility that the primary injury may involve the entire pulmonary vasculature simultaneously instead of primarily affecting the veins and the arteries only secondarily (20). Finally, since the WHO classification, two other entities, *primary pulmonary arteritis and hemangiomatosis*, have been recognized as possible causes of clinical primary pulmonary hypertension (1,14).

As it became evident in the course of reviewing material submitted to the National Registry of Primary Pulmonary Hypertension that the WHO classification needed revision, the classification of histopathological subsets shown in Table 1 was adopted for the analysis of cases referred to the Registry (11).

TABLE 2 HISTOLOGICAL TYPES OF HYPERTENSIVE VASCULAR DISEASE AMONG 38 AUTOPSIES IN THE REGISTRY

Type	Incidence		Age		Sex ratio
	Number	%	Mean	Range	M/F
Primary pulmonary arteriopathy	33	87	37	6–66	11/22
Pulmonary veno-occlusive disease	5	13	28	11–43	3/2
Pulmonary capillary hemangiomatosis	0	—	—	—	—

INCIDENCE OF HISTOPATHOLOGICAL SUBSETS IN THE REGISTRY POPULATION

Table 2 summarizes the incidence and demographic features of the histopathological subsets in 38 autopsies of patients in the National Registry on Primary Pulmonary Hypertension. Cases were categorized histopathologically according to whether the predominant pathology affected the media or intima of 60 randomly selected muscular pulmonary arteries and arterioles, and according to the presence or absence of lesions in the pulmonary veins, venules, and capillaries. By limiting the analysis to autopsies, it was possible to take advantage of the opportunity of random sampling from different lobes and to establish unequivocally the primary nature of the pulmonary hypertensive disease by excluding any extrapulmonary cause of the disease.

Pulmonary arteriopathy was the predominant vascular hypertensive lesion in 33 of the 38 patients (87 percent) (Table 2). A similar experience has been reported in other large series by Wagenvoort (15,17) and Bjornsson and Edwards (1). Among the subsets of pulmonary arteriopathy, 20 patients (60 percent) had primary pulmonary arteriopathy with thrombotic and plexiform lesions; 10 (30 percent) showed only thrombotic lesions. Three patients (9 percent) had pulmonary artery medial hypertrophy and intimal fibrosis (Table 3).

TABLE 3 HISTOLOGICAL PATTERNS AMONG 33 CASES OF PRIMARY PULMONARY ARTERIOPATHY

Pattern	Incidence		Age		Sex
	Number	%	Mean	Range	
with plexiform lesions	14	42	29	15–52	F
	6	18	32	10–57	M
with thrombotic lesions	6	18	37	22–55	F
	4	12	40	35–44	M
with medial hypertrophy and intimal fibrosis	2	6	63	61–66	F
with isolated medial hypertrophy	1			6	M
with isolated arteritis	0	—	—	—	—

The incidence in the Registry of pulmonary hypertensive arteriopathy with thrombotic lesions which corresponds to the thromboembolic pulmonary arteriopathy reported by others (1,17), is less than that reported by Bjornsson and Edwards (1) in a retrospective study at the Mayo Clinic of 80 patients with primary pulmonary hypertension. In the Registry, the overall incidence of this form of arteriopathy was 30 percent, whereas in the Mayo Clinic study it was 56 percent. These discrepancies most likely stem from the stricter criteria adopted by the Registry for inclusion of patients in the study. The Registry results are closer to those of the Wagenvoorts who reported a 20 to 30 percent incidence of thromboembolic pulmonary hypertension (15,17). Bjornsson and Edwards argue that instead of being embolic in origin, this form of hypertensive arteriopathy is probably thrombotic (1). Whether thrombosis is the primary lesion or is secondary to intimal damage caused by the abnormal pulmonary hemodynamics remains to be resolved.

In the Registry the incidence of eccentric intimal lesions and thrombotic lesions in the arteriopathy with plexiform lesions was high. This high incidence also occurred in the Mayo Clinic study (1) in which, as indicated above, the eccentric intimal lesions and thrombosis were considered to be secondary to intimal damage. Virtually every case of "plexogenic pulmonary arteriopathy" had associated thrombotic lesions, a finding that has not been emphasized previously (1,15,17), and which should be kept in mind by pathologists evaluating lung biopsies where only few arteries are available for examination.

Quantitative analysis of the histopathological lesions in the pulmonary arteries of cases of "plexogenic arteriopathy" submitted to the Registry showed that plexiform lesions were present in fewer than 10 percent of the muscular arteries. However, the incidence of recanalized thromboemboli was less in the "plexogenic" than in the "thromboembolic" groups. As shown in Table 3, pulmonary arteriopathy with concentric laminar intimal fibrosis and plexiform lesions was almost exclusively found in young women. Although the reasons for this predilection are unknown, it appears that the presence of pulmonary arteriopathy with concentric laminar intimal fibrosis and plexiform lesions is associated with being young and female. In the Mayo study, this form of pulmonary hypertensive vascular disease was noted to be associated with a greater frequency of sudden death (1).

In the Registry, pulmonary veno-occlusive disease was found in 13 percent of cases that satisfied clinical criteria for primary pulmonary hypertension (Table 2); the vascular lesions were present in veins, arteries, and capillaries. As reported by Wagenvoort et al. (20), the presence of widespread arterial intimal lesions in pulmonary veno-occlusive disease suggests that this entity may be a syndrome resulting from multiple injuries to the *entire* pulmonary vascular tree rather than a single disease that inflicts its primary damage on the pulmonary venous circulation.

The Registry included no instance of either primary pulmonary arteritis or of pulmonary capillary hemangiomatosis.

LUNG BIOPSY IN THE DIAGNOSIS OF PRIMARY PULMONARY HYPERTENSION

Wagenvoort has written extensively on the use of lung biopsy in the diagnosis of pulmonary vascular disease (15,17). As in every biopsy procedure, benefits to the patient must be weighed against risks. In 25 patients with primary pulmonary hypertension who underwent open lung biopsy at the Hospital of the University of Pennsylvania between 1981 and 1987, five died 1 to 10 days after the procedure. However, in no instance could death be attributed to the procedure itself (Table 4).

For a lung biopsy to provide meaningful information, a number of prerequisites must be met:

1. Most important, the *clinician* should review with the pathologist, prior to the biopsy, the kind of information that is expected from the procedure and how the findings will influence patient management.
2. The *chest surgeon* should realize that vessels 500 μm in diameter must be included in the specimen. Accordingly, the biopsy should not be a thin sleeve of tissue removed from the edge of a lobe but rather a wedge-shaped piece of tissue about 2 × 2 × 1.5 cm.
3. The *pathologist* must be aware of the fact that assessment of pulmonary vascular pathology requires the lung tissue to be fixed in the distended state and the sections to be stained in order to demonstrate all of the vascular components. Several techniques are available to achieve these goals. With respect to ensuring proper fixation, our laboratory serially sections the tissue and fixes the tissue slices under vacuum. The entire specimen is sectioned and embedded for microscopic study since the blood vessels are not uniformly distributed within the pulmonary parenchyma. Stains to vi-

TABLE 4 DEATHS AFTER OPEN LUNG BIOPSY FOR THE DIAGNOSIS OF UNEXPLAINED PULMONARY HYPERTENSION

Age	Sex	PA pressures (mmHg) syst/diast/mean	PVR (dynes · sec/cm^5)	Days from biopsy to death	Cause of death
49	F	67/22/41	760	2	Apparent acute myocardial infarction while in SICU postbiopsy
17	F	100/44/60	1020	6	Variceal upper gastrointestinal bleed (portal hypertension secondary to portal vein thrombosis)
36	M	71/31/47	860	14	Progressive right heart failure—had recovered from biopsy and had been discharged postop day 11
24	F	112/54/79	2600	6	Stable right heart failure complicated by sudden bradyarrhythmia and hypotension
29	M	85/50/66	1230	5	Sudden ischemic-type chest pain with acute worsening of stable right heart failure while discharge plans were being finalized

sualize elastic tissue, connective tissue, and smooth muscle (such as the Verhoeff-van Gieson stain) are used to characterize the affected vessels and to localize the pathological changes. The pathologist should also note the number and types of vessels that are seen, the severity of the anatomical changes, and any associated pathology.

Morphometric measurements of wall thickness and of the layers of the vascular wall are powerful tools for correlating hemodynamic and pathological data (11,13). However, they require careful fixation of the lung specimens and time consuming measurements. Since this is not always feasible, semiquantitative estimates of severity and type of vascular damage can be made by any anatomic pathologist and have been found to provide useful correlation with hemodynamic changes (12). Grading of vascular lesions by the method of Heath and Edwards (6), which was originally developed for the assessment of hypertensive pulmonary lesions secondary to congenital heart defects, has not been validated for the assessment of vascular pathology in primary pulmonary hypertension (15).

Open lung biopsy in the evaluation of patients with primary pulmonary hypertension is of value in excluding the presence of other conditions that may influence therapeutic approaches and in providing an objective representation of the anatomical alterations in small vessels. Evaluation of the type and extent of pathological lesions remains the only rational approach to therapy in these patients who are notoriously difficult to manage.

ACKNOWLEDGMENTS

The original material on which this chapter is based was partially supported by contract #1-HR-14000 from the NHLBI and relied on the contribution of cases from medical centers in the Registry.

REFERENCES

1. Bjornsson J, Edwards WD: Primary pulmonary hypertension: a histopathologic study of 80 cases. Mayo Clin Proc 60:16–25, 1985.

2. Brenner O: Pathology of the vessels of the pulmonary circulation. Arch Intern Med 56:211–237, 457–497, 724–752, 976–1014, 1189–1241, 1935.

3. Edwards WD, Edwards JE: Clinical primary pulmonary hypertension. Three pathologic types. Circulation 56:884–888, 1977.

4. Fernie JM, Lamb D: A new method for quantitating the medial component of pulmonary arteries. Arch Pathol Lab Med 109:156–162, 1985.

5. Hatano S, Strasser T (eds): *Primary Pulmonary Hypertension. Reports on a WHO Meeting.* Geneva, World Health Organization, 1975.

6. Heath D, Edwards JE: The pathology of hypertensive pulmonary vascular disease. A description of six grades of structural changes in the pulmonary arteries with special reference to congenital cardiac septal defects. Circulation 18:533–547, 1958.

7. Kay MJ, Heath D: Pathologic study of unexplained pulmonary hypertension. Sem Respir Med 7:180–192, 1985.

8. Lopes de Faria J: Cor pulmonale in Manson's Schistosomiasis. Am J Pathol 30:167–193, 1954.

9. Magee F, Wright JL, Kay MJ, Peretz D, Donevan R, Churg A: Pulmonary capillary-hemangiomatosis. Am Rev Respir Dis 132:922–925, 1985.

10. Mecham RP, Whitehouse LA, Wrenn DS, Parks WC, Griffin GL, Senior RM, Crouch EC, Stenmark KR, Voelkel NF: Smooth muscle-mediated connective tissue remodeling in pulmonary hypertension. Science 237:423–437, 1987.

11. Palevsky HI, Weber KT, Pietra GG, Janicki JS,

Schloo BL, Rubin E, Fishman AP: Unexplained pulmonary hypertension: Vascular structure and responsiveness to vasodilator agents. (In preparation).

12. Pietra GG, Schloo BL: Pathology of primary pulmonary hypertension, in Bergofsky EH (ed), *Abnormal Pulmonary Circulation*. New York, Churchill Livingstone, 1986, pp 265–282.

13. Rabinovitch M, Keane JF, Norwood WI, Castaneda AR, Reid L: Vascular structure in lung tissue obtained at biopsy correlated with pulmonary hemodynamic findings after repair of congenital heart defects. Circulation 4 : 655–667, 1984.

14. Wagenvoort CA: Capillary haemangiomatosis of the lung. Histopathology 2 : 401–406, 1978.

15. Wagenvoort CA: Lung biopsy specimens in the evaluation of pulmonary vascular disease. Chest 77 : 614–625, 1980.

16. Wagenvoort CA: Grading of pulmonary vascular lesions. A reappraisal. Histopathology 5 : 595–598, 1981.

17. Wagenvoort CA, Wagenvoort N: Primary pulmonary hypertension. A pathologic study of the lung vessels in 156 clinically diagnosed cases. Circulation 42 : 1163-1184, 1970.

18. Wagenvoort CA, Wagenvoort N: The pathology of pulmonary veno-occlusive disease. Virchows Arch A Path Anat Histol 364 : 69–79, 1974.

19. Wagenvoort CA, Wagenvoort N (eds): Unexplained plexogenic pulmonary arteriopathy: Primary pulmonary hypertension, in *Pathology of Pulmonary Hypertension*. New York, John Wiley & Sons, 1977, pp 119–142.

20. Wagenvoort CA, Wagenvoort N, Takahashi T: Pulmonary veno-occlusive-disease: Involvement of pulmonary arteries and review of the literature. Hum Pathol 16 : 1033–1041, 1985.

21. Widgren S, Kapanci Y: Menocilbedingte pulmonale Hypertonie. Vorläufige morphologische Ergebnisse über 8 pathologisch-anatomisch untersuchte Fälle. Z Kreislauf-Forsch 59 : 924–930, 1970.

Paul S. Levy, Sc.D.

Stuart Rich, M.D.

Janet Kernis, M.P.H.

35 ─────────────────

Mortality Follow-Up of Primary Pulmonary Hypertension

The Patient Registry for the Characterization of Primary Pulmonary Hypertension (PRPPH) enrolled over 200 patients diagnosed as having primary pulmonary hypertension at 35 clinical centers throughout the United States between July 1, 1981 and September 30, 1985. A previous report describes in detail the methods used in the PRPPH and the major findings of the baseline diagnostic examination (2). This present report presents the findings as of February 1, 1987 on the mortality follow-up of these patients.

METHODS

Subjects

Between July 1, 1981 and September 30, 1985, 192 patients were enrolled in the PRPPH. These subjects had primary pulmonary hypertension without evidence of cirrhosis of the liver, collagen vascular disease, or intravenous drug abuse, and they were followed for vital status (alive or dead) at 6-month intervals. For each subject who died during the follow-up period, a cause of death form was completed at the clinical center where the subject was enrolled and sent to the Data and Coordinating Center for analysis. As of February 1, 1987, 96 of these 192 patients were still alive and 95 were dead.

Survival Analysis

Actuarial methods based on standard life table analysis as well as those based on Kaplan-Meier statistics were used to estimate parameters of the survival distribution (1). The proportional hazards model (i.e., Cox regression) (1) was used to examine relationships between survival and selected demographic, medical history, pulmonary function, and hemodynamic variables measured at the baseline examination.

Cause of Death Analysis

Of the 95 subjects who were dead as of February 1, 1987, 82 had cause of death forms completed. Of these, 27 (32.9 percent) were classified as sudden death, 42 (51.2 percent) as right ventricular failure, and 13 (15.9 percent) as other causes. Differences between those having sudden death and those dying from right ventricular failure with respect to demographic, medical history, hemodynamic, and pulmonary function variables were examined for statistical significance by Wilcoxon or Chi-squared tests where appropriate.

RESULTS

Survival Analysis

The 192 patients involved in the follow-up and survival experience contributed 373 person years of follow-up. Of the 192 patients, 111 (58.1 percent) were followed for at least 1 year; 80 (41.9 percent) for at least 2 years; 45 (23.6 percent) for at least 3 years; 22 (11.5 percent) for at least 4 years, and 8 (4.2 percent) for at least 5 years. The estimated mean survival was 2.65 years and the estimated median survival was 2.5 years. The estimated percentage surviving at least 1 year was 67 percent, at least 3 years was 46 percent, and at least 5 years was 28 percent.

The risk of mortality was significantly higher among those patients classified in New York Heart Association (NYHA) functional class III or IV than among those classified in the NYHA functional class I or II (p < .04). Presence of Raynaud's phenomenon was also significantly associated with increased risk of mortality (p < .05). Hemodynamic variables significantly associated with increase in mortality were elevated mean right atrial pressure (p < .0001), elevated mean pulmonary artery pressure (p < .002), and decreased cardiac index (p < .001). Likewise, variables derived from these hemodynamic measurements (e.g., elevated mean pulmonary and systemic vascular resistances, decreased stroke volume index) were also significantly related to mortality. None of the pulmonary function tests were significantly associated with mortality. The only other variable significantly associated with mortality was systemic arterial P_{CO2} (low levels associated with increased risk of mortality; p < .04).

For those patients classified as dying of right ventricular failure and those classified as having sudden deaths, mean levels of selected demographic, hemodynamic, and pulmonary function test variables did not differ significantly.

DISCUSSION

The major findings of this mortality follow-up analysis are that the variables significantly associated with increased mortality are the hemodynamic variables measured at the baseline examination: those patients who were most compromised hemodynamically at the baseline examination were at greatest risk of mortality. None of the pulmonary function tests, medical history, or demographic variables seemed to have good prognostic value with respect to survival. Among those who died, there also appeared to be no relationship between the level of any of the baseline variables and the cause of death (right ventricular failure or sudden death).

REFERENCES

1. Lee E: *Statistical Methods for Survival Analysis.* Belmont, CA, Lifetime Learning Publication, 1980.

2. Rich SR, Dantzker DR, Ayres SM, Bergofsky EH, Brundage BH, Detre KM, Fishman AP, Goldring RM, Groves BM, Koerner SK, Levy PC, Reid LM, Vreim CE, Williams GW: Primary pulmonary hypertension: A national prospective study. Ann Intern Med 107:216–223, 1987.

PART FIVE

Treatment of Pulmonary Hypertension

Lewis J. Rubin, M.D.

36

Vasodilator Therapy (General Aspects)

The management of patients with systemic hypertension or left ventricular failure has been substantially improved by the development of potent vasodilators. By reducing systemic vascular resistance, these agents decrease left ventricular afterload and improve left ventricular function. In recent years, the same approach has been used to treat patients with pulmonary hypertension and right ventricular failure. This chapter will review the general aspects of vasodilator therapy for pulmonary hypertension, including the rationale for their use and the questions which remain unanswered concerning their role.

Pulmonary hypertension is not a disease, per se, but rather a hemodynamic abnormality which is shared by a variety of disease states. Some of these conditions, such as primary pulmonary hypertension (PPH), produce elevations in pulmonary artery pressure by directly attacking the resistance vessels; others, such as chronic obstructive airways disease, produce pulmonary hypertension indirectly through the effects of derangements in airflow and gas exchange on the vasculature. Diseases such as recurrent thromboembolism or pulmonary fibrosis produce obstruction or destruction of the vasculature. Regardless of the pathogenesis of pulmonary hypertension, the increased pressure in the pulmonary circulation results in a progressive inability of the right ventricle to sustain its output, and frequently leads to right ventricular failure and death. Although the severity of pulmonary hypertension differs in these various clinical states, prognosis in these diseases has been correlated with the ability of the right heart to sustain its output: mortality from cor pulmonale secondary to chronic obstructive airways disease has been correlated with oxygen delivery (the product of cardiac output and the oxygen content of arterial blood) (9) and pulmonary vascular resistance (the relationship between the pulmonary vascular pressure gradient and the pulmonary blood flow) (4); survival in PPH is shortened by the presence of right ventricular failure (15). Accordingly, interventions which might reduce right ventricular afterload, thereby preserving or improving right ventricular function in pulmonary hypertension, could be potentially useful.

A variety of systemic vasodilators have been shown to decrease in experimental animals in which vasoconstriction has been induced by acute or chronic hypoxic ventilation or by the infusion of vasopressor substances (10,12,20,21). These observations lend support to the concept that pulmonary hypertension can be treated pharmacologically using vasodilator agents when the increase in pulmonary vascular resistance is produced by a vasoconstrictive stimulus.

The case for vasoconstriction in clinical forms of chronic pulmonary hypertension rests largely on pathological studies of the pulmonary vasculature. Wagenvoort (19) observed the frequent finding of medial hypertrophy of small pulmonary arteries and muscularization of pulmonary arterioles in the lungs of patients with PPH. He suggested that vasoconstriction was an early feature of PPH and that it ultimately led to more severe vascular obliteration. Patients with chronic hypoxic lung disease have comparable pathological findings that are much less marked (18). In contrast, conditions such as recurrent thromboembolic disease, granulomatous lung disease, or severe interstitial disease with fibrosis are associated with obliteration or obstruction of the vasculature, with little pathological evidence to support a vasoconstrictive process (18).

Although clinical experience using vasodilator therapy in pulmonary hypertension has been limited and largely anecdotal, several observations have suggested that this approach has the potential for improving the clinical state of some patients. For example, reports of marked reduction in pulmonary artery pressure, accompanied by increase in cardiac output and sustained improvement in symptoms, do suggest that vasodilator therapy can be of therapeutic benefit. Reversal of echocardiographic and electrocardiographic signs of right ventricular hypertrophy with chronic therapy have also been reported in individuals treated for prolonged periods (5,8,14). Vasodilators have also been shown to improve right ventricular function—at least acutely (3,16,17).

The enthusiasm generated by these reports has been tempered by others indicating that vasodilators given to patients who seemed to be similar either had no beneficial effect or elicited serious adverse effects (13). The hazards of vasodilators in pulmonary hypertension are discussed in another chapter (see chapter by Palevsky). However, the contrasting results from the use of vasodilators in pulmonary hypertension raises questions that are pertinent at this juncture.

DEFINITION OF A "BENEFICIAL" RESPONSE TO THERAPY

Most investigators would agree that a sustained decrease in pulmonary artery pressure accompanied by an unchanged or increased cardiac output and oxygen delivery and an unchanged systemic blood pressure is beneficial; however, this response is relatively infrequent. Oppositely, an increased pulmonary artery pressure or a fall in systemic blood pressure that evokes symptoms would be considered deleterious. The most frequent response to vasodilators, particularly in patients with PPH, is an increase in cardiac output and oxygen delivery while

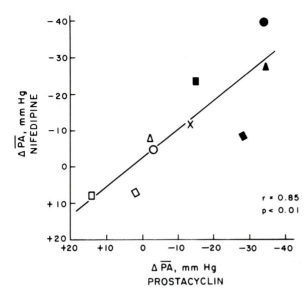

Figure 1: Correlation in nine patients between the absolute change from baseline in mean pulmonary artery pressure with prostacyclin and the absolute change from baseline in mean pulmonary artery pressure with sublingual nifedipine administration. Reproduced from Barst [1].)

pulmonary arterial pressure either remains unchanged or decreases minimally. Although these changes have been associated with improved right ventricular function and exercise tolerance, many believe that increasing flow without reducing pressure need not be "beneficial"; indeed, it may actually be deleterious because ventricular work is increased.

IDENTIFICATION OF THE PULMONARY HYPERTENSIVE PATIENTS WHO ARE THE BEST CANDIDATES FOR A THERAPEUTIC TRIAL WITH VASODILATORS

Because the efficacy of vasodilator therapy for pulmonary hypertension is as yet unproven, this approach should be regarded as investigational. Although chronic obstructive airways disease is frequently associated with pulmonary hypertension, hemodynamic improvement often follows the use of an aggressive conventional regimen directed at improving airflow and alveolar ventilation. Supplemental oxygen is the only therapeutic modality which has been shown to prolong survival in chronic obstructive airways disease although the hemodynamic changes that it elicits are often modest.

Although primary pulmonary hypertension (PPH) is a rare disease, most of the published literature dealing with vasodilators in pulmonary hypertension has focused on this disorder, perhaps because of its dismal prognosis if untreated. In theory, individuals with PPH in which medial hypertrophy is the predominant vascular lesion would be expected to have the best response, while those in whom more advanced lesions predominate, e.g., concentric intimal fibrosis or plexiform lesions, would be more apt to have the least response. Lupi-Herrera et al. (11) supported this concept by the finding that subjects with the least severe hemodynamic alterations were the most likely to respond to hydralazine with substantial reductions in pulmonary vascular resistance.

Several investigators have advocated evaluating an individual's vascular responsiveness acutely with a potent, short-acting, titratable agent prior to embarking on therapy with an oral agent. Correlations have been demonstrated between the responses to prostacyclin (prostaglandin I_2, PGI_2) and both hydralazine and nifedipine (1) (Fig. 1). This approach minimizes the risk of prolonged, or life-threatening, adverse experiences which have followed the use of other, less controllable, agents in nonresponsive subjects.

THE CHOICE OF OPTIMAL AGENT AND OPTIMAL DOSES

The optimal vasodilator would be one with consistent, selective pulmonary vascular effects; unfortunately, no selective or even preferential pulmonary vasodilator agent has yet been identified. To date, the calcium channel blockers nifedipine and diltiazem have been the most widely used agents; but these agents have systemic vascular effects as well.

There is no "safe" dose of a vasodilator in pulmonary hypertension, since adverse effects have been noted in some patients even after receiving relatively low doses. A recent report by Rich and Brundage (14) has suggested that large doses of calcium channel blockers may be required to achieve significant hemodynamic effects in PPH. While this observation is exciting, it awaits confirmation in larger studies, particularly because of the risks of high-dose vasodilator therapy in these hemodynamically fragile individuals.

THE EFFECTS OF VASODILATOR THERAPY ON THE NATURAL HISTORY AND SURVIVAL OF PULMONARY HYPERTENSION

There have not yet been any clinical trials designed to evaluate the effects of therapy on survival. Thus, the effects of therapy on the natural history of pulmonary hypertension remain unclear despite occasional impressive hemodynamic and clinical responses. An additional frustrating problem is the patient who manifests dramatic hemodynamic responses to acute testing but loses this effect in the course of chronic therapy. Presumably, this is due to progression of disease, although tachyphylaxis is also possible.

Regardless of whether vasodilators prolong survival, they may be useful in the short-term management of hemodynamic deterioration. Higenbottam et al. (7) have used prostacyclin administered by continuous intravenous infusion to sustain deteriorating PPH patients in anticipation of eventual heart-lung transplantation; others have used prostacyclin to increase oxygen delivery in patients with pulmonary hypertension and the adult respiratory distress syndrome (2).

The potential of modifying pulmonary vascular disease using pharmacological agents remains appealing, despite the pitfalls documented in the literature. However, the validity of this approach is still unproven, and many questions concerning the use of vasodilators remain unanswered. The answers to these questions will have to be sought in multicenter studies.

REFERENCES

1. Barst RJ: Pharmacologically induced pulmonary vasodilatation in children and young adults with primary pulmonary hypertension. Chest 89 : 497–503, 1986.

2. Bihari D, Smithies M, Gimson A, Tinker J: The effects of vasodilation with prostacyclin on oxygen delivery and uptake in critically ill patients. N Engl J Med 317 : 397–403, 1987.

3. Brent BN, Berger HJ, Matthay RA, Mahler D, Pytlik L, Zaret BL: Contrasting acute effects of vasodilators (nitroglycerin, nitroprusside, and hydralazine) on right ventricular performance in patients with chronic obstructive pulmonary disease and pulmonary hypertension: A combined radionuclide-hemodynamic study. Am J Cardiol 51 : 1682-1689, 1983.

4. Burrows B, Kettel LJ, Niden AH, Rabinowitz M, Diener DF: Patterns of cardiovascular dysfunction in chronic obstructive lung disease. N Engl J Med 286 : 912–917, 1972.

5. Chan NS, McLay J, Kenmure ACF: Reversibility of primary pulmonary hypertension during six years of treatment with oral diazoxide. Br Heart J 57 : 207–209, 1987.

6. DeFeyter PJ, Kerkkamp HJ, deJong JP: Sustained beneficial effect of nifedipine in primary pulmonary hypertension. Am Heart J 105 : 333–334, 1983.

7. Higenbottam T, Wheeldon D, Wells F, Wallwork J: Long-term treatment of primary pulmonary hypertension with continuous intravenous epoprostenol (prostacyclin). Lancet 1 : 1046-1047, 1984.

8. Kambara H, Fujimoto K, Wakabayashi A, Kawai C: Primary pulmonary hypertension: Beneficial therapy with diltiazem. Am Heart J 101 : 230–232, 1981.

9. Kawakami Y, Kishi F, Yamamoto H, Miyamoto K: Relation of O_2 delivery, mixed venous oxygenation, and pulmonary hemodynamics to prognosis in chronic obstructive pulmonary disease. N Engl J Med 308 : 1045-1049, 1983.

10. Kennedy T, Summer W: Inhibition of hypoxic pulmonary vasoconstriction by nifedipine. Am J Cardiol 50 : 864–868, 1982.

11. Lupi-Herrera E, Sandoval J, Seoane M, Bialostozky D: The role of hydralazine therapy for pulmonary arterial hypertension of unknown cause. Circulation 65 : 645–650, 1982.

12. McMurtry IF, Davidson AB, Reeves JT, Grover RF: Inhibition of hypoxic pulmonary vasoconstriction by calcium antagonists in isolated rat lungs. Circ Res 38 : 99–104, 1976.

13. Packer M, Greenberg B, Massie B, Dash H: Deleterious effects of hydralazine in patients with pulmonary hypertension. N Engl J Med 306 : 1326–1331, 1982.

14. Rich S, Brundage BH: High-dose calcium channel-blocking therapy for primary pulmonary hypertension: evidence for long-term reduction in pulmonary arterial pressure and regression of right ventricular hypertrophy. Circulation 76 : 135–141, 1987.

15. Rich S, Levy PS: Characteristics of surviving and nonsurviving patients with primary pulmonary hypertension. Am J Med 76 : 573–578, 1984.

16. Rubin LJ, Handel F, Peter RH: The effects of oral hydralazine on right ventricular end-diastolic pressure in patients with right ventricular failure. Circulation 65 : 1369–1372, 1982.

17. Rubin LJ, Nicod P, Hillis LD, Firth BG: Treatment of primary pulmonary hypertension with nifedipine. Ann Intern Med 99 : 433–438, 1983.

18. Taylor WE: Pathology of pulmonary heart disease, in Rubin LJ (ed), *Pulmonary Heart Disease.* Boston, Martinus Nijhoff, 1984, pp 65–105.

19. Wagenvoort CA, Wagenvoort N: Primary pulmonary hypertension. A pathologic study of the lung vessels in 156 clinically diagnosed cases. Circulation 42 : 1163–1184, 1970.

20. Weir EK, Chidsey CA, Weil JV, Grover RF: Inhibition of hypoxic pulmonary vasoconstriction by calcium antagonists in isolated rat lungs. Circ Res 38 : 99–104, 1976.

21. Young TE, Lundquist LJ, Chesler E, Weir EK: Comparative effects of nifedipine, verapamil, and diltiazem on experimental pulmonary hypertension. Am J Cardiol 51 : 195–200, 1983.

E. Kenneth Weir, M.D.

37 ———————————————

Acute Vasodilator Testing and Pharmacological Treatment of Primary Pulmonary Hypertension

Primary pulmonary hypertension is the term commonly used to describe pulmonary hypertension in which the etiology cannot be defined by clinical means, such as pulmonary function tests, ventilation-perfusion scans, cardiac catheterization, or pulmonary angiography. Although the condition seems fairly uniform from a clinical standpoint, it is clear from autopsy and lung biopsy that primary pulmonary hypertension is histologically diverse.

HISTOLOGICAL SUBSTRATE FOR VASODILATOR THERAPY

A number of different elements contribute to the increase in pulmonary vascular resistance in an individual patient. These include vasoconstriction, intimal proliferation and fibrosis (both concentric and eccentric), thrombosis in situ and/ or thromboembolism of the small pulmonary arteries, and occasionally veno-occlusive disease. Although histological appearances have been divided into separate groups (see Chapter 34) (Table 1), it is uncertain whether the histological groups indicate entirely distinct diseases or whether they are parts of the spectrum of one disease.

Because of our present lack of knowledge concerning etiology, treatment is empirical. Because thrombosis in situ or thromboembolism may be present in conjunction with plexogenic arteriopathy (3,11,55), anticoagulation is probably appropriate whatever the histological substrate, in the absence of specific contraindications (see Chapter 38) (11).

TABLE 1 HISTOLOGICAL CHARACTERISTICS OF PRIMARY PULMONARY HYPERTENSION

	Wagenvoort & Wagenvoort (55)	Bjornsson & Edwards (3)
Number of cases	156	80
Thromboembolic	20%	56%
Plexogenic	71%	28%
Veno-occlusive	3%	6%
Other	6%	10%

IMPORTANCE OF PULMONARY VASCULAR TONE

The use of vasodilators in primary pulmonary hypertension presupposes that pulmonary vascular tone plays a significant part in the elevated pulmonary vascular resistance of at least some patients. It is not known whether the first functional derangement in primary pulmonary hypertension occurs in the smooth muscle or the endothelium of the small pulmonary arteries. If the initial change is severe and prolonged vasoconstriction, followed by intimal damage and ultimately by the development of plexogenic arteriopathy (58), the potential benefit of vasodilators is clear. Alternatively, if the primary abnormality is in the endothelial cells (1), proliferating endothelial cells might cause vasoconstriction either by releasing a constrictor substance or by interaction with platelets to increase production of thromboxane A_2, or damaged endothelium might fail to produce a vasodilator substance, such as prostacyclin or endothelium-derived relaxing factor. A third possibility is in vessels with thickened intima, where normal pulmonary vascular tone might reduce the lumen of the vessel. Whatever the pathophysiological sequence, a reduction in the tone of the small pulmonary arteries could be beneficial.

GOAL OF VASODILATOR THERAPY

If the only abnormality at the time of diagnosis were vasoconstriction, then effective vasodilator therapy might be able to restore normal pulmonary arterial pressure and vascular resistance and prevent progression. To date, there is little evidence that this can be achieved. In the few patients in whom prolonged improvement has occurred, the possibility exists that they represent spontaneous remission. In a small number of patients, to whom vasodilators have been given, withdrawn, and restarted over a period of years (6), the impressive results suggest that vasodilators may occasionally be of long-term benefit (Fig. 1).

Most investigators examining the use of vasodilators have made reduction in pulmonary artery pressure their principal goal. However, the reduction achieved has usually been modest and the severity of pulmonary hypertension, in terms of pulmonary artery pressure at the time of diagnosis, has not correlated with survival (12,20). Cardiac index seems to give the best indication of survival; right ventricular end-diastolic pressure is also helpful. It may be that, late in the course of the disease, right ventricular function is the critical factor in determining survival. Although a low cardiac index is a bad prognostic sign, an increase in cardiac index associated with vasodilator therapy need not be beneficial unless right ventricular end-diastolic pressures were to fall concomitantly. Currently, the best hemodynamic response to a vasodilator seems to be a decrease in pulmonary arterial pressure coincident with an increase in cardiac index.

CHANGES IN PULMONARY VASCULAR RESPONSIVENESS TO VASODILATORS OVER TIME

It is generally believed that in the early stages of the disease, regardless of whether the initial lesion is in the intima or smooth muscle, vasoconstriction is often present and that it may be reduced by vasodilator therapy. Later in the course of the disease, intimal fibrosis, or fibrosis in the hypertrophied media, presumably prevents vasodilation. This idea was clearly stated by Samet et al. in 1960, in relation to the responses of two patients to the infusion of acetylcholine into the right ventricular outflow tract: "The magnitude of the fall in pulmonary arterial pressure in M. J. Hol. suggests that the vasoconstrictive factor was of primary importance in the maintenance of the pulmonary arterial hypertension, and is in keeping with the thesis that the disease process was less advanced than in L. Fen. In the latter patient, the degree of pulmonary hypertension and the more limited response to infusion of acetylcholine are both probably due to the

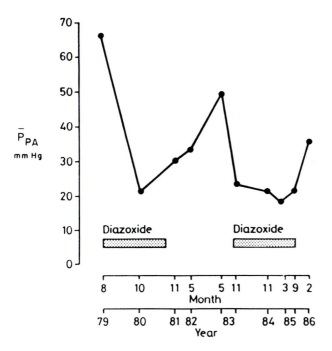

Figure 1: Changes in mean pulmonary arterial pressure (P_{PA}) over 6.4 years in a 32-year-old woman with primary pulmonary hypertension. Diazoxide was administered for two periods during the 6.5 years. (Reproduced from Chan et al. [6].)

superimposition of pulmonary vascular disease upon the vasoconstrictive factor" (53).

Three years later, a paper by Samet and Bernstein (52) found that pulmonary arterial pressure and vascular resistance had increased substantially in M. J. Hol. and that pulmonary vascular reactivity to acetylcholine was lost. The concept of progression and loss of response has been supported in a recent study by Barst (2): in patients with primary pulmonary hypertension, both prostacyclin and nifedipine produced a greater decrease in pulmonary arterial pressure in younger patients than in older patients ($p < 0.01$).

ACUTE TRIAL OF VASODILATORS

It is evident from the preceding discussion that the response to vasodilators is likely to be extremely variable. In some patients, vasoconstriction predominates and may be responsive whereas in others thrombosis or intimal fibrosis predominates with little vasoconstriction. Some patients are relatively early in the course of their disease and others late. The acute administration of vasodilators accompanied by hemodynamic monitoring helps to identify those patients in whom vasoconstriction is an important factor. Ideally, acute vasodilator trials should provide information about (1) the presence or absence of vasoconstriction and, thus, the likelihood of a response to chronic vasodilator therapy; (2) the presence or absence of fixed structural pulmonary vascular changes; (3) prognosis; and (4) the safety of administering vasodilators.

Acute Testing and Chronic Responses

The acute trial is quite accurate in predicting which patients will show longer term improvement. In a review of 117 published vasodilator trials, Reeves et al. found that in 45 percent of patients the pulmonary vascular resistance was reduced by 30 percent or more (39). Follow-up of at least 3 months was available in all patients: chronic clinical or hemodynamic improvement was reported in only 6 percent of those who underwent an acute decrease in resistance less than 30 percent, whereas 62 percent of those with 30 percent decrease in resistance showed improvement (Fig. 2). Those in whom improvement was maintained during chronic vasodilator therapy also tended to have the greater acute responses.

The Presence or Absence of Fixed Structural Pulmonary Vascular Changes

Although Samet et al. had suggested that the absence of a vasodilator response to acetylcholine might be attributable to more advanced pulmonary vascular disease (53), the lack of a response could also signify endothelial injury or dysfunction rather than fixed obstruction to flow. Acetylcholine is now known to cause relaxation by way of an endothelium-dependent relaxing factor. Theoretically, it should be possible to distinguish between obstruction and endothelial injury by

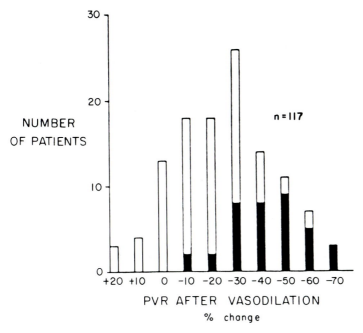

Figure 2: Comparison of acute and longer term (greater than 3 months) changes in pulmonary vascular resistance induced by vasodilators in 117 patients. The patients who had favorable long-term responses (shaded bars) tended to have the largest acute reductions (open bars) in pulmonary vascular resistance. (Reproduced from Reeves et al. [39].)

comparing the hemodynamic changes caused by acetylcholine with those elicited by a vasodilator, such as nitroglycerin, that acts directly on the vascular smooth muscle.

There is relatively little information linking pulmonary vasodilator responses to morphology. In 1969, Rao et al. found a close correlation between excellent acute responses to acetylcholine, tolazoline, and isoproterenol with histological evidence of marked medial hypertrophy on the one hand and minimal intimal fibrous thickening of the small pulmonary arteries on the other (38). More recently, the pulmonary vascular morphology obtained on lung biopsy of 12 patients was correlated with their hemodynamic responses to vasodilators (34). No patient who had an intimal area greater than 15 percent of the vascular cross-sectional area or an intima/wall thickness ratio greater than 0.2 was responsive to any vasodilator agent. A thickened media, in conjunction with a normal or near-normal intima, favored the possibility of responsiveness to pulmonary vasodilators. This concept is illustrated in Figure 3. Although histology may help to predict the response to vasodilators, it does not follow that the absence of a vasodilator response necessarily implies considerable intimal thickening since fibrosis in the media may also limit vasodilatation. More studies are needed to define the precision with which pulmonary vasodilator responses can predict pulmonary vascular morphology.

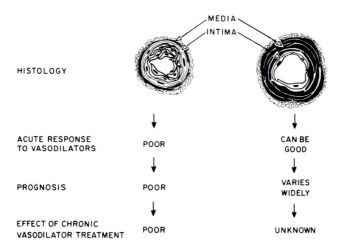

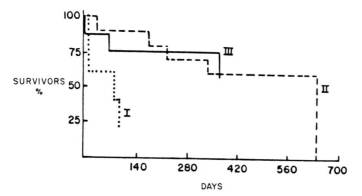

Figure 3: Schematic representation of effects of intimal thickening (left) and of intimal thickening in one small pulmonary artery and medial thickening (right) on vasodilator responses. Indicated are the known correlations between morphology, prognosis as well as the acute and chronic responses to vasodilators (34,35,38,39,41).

The Acute Response to Vasodilators as a Guide to Prognosis

Rich et al. tried to determine whether a "favorable" acute response to nifedipine or hydralazine (greater than 20 percent fall in pulmonary vascular resistance) would indicate a better clinical course over the next 2 years (41). Eighteen patients who showed favorable responses acutely survived longer on average than five patients who did not (Fig. 4). Chronic treatment with vasodilators did not

Figure 4: Correlation between acute response to vasodilators and longer term prognosis. Kaplan-Meier estimate of survival in patients with primary pulmonary hypertension. Group I: *non-responders;* acute pulmonary vascular resistance response to nifedipine or hydralazine less than 20 percent reduction (n = 5). Group II: *acute responders not given long-term vasodilators* (n = 9). Group III: *acute responders given long-term vasolidaltors* (n = 9). In this randomized study, long-term vasodilator treatment did not alter survival. (Reproduced from Rich et al. [41].)

appear to improve survival. However, the number of patients was small and the patients were not randomized to treatment or no treatment. These results are compatible with the conclusions of Reeves et al. They reported that 62 percent of patients in whom pulmonary vascular resistance decreased by more than 30 percent in response to the acute administration of a vasodilator improved during chronic treatment, whereas only 6 percent of those who did not respond to the acute trial improved chronically (39).

One additional study helps to complete the triangle of reactivity, prognosis, and morphology (35). Fifteen patients with primary pulmonary hypertension underwent lung biopsy and were followed on the average for 22 months. They were then characterized as either stable or improved (n = 6), or worse or dead (n = 9). The single morphometric feature of the small pulmonary arteries which differed significantly between the two groups was the fraction of the cross-sectional area of the arterial wall occupied by the intima: $10.1 \pm 7.7\%$ in those doing well and $25.6 \pm 15.8\%$ in those doing poorly. In these relatively small groups, there was no difference in baseline hemodynamics or in the response to vasodilators.

Taking into account the information reviewed above, it seems likely that the acute response to vasodilators does give an indication of the underlying morphology. Moreover, these functional and structural facets of the pulmonary vasculature together play a large part in determining prognosis (Fig. 3).

Safety of the Acute Testing of Vasodilators

The risk of right heart catheterization in primary pulmonary hypertension patients is low. No deaths related to the diagnostic catheterization occurred in the 187 patients reported by the Registry (42). Nor were there any long-term sequelae. In the course of 417 vasodilator trials recorded by the National Registry on Primary Pulmonary Hypertension there were two deaths, giving a mortality rate of less than 0.5 percent. This recent experience stands in contrast to impressions that may be gained from uncritical reading of retrospective studies (45). The older reviews can be criticized not only on the basis of nonuniform patients and protocols and of inconsistent statistical approach but also with respect to the relevance today of experiences with cardiac catheterization that date back more than 30 years.

Although the risk of death associated with the acute testing of vasodilators in patients with primary pulmonary hypertension can be stated fairly accurately, the effect of chronic vasodilator treatment on quality of life and survival is still uncertain. There is little question that in some patients vasodilators can greatly improve functional capacity. However, whether longevity is increased is unsettled and awaits a controlled clinical trial. As a result of the accumulated experience with a number of vasodilators, documented by the National Registry on Primary Pulmonary Hypertension, the way has been paved for investigators to agree to trials of particular agents and on protocols.

Hemodynamic Responses to the Acute Use of Vasodilators

Almost all the vasodilators used in patients with primary pulmonary hypertension were developed for the treatment of systemic hypertension. Consequently,

TABLE 2 HEMODYNAMIC RESPONSES TO THE ACUTE TRIAL OF VASODILATORS

Drug and reference	Number of patients	Cardiac output % change	PA pressure % change	TPR or PVR % change	SYS pressure % change
Captopril					
Rich (44)	4	+10	+5	−4	−10
Ikram (18)	5	0	−15	−11	−22
Leier (22)	5	+18	−2	+2	—
Diazoxide					
Wang (56)	3	+78	−14	−52	−23
Honey (17)	9	+74	−4	−44	−26
Hydralazine					
Lupi-Herrera (26)	12	+55	+3	−23	—
Responders*	6	+69	−8	−43	—
Packer (31)	11	+35	0	−30	−13
Fisher (9)	5	+33	+2	−24	−26
Rich (41)	16	+30	0	−20	—
Groves (13)	7	+54	+2	−33	−15
Isoproterenol					
Daoud (7)	6	+47	+10	−23	−5
Lupi-Herrera (26)	5	+55	−17	−33	−6
Nifedipine					
Mohiuddin (28)	6	+34	−20	−38	−10
Rubin (47)	9	+47	−3	−36	−14
Packer (31)	11	+7	−23	−38	−20
Olivari (29)	7	+31	−14	−35	−14
Fisher (9)	5	+7	−14	−22	−16
Rich (41)	23	+29	−4	−22	—
Barst (2)	9	+21	−18	−32	−14
Responders*	5	+24	−28	−48	−17
High Dose Nifedipine/ Diltiazem					
Rich (40)	13	+22	−30	−43	−15
Responders*	8	+41	−43	−60	−12
Nitroglycerin					
Pearl (36)	9	+28	−15	−40	−15
Nitroprusside					
Fuleihan (10)	7	+29	−8	−26	−11
Phentolamine					
Levine (23)	4	+25	−4	−28	—
Prostacyclin					
Guadagni (14)	4	+26	−30	−47	−33
Rubin (46)	7	+56	−11	−43	−14
Groves (13)	7	+77	−7	−44	−15
Barst (2)	9	+41	−18	−47	−9
Responders*	5	+38	−31	−58	−5
Jones (19)	10	+18	−4	−19	−14
Verapamil					
Landmark (21)	9	+14	−11	−4	—
Packer (31)	12	−12	−25	−20	−15

PA: pulmonary arterial; SYS: systemic arterial; TPR: total pulmonary resistance.
*Responders: a subset singled out as having a good hemodynamic response to the vasodilator.

it is not surprising that a reduction in systemic arterial pressure occurs during acute vasodilator trials. In fact, the dose of vasodilator administered is often titrated up until a predetermined fall in systemic pressure is observed. At present, with the exception of oxygen, none of the available vasodilators are selective for the pulmonary circulation. Moreover, the acute administration of oxygen rarely has a significant effect on pulmonary arterial pressure in primary pulmonary hypertension.

Three general categories of hemodynamic responses can follow the administration of vasodilators; one of these is potentially beneficial whereas two could be dangerous. The "good" category is represented by the patient in whom both pulmonary and systemic arterial beds dilate, cardiac output increases, and a significant decrease occurs in pulmonary arterial pressure associated with a small fall in systemic arterial pressure. The second category is illustrated by the patient in whom systemic vasodilatation occurs, but cardiac output cannot increase because of fixed pulmonary vascular obstruction. Under these circumstances, systemic arterial pressure can fall precipitously (30). The third category is typified by the individual in whom cardiac output increases in response to systemic vasodilatation, but inadequate pulmonary vasodilatation leads to even more severe pulmonary hypertension (49).

The mean responses reported for most of the commonly used vasodilators are given in Table 2. The "average" response is an increase in cardiac output of about 30 percent, a similar decrease in pulmonary vascular resistance, and a relatively small decrease in pulmonary and systemic arterial pressure. The earlier discussion pointed out that the "average" response is less important than the ability to identify "responders," i.e., those who might benefit from long-term vasodilator therapy. The hemodynamics of small groups of such responders are also shown in Table 2.

Are All Vasodilators Equally Effective When Given Acutely?

Comparison of vasodilators on the basis of the published reports is difficult because there are no randomized data, and only occasional papers compare one agent with another in the same group of patients. However, some agents do appear to be less effective, or more likely to have serious side effects, than others. For example, the usual reductions in pulmonary arterial pressure and resistance induced by captopril and verapamil are small compared to those achieved with other agents; also, the negative inotropic effects of verapamil can depress right ventricular function with serious consequences (32). Isoproterenol has the advantages that it can be titrated easily and almost invariably increases cardiac output; unfortunately, pulmonary arterial pressure often increases along with the increase in cardiac output (16). Therefore, the use of isoproterenol in acute testing is less popular now than a few years ago.

In four studies involving the same patients, the acute hemodynamic effects of hydralazine have been compared to those of calcium blockers or prostacyclin administration (2,9,13,41). The acute administration of hydralazine tends to increase cardiac output more, and to reduce systemic vascular resistance further, than does nifedipine. But, unlike nifedipine, it seldom decreases pulmonary arterial pressure. In one study, nifedipine decreased pulmonary arterial pressure

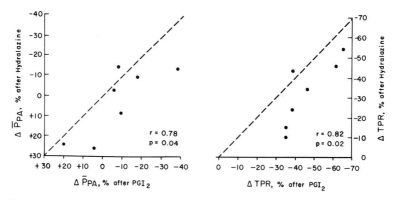

Figure 5: Correlation between the percentage decreases in pulmonary arterial pressure (PPA) and total pulmonary resistance (TPR) caused by hydralazine and prostacyclin (PGI₂) in seven patients with primary pulmonary hypertension. (Reproduced from Groves et al. [13].)

in four out of five patients whereas hydralazine only reduced pressure in one (9). Although right atrial pressure did not increase following nifedipine in that trial, it has done so in others (31).

As may be seen in Figure 5, the hemodynamic responses to hydralazine and prostacyclin are similar in individual patients (13). However, prostacyclin caused a greater decrease in total pulmonary resistance. On the average, neither agent produced a significant decrease in pulmonary arterial pressure. But, in three of the seven patients, pulmonary arterial pressure decreased by more than 10 mmHg. Thus, the overall hemodynamic response to hydralazine does not seem to be quite as favorable as the responses to prostacyclin and nifedipine. A close correlation between the magnitude of the pulmonary vasodilator responses to prostacyclin and nifedipine has also been demonstrated in nine young patients with primary pulmonary hypertension (2).

PROSTACYCLIN AS A GUIDE TO VASODILATOR THERAPY

Prostacyclin seems to be an excellent agent for acute vasodilator testing since the dose can be rapidly titrated against the hemodynamic response and the half-life is very short. The fact that the duration of action is short is advantageous in terms of reducing the length of any systemic hypotension that might ensue, but bad in that chronic therapy requires continuous intravenous infusion. If prostacyclin is effective acutely, it is important to identify an oral agent which, if administered chronically, might be able to sustain pulmonary vasodilatation.

In a recent comparison of vasodilators, 10 patients with primary pulmonary hypertension were tested using an average of five agents per patient (33). The agents were acetylcholine, hydralazine, isoproterenol, nifedipine, nitroglycerin, nitroprusside, phentolamine, and prostacyclin. In 6 of the 10, the greatest vasodilator responses were achieved by prostacyclin; no patient showed a substantial vasodilator response to one of the other agents without also exhibiting a favorable response to prostacyclin.

Another study examined the efficacy of diltiazem, hydralazine, isoproterenol,

TABLE 3 HEMODYNAMIC RESPONSES TO THE CHRONIC USE OF VASODILATORS

Drug and reference	Number of patients	Months of administration	Cardiac output % change	PA pressure % change	TPR or PVR % change
Captopril					
Leier (22)	4	3	0	+3	+6
Diazoxide					
Wang (56)	1		+52	−11	−39
Honey (17)	5	1–3	+97	−20	−60
Hall (15)	1	15	+11	−60	−67
Hydralazine					
Rubin (48)	4	3–6	+68	−12	−52
Isoproterenol					
Daoud (7)	1	24	+42	−11	−39
Lupi-Herrera (26)	1	36	+33	−68	−81
Pietro (37)	1	48	+132	−30	−70
Nifedipine					
Rubin (47)	6	4–14	+39	−7	−37
Saito (51)	1	30	+12	−45	−51
DeFeyter (8)	1	6	+19	−45	−63
Lunde (25)	1	16	+9	−39	−48
Olivari (29)	4	3–10	+29	−16	−31
High Dose Nifedipine/ Diltiazem					
Rich (40)	5	12	+71	−34	−64
Phentolamine					
Ruskin (50)	1	7	+4	−22	−23
Thromboxane SI					
Rich (43)	10	3	−3	−10	−23
Verapamil					
Packer (31)	1	3	−10	−12	−17

PA: pulmonary arterial; TPR: total pulmonary resistance; PVR: pulmonary vascular resistance; Thromboxane SI: thromboxane synthetase inhibitor.

nitroglycerin, phentolamine, and prostacyclin in 13 patients (54). In three of the patients, none of these agents was effective. Prostacyclin was the only vasodilator which caused a significant reduction in pulmonary vascular resistance in all of the remaining 10 patients; it also produced the greatest mean fall in resistance (40% ± 15 SD). If other acute comparisons confirm the sensitivity of the prostacyclin challenge in detecting the potential for vasodilatation, the initial workup of these patients could be considerably simplified. At present, prostacyclin is the front-runner for the best acute vasodilator (24).

THE CHRONIC HEMODYNAMIC CHANGES INDUCED BY VASODILATORS

The data discussed earlier show that the acute hemodynamic responses to vasodilators provide information about the long-term prognosis of primary pulmonary hypertension patients and may give a clue to the underlying histology. It has not been demonstrated in prospective, controlled studies that the chronic use of vasodilators prolongs life. Indeed, it has been suggested that in some patients life may actually be shortened by the hazards of vasodilatation (45). A good chronic pulmonary vascular response to vasodilators appears to be very unlikely in the absence of a significant acute fall in pulmonary vascular resistance induced by the initial trial of vasodilators (Fig. 2) (39). If chronic vasodilator therapy is limited to those who do respond acutely, risks will be reduced and potential benefits will be enhanced.

Table 3 shows the chronic hemodynamic responses reported for vasodilators. Unfortunately, since different vasodilators have not been compared over long periods in the same group of patients, the data are not strictly comparable. However, the overall hemodynamic effects of captopril, a thromboxane synthetase inhibitor (CGS 13080), and verapamil do not appear to be very favorable. The long-term administration of isoproterenol is occasionally associated with improved hemodynamics (37), but its use is often limited by the occurrence of palpitations and tremor. Intolerable side effects have been reported by some patients during the administration of virtually every vasodilator now in use (5,17,30,32). Tachyphylaxis may occur during short (57) or long-term (19,23) treatment. Chronic infusions of prostacyclin can be quite successful in improving exercise tolerance, but septicemia and ascites have been troublesome complications (19). The combined use of more than one vasodilator may increase the therapeutic action of these agents while reducing the side effects (43).

A Long-Term Controlled Trial?

Because of the potential complications and side effects associated with vasodilator treatment, a controlled trial is needed to determine whether chronic therapy is

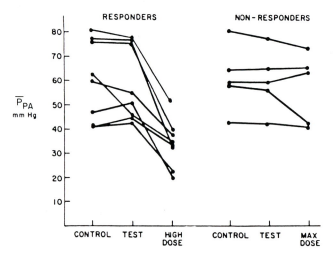

Figure 6: High-dose calcium channel blocking therapy. In some patients who are unresponsive to conventional doses (nifedipine 20 mg or diltiazem 60 mg, p.o.), higher doses sometimes succeed in reducing pulmonary arterial pressures. For high-dose therapy, conventional dose was repeated hourly for up to 12 hr until there occurred either a 50 percent decrease in pulmonary vascular resistance and a 33 percent fall in mean pulmonary arterial pressure (responders), or adverse effects (nonresponders). (Modified after Rich & Brundage [40].)

beneficial in a significant percentage of primary pulmonary hypertension patients. Certain agents seem to be likely candidates for a controlled trial. For example, even though experience with nifedipine has not been entirely favorable (31), the bulk of the evidence seems promising (8,25,29,43,47,51). Using doses of nifedipine as high as 40 mg/6 hr, Mohiuddin et al. reduced mean pulmonary arterial pressure and total pulmonary resistance in each of six patients who had not responded acutely to hydralazine, diazoxide, or terbutaline (28). Recently, Rich and Brundage, using even higher doses of nifedipine or an equivalent dose of diltiazem, reported excellent short- and long-term hemodynamic results in a majority of the patients studied (Fig. 6) (40). Overall, the experience with nifedipine appears more favorable than with other vasodilators. Consequently, a calcium channel blocker, other than verapamil, would be one logical choice for use in a controlled trial.

CONCLUSION

As vasoconstriction probably contributes to the pulmonary hypertension of most patients with primary pulmonary hypertension at some stage in the course of their disease, vasodilators offer a logical approach to therapy. However, it remains to be seen whether vasodilator therapy actually alters prognosis (41). Acute testing can identify those patients who show a significant pulmonary vasodilator response and would be suitable for chronic treatment. In using vasodilators, it should be remembered that many have other effects, such as the inhibition of platelet aggregation or the inhibition of cell proliferation, which might be important interventions in primary pulmonary hypertension. It is also important to keep in mind other forms of treatment such as anticoagulation and supplementary oxygen. In one review, the only feature associated with a high incidence of sudden death in primary pulmonary hypertension patients was a low systemic arterial oxygen tension (20). Home oxygen has been found to improve longevity in children with the Eisenmenger complex (4) but has not been assessed in primary pulmonary hypertension. Major advances in the treatment of primary pulmonary hypertension will require a better understanding of the underlying pathophysiology.

ACKNOWLEDGMENTS

I am very grateful to Ms. Judy Burrichter for her help in the preparation of this manuscript.

REFERENCES

1. Anderson EG, Simon G, Reid L: Primary and thrombo-embolic pulmonary hypertension: a quantitative pathological study. J Pathol 110:273–293, 1973.

2. Barst RJ: Pharmacologically induced pulmonary vasodilatation in children and young adults with primary pulmonary hypertension. Chest 89:497–504, 1986.

3. Bjornsson J, Edwards W: Primary pulmonary hypertension: a histopathologic study of 80 cases. Mayo Clin Proc 60:16–25, 1985.

4. Bowyer JJ, Busst CM, Denison DM, Shinebourne EA: Effect of long term oxygen treatment at home in children with pulmonary vascular disease. Br Heart J 55:385–390, 1986.

5. Buch J, Wennevold A: Hazards of diazoxide in pulmonary hypertension. Br Heart J 46:401–403, 1981.

6. Chan NS, McLay J, Kenmure AC: Reversibility of primary pulmonary hypertension during six years of treatment with oral diazoxide. Br Heart J 57:207–209, 1987.

7. Daoud FS, Reeves JT, Kelly DB: Isoproterenol as a potential pulmonary vasodilator in primary pulmonary hypertension. Am J Cardiol 42:817–822, 1978.

8. DeFeyter PJ, Kerkkamp HJ, de Jong JP: Sustained beneficial effect of nifedipine in primary pulmonary hypertension. Am Heart J 105:333–334, 1983.

9. Fisher J, Borer JS, Moses JW, Goldberg HL, Niarchos AP, Whitman HH, Mermelstein M: Hemodynamic effects of nifedipine versus hydralazine in primary pulmonary hypertension. Am J Cardiol 54:646–650, 1984.

10. Fuleihan DS, Mookherjee S, Potts JL, Obeid AI, Warner RA, Eich RH: Sodium nitroprusside: a new role as a pulmonary vasodilator. Am J Cardiol 43:405, 1979 (abstract).

11. Fuster V, Steele PM, Edwards WD, Gersh BJ, McGoon MD, Frye Primary pulmonary hypertension: natural history and the importance of thrombosis. Circulation 70:580–587, 1984.

12. Glanville AR, Burke CM, Theodore J, Robin ED: Primary pulmonary hypertension: length of survival in patients referred for heart-lung transplantation. Chest 91:675–681, 1987.

13. Groves BM, Rubin LJ, Frosolono MF, Cato AE, Reeves JT: A comparison of the acute hemodynamic effects of prostacyclin and hydralazine in primary pulmonary hypertension. Am Heart J 110:1200–1204, 1985.

14. Guadagni DN, Ikram H, Maslowski AH: Haemodynamic effects of prostacyclin (PGI_2) in pulmonary hypertension. Br Heart J 45:385–388, 1981.

15. Hall DR, Petch M: Remission of primary pulmonary hypertension during treatment with diazoxide. Br Med J 282:1118, 1981.

16. Hermiller JB, Bambach D, Thompson MJ, Huss P, Fontana ME, Magorien RD, Unverferth DV, Leier CV: Vasodilators and prostaglandin inhibitors in primary pulmonary hypertension. Ann Intern Med 97:480–489, 1982.

17. Honey M, Cotter L, Davies N, Denison D: Clinical and haemodynamic effects of diazoxide in primary pulmonary hypertension. Thorax 35:269–276, 1980.

18. Ikram H, Maslowski AH, Nicholls MG, Espiner EA, Hull FT: Haemodynamic and hormonal effects of captopril in primary pulmonary hypertension. Br Heart J 48:541–545, 1982.

19. Jones DK, Higenbottam TW, Wallwork J: Treatment of primary pulmonary hypertension with intravenous epoprostenol (prostacyclin). Br Heart J 57:270–278, 1987.

20. Kanemoto N: Natural history of pulmonary hemodynamics in primary pulmonary hypertension. Am Heart J 114:407–413, 1987.

21. Landmark K, Refsum AM, Simonsen S, Storstein O: Verapamil and pulmonary hypertension. Acta Med Scand 204:299–302, 1978.

22. Leier CV, Bambach D, Nelson S, Hermiller JB, Huss P, Magorien RD, Unverferth DV: Captopril in primary pulmonary hypertension. Circulation 67:155–161, 1983.

23. Levine TB, Rose T, Kane M, Weir EK, Cohn JN: Treatment of primary pulmonary hypertension by alpha adrenergic blockade. Circulation 62:III–26, 1980 (abstract).

24. Long WA, Rubin LJ: Prostacyclin and PGE_1 treatment of pulmonary hypertension. Am Rev Respir Dis 136:773–776, 1987.

25. Lunde P, Rasmussen K: Long-term beneficial effect of nifedipine in primary pulmonary hypertension. Am Heart J 108:415–416, 1984.

26. Lupi-Herrera E, Bialostozky D, Sobrino A: The role of isoproterenol in pulmonary artery hypertension of unknown etiology (primary). Chest 79:292–296, 1981.

27. Lupi-Herrera E, Sandoval J, Seoane M, Bialostozky D: The role of hydralazine therapy for pulmonary arterial hypertension of unknown cause. Circulation 65:645–650, 1982.

28. Mohiuddin SM, Esterbrooks D, Saenz A, O'Donahue W, Mooss AN, Sketch MH, Runco V: Hemodynamic effects of nifedipine in severe primary pulmonary hypertension. Circulation 64:IV–297, 1982 (abstract).

29. Olivari MT, Levine TB, Weir EK, Cohn JN: Hemodynamic effects of nifedipine at rest and during exercise in primary pulmonary hypertension. Chest 86:14–19, 1984.

30. Packer M, Greenberg B, Massie B, Dash H: Deleterious effects of hydralazine in patients with pulmonary hypertension. N Engl J Med 306:1326–1331, 1982.

31. Packer M, Medina N, Yushak M: Adverse hemodynamic and clinical effects of calcium channel blockade in pulmonary hypertension secondary to obliterative pulmonary vascular disease. J Am Coll Cardiol 4:890–901, 1984.

32. Packer M, Medina N, Yushak M, Wiener I: Detrimental effects of verapamil in patients with primary pulmonary hypertension. Br Heart J 52:106–111, 1984.

33. Palevsky HI, Fishman AP: Comparison of acute hemodynamic responses to prostacyclin with standard vasodilators in patients with primary pulmonary hypertension. Chest 93:179S, 1988.

34. Palevsky HI, Schloo BL, Pietra GG, Fishman AP: A potential new role for open lung biopsies in the evaluation of unexplained pulmonary hypertension. Am Rev Respir Dis 131:A401, 1985 (abstract).

35. Palevsky HI, Schloo BL, Pietra GG, Fishman AP: The relationship between morphometry and clinical course in patients with unexplained pulmonary hypertension. Clin Res 34:728A, 1986 (abstract).

36. Pearl RG, Rosenthal MH, Schroeder JS, Ashton JPA: Acute hemodynamic effects of nitroglycerin in pulmonary hypertension. Ann Intern Med 99:9–13, 1983.

37. Pietro DA, LaBresh KA, Shulman RM, Folland ED, Parisi AF, Sasahara AA: Sustained improvement in primary pulmonary hypertension during six years of treatment with sublingual isoproterenol. N Engl J Med 310:1032–1034, 1984.

38. Rao BNS, Moller JH, Edwards JE: Primary pulmonary hypertension in a child: response to pharmacologic agents. Circulation 40:583–587, 1969.

39. Reeves JT, Groves BM, Turkevich D: The case for treatment of selected patients with primary pulmonary hypertension. Am Rev Respir Dis 134:342–346, 1986.

40. Rich S, Brundage BH: High-dose calcium channel-blocking therapy for primary pulmonary hypertension: evidence for long-term reduction in pulmonary arterial pressure and regression of right ventricular hypertrophy. Circulation 76:135–141, 1987.

41. Rich S, Brundage BH, Levy PS: The effect of vasodilator therapy on the clinical outcome of patients with primary pulmonary hypertension. Circulation 71:1191–1196, 1985.

42. Rich S, Dantzker DR, Ayres SM, Bergofsky EH, Brundage BH, Detre KM, Fishman AP, Goldring RM, Groves BM, Koerner SK, Levy PC, Reid LM, Vreim CE, Williams GW: Primary pulmonary hypertension. A national prospective study. Ann Intern Med 107:216–223, 1987.

43. Rich S, Hart K, Kieras K, Brundage B: Thromboxane synthetase inhibition in primary pulmonary hypertension. Chest 91:356–360, 1987.

44. Rich S, Martinez J, Lam W, Rosen KM: Captopril as treatment for patients with pulmonary hypertension: problem of variability in assessing chronic drug treatment. Br Heart J 48:272–277, 1982.

45. Robin ED: The kingdom of the near-dead: the shortened unnatural life history of primary pulmonary hypertension. Chest 92:330–334, 1987.

46. Rubin LJ, Groves BM, Reeves JT, Frosolono M, Handel F, Cato AE: Prostacyclin-induced acute pulmonary vasodilation in primary pulmonary hypertension. Circulation 66:334–338, 1982.

47. Rubin LJ, Nicod P, Hillis LD, Firth BG: Treatment of primary pulmonary hypertension with nifedipine. Ann Intern Med 99:433–437, 1983.

48. Rubin LJ, Peter RH: Oral hydralazine therapy for primary pulmonary hypertension. N Engl J Med 302:69–74, 1980.

49. Rubino JM, Schroeder JS: Diazoxide in the treatment of primary pulmonary hypertension. Br Heart J 42:362–363, 1979.

50. Ruskin JN, Hutter AM: Primary pulmonary hypertension treated with oral phentolamine. Ann Intern Med 90:772–774, 1979.

51. Saito D, Haraoka S, Yoshida H, Kusachi S, Yasuhara K, Nishihara M, Fukuhara J, Hagashima H: Primary pulmonary hypertension improved by long-term oral administration of nifedipine. Am Heart J 105:1041-1042, 1983.

52. Samet P, Bernstein WH: Loss of reactivity of the pulmonary vascular bed in primary pulmonary hypertension. Am Heart J 66:197–199, 1963.

53. Samet P, Bernstein WH, Widrich J: Intracardiac infusion of acetylcholine in primary pulmonary hypertension. Am Heart J 60:433–439, 1960.

54. Simonneau G, Herve P, Petitpretz P, Girad P, Salmeron S, Escourrou P, Baudoin C, Nebout T, Duroux P: Detection of a reversible component in primary pulmonary hypertension: value of prostacyclin acute infusion. Am Rev Respir Dis 133:A223, 1986 (abstract).

55. Wagenvoort CA, Wagenvoort N: Primary pulmonary hypertension: a pathologic study of the lung vessels in 156 clinically diagnosed cases. Circulation 42:1163-1184, 1970.

56. Wang SW, Pohl JE, Rowlands DJ, Wade EG: Diazoxide in treatment of primary pulmonary hypertension. Br Heart J 40:572–574, 1978.

57. Wood BA, Tortoledo F, Luck JC, Fennell WH: Rapid attenuation of response to nifedipine in primary pulmonary hypertension. Chest 82:793–794, 1982.

58. Yamaki S, Wagenvoort CA: Comparison of primary plexogenic arteriopathy in adults and children. Br Heart J 54:428–435, 1985.

Marc Cohen, M.D.
Valentin Fuster, M.D.
William D. Edwards, M.D.

38 _____

Anticoagulation in the Treatment of Pulmonary Hypertension

Since primary pulmonary hypertension was first described in detail by Dresdale et al. (7), there has been an impressive array of small studies describing a beneficial response to one or another vasodilator drug. However, even the most recent reports (20,27,28), which describe short-term improvement in pulmonary hemodynamics and exercise tolerance after vasodilator therapy, indicate that long-term survival is not improved. In fact, the only study to date which shows a beneficial effect of medical therapy on survival in a large population of carefully screened patients with primary pulmonary hypertension, the Mayo Clinic study (12), suggests that anticoagulation may be effective in prolonging life.

RETROSPECTIVE MAYO CLINIC STUDY

In order to obtain a better understanding of the natural history and possible pathogenetic mechanisms of the disease, a long-term retrospective follow-up study was made of 120 patients with primary pulmonary hypertension—diagnosed by strict clinical and hemodynamic criteria. The results suggest that thrombosis and anticoagulant therapy may have an important role in this disease.

Patient Population

The study population consists of 120 cases of primary pulmonary hypertension diagnosed at the Mayo Clinic between the years 1955 and 1977. All patients had

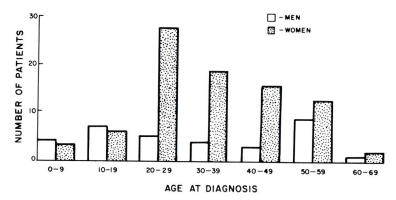

Figure 1: Age distribution of 33 males and 98 females at the time that the diagnosis of primary pulmonary hypertension was made. (Modified after Fuster et al. [12].)

a follow-up of at least 5 years unless death supervened. The median follow-up period was 14 years and the longest was 27 years. Recurrent thromboembolic disease was excluded by pulmonary angiography in 36 patients and at autopsy in 56 patients. In the remaining patients, careful history and physical examination did not suggest thromboembolic disease.

There were 33 males (27 percent) and 87 females (73 percent) (Fig. 1) with a mean age of 34 years at the time of initial presentation to the Mayo Clinic. The median interval from the initial symptoms to the clinical and hemodynamic diagnosis of primary pulmonary hypertension was 1.9 years. The most common clinical features were exertional dyspnea (75 percent); loud second heart sound (98 percent); radiographic abnormalities (95 percent) in the form of cardiomegaly or prominent central pulmonary arteries; and electrocardiographic abnormalities (95 percent) in the form of right ventricular hypertrophy, right axis deviation, or a large P wave. Exertional dizziness or syncope (30 percent), exertional chest pain (8 percent), and ankle swelling (8 percent) were additional less common symptoms.

Cardiac catheterization revealed peak systolic pulmonary artery pressure higher than 50 mmHg in all patients, a cardiac index less than 2.5 L/min/m² in 85 patients (71 percent), and in 113 patients (94 percent), a total pulmonary vascular

TABLE 1 HEMODYNAMIC FEATURES AT DIAGNOSIS

	Mean	Range
Pulmonary artery pressure (mmHg)		
Peak	98	53–208
Mean	64	36–120
Pulmonary index (L/min/m²)	2.2	0.7–5.0
Total pulmonary resistance (U/m²)	33	11–95
Right ventricular end-diastolic pressure (mmHg)	13	2–30
Systemic arterial saturation (%)	91	42–99
Pulmonary arterial saturation (%)	60	20–80

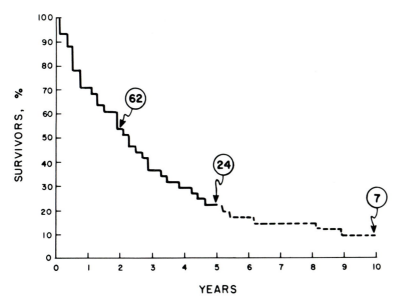

Figure 2: Duration of survival of 115 patients with primary pulmonary hypertension who underwent diagnostic catheterization. Circles enclose numbers of living patients under observation at 2, 5, and 10 years, respectively. (Reproduced from Fuster et al. [12].)

resistance greater than 15 Wood units/m²; total pulmonary vascular resistance was calculated as mean pulmonary pressure divided by the cardiac index. Systemic arterial oxygen saturation less than 90 percent was observed in 32 patients (27 percent). Clearly, by the time patients with primary pulmonary hypertension present for examination, their disease is far advanced.

Pulmonary angiography showed abnormalities in 30 of the 36 patients in whom it was performed (83 percent). The main pulmonary arteries and their primary branches were dilated, and the distal branches were pruned and quite tortuous. No embolic occlusions was demonstrated angiographically.

Clinical Course, Prognostic and Therapeutic Factors

During the follow-up period, 112 patients (93 percent) had died (Fig. 2). The median interval from diagnosis to death was 1.9 years (range 0–16 years); more than 75 percent of the deaths occurred within the first 5 years after diagnosis. Death was associated with right cardiac failure in 71 patients; pulmonary arterial dissection with tamponade in 1; and minor surgery in 1. In 18 patients, the cause of death could not be determined. A number of clinical and hemodynamic variables were tested for prognostic importance by univariate and stepwise multivariate analysis for the group as a whole who survived diagnostic cardiac catheterization (115 patients). Univariate analysis identified total pulmonary vascular resistance, arterial oxygen saturation, and anticoagulant therapy as strong prognostic variables.

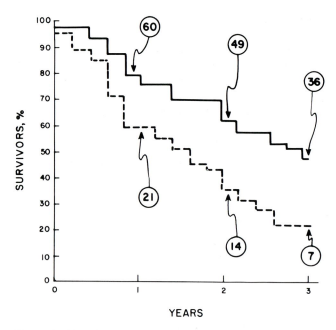

Figure 3: Duration of survival with and without anticoagulant therapy in primary pulmonary hypertension. The survival rate was better among the 78 patients who received oral anticoagulants (upper line) than among the 37 who did not (lower line) (P = 0.02, log rank test). Circles enclose numbers of patients living at the end of each year. (Reproduced from Fuster et al. [12].)

Impact of Anticoagulant Therapy

To evaluate the prognostic and therapeutic effect of anticoagulants, the survivorship of the 78 anticoagulated patients was compared with that of the 37 who received no anticoagulants. Patients were considered as being "anticoagulated" if coumadin therapy was begun within the first 12 months after diagnosis. The group treated with anticoagulants had a statistically significant improvement in survivorship compared to the group of patients who did not receive anticoagulants during their follow-up (Fig. 3). There were no significant differences between the two groups with regard to other clinical or hemodynamic variables that could account for the difference in survivorship. Stepwise multivariate analysis identified arterial oxygen saturation and anticoagulant therapy as the only two independent variables that had prognostic significance.

It should be realized that even among patients receiving anticoagulant therapy, the mortality rate was high. In almost all patients in this study, the disease had already progressed to an advanced stage. As mentioned above, 94 percent of patients presented with a pulmonary vascular resistance of 15 Wood units or greater. In some, symptoms had been present for a long time prior to diagnosis; in others, the course was insidious. Therefore, intervention with anticoagulant therapy was started too late, since it must be started early in the course of primary pulmonary hypertension if it is to be effective.

Limitations of the Mayo Clinic Study

For several reasons, the effect of oral anticoagulant therapy on outcome was somewhat difficult to assess in the retrospective Mayo Clinic study. First, in many patients, treatment was begun at various intervals after diagnosis, and specific reasons for initiating or withholding therapy were not uniform. To minimize this bias, we defined anticoagulated patients as those whose therapy with anticoagulants was started within the first year after diagnosis. Second, even among patients receiving anticoagulant therapy, the mortality rate was high. Nevertheless, univariate and multivariate analysis did show a significant beneficial effect of anticoagulant therapy on overall survival. This improved survival was noted in patients in both major pathological groups, i.e., small vessel thromboembolic pulmonary hypertension or plexogenic pulmonary arteriopathy (see below), who were treated with anticoagulants. The number of patients treated within each pathological subtype was too small to assess whether anticoagulant therapy has more effect on the small vessel thromboembolic pulmonary hypertension than on plexogenic pulmonary arteriopathy.

EARLIER STUDIES AND CASE REPORTS SUPPORTING ANTICOAGULATION

In the late 1940s and early 1950s, several studies suggested that thrombosis may play a prominent role in the pathogenesis of primary pulmonary hypertension. Experimental studies in animals by Harrison (15,16) and by Barnard (1), using repeated intravenous injections of small clots or of thromboplastin, indicated that these small emboli could trigger arterial reaction in which the intima was markedly thickened. Indeed, Barnard suggested that, "The lesions of experimental thromboembolic arteriosclerosis using fibrin prepared in vitro correspond closely with those described and illustrated in human cases of primary pulmonary hypertension . . ."(1).

Shortly thereafter, Wood (36) described two patients in whom severe pulmonary hypertension and right ventricular failure appeared several months after pregnancy; continuous anticoagulant therapy caused regression of the patients' signs and symptoms. A similar instance of obliterative pulmonary hypertension that appeared insidiously several months after pregnancy was described by Wilcken et al. (35): using serial cardiac catheterizations, they found a significant drop in pulmonary vascular resistance after 18 months of continuous anticoagulation. However, the reports of Wood and of Wilcken provided neither pulmonary angiographic nor pathological data concerning the presence, or absence, of gross (as contrasted with microscopic) proximal pulmonary emboli.

Several clinicopathologic studies in 1957 suggested a role for microscopic thrombosis in some patients with primary pulmonary hypertension. Kuida et al. (21) described four patients with idiopathic pulmonary hypertension: two had evidence of microscopic thrombi; one of the two had thrombus in association with an arteritis. Shepherd et al. (29) reviewed 10 cases, several of which demonstrated bland intraluminal thrombi or thrombi overlying areas of arteritis. In 11 patients with primary pulmonary hypertension, Evans et al. (10) found thrombosis of segmental and smaller arteries to be relatively common at autopsy. However, their failure to find evidence of thrombi in some of these patients raised questions about the role of thrombosis in this disease. Skepticism regarding the role of thrombosis was reinforced by the observations of Sleeper et al. who, on serial cardiac catheterizations, found an inexorable progression of the disease regardless of the medical regimen, including anticoagulation (30).

In 1963, Goodwin et al. described a group of 19 patients with obliterative pulmonary hypertension (14). Eleven of the 19 patients presented with clinical suspicion of acute pulmonary embolism whereas the other eight patients experienced an insidious onset in the form of idiopathic pulmonary hypertension. At autopsy, several patients in both groups only had thrombotic occlusion of the smaller pulmonary arteries and arterioles. Anticoagulation did not seem to be of any therapeutic benefit.

Further debate concerning the role of thrombosis in primary pulmonary hypertension was fostered by the clinicopathologic observations of Walcott et al. in 23 patients (33). Ten of their patients had clear-cut evidence of thromboembolic changes in small pulmonary arteries (< 4 mm). However, the authors did not interpret these changes to be extensive enough to account for the level of pulmonary hypertension. Moreover, therapy with anticoagulation did not seem to have any dramatic beneficial result.

In contrast to these studies, more recent reports have suggested a therapeutic role for anticoagulation. In 1976, Bourdillon and Oakley described dramatic regression of primary pulmonary hypertension in a teenage girl (5). Even though thromboembolic disease of large pulmonary vessels was excluded by pulmonary angiography and lung scanning, the patient was maintained on full dose anticoagulation. Over an 8-year period that entailed serial cardiac catheterizations, significant regression of the severe pulmonary hypertension occurred. Interestingly, despite improvement while on anticoagulants, the authors stated, "It is unlikely that the anticoagulants were directly relevant to the patient's recovery. . . ." Based on extensive pathological examination of the chambers of the heart and lungs in patients with pulmonary hypertension of varied etiologies, James advanced the hypothesis that discrete mural thrombi in the antral portion of the right atrium could be the source for chronic microemboli to the lungs (19).

In 1986, Cohen and Fuster (6) described a patient with "primary" pulmonary hypertension in whom open lung biopsy showed microscopic thromboemboli even though a lung scan had excluded gross pulmonary embolism. Serial cardiac catheterization while on full dose anticoagulation therapy for 2½ years revealed regression of the pulmonary hypertension. However, the three recent case studies just mentioned (5,6,19), which suggest a major role for thrombosis and anticoagulation, are only isolated reports. To be convincing, pathological studies in a large series of patients will be required.

HISTOPATHOLOGY OF PRIMARY PULMONARY HYPERTENSION: PREVALENCE OF THROMBOSIS IN THE SMALL PULMONARY ARTERIES

To date, several large scale histopathological studies involving more than 50 patients with primary pulmonary hypertension have been published (4,8,12,25,32). We will now briefly discuss these studies, focusing on the prevalence of thrombosis in the small pulmonary arteries.

The first large series was reported by Wagenvoort and Wagenvoort (32). Lung tissue from 156 patients with primary pulmonary hypertension was analyzed. Most patients were found to have the triad of medial hypertrophy, laminar intimal fibrosis, and plexiform lesions. However, in 31 of the 156 patients (20 percent), organized thrombi were found within small pulmonary arteries. Moreover, thrombotic occlusions were found in six of the patients in the "plexogenic" group. The patient population with thrombotic occlusions was attributed to probable embolic disease and to "true" primary pulmonary hypertension. However, in 1984 and 1985, two studies presented detailed autopsy data on patients who clearly had no evidence of proximal pulmonary embolic disease (4,12). In the Mayo Clinic study, the major histological feature in 57 percent of the autopsy lung specimens was thrombosis; in 38 percent of the autopsies, plexogenic arteriopathy was the main feature. In 80 patients with primary pulmonary hypertension, Bjornsson and Edwards (4) observed at least three distinct histological subtypes: 58 percent demonstrated small vessel thromboembolic disease; 28 percent demonstrated plexogenic arteriopathy; the remaining 16 percent showed isolated medial hypertrophy, arteritis, or pulmonary venous disease. Patients with plexiform lesions often had platelet-fibrin thrombi lining the small vascular channels within the plexiform lesions. Moreover, patients who had pulmonary venoocclusive disease at autopsy were characterized by organized or, on rare occasion, fresh thrombi in the pulmonary venules and veins.

The most recent large scale pathological study is the prospective study sponsored by the National Heart, Lung, and Blood Institute (see chapter by Pietra). In lung tissue obtained from 94 patients, both plexiform arteriopathy and thrombotic arteriopathy was found in the majority of cases (25). In fact, the designation of predominant thrombotic arteriopathy was made in 41 of the 94 patients. The observation of plexiform and/or thrombotic disease in patients with primary pulmonary hypertension substantiates the subtype designation promoted by the World Health Organization (17), and by Edwards and Edwards (8), which indicates that even in the absence of gross pulmonary embolism, there is a thrombotic component in a large fraction of patients with primary pulmonary hypertension. Lastly, histological analysis of 12 patients with coexistent pulmonary and portal hypertension has disclosed thrombosis in the small pulmonary arteries of 8 of the 12 patients (9).

The etiology of the thrombotic process is unknown. In those cases where both elastic (pulmonary vessels larger than several millimeters in diameter) and muscular pulmonary arteries are involved, the thrombotic process is probably embolic in origin. However, macroscopic venous thromboembolism is unlikely to explain the commonly observed pattern in primary pulmonary hypertension in which only the small (less than 1 mm), muscular arteries contain thrombi. The pathogenesis in these cases may have been due to microemboli, possibly from the right atrium (19) or from the pelvis. Events surrounding menstruation may initiate an insidious process; pelvic microthrombi may form at this time and embolize to the lung; or in women with hyperreactive muscular pulmonary arteries, the hormonal environment associated with menstruation may induce prolonged pulmonary vasoconstriction. Alternatively, the pulmonary thromboses may have occurred in situ and due to some abnormality in arterial wall-coagulation interaction.

But even though either, or both, mechanisms may be involved in the pathogenesis of pulmonary hypertension in women, the process in men and young children is more difficult to explain. In 1973, Inglesby et al. (18) reported that in 7 of 10 patients with familial primary pulmonary hypertension, there was an abnormally high level of antiplasmin, suggesting a primary defect in fibrinolysis in this disease. However, several years later, Tubbs et al. (31) reported no deficiency in any of the fibrinolytic proteins in familial primary pulmonary hypertension. Nonetheless, the possibility remains that a defect in fibrinolysis is a mechanism of this disease (11).

It is conceivable that a primary abnormality of the muscular pulmonary arteries (such as hyperreactivity with vasospasm) could produce fibrinoid necrosis and plexiform lesions in one person and in situ thrombosis in another. Moreover, it is possible that platelets may contribute to the progression of primary pulmonary hypertension, either directly by luminal obstruction or indirectly by release of platelet-derived smooth muscle growth factor. In fact, in an elegant experimental model of pulmonary microembolism, Mlczoch et al. (23) observed that the pulmonary hypertension seen after embolization was not only the result of mechanical luminal obstruction but also the result of vasoconstrictive substances released into the pulmonary circulation by platelets: dogs deprived of functional platelets had much lower pulmonary arterial pressures after glass beads were embolized than did their counterparts with intact platelets. The role of antiplatelet agents in human pulmonary hypertension has yet to be explored.

PULMONARY THROMBOSIS IN CONGENITAL HEART DISEASE

Thrombosis within the small pulmonary arteries of patients suffering from congenital heart disease may aggravate the pulmonary hypertension already triggered by increased flow, pressure, or hypoxia. As early as 1958, Best and Heath (3) described seven patients with cyanotic congenital heart disease, five of whom had secondary polycythemia. Multiple microscopic pulmonary thrombi were observed in four of the five with polycythemia. In 1975, Waldman et al. (34) observed a shortened platelet survival time in hypoxemic patients with congenital heart disease. However, no evidence for disseminated intravascular coagulation was documented. In contrast, Levin et al. (22) showed that 8 of 23 infants with persistent pulmonary hypertension had extensive platelet-fibrin thrombi in the small pulmonary arteries. Newfeld et al. (24) examined autopsy and lung biopsy tissue in 101 children with transposition of the great arteries: in 20 to 30 percent of the children, microthrombi were found, regardless of whether the ventricular septum was intact or not. Bermen et al. (2) made a similar observation in a child dying after a Mustard operation.

Two recent investigations in patients with congenital heart disease and pulmonary hypertension (13,26) have focused attention on abnormalities in the Von Willebrand factor secreted by the endothelial cells. Both studies observed an increased amount of circulating Von Willebrand antigen without a commensurate increase in the biological activity. In addition, changes in the multimeric pattern of the large protein were noted in patients with pulmonary hypertension compared to the patients with normal pulmonary pressures. Abnormalities in Von Willebrand factor may result in abnormal platelet-vessel wall interactions in the pulmonary circulation which may result in intravascular thrombosis or release of platelet-derived vasoactive compounds.

Finally, it is probable that intravascular thrombosis occurs in the end stage of cyanotic congenital heart disease. The risk/benefit ratio of anticoagulation in such patients remains to be determined.

LIMITATIONS AND FUTURE CONSIDERATIONS

The pathological studies cited above strongly suggest that thrombosis is an important contributing mechanism in the pathogenesis of primary pulmonary hypertension and possibly in other causes of pulmonary hypertension. Although antithrombotic therapy with anticoagulants did seem to be efficacious in some of the studies mentioned, extrapolation to the general population with primary or secondary pulmonary hypertension must be made with caution. Many questions remain unanswered. What is the basis of the thrombosis? Is it due to microemboli or does it arise in situ? Is there a significant role for thrombosis and anticoagulation in patients with predominantly plexogenic arteriopathy? It is possible that all patients with pulmonary hypertension may benefit from anticoagulant therapy probably because of prevention of complicating secondary thrombi. One lesson is clear: if any therapeutic modality is to be effective in primary pulmonary hypertension, it must be started early in the course of the disease.

REFERENCES

1. Barnard PJ: Thrombo-embolic primary pulmonary arteriosclerosis. Br Heart J 16:93–100, 1954.

2. Berman W Jr, Whitman V, Pierce WS, Waldhausen JA: The development of pulmonary vascular obstructive disease after successful Mustard operation in early infancy. Circulation 58:181–185, 1978.

3. Best PV, Heath D: Pulmonary thrombosis in cyanotic congenital heart disease without pulmonary hypertension. J Pathol Bacteriol 75:281–291, 1958.

4. Bjornsson J, Edwards WD: Primary pulmonary hypertension: A histopathologic study of 80 cases. Mayo Clin Proc 60:16–25, 1985.

5. Bourdillon PD, Oakley CM: Regression of primary pulmonary hypertension. Br Heart J 38:264–270, 1976.

6. Cohen M, Edwards WD, Fuster V: Regression in thromboembolic type of primary pulmonary hypertension during 2½ years of antithrombotic therapy. J Am Coll Cardiol 7:172–175, 1986.

7. Dresdale DT, Schultz M, Michtom RJ: Primary pulmonary hypertension. I. Clinical and hemodynamic study. Am J Med 11:686–694, 1951.

8. Edwards WD, Edwards JE: Clinical primary pulmonary hypertension: Three pathologic types. Circulation 56:884–888, 1977.

9. Edwards BS, Weir EK, Edwards WD, Ludwig J, Dykoski RK, Edwards JE: Coexistent pulmonary and portal hypertension: Morphologic and clinical features. J Am Coll Cardiol 10:1233–1238, 1987.

10. Evans W, Short DS, Bedford DE: Solitary pulmonary hypertension. Br Heart J 19:93–116, 1957.

11. Fuchs J, Mlczoch J, Niessner H, Lechner K: Abnormal fibrinolysis in primary pulmonary hypertension. Eur Heart J 2:A168, 1981.

12. Fuster V, Steele PM, Edwards WD, Gersh BJ, McGoon MD, Frye RL: Primary pulmonary hypertension: Natural history and the importance of thrombosis. Circulation 70:580–587, 1984.

13. Geggel RI, Carvalho AC, Hoyer LW, Reid LM: Von Willebrand factor abnormalities in primary pulmonary hypertension. Am Rev Respir Dis 135:294–299, 1987.

14. Goodwin JF, Harrison CV, Wilcken DEL: Obliterative pulmonary hypertension and thrombo-embolism. Br Med J 1:701–711; 777–783, 1963.

15. Harrison CV: Experimental pulmonary arteriosclerosis. J Path Bact 60:289–293, 1948.

16. Harrison CV: Experimental pulmonary hypertension. J Path Bact 63:195–200, 1951.

17. Hatano S, Strasser T (eds): Primary pulmonary hypertension: Report on a WHO meeting. Geneva, World Health Organization, 1975.

18. Inglesby TV, Singer JW, Gordon DS: Abnormal fibrinolysis in familial pulmonary hypertension. Am J Med 55:5–14, 1973.

19. James TN: Thrombi in antrum atrii dextri of human heart as clinically important source for chronic microembolisation to lungs. Br Heart J 49:122–132, 1983.

20. Jones DK, Higenbottam TW, Wallwork J: Treatment of primary pulmonary hypertension with intravenous epoprostenol (prostacyclin). Br Heart J 57:270–278, 1987.

21. Kuida H, Dammin GJ, Haynes FW, Rapaport E, Dexter L: Primary pulmonary hypertension. Am J Med 23:166–182, 1957.

22. Levin DL, Weinberg AG, Perkin RM: Pulmonary microthrombi syndrome in newborn infants with unresponsive persistent pulmonary hypertension. J Pediatr 102:299–303, 1983.

23. Mlczoch J, Tucker A, Weir EK, Reeves JT, Grover RF: Platelet-mediated pulmonary hypertension and hypoxia during pulmonary microembolism: Reduction by platelet inhibition. Chest 74:648–653, 1978.

24. Newfeld EA, Paul MH, Muster AJ, Idriss FS: Pulmonary vascular disease in complete transposition of the great arteries: A study of 200 patients. Am J Cardiol 34:75–82, 1974.

25. Pietra GG, Edwards WD, Kay JM: The spectrum of pulmonary arterial lesions in patients with primary pulmonary hypertension (abstract). International Conference on Primary Pulmonary Hypertension, 1987. Sponsored by the Division of Lung Diseases, National Heart, Lung, and Blood Institute.

26. Rabinovitch M, Andrew M, Thom H, Trusler GA, Williams WG, Rowe RD, Olley PM: Abnormal endothelial factor VIII associated with pulmonary hypertension and congenital heart defects. Circulation 76:1043–1052, 1987.

27. Rich S, Brundage BH: High dose calcium channel-blocking therapy for primary pulmonary hypertension: Evidence for long-term reduction in pulmonary arterial pressure and regression of right ventricular hypertrophy. Circulation 76:135–141, 1987.

28. Rich S, Brundage BH, Levy PS: The effect of vasodilator therapy on the clinical outcome of patients with primary pulmonary hypertension. Circulation 71:1191–1196, 1985.

29. Shepherd JT, Edwards JE, Burchell HB, Swan HJC, Wood EH: Clinical, physiological, and pathological considerations in patients with idiopathic pulmonary hypertension. Br Heart J 19:70–82, 1957.

30. Sleeper JC, Orgain ES, McIntosh HD: Primary pulmonary hypertension: Review of clinical features and pathologic physiology with a report of pulmonary hemodynamics derived from repeated catheterization. Circulation 26:1358-1369, 1962.

31. Tubbs RR, Levin RD, Shirey EK, Hoffman GC: Fibrinolysis in familial pulmonary hypertension. Am J Clin Pathol 71:384–387, 1979.

32. Wagenvoort CA, Wagenvoort N: Primary pulmonary hypertension: A pathologic study of the lung vessels in 156 clinically diagnosed cases. Circulation 42:1163–1184, 1970.

33. Walcott G, Burchell HB, Brown AL: Primary pulmonary hypertension. Am J Med 49:70–79, 1970.

34. Waldman JD, Czapek EE, Paul MH, Schwartz AD, Levin DL, Schindler S: Shortened platelet survival time in cyanotic heart disease. J Pediatr 87:77–79, 1975.

35. Wilcken DEL, MacKenzie KM, Goodwin JF: Anticoagulant treatment of obliterative pulmonary hypertension. Lancet 2:781–783, 1960.

36. Wood P: *Diseases of the Heart and Circulation*, 2nd ed. London, Eyre and Spottiswoode, 1956.

Tim W. Higenbottam, M.D.

39

The Criteria and Preparation for Heart-Lung Transplantation

Successful human lung transplantation is still in its infancy compared with other forms of organ transplantation. While still at an innovative stage, the risks are comparatively greater and the resources more scarce. For these reasons, the criteria for patient selection are restrictive. This is to minimize the risks and to ensure, as far as possible, a successful outcome. With increasing experience, it will be possible to relax these restrictions, as has been the case with other forms of transplantation. Much of what will be described in this chapter represents only the initial steps toward the establishment of lung transplantation in clinical practice.

HISTORICAL PERSPECTIVE

To understand both the limits and potential for lung transplantation, it is important to have some understanding of the stages of development through which it has passed over the last 30 years.

Much of the early experience with lung transplantation was not encouraging (28). An important problem was the failure of healing of the anastomosis between donor and recipient airways. In part, the explanation was the need to use, during perioperative stage, high-dose corticosteroids as an immunosuppressant. This not only delayed healing but also predisposed to infection. Better healing was achieved with the introduction of the immunosuppressant cyclosporine in 1979, which largely erased the need for high-dose steroids after transplantation (3).

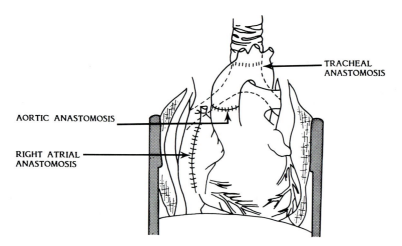

Figure 1: Schematic drawing of the heart-lung transplant operation at completion. The donor heart is anastomosed at the right atrium and ascending aorta. The donor lungs are anastomosed about 1.4 cm above the carina.

Failure of the anastomosis to heal also reflected the difficulty in re-establishing an arterial blood supply to the lower end of the trachea and main bronchus. Using a primate model, Reitz et al. (24) developed the 'en-bloc' heart and lung transplant operation. The trachea of the recipient was anastomosed, one to two rings of trachea above the carina to the lower end of the donor trachea (Fig. 1). Reitz and his colleagues were able to demonstrate that mediastinal collaterals, in particular those from the coronary arteries of the donor heart, extended to supply the lower trachea and main bronchial arteries. This 'en-bloc' heart-lung transplant, with cyclosporine was successful first in primates and then was used clinically in man (24)

The Toronto Transplantation Group re-explored single lung transplantation. To improve revascularization of the donor bronchus after transplantation, omentum was mobilized and 'wrapped' around the bronchial anastomosis (27). To date, clinical results using this technique have been encouraging.

Attempts have been made to transplant both lungs without the heart, but these efforts have failed to achieve adequate healing of the tracheal anastomosis leading to dehiscence or tracheal stenosis. This serves to emphasize the importance of the original observations of Reitz et al. on the value of the mediastinal collaterals in revascularizing the donor bronchi and trachea.

THE DONOR OPERATION AND SELECTION

The donor operation has been previously described in detail (24). Three important areas will be covered in the course of this discussion: lung preservation, distant hospital organ procurement, and avoidance of donor acquired infections.

Lung Preservation

Success in transplanting any organ is determined by the initial graft function. For lung transplantation where no alternative postoperative support is available, it is vital that the grafted lungs function immediately. For this reason, much experimental effort has been expended to preserve optimally the lungs for transplantation. Broad guidelines have emerged, namely, to keep the lungs inflated, to chill them to 4°C, and to perfuse the pulmonary vascular bed with solutions of an intracellular electrolyte composition also containing albumin or whole blood (9). Experimental application of these principles limits ischemic lung injury and prevents the so-called "reimplantation" response which can follow transplantation and shares many pathophysiological features with adult respiratory distress syndrome.

Despite these advances in lung preservation, most centers were initially reluctant to extend the ischemic times of the donor lungs beyond one hour. Donors were, therefore, transported to the recipient's hospital. The donor and recipient operations were then performed in adjoining operating rooms. While this practice was clinically successful, it limited considerably the number of donor referrals and so impeded progress of lung transplantation.

Distant Hospital Organ Procurement

To extend the donor lung ischemic time in order to enable procurement of organs from distant hospitals, a number of "long-term" preservation systems have been developed. The most complicated, developed in Pittsburgh, is an isolated heart-lung block where the lungs are artificially ventilated, and the beating heart perfuses the lungs (7). Harefield Hospital in Great Britain puts the donor on cardiopulmonary bypass to cool quickly the donor organs. At Papworth Hospital, the donor is pretreated with a vasodilator, intravenous prostacyclin (PGI$_2$), and a simple single flush with a standard perfusion solution (8,29). All these techniques

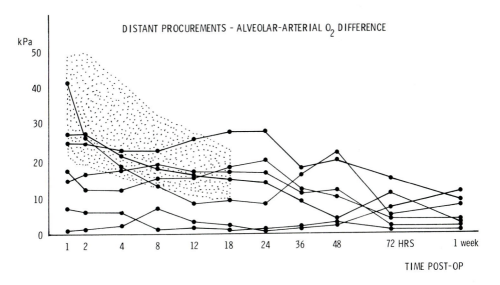

Figure 2: The individual values for alveolar-arterial oxygen difference (kPa) in patients to receive organs through distant hospital procurement. Ischemic times average 110 min; the longest was 3.5 hr. The postoperative values are shown up to 1 week. The hatched area represents mean ± 2 S.D. of the postoperative alveolar-arterial oxygen difference in 13 patients who underwent cardiopulmonary bypass for coronary artery disease.

give good results and have extended ischemic times beyond 4 hr. Our system gives comparable postoperative gas exchange to routine cardiopulmonary by-pass patients (Fig. 2). As donor lungs and hearts can now be obtained from distant hospitals, donor referrals have increased. In the United Kingdom and Europe, the number of donors does not appear to be a limiting factor in lung transplantation.

Donor Selection

The criteria for accepting a donor for heart-lung transplantation are now well established (Table 1); most are self-explanatory. Similar criteria also apply to single lung transplants.

Along with matching our donors and recipients for class I or ABO blood group antigens, the size of the donor lungs are matched to the size of the recipient's thoracic cavity. If donor lungs are too large, atelectasis and intrapulmonary right-to-left shunting occurs. Various methods are used to match the size of donor lungs to recipient's thoracic cavity. At Papworth Hospital, we have adopted a simple radiographic technique, comparing the vertical height of the thoracic vertebrae of donor and recipient (8).

TABLE 1 CRITERIA FOR SELECTION OF HEART-LUNG DONORS

Age < 35 years
ABO compatibility
Clear chest radiograph
No respiratory infection
Close size match to lung volume of the recipient
Arterial P_{O_2} > 45 mmHg on 100% O_2
Low peak inspiratory pressure at normal tidal volumes
No major chest trauma
Short period of ventilation

Screening for Donor Diseases

Following the development of fatal primary cytomegalovirus (CMV) pneumonitis in recipients who preoperatively were negative for CMV on serology but received organs from CMV positive donors (14), we now pretest the donor serology for CMV which forms part of our HIV serological testing program. Now, CMV nega-tive recipients only receive organs from CMV negative donors. This is similar to the practice in bone marrow transplantation and has avoided further deaths from CMV (14).

PATIENTS SUCCESSFULLY TREATED BY LUNG TRANSPLANTATION

The combined heart-lung transplant offers an ideal surgical solution to those in-tractable diseases where both lungs and heart are involved (Table 2). In most cases, patients present with either primary or secondary pulmonary hypertension. Initially, heart-lung transplantation was used to treat Eisenmenger's syndrome and primary pulmonary hypertension (2). It has subsequently been extended to treat primary lung disease associated with secondary pulmonary hypertension (21), including cystic fibrosis (16,25).

Single lung transplantation, considered unsuitable for treating emphysema or suppurative lung disease, has been used successfully to treat cryptogenic fibrosing alveolitis (27). It has been argued that single lung transplantation may also be useful in the treatment of primary pulmonary hypertension although experimental evidence in support of this claim is unavailable.

TABLE 2 INDICATIONS FOR HEART-LUNG TRANSPLANTATION

Cardiopulmonary
 Congenital heart disease with pulmonary hypertension (Eisenmenger's syndrome)
 Acquired heart disease with right ventricular failure and increased pulmonary vascular resistance
Pulmonary
 Primary pulmonary hypertension
 Cryptogenic fibrosing alveolitis
 End-stage chronic obstructive pulmonary disease and emphysema
 Cystic fibrosis

Criteria for Patient Selection

The present criteria in selecting patients for heart-lung transplantation reflect the innovative stage of development of this form of surgery (Table 3). There is as yet no 10-year survival data; for this reason, transplantation is offered only to those patients with end-stage disease and for whom alternative therapy is unlikely to be helpful. Clearly, such general guidelines do not apply to all patients, and in certain diseases prognosis may be more accurately predicted. These will be dealt with later.

Currently, heart-lung transplantation is restricted to patients between the ages of 10 and 49 years. Whether to perform heart-lung transplantation on children between 5 and 9 years of age is being considered in the United Kingdom by a committee of the Royal College of Surgeons.

In the early development of heart-lung transplantation, previous thoracic surgery was considered a contraindication. This reflected the hazards of postoperative chest wall bleeding, which was a major cause of fatality in early series (2).

TABLE 3 CRITERIA FOR SELECTION OF PATIENTS FOR HEART-LUNG TRANSPLANTATION

 Age > 10 < 49 years
 No systemic illness
 No severe secondary organ failure
 No previous major cardiothoracic surgery
 No high-dose corticosteroids

With increasing experience, this has become less of a problem. As a result, patients who have had previous mediastinotomy for corrective cardiac surgery and those who have had lung biopsies or lobectomies are now being considered for heart-lung transplantation (12). Previous surgery to the pleura, pleurodesis, or pleurectomy, however, remain contraindications along wth sepsis outside the lungs.

Multiple, simultaneous organ transplantation is becoming possible. In 1987, transplantation of heart, lungs, and liver was performed at our institute on a patient with primary biliary cirrhosis and pulmonary hypertension (30). Well-controlled insulin-dependent diabetes mellitus is no longer a contraindication.

As with any innovative treatment where risks are greater than more established therapy, a patient must have a positive attitude to transplantation. Sound social and family background are also positive assets.

PREOPERATIVE INVESTIGATIONS

Patients are admitted to hospital for a 4-day period during which time they become acquainted with the staff and the transplant unit. Their suitability for transplant surgery is assessed and physiological measurements performed to gauge prognosis.

A routine series of investigations are performed. These studies provide information on the patient's ABO blood group, the status of their CMV and toxoplasma serology. Liver and renal function are assessed. A chest radiograph is used to gauge cardiac dilatation, and an electrocardiogram is performed to assess right ventricular hypertrophy. Urine and sputum are cultured for bacterial pathogens.

Adequacy of the respiratory musculoskeletal system is assessed by simple spirometry and measurement of total lung capacity (TLC) and residual volume (RV) using a whole body plethysmograph. Since immediate postoperative care involves early removal of assisted ventilation, usually within 24 hr, we also measure the patient's ventilatory response to rebreathing carbon dioxide using a modified Read method (22). We have found this practice useful in predicting those patients in hypercapnic respiratory failure who may require prolonged assisted ventilation after the operation (16).

Prognostic Measurements

For Eisenmenger's syndrome and pulmonary hypertension secondary to cardiac disease, we have used a reduction in 12-min walking distance, a test of exercise tolerance, of less than 300 meters as an inclusion criterion for transplantation. In addition, arterial oxygen tension (Pa_{O_2}) less than 60 mmHg is used. Symptoms of syncope and angina are also considered important prognostic indicators.

In primary pulmonary hypertension, a reduced cardiac index and a mixed venous oxygen saturation ($S\bar{v}_{O_2}$) less than 63 percent are considered inclusion criteria for transplantation (6). The height of the mean pulmonary artery pressure ($\bar{P}pa$) offers less prognostic value.

Primary lung disease poses a difficulty in gauging prognosis. Broadly speaking, a forced expired volume in one second (FEV$_1$) less than 28 percent predicted and/or a single breath capacity for carbon monoxide (DL$_{CO}$) less than 64 percent have been used (17). In cystic fibrosis, these values correlate with exercise-induced arterial oxygen desaturation. For certain diseases which progress rapidly, e.g., histiocytosis X and sarcoid, we have monitored the decline in function on therapy, accepting the patient when the above levels of FEV$_1$ and DL$_{CO}$ have been achieved. As the prognosis of primary lung disease is greatly affected by the development of secondary pulmonary hypertension (1), clinical signs of such a development are monitored using, among other methods, echocardiograms with Doppler assessment. At present, these patients do not undergo right heart catheterization.

If after the period of evaluation the patient is determined to be a suitable candidate for heart-lung transplantation, a place on the waiting list is offered. Currently, the median waiting period is 10 months, with a range extending from one week to 35 months. Patients wait until a suitable donor is found, matching them in size, ABO blood group and CMV status. At present, the major cause for delay in the United Kingdom is the scarcity of surgical, medical and nursing resources.

From these observations, it is understood that heart-lung transplantation is *not* considered as an emergency treatment for patients who are critically ill, e.g., with respiratory failure requiring continuous assisted ventilation.

Care of the Patient Awaiting Heart-Lung Transplantation

During the early phase of the development of heart-lung transplantation, the average waiting period could be as long as 18 months. As a result, up to 20 percent of our patients on the waiting list died before surgery became available. To overcome this problem, we have initiated palliative treatment of patients in an attempt to improve quality of life and prolong survival.

Conventional treatment has been optimized for patients with Eisenmenger's syndrome and chronic lung disease, including long-term continuous oxygen therapy (19).

Long-Term Intravenous Infusion of Prostacyclin

In primary pulmonary hypertension, we have attempted to optimize vasodilator therapy. Each patient considered for heart-lung transplantation has undergone an acute trial of prostacyclin (PGI$_2$) as a prelude to long-term infusion (23).

The clinical trial of PGI$_2$ is performed during a routine right heart catheterization. After an 8-hr fast, the patient is sedated with diazepam, and a triple lumen floatation catheter is inserted through the internal jugular vein. Under fluoroscopic control, the catheter tip is positioned in the pulmonary artery. Following baseline measurements performed in triplicate at rest, an intravenous infusion of PGI$_2$ is started in a peripheral vein. Dosage is increased at increments of 2 ng/Kg/min every 10 min until either the mean systemic artery pressure ($\bar{P}a$) or pulmonary vascular resistance (PVR) falls by 20 percent. An increase in cardiac output ($\dot{Q}$) of 30 percent without a rise in mean pulmonary artery pressure ($\bar{P}pa$)

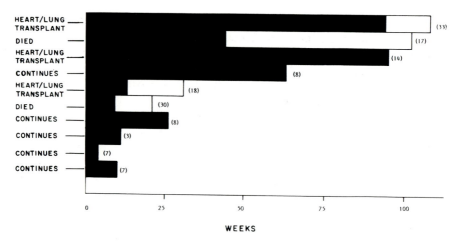

Figure 3: Block diagram showing the duration of treatment of our first 10 patients with pulmonary hypertension treated with a continuous infusion of prostacyclin. The shaded rows represent the length of time PGI_2 infusion effected an increase in exercise tolerance. The dose of PGI_2 in ng/Kg/min is shown together with the outcome of treatment.

and a 20 percent rise in mixed venous oxygen saturation ($S\bar{v}_{O_2}$) are also recorded as useful responses. The PGI_2 infusion is gradually reduced to zero over 15 min, and the patient is returned to the ward after removal of the pulmonary artery catheter and arterial line.

On the ward, the PGI_2 infusion is started again at a dose of 2 ng/Kg/min below the maximal dose achieved during the catheter study. Arterial blood pressure is monitored in a conventional fashion.

The PGI_2 infusion is continued for one week. Improvement of the patient's clinical condition is usually obvious. Objective measurements of an increase in the maximal rate of oxygen consumption ($\dot{V}_{O_2}$) during a progressive exercise test (5) or an increase in the 12-min walking distance are used to decide whether to continue PGI_2 for a prolonged period. Long-term PGI_2 is administered through a subcutaneous tunneled line inserted into the subclavicular vein; the continuous PGI_2 infusion is delivered using an electrical syringe pump.

Patients have continued with this therapy for up to 3 years although the initial improvement usually lasts only 3 to 6 months, after which transplantation is usually required (Fig. 3). Complications have included infected lines and mechanical failures of the infusion system (15). However, this therapeutic approach has afforded patients a reasonable quality of life while awaiting surgery.

THE FUTURE OF TRANSPLANTATION

Current Issues

Several areas remain where further developments and research are needed. Initially, it was believed that with the combined heart-lung operation, rejection could be monitored by endomyocardial biopsy (24). This is an established technique in cardiac transplantation. However, both in vivo (4) and in clinical practice (18), the lungs reject independently from the heart. Indeed, cardiac rejection appears uncommon (13). As a result of reliance on clinical criteria to diagnose rejection in early series of patients, chronic lung rejection in the form of a disabling obliterative bronchiolitis has been common (2).

To overcome this lack of diagnostic precision, we have used transbronchial lung biopsy to repeatedly obtain lung tissue for histology (10,11,26). Indications for biopsy include a fall in forced expired volume in one second (FEV_1) (20). This appears to offer a sensitive guide to rejection and enables the efficacy of treatment with augmented immunosuppression to be monitored (Fig. 4). With this technique and perhaps the use of bronchoalveolar lavage (BAL) to assess lymphocyte reactivity (7), it may be possible to limit the long-term problem of obliterative bronchiolitis.

The survival rate and quality of life following heart-lung transplantation remain unknown. Until the 10-year survival is known, only a cautious extension of the criteria for patient selection will be possible. In the future, it may be decided to accept as candidates for heart-lung transplantation those patients who have a reasonable chance of survival despite living greatly restricted lives.

Heart-lung transplantation remains expensive, at least twice the cost of cardiopulmonary bypass for coronary artery grafting and approximately $2,000

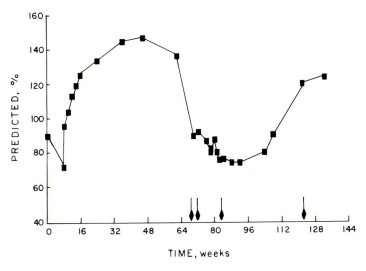

Figure 4: This illustration shows the value of the measurement of forced expired volume in one second (FEV_1) in determining the need for transbronchial lung biopsy in a heart-lung transplant patient. The initial fall in FEV_1 was associated with rejection seen on histology. Biopsy was performed at the point indicated by the arrow. No initial response to "pulsed" 3 days of augmented immunosuppression occurred. Two further biopsies show rejection. However, after the third "pulse," low dose prednisolone was continued for 9 months, FEV_1 returned to normal, and the final biopsy was normal.

more than heart transplantation. As with all expensive procedures, the cost to society through increased medical insurance must be weighed against the potential benefits of heart-lung transplantation. But, if heart-lung transplantation develops in an equivalent manner to the transplantation of other organs, the cost of the procedure will inevitably fall.

REFERENCES

1. Bishop JM, Cross KM: Physiological variables and mortality in patients with various categories of chronic respiratory disease. Bull Eur Physiopathol Respir 20:495–500, 1984.

2. Burke CM, Theodore J, Baldwin JC, Tazelaar HD, Morris AJ, McGregor C, Shumway NE, Robin ED, Jamieson SW: Twenty-eight cases of human heart-lung transplantation. Lancet 1:517–519, 1986.

3. Calne RY, Rolles K, White DJ, Thiru S, Evans DB, McMaster P, Dunn DC, Craddock GN, Henderson RG, Aziz S, Lewis P: Cyclosporin A initially as the only immunosuppressant in 34 recipients of cadaveric organs: 32 kidneys, 2 pancreases, and 2 livers. Lancet 2:1033–1036, 1979.

4. Cooper DK, Novitzky D, Rose AG, Reichart BA: Acute pulmonary rejection precedes cardiac rejection following heart-lung transplantation in a primate model. J Heart Transplant 5:29–31, 1986.

5. D'Alonzo GE, Gianotti L, Dantzker DR: Noninvasive assessment of hemodynamic improvement during chronic vasodilator therapy in obliterative pulmonary hypertension. Am Rev Respir Dis 133:380–384, 1986.

6. Fuster V, Steele PM, Edwards WD, Gersh BJ, McGoon MD, Frye RL: Primary pulmonary hypertension: natural history and importance of thrombosis. Circulation 70:580–587, 1984.

7. Griffith BP, Hardesty RL, Trento A, Paradis IL, Duguesnoy RJ, Zeevi A, Dauber JH, Dummer JS, Thompson ME, Gryzan S, Bahnson HT: Heart-lung transplantation: Lessons learned and future hopes. Ann Thorac Surg 43:6–16, 1987.

8. Hakim M, Higenbottam TW, Bethune D, Cory-Pearce R, English TA, Kneeshaw J, Wells FC, Wallwork J: Selection and procurement of combined heart and lung grafts for transplantation. J Thorac Cardiovasc Surg 95:474–479, 1988.

9. Haverich A, Scott WC, Jamieson SW: Twenty years of lung preservation—A review. J Heart Transplant 4:234–240, 1985.

10. Higenbottam T, Stewart S, Penketh A, Wallwork J: Transbronchial lung biopsy for the diagnosis of rejection in heart-lung transplant patients. Transplantation 46:532–539, 1988.

11. Higenbottam T, Stewart S, Wallwork J: Transbronchial lung biopsy for the diagnosis of rejection and infection of heart-lung transplant patients. Transplant Proc 20:767–769, 1988.

12. Hutter JA, Despins P, Higenbottam TW, Stewart S, Wallwork J: Heart-lung transplantation: better use of resources. Am J Med 85:4–11, 1988.

13. Hutter JA, Higenbottam TW, Stewart S, Wallwork J: Routine endomyocardial biopsy is redundant in heart-lung recipients. J Heart Transplant. In Press.

14. Hutter JA, Scott JP, Wreghitt T, Stewart S, Higenbottam TW, Wallwork J: The importance of cytomegalovirus in heart-lung transplantation recipients. Chest. In Press.

15. Jones DK, Higenbottam TW, Wallwork J: Treatment of primary pulmonary hypertension with intravenous epoprosterol (prostacyclin). Br Heart J 57:270–278, 1987.

16. Jones DK, Higenbottam TW, Wallwork J: Successful heart-lung transplantation for cystic fibrosis. Chest 93:644–645, 1988.

17. Lebecque P, Lapierre JG, Lamarre A, Coates AL: Diffusion capacity and oxygen desaturation effects on exercise in patients with cystic fibrosis. Chest 91:693–697, 1987.

18. McGregor CG, Baldwin JC, Jamieson SW, Billingham ME, Yousem SA, Burke CM, Oyer PE, Stinson EB, Shumway NE: Isolated pulmonary rejection after combined heart-lung transplantation. J Thorac Cardiovasc Surg 90:623–636, 1985.

19. Nocturnal Oxygen Therapy Trial Group. Continuous or nocturnal oxygen therapy in hypoxemic chronic obstructive lung disease: a clinical trial. Ann Intern Med 93:391–398, 1980.

20. Otulana BA, Higenbottam TW, Hutter J, Wallwork J: Close monitoring of lung function in heart-lung transplants allow detection of pulmonary infection and rejection (Abstract). Am Rev Respir Dis 137:P245, 1988.

21. Penketh AR, Higenbottam TW, Hakim M, Wallwork J: Heart and lung transplantation in patients with end stage lung disease. Br Med J 295:311–314, 1987.

22. Read DJ: A clinical method for assessing the

ventilatory response to carbon dioxide. Australas Ann Med 16:20–32, 1967.

23. Reeves JT, Groves BM, Turkevich D: The case for treatment of selected patients with primary pulmonary hypertension. Am Rev Respir Dis 134: 342–346, 1986.

24. Reitz BA, Burton NA, Jamieson SW, Bieber CP, Pennock JL, Stinson EB, Shumway NE: Heart and lung transplantation. Autotransplantation and allo-transplantation in primates with extended survival. J Thorac Cardiovasc Surg 80:360–371, 1980.

25. Scott JP, Higenbottam TW, Hutter J, Hodson M, Stewart S, Penketh AR, Wallwork J: Heart-lung transplantation for cystic fibrosis. Lancet 2:192–194, 1988.

26. Stewart S, Higenbottam TW, Hutter JA, Pen-keth ARL, Zebro TJ, Wallwork J: Histopathology of transbronchial biopsies in heart-lung transplantation. Transplant Proc 20:764–766, 1988.

27. Toronto Lung Transplant Group. Unilateral lung transplantation for pulmonary fibrosis. N Engl J Med 314:1140–1145, 1986.

28. Veith FJ: Lung transplantation. Surg Clin North Am 58:357–364, 1978.

29. Wallwork J, Jones K, Cavarocchi N, Hakim SM, Higenbottam TW: Distant procurement of organs for clinical heart-lung transplantation using a single flush technique. Transplantation 44:654–658, 1987.

30. Wallwork J, Williams R, Calne RY: Transplantation of liver, heart, and lungs for primary biliary cirrhosis and primary pulmonary hypertension. Lancet 2:182–185, 1987.

CONTRIBUTORS

Steven M. Albelda, M.D.
Assistant Professor of Medicine, Cardiovascular-Pulmonary Division,
Department of Medicine, University of Pennsylvania School of Medicine;
Associate Scientist, Wistar Institute, Philadelphia, Pennsylvania

William E. Benitz, M.D.
Assistant Professor of Pediatrics, Division of Neonatal and Developmental
Medicine, Department of Pediatrics, Stanford University School of Medicine,
Stanford, California

Edward H. Bergofsky, M.D.
Head, Pulmonary-Critical Care Division, Department of Medicine, State
University of New York at Stony Brook, Stony Brook, New York

Kenneth L. Brigham, M.D.
The Joe and Morris Werthan Professor of Investigative Medicine, Director,
Center for Lung Research and Division of Pulmonary Medicine, Vanderbilt
University School of Medicine, Nashville, Tennessee

D. Leslie Brown, Ph.D.
Clinical Research Division, Wellcome Research Laboratories, Research Triangle
Park, North Carolina; Department of Pediatrics, University of North Carolina
at Chapel Hill, Chapel Hill, North Carolina

Bruce H. Brundage, M.D.
Professor of Medicine, Chief, Section of Cardiology, Department of Medicine,
University of Illinois at Chicago, Chicago, Illinois

Sidney Cassin, Ph.D.
Department of Physiology, College of Medicine, University of Florida,
Gainesville, Florida

Janice T. Coflesky, Ph.D.
Research Associate, Department of Physiology and Biophysics, College of
Medicine, University of Vermont, Burlington, Vermont

Marc Cohen, M.D.
Assistant Professor of Medicine, Division of Cardiology, Department of
Medicine, The Mount Sinai Medical Center, New York, New York

Isabel Coma-Canella, M.D.
Coronary Care Unit, Hospital La Paz, Madrid, Spain

David R. Dantzker, M.D.
Professor of Medicine, Director, Pulmonary Division, Department of Internal
Medicine, University of Texas Health Science Center, Houston, Texas

Christopher A. Dawson, Ph.D.
Professor of Physiology, Department of Physiology, Medical College of
Wisconsin; Research Service, Clement J. Zablocki VA Medical Center,
Milwaukee, Wisconsin

William D. Edwards, M.D.
Consultant, Division of Pathology, Mayo Clinic and Mayo Foundation; Associate
Professor of Pathology, Mayo Medical School, Rochester, Minnesota

C. Gregory Elliott, M.D.
Associate Profesor of Medicine, University of Utah School of Medicine; Medical
Director, Respiratory Care, LDS Hospital, Salt Lake City, Utah

John N. Evans, Ph.D.,
Associate Professor, Department of Physiology and Biophysics, College of
Medicine, University of Vermont, Burlington, Vermont

Anthony P. Farrell, Ph.D.
Associate Professor, Department of Biological Sciences, Simon Fraser
University, Burnaby, British Columbia, Canada

Jeffrey D. Fisher, M.D.
Clinical Associate Professor of Medicine, Division of Cardiology, New York
Hospital—Cornell University Medical Center, New York, New York

Alfred P. Fishman, M.D.
William Maul Measey Professor of Medicine, Director, Cardiovascular-
Pulmonary Division, Hospital of the University of Pennsylvania, Philadelphia,
Pennsylvania

Bruce A. Freeman, Ph.D.
Associate Professor of Anesthesiology and Biochemistry, Departments of
Anesthesiology and Biochemistry, University of Alabama at Birmingham,
Birmingham, Alabama

Valentin Fuster, M.D.
Arthur M. & Hilda A. Master Professor of Medicine, Chief, Division of
Cardiology, Department of Medicine, The Mount Sinai Medical Center, New
York, New York

Joan Gil, M.D.
Professor of Pathology, Department of Pathology, Mount Sinai School of
Medicine, New York, New York

Miguel A. Gomez Sanchez, M.D.
Cardiology Service, Hospital Primero de Octubre, Madrid, Spain

Robert F. Grover, M.D., Ph.D.
Professor Emeritus of Medicine, Cardiovascular-Pulmonary Research
Laboratory, University of Colorado Health Sciences Center, Denver, Colorado

Bertron M. Groves, M.D.
Associate Professor of Medicine, Director, Cardiac Catheterization Laboratory,
University of Colorado Health Sciences Center, Denver, Colorado

Hans Peter Gurtner, M.D.
Professor of Medicine, Head, Section of Cardiology, Department of Internal
Medicine, University of Bern School of Medicine, Inselspital, Bern, Switzerland

Katherine A. Hajjar, M.D.
Assistant Professor of Pediatrics and Medicine, Cornell University Medical
College, New York, New York

Michael A. Heymann, M.D.
Professor of Pediatrics and Obstetrics, Gynecology, and Reproductive Sciences,
Senior Staff Member, Cardiovascular Research Institute, University of
California, San Francisco, San Francisco, California

Tim W. Higenbottam, M.D.
Director, Respiratory Physiology Department, Papworth Hospital, Cambridge,
England

Alice R. Johnson, Ph.D.
Department of Biochemistry, University of Texas Health Center at Tyler,
Tyler, Texas

María José Mestre de Juan, M.D.
Department of Anatomic Pathology, Hospital Primero de Octubre, Madrid,
Spain

Janet Kernis, M.P.H.
Research Specialist, Epidemiology and Biometry Program, School of Public
Health, University of Illinois at Chicago, Chicago, Illinois

Spencer K. Koerner, M.D.
Professor of Medicine, Director, Division of Pulmonary Medicine, Cedars-Sinai
Medical Center, Los Angeles, California

Michael I. Kotlikoff, V.M.D., Ph.D.
Assistant Professor of Pharmacology, Department of Animal Biology, School of

Veterinary Medicine, Cardiovascular-Pulmonary Division, University of Pennsylvania School of Medicine, Philadelphia, Pennsylvania

Paul S. Levy, Sc.D.
Professor and Director, Epidemiology and Biometry Program, School of Public Health, University of Illinois at Chicago, Chicago, Illinois

Susan L. Lindsay, M.B.B.S
Visiting Professor of Anesthesiology, Departments of Anesthesiology and Biochemistry, University of Alabama at Birmingham, Birmingham, Alabama

John H. Linehan, Ph.D.
Professor of Physiology, Department of Mechanical Engineering, Marquette University, Milwaukee, Wisconsin

Walker A. Long, M.D.
Senior Clinical Research Scientist, Clinical Research Division, Wellcome Research Laboratories, Research Triangle Park, North Carolina; Department of Pediatrics, University of North Carolina at Chapel Hill, Chapel Hill, North Carolina

Jose López-Sendón, M.D.
Coronary Care Unit, Hospital La Paz, Madrid, Spain

James E. Loyd, M.D.
Assistant Professor of Medicine, Vanderbilt Center for Lung Research, Department of Medicine, Vanderbilt University School of Medicine, Nashville, Tennessee

Michael Magno, Ph.D.
Assistant Professor, Department of Physiology and Biophysics, Hahnemann University, Philadelphia, Pennsylvania

Kenneth M. Moser, M.D.
Professor of Medicine, Director, Pulmonary and Critical Care Medicine, University of California, San Diego School of Medicine, UCSD Medical Center, San Diego, California

Ralph L. Nachman, M.D.
Professor of Medicine, Chief, Division of Hematology-Oncology, Cornell University Medical College, New York, New York

John H. Newman, M.D.
Associate Professor of Medicine, Vanderbilt Center for Lung Research, Department of Medicine, Vanderbilt University School of Medicine, Nashville, Tennessee

Harold I. Palevsky, M.D.
Assistant Professor of Medicine, Cardiovascular-Pulmonary Division, Hospital of the University of Pennsylvania, Philadelphia, Pennsylvania

Andrew J. Peacock, M.D.
Visiting Research Scholar, from the University of Southampton, Southampton, United Kingdom

Robert H. Peter, M.D.
Professor of Medicine, Department of Medicine, Duke University Medical Center, Durham, North Carolina

Giuseppe G. Pietra, M.D.
Professor of Pathology, Department of Pathology and Laboratory Medicine, Hospital of the University of Pennsylvania, Philadelphia, Pennsylvania

Daniel A. Pietro, M.D.
Assistant Professor of Medicine, VA Medical Center, West Roxbury, Massachusetts

John T. Reeves, M.D.
Professor of Medicine, Cardiovascular Pulmonary Research Laboratory, Division of Cardiology, University of Colorado School of Medicine, Denver, Colorado

Lynne M. Reid, M.D.
S. Burt Wolbach Professor of Pathology, Harvard Medical School; Pathologist-in-Chief, The Children's Hospital, Boston, Massachusetts

Stuart Rich, M.D.
Associate Professor of Medicine, Associate Chief, Section of Cardiology, Department of Medicine, University of Illinois College of Medicine at Chicago, Chicago, Illinois

Sharon I.S. Rounds, M.D.
Associate Professor of Medicine, Department of Medicine, Brown University; VA Medical Center, Providence, Rhode Island

Lewis J. Rubin, M.D.
Head, Pulmonary Division, Associate Professor of Medicine and Physiology, University of Maryland School of Medicine, Baltimore, Maryland

Una S. Ryan, Ph.D.
Professor of Medicine, Department of Medicine, University of Miami School of Medicine, Miami, Florida

Scott J. Soifer, M.D.
Associate Professor of Pediatrics, Associate Staff Member, Cardiovascular Research Institute, University of California, San Francisco, San Francisco, California

Andrew P. Somlyo, M.D.
Director, Pennsylvania Muscle Institute, Professor of Physiology and Pathology, University of Pennsylvania School of Medicine, Philadelphia, Pennsylvania

Avril V. Somlyo, Ph.D.
Research Professor of Physiology, University of Pennsylvania, School of Medicine, Philadelphia, Pennsylvania

Kurt R. Stenmark, M.D.
Assistant Professor of Pediatrics, University of Colorado School of Medicine, Denver, Colorado

Dragoslava Vesselinovitch, M.S., D.V.M.
Research Associate (Professor of Pathology), Department of Pathology, University of Chicago, Chicago, Illinois

Carol E. Vreim, Ph.D.
Associate Director, Division of Lung Diseases, National Heart, Lung and Blood Institute, National Institutes of Health, Bethesda, Maryland

C.A. Wagenvoort, M.D.
Emeritus Professor of Pathology, University of Amsterdam; Honorary Consultant Pathologist, Erasmus University; Department of Pathology, Erasmus University Rotterdam, Rotterdam, The Netherlands

E. Kenneth Weir, M.D.
Professor of Medicine, University of Minnesota; Department of Medicine, Minneapolis VA Medical Center, Minneapolis, Minnesota

Robert W. Wissler, M.D., Ph.D.
Distinguished Service Professor, Program Director, Multicenter Cooperative Study of the Pathobiological Determinants of Atherosclerosis in Youth, Department of Pathology, University of Chicago, Chicago, Illinois

INDEX

Acetylcholine
  endothelium, vasoactive effects on, 75–76, 226
  and fetal pulmonary vascular resistance, 162,
      165, 376
  lungfish, vasoactive effects in, 23
  in muscle relaxation, 58–59, 60
  and neonatal pulmonary vascular resistance, 318
  and pulmonary vascular tone, 111, 112
  in vasodilator therapy, 487–89, 494
  and vessel wall metabolism, 64
Acidemia, 372, 381
Acidosis, 113–15, 336–37, 378
  lactic, 361
Acinus, 264
Actin filaments, 35–37, 179
Actin phenotypes, 65–66
Adenine nucleotides, 70, 226
Adenosine, 104
Adenosine diphosphate (ADP), 70
Adenosine monophosphate (AMP), 70, 183
Adenosine triphosphate (ATP)
  and endothelial cell prostaglandin production, 120
  lung metabolism of, 70
  in smooth muscle contraction, 37, 75
Adenosine triphosphatease (ATPase)
  myosin, 35–37
  sites of activity, 71
Adrenaline, 321
Adrenergic innervation
  and hypoxic pressor response, 125, 321
  species differences, 133–34, 321
Adult respiratory distress syndrome (ARDS)
  endothelial cell in, 80
  endothelial injury in, 173
  oxygen radicals and, 227
  oxygen therapy, 482
  pulmonary vascular permeability in, 100
Adventitia
  calf, illus. 317
  cells
    DNA synthesis in hyperoxia, 65
    elastin production, 176

collagen in, 273
  damage to, 268, 463–64
  fibroblasts, 261
    damage from hyperoxia, 273–74
    damage from hypoxia, illus. 267, 268
    hyperplasia in, 264, 265
    protein synthesis, 318
  hypoxia and, 124, 316
  lesions, in, 459–60
  neonatal, 316, 379
Afferent stimulation, 135
Age
  of primary pulmonary hypertension registry
      patients, 452, 468
  and pulmonary veno-occlusive disease, 344
Agenesis, pulmonary artery, 425
Agonists, endothelial cells and, 75–78
Air-breathing fishes
  hemodynamics, 22, 23, 27, 28
  pulmonary circulation, 17, 18, illus. 19
Air-breathing organ (ABO), 17, illus. 19
  blood flow to, 18, 22, 23, 28
Airway smooth muscle, 155
Airways obstruction, 454–55
Albumin
  clearance of, illus. 178, illus. 181
  endothelial permeability to, 177
  endothelium-derived relaxing factor and, 122
  in vascular perfusion, 513
Alcohol abuse, 364
Alkaline phosphatase, 363
Alkalosis, 114–15, 454, 455
Allograft rejection, 462
Alpha₁-antiproteinase deficiency, 311
Alpha blockade, 135
Alpha receptors, 135
Altitude
  chronic mountain sickness, 296–97
  and chronic pulmonary hypertension, 124–25,
      265, 283–98
  and familial pulmonary hypertension, 310–11
  and hypoxic pressor response, 113–14

Altitude (*continued*)
  and initial tone, 111
  and postnatal hypoxia, 315–18
  and primary pulmonary hypertension registry patients, 449
  and right ventricular hypertrophy, 319, 324
Alveolar-arterial oxygen difference, 513
Alveolar capillaries
  damaged, *illus.* 103, *illus.* 340
  normal function of, 3, 9
  and wedge pressure, 42
Alveolar edema, *illus.* 340
Alveolar hyperventilation, 400
Alveolar hypoventilation, 124, 295, 399–400
Alveolar hypoxia
  and capillary pressure, 99
  causes of, 335
  and oxygen saturation, *illus.* 113
  and pulmonary pressor response, 112
  and pulmonary vasoconstriction, 95, 96, 98, 140, 158
    attenuation of, 157–58
    species differences, 133, 310
  and vascular lesions, 336–37
Alveolar wall
  blood supply to, 261, 264
  gas exchange in, 3
hexagonal network of, 5–8
  normal function of, 9–13
  thinning of, 275
Alveoli
  air pressure in, 9, 12–14
  development of, 373–74
  distension of, and vascular resistance, 378
  ducts, 266
  epithelial cell, 274
  interstitium, 8
  macrophages, 102, *illus.* 465
  monocrotaline damage to, 321
  oxygen tension (PA_{O_2}), 46, 47, 49, 319
    and hypoxia, 112, 283, 287
    pulmonary vascular bed, effects on, 273
  resistance, 113
  ventilation, 162, 293, 481
Alveolitis, cryptogenic fibrosing, 515
Amines, 70, 378. *See also* Norepinephrine
Amino acid, 223
Aminorex, 334, 336, 361, 385, 437, 441–42
  pulmonary hypertension, 397–409
Amphibians, 18, 25, 27
  anuran, 17, *illus.* 19
  larvae, *illus.* 19, 24–25, 27
Amplification, endothelial, 80
Anaphylatoxin metabolism, 72
Anaphylaxis, 121
Anastamosis, 511–12
Anesthesia, 114, 115
Aneurysmal dilations, *illus.* 424
Angina, 516

Angiogenesis, 206, 209
Angiogram
  embolic occlusion, *illus.* 415, *illus.* 422
  thrombus, *illus.* 423, *illus.* 424, *illus.* 432
Angiography, 413, 425, 426
  in primary pulmonary hypertension registry, 445, 447–48, 449, 456, 502
Angiomatoid lesions, 277–78, 404, 416
Angioscopy, 425–26
Angiotensin, 96–97
Angiotensin I
  conversion to angiotensin II, 70–72, 104
Angiotensin II
  conversion from angiotensin I, 70–72, 104
  stimulation of platelet-activating factor production, 378
  stimulation of prostaglandin production, 124, 377
  vascular reactivity to, 60
  as vasoconstrictor, 95, 209
Angiotensin converting enzyme (ACE), 70–72, 75, 104, 174–75, 321
Aniline, 387
Animal models, 315–25
ANOVA, 355
Anoxia, *See* Hypoxia
Antibiotics, 219, 372
Antibodies
  antinuclear (ANA), 448, 454
    serologies, 357, 358
  bradykinin, 157
Anticoagulant therapy, 485, 497, 504–6
  in aminorex hypertension, 408
  in pulmonary veno-occlusive disease, 344
  in thromboembolic hypertension, 415, 426
Anticoagulation. *See also* Heparin
  endothelial cell mechanisms, 231–34
Antigen-antibody reaction, 178
Antineoplastic agents, 219
Antinuclear antibodies (ANA), 448, 454
  in cirrhosis with pulmonary hypertension, 363
  serologies, 357, 358
Antioxidants, 217, 223
Antiplasmin, 507–8
Antithrombin, 191
Antithrombin III
  deficiency, 311, 414–415
  heparin mediation, 188, 189, 199, 232
ANTU (α-naphthylthiourea), 60, 75
Aorta
  blood pressure, 137, 153
  chemoreceptors in, 140–41
  smooth muscle in, 31
Aortic atherosclerosis, 252
Aortic stenosis, 427
Apnea
  in intermittent air breathers, 17, 18, 20–22, 26, 29
  nervous system and, 136, 137
Appetite suppressants, 402, 466–67. *See also* Aminorex

Arachidonic acid. *See also* Leukotrienes; Prosta-
    glandins; Thromboxanes
  cyclooxygenase, reaction with, 224
  endothelial cell release of, 175, 180
  and leukotriene synthesis, 225
  lipoxygenase products of, 97, 100
  metabolites of, 60–64,67, 183, 222, 378
    and cell proliferation, 209
    and hypoxic pressor response, 121
  platelet-derived growth factor and, 203
  and prostaglandin generation, 72, 116, 162, 174
  and pulmonary vascular resistance increase, 165,
    166
  sites of action of inhibitors, *illus.* 168
  in toxic oil syndrome, 388
Arrhythmias, 427
Arterial hypocapnia, 400
Arterial hypoxemia, 360, 400, 427, 454, 455
Arterial hypoxia, 248
Arterialization of veins, 345, *illus.* 347, 349, 465
Arteries, 4. *See also* Pulmonary arteries
  blood gas, 419
  blood pressure, perinatal, 374–76
  bronchial, 261, 337, 418
  carbon dioxide pressure, 162, 164, 324, 406, 474
  compliance, 51, 53, 57
  dilation of, *illus.* 328, 329, 330
  injury to, 190, *illus.* 266
  intima, 198, 463
  media, 198, 463
  mural thrombosis in, 248
  muscularization of in persistent pulmonary hy-
    pertension of the newborn, 373–74, 379
  neonatal, 278–79
  oxygen pressure, 162, 372, 516
    exercise and, 419
    in toxic oil syndrome, 392
  oxygen saturation, 293, 296, 503
  pH, 162, 164
  pulmocutaneous, 25
  recanalization of, 345
  renal, 319
  resistance, 263–64, 479
  wall tension, 248
  wedge pressure, 42–45
Arteriography, bronchial, 426
Arterioles, *illus.* 4, 6
  calf, *illus.* 317
  hypoxia and, 113
  intra-acinar, 460
  muscular pulmonary, 460
  pulmonary, muscularization of
    in plexogenic pulmonary arteriopathy, 333, 336
    in primary pulmonary hypertension, *illus.* 460,
      480
    in seconary pulmonary hypertension, *illus.*
      328, 329
Arteriovenous shortcuts, 11–13
Arteritis, *illus.* 335, 336, 345, 463

histopathological features, 466
  primary pulmonary, 459, 467
  in primary pulmonary hypertension, 505, 507
Ascites, 324, 496
Asphyxia, 381
Aspiration, blood, 372
Aspirin, 224–25, 379
Atelectasis, 514
Atherogenesis
  endothelial cells and, 64
  in the pulmonary artery, 245–54
Atheromas, 187, *illus.* 330
Atherosclerosis, 222, 331
  aortic, 252
  blood flow and, 253
  emphysema and, 252, 253–54
Atrial septal defect, 54, 334, 427
Atropine
  and acetylcholine response, 59
  and bronchial vascular resistance, 154, 155
  injections of, 22, 25
  and pulmonary arterial pressure, 142
  vasodilation, effect on, 135
Autocrine secretion, 211, 235, 238
Autoimmune disease, 245
Autonomic nervous system
  and fetal vascular tone, 164–65
  and pulmonary circulation, 134–35
  and pulmonary hypertension, 321
  and pulmonary vascular resistance, 109, 111
Autooxidation, 220
Autopsy, 307
Azathioprine, 344
Azotemia, 355

Back perfusion, 426
Bacteria, 79, 95, 221
Baroreceptor influences, 136
Basic fibroblast growth factor (bFGF), 271
Beta blockade, 133, 135
Beta receptors, 135
Bilirubin, 363
Bimodal air breathers, 17, 28
Biopsy
  bronchial, 446
  endomyocardial, 518–19
  lung, 341, 344, 427
    and heart-lung transplantation, 516, 519
    in primary pulmonary hypertension registry,
      446, 447, 448, 449, 470–71
Blood. *See also* Coagulation; Erythrocytes;
    Leukocytes
  aspiration, 372
  cholesterol, 249
  clotting factors, 231
  gas, arterial, 419
  in heart-lung transplantation, 513
  lipid, 245
  pH, 73, 114, 162

Blood (*continued*)
pressure
lungs and, 72
perinatal arterial, 374–76
quality, lungs and, 69
transfusion, 381
viscosity
hematocrit concentration and, 46, 381
hypoxia and, 289
and mechanical energy balance, 45, 46
and resistance, 297, 376, 380
Blood flow
and atherosclerosis, 253
bronchial, 153, 512
capillary, 14, 28–29
central nervous system and, 132, 144
distribution in lungs, 96–98
exercise and, 288–89
fetal, 371, 374, 375–76
in fishes, 23
hematocrit concentration and, 297, 375
injury, 260, 276
in intermittent air breathers, 18–23, 25–28
and mechanical energy balance, 45–47
neonatal, 162, 377, 378, 379–80
oscillatory pressure-flow relations, 52–54
parenchymal, 419
in perfusion, 23, 376, 513
perinatal, 161
and resistance, 92
in toads, *illus.* 21
vascular pressure-flow curve, 47–51
velocity, 14, 54
Blood pressure. *See* Pulmonary arterial blood
pressure
Bone, 207
marrow transplantation, 514
Bradycardia
chemoreceptor influences, 140–41
cholinergic mediation of, 22, 27, 28
in crocodiles, 26
Bradykinin
activation of ionic currents, 78
antibodies, 157
and endothelial membrane, 179, 180
endothelial metabolism of, 70–72, 75, 104
and endothelial prostacyclin formation, 175, 180
and fetal pulmonary vascular resistance, 162,
165, 376, 377, 378
and initial tone, 111
receptors, 77
and vascular relaxation, 226
Brain. *See also* Central nervous system
hypoxia of, 140
microcirculation, 233
pulmonary circulation regulation, 133, 142–45
Branch stenosis, 425
Brisket disease, 310
Bronchi, compression of, 330

Bronchial biopsy, 446
Bronchial circulation, 3, 4, 116, 151–58
arteries, 261, 337, 418
arteriography, 426
blood flow, 153, 512
vascular resistance, 153 *illus.* 154, 157
vasoconstriction, 155, 157—58, 226
vasodilation, 155, 156–57, 158
veins, 337, 345
Bronchiolitis, obliterative, 519
Bronchitis, chronic, 336
Bronchoalveolar fluid, 121–23, 519
Bronchopulmonary dysplasia, 323
Bullfrog, 20
Burroughs Wellcome Co., xiv

Cachectin, 208
Calcium
Ca^{2+}
activation of smooth muscle contraction, 31,
32–37, 118, 119
in endothelial signal transduction, 77–78, 79
intracellular, 123
^{45}Ca, 78
extracellular, 87
and hypoxic pressor response, 116, 118
ionophore, 64, 75, 77–78
Calcium channel blockers
in vasodilator therapy, 448, 482, 497
Caldesmon, 35–37
Calmodulin, 35
Calves, newborn, 315–18
Capillaries
alveolar
damaged, *illus.* 103, *illus.* 340
normal function of, 3, 9
and wedge pressure, 42
blood flow in, 28–29
endothelial cells, 206
permeability, 100–101, 122–23
pre- and postcapillary segments, 261
pulmonary, 3, 5–8
pressure, 42, 44, 99–100, 390
in pulmonary veno-occlusive disease, *illus.* 465
recruitment and derecruitment of, 9
rabbit, *illus.* 10, *illus.* 12
Capillary hemangiomatosis, 466, 469
Captopril, 492, 493, 495
Carbachol, 35
Carbon dioxide
in chronic obstructive airways disease, 295, 296,
298
end-tidal concentration, 137, 139–140
pressure, arterial, 162, 164, 324, 406, 474
pulmonary pressor response, 114, 115
Carbonic anhydrase, 71, 73
Carbon monoxide, 419
Carboxypeptidase N (CPN), 71, 72
Carcinoid syndrome, 362–63

Cardiac catheterization, 444–45, 448, 449, ^56, 491
Cardiac index, 367, 487, 502, 516
Cardiac output, (Q̇). *See also* Blood flow
   altitude and, 287–88, 295
   brain regulation of, 146
   fetal, 374, 375
   in hepatic cirrhosis, 367–68
   and impedance plethysmography tests, 420–21
   and lung injury, 260
   neural stimulation and, 139, 140, 141, 142, 143, 144
   in primary pulmonary hypertension registry patients, 453, 455
   and pulmonary circulation, 57, 104, 222
   and pulmonary vascular resistance, 41–42, 51
   surgery and, 429
   vasodilator therapy, response to, 480–81, 493, 517–18
Cardiac shunts, congenital, 334–36, 341
Cardiomegaly, 373, 502
Cardioplegia, 427
Cardiopulmonary bypass, 413, 421, 514, 519
Carotid body
   baroreceptors, 136
   and bronchial circulation, 155
   chemoreceptors, 140–42, 153–54, 156, 158
   and ventilation, 115
Carrageenan, 323
Cats, 4, 133, 142
Cattle, 113, 293, 310
Cells. *See also* Endothelial cells; Smooth muscle cells
   adventitial
      DNA synthesis in hyperoxia, 65
      elastin production, 176
   hyperplasia, 65
   hypertrophy, 65
   immunocompetent, 80
   injury to, 259–60
   lysis, 176, 181, 221, 223
   mesenchymal, 209
   metabolism of, 120, 123,
   mutation of, 223
   myeloid, 203
   pH of, 203
   proliferation, 201
      endothelial cell mediation of, 64–65
      inhibition of, 208
      polypeptide growth factors and, 202, 205–6, 207, 210
      hypoxia and, 320
   replication of, 179
   sustenacular, 116
Central nervous system regulation of primary circulation, 131–46
C-fos protooncogene, 80
cGMP. *See* Cyclic guanosine 3′5′-monophosphate
Chemodenervation, 141
Chemoreceptors
   aortic, 140–41

carotid body, 140–42, 153–54, 156, 158
   laryngeal, 138–39
   systemic arterial, 153–54, 157–58
Chemotherapy, 350
Chest pain, 400, 453, 502
Chickens, 324
Cholesterol
   blood, 249
   catabolism, 254
   esters, 246
   hypercholesterolemia, 248, 249, 254
Cholinergic inhibition, 28
Cholinergic innervation, 133–34
Cholinergic vasoconstriction, 24, 28
Chondrocytes, 206
Chondroitinase, 195, 197
Chondroitin proteoglycan, 198
Chondroitin sulfate, 192
^{51}Chromium release, 179, 180–81, 182, 183
Chronic bronchitis, 336
Chronic hypoxic ventilation, 480
Chronic lung disease, 517
Chronic mountain sickness, 124, 296–97, 310, 311
Chronic obstructive airways disease, 283, 295, 296
   and pulmonary hypertension, 297, 479, 481
Chronic pulmonary hypertension. *See also* Secondary pulmonary hypertension
   animal models, 315–25
   of vascular origin (CPHVO), 397–99
Cirrhosis, hepatic
   and hypoxic pressor response, 114
   with pulmonary hyptertension, 353, 359–68, 385, 398, 438
Closing pressures, 49–51
Clubbing, 360, 453
Coagulation
   clotting factors, 231
   disorders, 311
   endothelial cell modulation of, 231–34, 237–40
   endothelial damage and, 350–51
   procoagulant molecules, 176
   thrombin and, 209, 211
Collagen diseases, 353–58, 398, 438, 446–47
Collagen production
   adventitial fibroblast, 265, 273
   in chronic pulmonary hypertension, 124, 318, 320
   platelet-derived growth factor stimulation of, 206
   smooth muscle cell, in atherogenesis, 246
Colony stimulating factors, 80, 203
Communication, vascular cell, 175, 179
Compensation, primary pulmonary hypertension registry, 449
Compliance, arterial, 51, 53, 57
Computed axial tomography (CAT), 426
Computer database, 437–38
Computer programs, 79
Concentric intimal fibroelastosis (CIF), laminar, 307
   lesions, 309

Concentric laminar intimal fibrosis
  histopathological features, 466, 467, 469
  lesions, *illus.* 334–35, 336, 461, 462, 466
C1q, 79
Congenital cardiac shunts, 334–36, 341
Congenital heart defects, 303, 466–67
Congenital heart disease, 245, 444. *See also* Eisen-
    menger's syndrome
  cyanotic, 508–9
  and heart-lung transplantation, 515
  lesions, 260, 462
  nervous system and, 145
  open lung biopsy in, 341
  and persistent pulmonary hypertension of the
    newborn, 372
  and vascular remodeling, 264
Congestive pulmonary vasculopathy, 338
Contraceptives, oral, 385, 453
Contractile cell, 261, 263
Contraction, smooth muscle, 31–37
Cooperativity, 37
Copper
  Cu^{2+}, in Fenton reaction, 218
  metabolism, 311
Corner capillaries, 11–13
Coronary angiography, 426
Coronary artery
  atherosclerosis, 249, 252
  bypass, 427
Coronary sinus, *illus.* 331, 333
Cor pulmonale, 283
  chronic, 145
  chronic obstructive airways disease and, 296, 479
  and primary pulmonary hypertension, 438
  in scleroderma, 353
Corticosteroids, 209, 511
Cough, 9–11, 418
Coumadin, 421, 428, 504
Crinopexy, 211
Crocodiles, 18, 25–27
Crossbridge cycling, 32, 37
Cryptogenic fibrosing alveolitis, 515
C3 receptors, 176
Cyanosis, 344, 371, 400
Cyanotic congenital heart disease, 508–9
Cyclic guanosine 3′5′-monophosphate (cGMP)
  endothelium and, 58, 59, 122
  oxygen radicals and, 120
Cyclooxygenase
  inhibition, 222, 224–25
    and cytotoxicity, 183
    and pulmonary vascular resistance, 92–96,
      97–98
  inhibitors
    and bronchial vasodilation, 152, 155
    and ductus arteriosus, 319
  and oxygen radicals, 226
  pathways, 121, 167, 168
  reaction with arachidonate, 224

Cyclosporine, 511, 512
Cystic fibrosis, 146, 311, 323, 515
Cytochrome P_{450}, 119
Cytokines, 80, 104, 173, 183, 208–9, 211
Cytolysis, 176, 181, 221, 223
Cytomegalovirus pneumonitis, 514
Cytosolic effects of oxygen, 224
Cytotoxicity, 179–83, 218, 223

Data requirements, 437–38, 444–45
Debrisoquine, 403
Demographics, of primary pulmonary hypertension
    registry, 452–53, 468
Dermatan sulfate, 192
Desmin, 66
Dexamethasone, 323
Dextran sulfate, 190–91, 192
Diabetes, 245, 247, 361
Diabetes mellitus, 228, 516
Diacylglycerol (DAG), 32, 77, 204, 205
Diagnosis, primary pulmonary hypertension,
    447–48, 465–67, 470–71
Diazepam, 517
Diazoxide, 487, 492, 495
Dibenamine, 165
Dietary pulmonary hypertension, 361, 385, 394, 409
Dietary pulmonary vasculopathy, 337–38
Di-homo-gamma-linolenic acid, 165
Diisopropylfluorophosphate (DFP), 237
Dilation. *See* Vasodilation
Dilation (dilatation) lesions, *illus.* 276, 464
  in aminorex hypertension, 404
  pulmonary arterial, *illus.* 335, 336, 464
Diltiazem, 494–95, 497
Disease
  and bronchial circulation, 151
  and hypoxic pressor response, 114
Dismutation, 218
Distensible vessels, 50–51
DNA
  oxygen radicals and, 223, 224
  synthesis, 65, 203
Dogs, 113, 133, 136, 142, 152, 506
Dopamine, 23, 70
Down's syndrome, 334
Drug abuse, 353, 446–47
Drugs
  endothelial metabolism of, 73–75
  hydroxylation of, 403–4
Ductus arteriosus
  in amphibian larvae, 24–25
  closing of, 279–80, 375
  constriction of, 379
  in fetus, 161, 315, 374
  hypoxia and, 116, *illus.* 117
  pressure and, 319
  shunts through, 316, 334, 372
Ductus Botalli, 23
Dysplasia, bronchopulmonary, 323

Dyspnea
    in aminorex pulmonary hypertension, 400
    in cirrhosis with pulmonary hypertension, 362
    in collagen vascular disease, 355
    in primary pulmonary hypertension, 453, 455, 502
    in pulmonary hypertension with hepatic cirrhosis, 364
    in pulmonary veno-occlusive disease, 338, 344
    in thromboembolic pulmonary hypertension, 417–18, 421

Eccentric intimal fibrosis (EIF), 307, *illus.* 332, 337, 338, *illus.* 339, *illus.* 340, 466, 467
    lesions, 309, 461–62, 469
Echocardiography, 419
Ectonucleotidases, 70
Edema. *See also* Pulmonary edema
    alveolar, *illus.* 340
    in cirrhosis with pulmonary hypertension, 362
    endothelial cell, 264
    hyperoxia and, 273
    interstitial, 344, 345, 348, 349
    leg, 453
    in primary pulmonary hypertension, 455
Eicosanoids. *See also* Leukotrienes; Prostaglandins; Thromboxanes
    arachidonic acid and, 224
    perinatal pulmonary circulation, effects on, 165–68
    synthesis of, 183, 226
Eicosapentanoic acid, 167
Eicosatetraenoic acid. *See* Arachidonic acid
Eisenmenger's syndrome, 353, 497, 515, 516, 517
Elastic pulmonary arteries
    damage to, 329, *illus.* 330, 331, 460
    obstruction of, 333
Elastin
    adventitial cell production of, 124, 176, 318
    hyperoxia and, 273
    in pulmonary artery, *illus.* 36, *illus.* 317
    smooth muscle cells and, 246
Electrical stimulation
    effect on bronchial vasodilation, 155
    effect on pulmonary hypertension, 133
    effect on pulmonary pressure, 137, 138–40, 143–45
    effect on pulmonary vascular tone, 134–35
    effect on pulmonary vasoconstriction, 132
Electromechanical coupling
    in excitation-contraction, 31–32, 33
    in hypoxic pressor response, 118, 119
Emboli, *illus.* 422. *See also* Thromboemboli
    resolution of, 414, *illus.* 415, 417
Embolic pulmonary arteriopathy, 333
Emphysema
    and atherosclerosis, 252, 253–54
    and hypertension, 337
    and lung transplantation, 515
    mortality, at altitude, 297

Endocrine system, 211
Endogenous substances, metabolism by endothelium, 69–73
Endomyocardial biopsy, 518–19
Endoplasmic reticulum, 77
Endothelial cells, 261, 410
    amplification, 80
    damage to
        antibody, *illus.* 180
        ANTU, *illus.* 74
        atherosclerosis, 245, 246, 247
        in cell culture, 173–83
        and heparan sulfate production, 195–99, 232
        hypertrophy, 271
        hypoxia, 86–87, 267, 268
        mechanisms of, 176
        monocrotaline, 321
        plexiform lesion, 463
        pulmonary hypertension with cirrhosis, 361, 362
        pulmonary veno-occlusive disease, 351
        thromboembolic pulmonary hypertension, 414
        and vascular tone, 486
    endothelium-derived relaxing factor production, 58
    hyperoxia and, 273–74
    interleukin-1 and, 208, 237
    lysis, 212
    migration and replication, 174
    modulation of coagulation and fibrinolysis, 231–41
    neonatal, 378, 379
    oxygen radicals and, 222, 226
    permeability, 177–79, 181
    production of vasomotor mediators, 80, 96, 103–4, 122–23, 486
    proliferation
        cytokines and, 208
        inhibition of, 210
        polypeptide growth factors and, 205, 206, 207, 270
        and pulmonary hypertension, 212–13
        regulation of, 201, 203, 268–69
        and vasoconstriction, 486
    purine receptors, 70
    smooth muscle cells and, 57–67
    transduction of oxygen, 85
    and vascular restriction, 264
Endothelin, 85, 87–88, 112, 116, 117, 122
Endothelium
    barrier function of, 177–79
    damage to, 394
    hypoxia and, 124
    of pulmonary veins, 349
    as a regulatory surface, 69–75
    as transducing surface, 75–80
    and vascular tone, *illus.* 117
Endothelium-dependent contracting factor (EDCF), 162
Endothelium-derived relaxing factor (EDRF)
    anticoagulation, 233

Endothelium-derived relaxing factor (*continued*)
 production of, 58, 64, 77, 92
  purine receptors and, 70
 properties and components of, 226–27
 and vascular resistance, 162
 and vascular tone, 67, 111, 112
 as vasodilator, 76, 122
Endotoxemia, 99, 102, 103, 274–75
Endotoxin
 and atherogenesis, 247
 endothelial cell activation, 212
 and endothelial interleukin-1 production, 104, 238
 and hypoxic vasoconstrictor response, 97
 and leukocyte adhesion, 240
 and pulmonary edema, 99–100
 and pulmonary hypertension, 100, 102, 260, 323
End-stage chronic obstructive pulmonary disease, 515
Englebreth-Holm-Swarm tumor, 197, 198
Enkephalin metabolism, 72
Environmental agents, 219
Enzymes, 119, 220
 proteolytic, 60
Eosinophils, 226, 387–88
Epidermal growth factor (EGF), 202, 207
Epinephrine, 70, 165. *See also* Norepinephrine
Epithelial cells, 206, 207
 alveolar, 274
Erythrocytes, 224, 294, 381
Erythropoiesis, 294
Erythropoietin, 119
Estradiol, 294
Estrogens, 114
Ethanol, 195
Ethchlorvynol, 178–79
Eukaryotic cells, 221
Evolution, 27–28, 29
Exercise
 and gas exchange, 289
 intolerance, 400
 and oxygen pressure, 419
 and pulmonary arterial pressure, 287–88,
  illus. 290, 310–11
 and pulmonary vascular resistance, *illus.* 93
 and vasoconstriction, 291
Extra-alveolar vessels, 46

Factor V, 231, 238
Factor Va, 233
Factor VIIa, 238
Factor VIIIa, 233–34
Factor VIII-related antigen, 277
Factor IXa, 233
Factor X, 231, 238
Factor Xa, 233, 238, 240
Fahraeus effect, 46
Familial primary pulmonary hypertension, 302–11,
 507–8
Familial pulmonary veno-occlusive disease, 301

Fatigue, 344, 355, 417–18, 421, 453, 455
Fatty acids, 70, 223–24, 228
Femoral vein, 426
Fenton reaction, 218, 220
Ferruginization, 463
Fetal gas, 163, 165
Fetus
 central nervous system, 131, 133
 ductus arteriosus, 116
 and hypoxia, 141
 lamb, 161–62, 163, 165
 lung expansion, 163
 lung smooth muscle, 319
 nutritional requirements, 161, 374
 pulmonary arterial pressure, 162, 164, 315, 316, 319
 pulmonary arteries, 264
 pulmonary arterioles, 319
 pulmonary circulation, 161–68, 373–78
 pulmonary vascular resistance, 162–64, 371, 373–74, 376
 pulmonary vasodilation, 163
Fibrin, 174, 233, 237
Fibrinogen, 179, 231, 277, 381
Fibrinoid degeneration, *illus.* 334–35, 336
Fibrinoid necrosis, 345, 463, 464, 508
Fibrinolysis, 240, 507–8
Fibrinolytic defects, 311
Fibrinolytic system, endothelial, 234–37
Fibroblast growth factors (FGF), 202, 203, 206, 271
Fibroblasts
 adventitial, 261
  hyperplasia in, 264, 265
  interstitial, 274
  proliferation in hyperoxia, *illus.* 267, 268, 273–74
  protein sythesis, 318
 in alveolar interstitium, 8
 and endothelial cells, 235
 hyperoxia and, 273
 interstitial, 273
 in intimal lesions, 201
 proliferation
  hypoxia and, 320
  inhibition of, 208
  polypeptide growth factors and, 203, 205–6, 207, 210
 and wall structure, 67
Fibronectin, 174, 179
Fibrosing mediastinitis, 426
Fibrosing pulmonary disease, 245–46
Fibrosing pulmonary vasculopathy, 337
Fibrosis, 179. *See also* Intimal fibrosis
 in aminorex pulmonary hypertension, 398
 cystic, 146, 311, 323, 515
 in elastic pulmonary arteries, 460
 in interstitium, 274, *illus.* 348, 419
 in media, 461
 in toxic oil syndrome, 387, 394

Fibrous septa, 464
Fishes, air breathing
    hemodynamics, 22, 23, 27, 28
    pulmonary circulation, 17, 18, *illus.* 19
Foam cells, 246–47, 248, 254. *See also* Macrophages
Fontan operation, 341
Foramen ovale, 316, 372, 375, 379, 427, 455
Foramen Panizzae, 25–26
Forced expired volume, 517
"Fos" protein, 205
Fulvine, 338

Gamma-interferon, 208–9
Gap junctional communication, 176
Gas exchange, 3, 15
    blood flow and, 96
    endothelial injury and, 173
    fetal, 161, 374
    growth rate and, 324
    neonatal, 162
    postoperative, 514
    and pulmonary hypertension, 289, 479
    vascular resistance and, 91, 92
Gender
    and chronic hypoxic pulmonary hypertension,
        294–95, 297–98
    and primary pulmonary hypertension, 302
    primary pulmonary hypertension registry
        patients, 452, 468
    and pulmonary veno-occlusive disease, 344, 350
Genetic factors
    in chronic hypoxic pulmonary hypertension, 113,
        285–87
    in familial primary pulmonary hypertension,
        304–5, 452–53
    heritable diseases, *illus.* 301, *illus.* 311
    in pulmonary arterial pressure, 309–11
    in pulmonary vascular reactivity, 294, 297
    in pulmonary veno-occlusive disease, 350
Geographic skewing in national registry, 449
Gills, 17, 18, 19, 28
    in amphibian larvae, 24–25
    in lungfish, 22–23
Glial cells, 206
Glomus cell, 116
Glucosamines, 187–89
Glucuronic acid, 187–89
Glutathione peroxidase, 223
Glycoproteins, 174
Glycosaminoglycans, 189, 196, 197, 232
Gnarly lungs, 111
Goats, 162, 165
G protein, 78
Granulocytes, 176
Granulocyte-macrophage colony-stimulating factor,
    174
Granulomatous lung disease, 480
Greenfield filter, 426, 427, 429
Growth control, gap junctions and, 176

Growth factors, 268. *See also specific factors*
    inhibition of, 209–10, 320–21
    and pulmonary hypertension, 201, 210–13
        cytokines, 208–9, 270
        polypeptide growth factors, 202–8
Growth rate, and pulmonary hypertension, 324
Guanosine triphosphate (GTP), 205
Guanylate cyclase, 58, 59, 122
Guinea pig, 34, 35

Harefield Hospital, 513
Hassell, John, 197–98
Hatfield family, 306
Heart. *See also* Cardiac output; Congenital heart
        disease; Shunting
    defects, congenital, 303, 466–67
    left atrial pressure, 41–42, 345
        endotoxin and, 100
        hypoxia and, 141
        laryngeal nerve stimulation and, 138–40
        postoperative, 427
    left atrium, 344
    left ventricular dysfunction, 332
    left ventricular failure, 145, 479
    lung and, 261
    palpitations, 453
    rate
        carotid body stimulation and, 153
        and hypoxia, 115–16
        turtle, *illus.* 21
    regurgitant murmurs, 453
    right atrial dilation, *illus.* 331, *illus.* 416
    right atrial pressure
        in diagnosis, 420–21
        in primary pulmonary hypertension registry
            patients, 453, 455, 474
    right atrium, 507
    right axis deviation, 502
    right heart catheterization, 517
    right heart failure, 310, 316
    right heart hypertrophy, 324
    right ventricle, resistance and, 91, 92
    right ventricular compliance, 332
    right ventricular dilation, *illus.* 331, *illus.* 416
    right ventricular failure
        in aminorex hypertension, 400, 404
        anticoagulant therapy, 505
        and heart-lung transplantation, 515
        in primary pulmonary hypertension, 455,
            474–75
        thromboembolism, 413, 416–17, 418
        vasodilator therapy, 479
    right ventricular function, 487, 493
    right ventricular hypertrophy
        altitude and, 319, 324
        in chronic pulmonary hypertension, 331–32
        in cirrhosis with pulmonary hypertension, 362
        decrease in, 320
        hematocrit and, 323

Heart (*continued*)
    hypoxia and, 319–20
    monocrotaline and, 322
    in primary pulmonary hypertension, 500
    thromboembolism, 413, 416
    vasodilator therapy, 480
    ventricular septal defect, 334
    ventricular septum, *illus.* 331, 332
Heart-lung transplantation, 228, 303, 518–20
    donor operation and selection, 512–15
    en-block, 512
    patient selection, 514–16
    preoperative investigations, 516–18
Hemangioendotheliomatosis, 459
Hemangiomatosis, 467
Hematocrit concentration
    and blood viscosity, 46, 381
    in chronic hypoxic pulmonary hypertension, 297
    in cirrhosis with pulmonary hypertension, 363
    gender and, 294–95, 297–98
    in persistent pulmonary hypertension of the
        newborn, 372
    polycythemia and, 289
    and pulmonary hypertension, 323, 324
    in pulmonary hypertension with cirrhosis, 364,
        366
    and resistance to blood flow, 297, 375
Hemodynamics
    of primary pulmonary hypertension, 455, 474,
        502–3
    responses to vasodilators, *illus.* 492, *illus.* 495
Hemoglobin
    in cirrhosis with pulmonary hypertension, 363
    in collagen vascular disease, 355
    endothelium-derived relaxing factor and, 122
    gender and, 294
    and oxygen radicals, 224
    in pulmonary hypertension with cirrhosis, 360,
        364, 366
Hemoptysis, 344, 418
Hemosiderin, 338
Hemosiderosis, *illus.* 348, 404
Heparan sulfate
    biochemistry, 187–89
    endothelial cell production of, 195–99, 232
    fibroblast growth factors and, 206
    vascular growth inhibition, 194–95, 210, 212
Heparin, 268
    angiogenesis inhibition, 209
    biochemistry, 187–89
    endothelial cell production of, 232
    fibroblast growth factors and, 206
    growth factor inhibition, 320–21, 323
    in surgery, 421, 428–29
    therapy, 415
    vascular growth inhibition, 189–94, 199–200,
        210, 274
Heparinase, 195–96
Heparin-antithrombin III system, 232

Hepatic cirrhosis. *See also* Liver and hypoxic
    pressor response, 114
    with pulmonary hypertension, 353, 359–68, 385,
        398, 438
Hepatic vein sclerosis, 363
Hepatic veno-occlusive disease, 338, 343, 350
Heritability. *See* Genetic factors
Hexagonal capillary network, *illus.* 6
Hexamethonium, 138, 142
High flow injury, 276–78
Histamine
    as bronchoconstrictor, 156, 226
    and endothelial membrane, 179
    promotion of cell replication, 268
    and prostaglandin formation, 175, 180, 377–78
    and pulmonary vascular resistance, 43, 44–45,
        99, 100, 165
    and pulmonary vascular tone, 111, 112
    as vasoconstrictor, 95, 96–97, 377
    as vasodilator, 165, 377
    and vessel permeability, 100–101
HIV serological testing, 515
Hoarseness, 331
Homocystinemia, 247
Hormonal stimulation, 176
Hospital of the University of Pennsylvania, 470
Humoral mediators, 91–92, 131
Hyalinosis, 398
Hyaluronic acid, 192
Hydralazine
    hemodynamic responses to, 492, 493–95
    and pulmonary vascular resistance, 481–82, 490
    and pulmonary veno-occlusive disease, 344
Hydrogen ions, 115, 378
Hydrogen peroxide (H_2O_2)
    biochemistry, 218, 219
    and hypoxic pressor response, 120–21
    production of, 220, 221, 222, 228
    sites of damage, 223, 224, 226
    stimulation of prostaglandin production, 177
12-Hydroperoxy-eicosatetraenoic acid (HPETE), 225
Hydroxy-eicosatetraenoic acids (HETE), 72–73,
       183, 225
Hydroxyl ($\cdot$OH)
    biochemistry, 218–19
    production of, 220, 221
    sites of damage, 223, 226
5-hydroxytryptamine (5-HT), 70
Hypercapnia, 114
Hypercapnic acidosis, 295, 298
Hypercholesterolemia, 248, 249, 254
Hyperemia, 158, 164
Hyperlipidemia, 248, 249, 253–54
Hyperoxia
    cell damage, 60, 267
    and endothelial cells, 65–66, 67, 177
    and vascular remodeling, 260, 271–74
Hyperplasia
    and pulmonary arterial wall, 65

and pulmonary vascular resistance, 288
and vascular remodeling, 264–65
Hyperpnea, 402
Hypertrophy. *See also* Medial hypertrophy
  cellular, and arterial wall, 65
  muscular, 416
  and vascular remodeling, 264–65
Hyperventilation
  in aminorex pulmonary hypertension, 400
  chronic hypoxia and, 293, 294, 297
  in embolism, 418
  in hepatic cirrhosis, 360
Hypobaric hypoxia, 267
Hypocalcemia, 372, 380
Hypocapnia
  in aminorex pulmonary hypertension, 400, 406
  in chronic hypoxia, 295
  in thromboembolic hypertension, 419
Hypoglycemia, 372, 380
Hypothalamus, 142
Hypothermia, 413, 427
Hypoventilation
  in aminorex pulmonary hypertension, 399–400
  chronic hypoxia and, 124, 293, 295–97
  and hypoxemia, 324
Hypoxemia
  in aminorex pulmonary hypertension, 400
  in chest radiograph, 373
  chronic hypoxia and, 124, 296, 297
  in chronic pulmonary hypertension, 316
  in hepatic cirrhosis, 360
  intrauterine, and hematocrit, 381
  in persistent pulmonary hypertension of the
      newborn, 379
  in primary pulmonary hypertension, 454, 455
  reperfusion lung injury and, 427
  and right ventricular hypertrophy, 324
  in thromboembolic hypertension, 419
  and vascular resistance, 376
Hypoxia
  acute
    effects on systemic vessels, 115
    lung injury and, 60
    and pulmonary vasoconstriction, 109–10, 140,
        480
    and vascular tone, 124
  alveolar
    and capillary pressure, 99
    causes of, 335
    and oxygen saturation, *illus.* 113
    and pulmonary pressor response, 112
    and pulmonary vasoconstriction, 95, 96, 98,
        140, 158
      attenuation of, 157
      species differences, 133, 310
    and vascular lesions, 336–37
  arterial wall and atherosclerosis, 248
  and bronchial circulation, 151–56, 157–58
  chemoreceptor influences, 140–42

chronic
  heparin and, 199–200
  and pulmonary vasoconstriction, 124–25, 480
  and endothelial cells, 64–65, 268
  and heparan sulfate, 198
  hypobaric, 267
  intrauterine, 279–80
  mixed venous, 112, *illus.* 113
  muscularization of pulmonary arterioles, 176
  and neonatal calves, 315–18
  and pulmonary vascular resistance, 289–91
  relative, 272–73
  systemic, and pulmonary vasoconstriction, 140
  in toxic oil syndrome, 392–93, 394
  and vascular remodeling, 260, 265–71, 273
Hypoxic pressor response. *See also*
      Vasoconstriction
  adrenergic innervation and, 125, 321
  heritable influences on, 309–11
  inhibition of, 167–68
  mechanisms of, 85–87, 117–23
  strength of, 113–14, 319–20
  systemic vessel hypoxia and, 115–16
  testing of, 109–10
Hypoxic pulmonary hypertension, chronic, 283–98,
      311, 319–21
Hypoxic pulmonary vasculopathy, 336–37

Ibuprofen, 98, 224–25
Idiopathic pulmonary fibrosis, 311
Idiopathic pulmonary hypertension, 276
Iduronic acid, 187–89
IgG proteins, 157
IgG receptors, 176
Iliac vein, 426
Immune complexes, 245, 247
Immunocompetent cells, 80
Immunological disorder, 350
Immunosuppressants, 511
Impedance plethysmography, 420–21
Indomethacin
  cyclooxygenase inhibition, 121, 224–25
  and ductus arteriosus, 280, 319, 379
  effect on cytotoxicity, 183
  effect on driving pressure, 322
  and pulmonary arterial pressure, 323
  and pulmonary vascular resistance, 92–93, 95,
      323, 377
Infants. *See* Newborn
Inferior vena cava, 426
Inflammatory mediators. *See also* Platelet activat-
      ing factor
  and cytotoxicity, 176, 179–83
Inflammatory response
  endothelial cell damage and, 212
  and endothelial cell function, 80
  granulomatous, 228
  in hyperoxia, 272
  interleukin and, 208

Inflammatory response (*continued*)
  macrophages in, 211
  neutrophils and, 221, 323
  oxygen radicals and, 221, 224
  and pulmonary hypertension, 95
Inflammatory vascular disease, 254
Inheritance. *See* Genetic factors
Initiation, 217. *See also* Oxygen radicals
Inositol 1,4,5-trisphosphate (InsP₃), 33
Inositol trisphosphate (IP₃), 77, 204
Input impedance, 52–54
Insulin-like growth factor 1 (IGF-1), 202, 203, 206–7
Interleukin-1 (IL-1)
  decrease of lung injury, 183
  endothelial cell activation of, 212, 238
  endothelial cell production of, 80, 104
  and fibroblast and smooth muscle cells, 274
  and leukocyte adhesion, 239–40
  and lymphoid cells, 203
  and plasminogen activator inhibitor, 239, 240–41
  pro-inflammatory effects, 208
Interleukin-2, 95, 203
Interleukin-6, 80
Intermittent air breathers, 17–29
International Society and Federation of Cardiology, 409
Interstitial cells, 8
Interstitial edema, 344, 345, 348, 349
Interstitial fibroblast, 274
Interstitial fibrosis, 274, *illus.* 348, 419
Interstitial lung disease, 357, 453, 480
Interstitium, 173
  alveolar, 8
  pulmonary, 99
Intima
  atheromas, 460
  endothelial cells, 261
  lesions, 201, 329–30
    in primary pulmonary hypertension, 459–60, 461–62
    in toxic oil syndrome, 387
  neointima, 427
  proliferation in, *illus.* 334–35, 336, 485
  smooth muscle cells, 247, *illus.* 263
    proliferation of, 189, 329–30
  thickening of, 489–91
Intimal fibroelastosis (CIF), laminar concentric, 307
  lesions, 309
Intimal fibrosis
  in aminorex hypertension, 404
  concentric laminar
    histopathological features, 466, 467, 469
    lesions, *illus.* 334–35, 336, 461, 462, 466
  eccentric, 307, *illus.* 332, 337, 338, *illus.* 339, *illus.* 340, 466, 467
    lesions, 309, 461–62, 469
  in primary pulmonary hypertension, 464, 468, 469, 507
  and pulmonary vascular resistance, 466, 485, 487

in pulmonary veins, 343, 344, *illus.* 346, *illus.* 347, 351
in toxic oil syndrome, 392–93
Intimal hyperplasia, 404
Intimal hypertrophy, 213, 466
Intrauterine hypoxia, 279–80
Ion fluxes, 119
Iron
  Fe²⁺, 218, 220
  Fe³⁺, 218, 220
Ischemia, 164, 380, 418, 513
Isoproterenol
  hemodynamic responses to, 392, 492, 493, 494–95, 496
  as vasodilator, 23, 489

Jamaican bush-tea, 338

Kidney, 12
  artery constriction, 319
  transplantation, 350
Kinase, myosin light chain (MLCK), 32, 33, 35–37
Kininase II, 70–72
Kininogen, 377

Lactic acidosis, 361
Lambs, 133
  fetal, 161–62, 163, 165
Lamellae, 22–23
Laryngeal nerve, 136, 330–31
  chemoreceptors, 138–39
  irritation, 146
  and pulmonary artery pressure, 137, 138–40
Laser flash photolysis, 37
Leg edema, 453
Lesions
  of the adventitia, 462
  in aminorex hypertension, 404
  angiomatoid, 276, 404, 416
  of the arterial wall, 463–64
  dilation, *illus.* 275, 464
    in aminorex hypertension, 404
    pulmonary arterial, 334, *illus.* 335, 464
  of the intima, 461–62
  in primary pulmonary hypertension, 459, 460–65
  in toxic oil syndrome, 387, 393–94
Leukocyte adhesion molecules (LAM), 237–38
Leukocytes
  adhesion of, 213, 239–40
  growth factors and, 207, 208, 212
  hyperoxia and, 272
  in leukotriene synthesis, 225
  mediator producing, 101–4
  platelet-activating factor and, 122–23
  polymorphonuclear (PMN)
    in arteritis, 461
    and endothelial injury, 176–77, 178, 181, 182–83
    and oxygen radicals, 221, 227–28
Leukotriene A₄ (LTA₄), 73, 225

Leukotriene B$_4$ (LTB$_4$), 72–73, 101–2, 180, 225, 226
Leukotriene C$_4$ (LTC$_4$), 61, 73, 95, 121–22, 162, 167, 225–26, 376
Leukotriene D$_4$ (LTD$_4$), 61, 73, 95–96, 162, 167–68, 225–26, 376
Leukotriene E$_4$ (LTE$_4$), 61, 73, 225
Leukotrienes
  as bronchoconstrictors, 225–26
  and endothelial damage, 60, 72–73, 178, 179
  as neonatal vasoconstrictor, 167–68
  production of, 72–73, 121–22, 183, 225–26
  and pulmonary vascular resistance, 95–97, 162
  and smooth muscle cell proliferation, 209
Life expectancy. *See* Mortality
Ligand (ATP)-gated channels, 32
Lineages Inc., 306
Lipids
  in atherosclerosis, 246–47, 248
  blood levels, 245
  hyperlipidemia, 248, 249, 253–54
  membrane, 223–24
Lipoproteins, 246, 247
  low density, 222, 224
Lipoxin, 227
Lipoxygenase
  inhibition of, 97, 225, 226
  pathway
    and hypoxic pressor response, 121, 167, 376
    and lipoxin, 227
Liver
  cirrhosis of
    and hypoxic pressor response, 114
    with pulmonary hypertension, 353, 359–68, 385, 398, 438
  and insulin-like growth factor, 206
  in thromboembolic pulmonary hypertension, 418
  transplantation of, 516
  vein sclerosis, 363
  veno-occlusive disease of, 338, 343, 350
Lobectomy, 516
Low density lipoproteins (LDL), 222, 224
Lung. *See also* Heart-lung transplantation
  biopsy, 341, 344, 427
    in primary pulmonary hypertension registry, 446, 447, 448, 449, 470–71
    and heart-lung transplantation, 516, 519
  blood circulation in, 96–98, 261
  development, 133, 134, 374
  edema, reperfusion, 427–28
  expansion, 163
  fetal, 163–64, 319, 374
  gnarly, 111
  and hypoxic pressor response, 110, 117
  injury, ischemic, 513
  interstitial spaces, 12
  lymph, 101
  neonatal, 162, 163–64, 263–64, 377–78
  perfusion, 91
    altitude and, 288
    alveolar, 12

  blood flow in, 23, 376, 513
  capillaries and, 9
  in diagnosis, 419–20
  in intermittent air breathers, 17, 18, 24
  in thromboembolic pulmonary hypertension, *illus.* 419
  and vasoconstriction, 96
  preservation, 512–13
  reperfusion injury, 427
  in a respirator, 14–15
  smooth muscle, fetal, 319
  tissue, in veno-occlusive disease, 345–48
  transplantation, 511–16
  ventilation
    carotid chemoreceptor stimulation and, 141
    in diagnosis, 419–20
    fetal, 163, 377
    and hypoxia, 115–16, 297–98, 480
    in intermittent air breathers, 18, 22, 24
    in newborns, 379
    and perinatal pulmonary circulation, 166
    and pulmonary vascular resistance, *illus.* 97
  ventilation-perfusion relationships, 91, 96, 158, 455
  vessel wall metabolism, 60–64
Lung cells, mediator production by, 101–4
Lung disease
  chronic, 517
  granulomatous, 480
  interstitial, 357, 453, 380
  intrinsic, 158
  parenchymal, 353, 358, 399–400
  primary, 515, 516–17
  suppurative, 515
Lungfishes, 17, 18, *illus.* 19, *illus.* 20, 22–23, 27
Lupus anticoagulant, 414–15
Lymphocytes
  adherence to basement membrane, 212
  in atherosclerosis, 246
  lymphokine release, 80
  lymphotoxin secretion, 208
  reactivity, 519
  vascular wall infiltration, 387, 392–93, 463
Lymphoid cells, 203
Lymphokines, 80
Lymphotoxin, 208

McCoy family, 306
Macrophages, 101
  alveolar, 102, *illus.* 340
  and granulomatous inflammation, 228
  and growth factors, 206, 207, 211
  lymphokine release, 80
  monocyte-derived, in atherosclerosis, 246–47
  pulmonary alveolar (PAMs), 220–21, 227
  pulmonary intravascular (PIM), 102–3
  in pulmonary venous hypertension, *illus.* 340, *illus.* 465
Malondialdehyde, 224
Mannitol, 228

"Mas" oncogene, 209
Mast cells, 101, 121, 189, 268, 394
    in fetuses, 377
Mayo Clinic, 469, 501, 505, 507
Mechanical energy balance, 45–47
Meclofenamate, 93, 97, 121
Meconium aspiration, 145, 279, 372
Media, *illus.* 460
    damage to, 463–64
    fibrosis in, 461
    hypoxia and, 124
    lesions in, 201, 459–60
    smooth muscle cells, 201, 247, 261, 263, 318
        and heparan sulfate, 194–95, 199
        neonatal, 381
    thickening of, vasodilators and, 489, 490
    vascular remodeling, 268, 379
Medial hypertrophy, 201, 272
    in aminorex pulmonary hypertension, 404
    in chronic pulmonary hypertension, 329,
        illus. 330, 338, *illus.* 340
    hyperoxia and, 273
    hypoxia and, 288
    in plexogenic pulmonary arteriopathy, *illus.* 334,
        335, 337, 467
    in primary pulmonary hypertension, 460–61, 466,
        468, 469, 480, 481, 507
    in pulmonary veno-occlusive disease, 345, 351,
        466
    in toxic oil syndrome, 393
Median sternotomy, 427
Mediastinitis, fibrosing, 426
Mediastinotomy, 516
Mediators
    from endothelium, 174
    humoral, 91–92, 131
    of hypoxic pressor response, 121–23
    lung production of, 101–4
    neurochemical, 116
Medulla, 133, 142–43
Melittin
    and arachidonate release, 180–81
    cytotoxicity, 182–83
    and endothelial cells, 175, 178, 179, 180
Membrane lipids, 223–24
MENOCIL, 397, 398
Menstruation, 507
Mephenytoin, 403
Mesenchymal cells, 209
Metabolism
    anaphylatoxin, 72
    cell, 120, 123
    of copper, 311
    of drugs, 403
    of endogenous substrates by endothelium, 69–73
    enkephalin, 72
    gap junctions and, 176
    vessel wall, 60–64
    of xenobiotic substances, 73–75

Methylene blue, 122
Methylprednisolone, 323
Microcirculation. *See also* Alveoli; Capillaries
    brain, 233
    pulmonary
        mediators in, 99–101
        neonatal, 278–79
        normal function of, 3–14, 261–63
        and pulmonary hypertension, 260, 280
Micropuncture studies, 113
Microthrombi, 454
Microthromboembolism, 372, 379
Microvascular endothelium, 175
Mitochondria, 34, *illus.* 36
    and Ca^{2+}, 36
    cytochrome oxidase, 119–20
    membranes, 123
    and oxygen radicals, 220
Mitogen (PDGF), 124
Mitogens, 195, 199
Mitosis
    in recovery from hyperoxia, 274
    smooth muscle cell, 179, 190
    in vascular remodeling, 267–71
Mitral stenosis
    and atherosclerosis, 249
    hypertensive vascular changes, 416
    and left bronchus, 330
    neurogenic component, 145
    and pulmonary artery pressure, 245
Mixed venous hypoxia, 112, *fig.* 113
Monocrotaline injury, 267
    hypertrophy, 271
    and pulmonary hypertension, 321–23, 324, 338
Monocytes, 206, 212, 246, 272
    intravascular, 102–3
Mormon church, 306
Morphometry of the Human Lung (Weibel), 8
Mortality
    in aminorex hypertension, 406–8
    in anticoagulant therapy, 504–5
    in emphysema, 297
    in familial hypertension, *illus.* 302
    in lung biopsy, 470
    in neonatal hypertension, 372
    in primary pulmonary hypertension, 408, 473–75
    in primary pulmonary hypertension and collagen
        vascular disease, 356, 358
    in Raynaud's phenomenon, 474
    surgery and, 430, 431
    vasodilator therapy and, 490–91
Muscular hypertrophy, 416
Muscularization
    of arteries
        in chronic pulmonary hypertension, 199
        in persistent pulmonary hypertension of the
            newborn, 373–74, 379
    of pulmonary arterioles
        hypoxia and, 176

in plexogenic pulmonary arteriopathy, 335, 337
in primary pulmonary hypertension, *illus.* 460, 480
in secondary pulmonary hypertension, 329, *illus.* 330
Mustard operation, 508
"Myc" protein, 205
Myeloid cells, 203
Myocardial cooling blanket, 427, 428
Myocardial dysfunction, 380
Myocardial function, 295
Myocardial infarction, 249, 418, 426
Myocytes, 332
Myofibroblasts, *illus.* 6, 8
  and intimal lesions, 329–30, 462
Myosin, 65
Myosin ATPase, 35–37
Myosin light chain kinase (MLCK), 32, 33, 35–37
Myosin light chain phosphorylation, 35–37, 87

National Heart, Lung, and Blood Institute, xiv, 437, 441, 442, 451, 507
National Institutes of Health, 409
National Registry on Primary Pulmonary Hypertension, 437–39, 441–43
  classifications, 459, 467
  collagen vascular disease in, 353
  data requirements, 444–45
  dilemmas of, 443–49
  familial pulmonary hypertension in, 302
  hepatic cirrhosis in, 359, 364
  patient characteristics, 357, 451–56, 468–69
  vasodilator trials, 491
Necrosis
  in aminorex hypertension, 404
  of endothelial cells, 264
  fibrinoid, 345, 463, 464, 508
  hyperoxia and, 260, 267, 271, 274
Neointima, 427
Neonatal omphalitis, 363
Neonate. *See* Newborn
Nerve growth factor, 203
Nerves
  peptidergic, 155
  phrenic
    activity, *illus.* 137, 140, 141
    injury, 427
    paralysis, 427
    paresis, 428
Nervous system, autonomic, 164–65, 321. *See also* Central nervous system
  blood flow and, 144
Neural cells, 203
Neurochemical mediators, 116
Neurotransmitters, 121
Neutral endopeptidase (NEP), 72
Neutropenia, 323
Neutrophils, 323
  accumulation of, indomethacin and, 95

and activating agents, 177
adhesion to endothelial cells, 239–40
endothelial modulation of, 73
and inflammatory response, 221, 323
leukotriene B_4 and, 226
leukotriene production, 101–2
and lung injury, 227
platelet-derived growth factor and, 206
and pulmonary edema, 176
Newborn. *See also* Persistent pulmonary hypertension of the newborn
  arterial CO_2 and pH, 164
  brain, 131
  growth of, and hypertension, 324
  lung, 162, 163–64, 264, 377–78
  normal pulmonary circulation, 133, 373–78
  pulmonary vascular resistance, 315, 316, 379, 380, 381
  transposition of the great vessels, 146
New York Heart Association, 452, 474
Nifedipine
  hemodynamic responses to, 492, 494, 495, 497
  and pulmonary artery pressure, 481–82, 488, 493
  and pulmonary vascular resistance, 490
Nitric oxide, 58, 76, 122, 226–27
Nitroglycerin, 392, 488–89, 492, 494–95
Nitroprusside, 492, 494
Nitrous acid, 189, 195–96, 197
Nitrovasodilators, 26
Norepinephrine, 70, 165, 254
N-sulfation, 188, 189
Nucleic acids, 223
5'-nucleotidase activity, 71
Nucleotides, adenine, 70, 226
Nutritional requirements, fetal, 161, 374

Obesity, 296, 298
Obliterative bronchiolitis, 519
Obliterative pulmonary hypertension, 311, 506
Obliterative vascular disease, 356–57
Observation, effects of, 443–44
Obstructive airways disease, chronic, 283, 295, 296
  and pulmonary hypertension, 297, 479, 481
Obstructive pulmonary disease, 245–46
Ohm's law, 45–46, 375
Oleoanilides, 361, 388
Oral contraceptives, 385, 453
Organ donation, 513–14
Orthodeoxia, 360
Osteoblasts, 206
Oxidative phosphorylation, 119–20
Oxygen. *See also* Hyperoxia; Hypoxia
  cytosolic effects of, 224
  delivery, 480–81, 482
  dissociation, *illus.* 113
  and endothelial cell injury, 58
  exercise and, 419
  and pulmonary artery pressure, 162, 265, 372, 516

Oxygen (*continued*)
    in toxic oil syndrome, 391, 392
    and pulmonary vascular resistance, 392
        concentration, 378
        inhalation, 318
        tension, 376
    saturation, 372, 419
        arterial, 293, 296–97, 503
    sensing site, 85–87
    sensors, 116, 118, 119–20
    therapy, 497, 517
    toxicity, 114
    as vasodilator, 493
Oxygen radicals
    and cell damage, 75, 79, 80, 217–28
        endothelial, 176–77
    and hypoxic pressor response, 120–21
    and thoracic radiation, 323

Papworth Hospital, 513, 514
Paracrine system, 211
Paraquat, 228
Parenchymal blood flow, 419
Parenchymal lung disease, 353, 358, 399–400
Particulates, endothelial cells and, 78–79
Pelvis, 507
Peptide histidine isoleucine (PHI), 155
Peptidergic nerves, 155
Peptides, 87. *See also* Cytokines; Growth factors
    vasoactive intestinal peptide (VIP), 111, 112, 155,
        226
Perfusates, 114
Perfusion lung scans, *illus.* 420, 421, 454, 456
Pericarditis, 427
Pericytes, 261, 262, 263, 275
    communication with endothelial cells, 176
    development into smooth muscle cells, 267–68,
        320, 373
    hypertrophy of, 265, 271
    proliferation in hyperoxia, 273–74
    proliferation in hypoxia, 269, 271
Peripheral pulmonary stenosis, 398
Permeability
    capillary, 100–101, 122–23
    endothelial cell, 177–79, 181
    microvascular, 60, 228
    vascular, 174
Peroxidase, 221, 226
Peroxidation, 223–24
Peroxides, 226
Persistent fetal circulation syndrome, 278, 371
Persistent pulmonary hypertension of the newborn,
        260, 371–73, 378–81
    animal models, 315–19
    central nervous system in, 145–46
    leukotrienes in, 167
    thrombi in, 508
    vascular remodeling in, 278–80
pH
    arterial, 162, 164

    blood, 73, 114, 162
    cytoplasmic, 203
    and pulmonary vascular resistance, 378
Phagocytosis, 78–79, 220–21
Pharmacological responses
    to aminorex, 402–3
    to endothelial cell damage, 58–60
    to hypoxia, 111–12
Pharmacomechanical coupling, 31–33
Phenformin, 361
Phenoxybenzamine, 135, 142
Phentolamine, 492, 494–95
Phlebitis, pulmonary, 345
Phorbol esters, 205
Phorbol myristate acetate (PMA), 177, 178, 181,
        221
Phosphatidyl-inositol bisphosphate (PIP$_2$), 33, 204
Phosphodiesterase, 205
Phospholipase A$_2$, 182–83
Phospholipase C, 32, 33
Phosphorylation
    myosin light chain, 35–37, 87
    oxidative, 119–20
    protein, 203, 204–5
Phrenic nerve
    activity, *illus.* 137, 140, 141
    injury, 427
    paralysis, 427
    paresis, 428
Pigs, 134, 137, 139, 140, 141, 143, 144
Placenta, 161, 374
Plaques, 246–47, 248, *illus.* 250–51, *illus.* 252
Plasmalemmal vesicles, 5
Plasmin, 233–34, 237
    antiplasmin, 507–8
Plasminogen, 237
Plasminogen activator inhibitor (PAI), 239, 240–41
Plasminogen activators, 234–36
Platelet-activating factor (PAF), 80
    endothelial damage and, 60, 173, 179, 181,
        182–83
    endothelial metabolism of, 73
    and leukocyte adhesion, 240
    production of, 92, 104, 122, 174
    and pulmonary vascular resistance, 162
    as vasoconstrictor, 122–23
    as vasodilator, 98, 122, 378
Platelet-derived growth factor (PDGF)
    endothelial production of, 174, 237–38, 240
    and fibroblasts, 210
    heparin inhibition of, 193, 320, 323
    and pulmonary hypertension, 205–6, 212
    and smooth muscle cells, 64
        proliferation, 67, 193, 202, 203–5, 240, 274
Platelet-derived growth factorlike protein
        (PDGFc), 269
Platelet heparitinase, 194–95
Platelets
    activation of, 240
    adhesion, 213

aggregation, 166, 174, 212, 226
endothelial receptors and, 76
granules, 206, 207–8
in hyperoxia, 272
in hypoxia, 508
metabolites of, 410
and plasminogen, 237
platelet-derived growth factor release, 67, 206
as thromboxane source, 103, 225
and vasoconstriction, 393, 394
Platypnea, 360
Pleural adhesions, 151
Pleural circulation, 3
Pleurisy, 418
Plexiform lesions
in aminorex hypertension, 404
in familial pulmonary hypertension, 307–9
in high flow injury, 277–78
in plexogenic pulmonary arteriopathy, 334,
illus. 335, 336
in primary pulmonary hypertension, 463–64, 466,
468, 469, 507, 508
in thromboembolic pulmonary hypertension, 416
in toxic oil syndrome, 393
Plexogenic pulmonary arteriopathy, 334–36, 353,
409–10, 454, 507
anticoagulant therapy, 485, 505
lesions of, 307, 309, 363, 404, 463, 465–67, 469
in primary pulmonary hypertension, 344, 357,
459, 486
Pneumonia, 114, 389, 393, 418
Poiseuille's law, 7, 46
Polycythemia
hypoxia and, 265, 289, 323
in infants, 146
and pulmonary hypertension, 296, 297
and pulmonary vascular resistance, 336–37
thrombi in, 508
Polymorphonuclear leukocytes (PMN)
in arteritis, 463
and endothelial injury, 176–77, 178, 181, 182–83
and oxygen radicals, 221, 228
Polypeptides, 70
growth factors, 202–8
Polysaccharides, 187–89, 190
Polyunsaturated fats, 124
Portal hypertension, 336, 359, 360, 361, 363
Positive end-expiratory pressure (PEEP) respira-
tor, 14–15
Postcapillary obstruction, 338–39
Prazosin, 392
Precapillary obstruction, 333–38
Precapillary pulmonary vascular resistance, 398
Pregnancy, 453, 505
and hypoxic pressor response, 114
use of prostaglandin inhibitors in, 379
Primary lung disease, 515, 516–17
Primary plexogenic arteriopathy, 350
Primary pulmonary arteritis, 459, 467
Primary pulmonary hypertension, 398, 400–401,

414. *See also* National Registry on Primary
Pulmonary Hypertension
clinical features, 453–55
definition of, 446–47
diagnosis of, 446–48, 465–67, 470–71
familial, 302–11, 507–8
in heart-lung transplantation, 515, 516
hemodynamic features, 353, 354–55, 455
histopathology, 459–70
mortality, 473–75
neural component of, 145, 146
open lung biopsy in, 341, 470–71
pulmonary vascular resistance in, 454, 502–3
and vascular remodeling, 275–76
vasodilator therapy, 479–82
acute, 485–95
anticoagulant, 505
chronic, 495–97
prostacyclin, 517–18
Progesterone, 294
Pronase®, 195
Propranolol, 135
Prostacyclin (PGI$_2$)
anticoagulation, 174, 227, 233
and blood flow, 174, 378
endothelial cell production of, 70, 72, 80, 96, 103,
176
bradykinin and, 75–76, 77, 180
inhibition of, 121
loss of, 222
melittin and, 175, 180
stimuli for, 179, 180, 183
hemodynamic responses to, 492, 493–95, 496
in lung transplantation, 513, 517–18
metabolites, endotoxin and, 94
and oxygen delivery, 482
and perinatal pulmonary circulation, 166–67
pulmonary artery accumulation of, in hyperoxia,
61–63
and pulmonary artery pressure, 481, 488
and pulmonary vascular resistance, 146, 318, 376,
377–78, 493–94
and vascular tone, 67, 111, 112
as vasodilator, 92, 97, 226
Prostaglandin D$_2$ (PGD$_2$), 101, 133, 233, 377
Prostaglandin E$_1$ (PGE$_1$), 72, 134, 166
Prostaglandin E$_2$ (PGE$_2$), 23, 61, 95, 101–2, 103,
165–66, 175, 376, 377
Prostaglandin F$_{2\alpha}$ (PGF$_{2\alpha}$) 58, 59, 95, 165–66
Prostaglandin H$_2$ (PGH$_2$), 175
Prostaglandins. *See also* Prostacyclin
angiogenic effect of, 209–210
and bronchial circulation, 152, 155–56
and ductus arteriosus, 116
lung degradation of, 72
and perinatal circulation, 165–67
production of
angiotensin II and, 124
endothelial damage and, 60, 183
oxygen radicals and, 224–26

Prostaglandins (*continued*)
    hydrogen peroxide and, 177
    and pulmonary vascular resistance, 162, 377
Prostanoids, 92–95, 96–97, 100. *See also*
    Prostaglandins
Protein C, 311, 414–15
Protein G, 78
Protein IgG, 157
Protein kinase C, 78, 79, 205
Protein kinases, 202–4
Protein S, 414–15
Proteins
    cytoskeletal, 178–79
    and oxygen radicals, 220, 223
    phosphorylated, 203, 204–5
    synthesis, 320
Proteoglycans, 189, 196
    in atherosclerosis, 246
    heparan sulfate, 197–98
    in intimal fibrosis, 462
Proteolytic enzymes, 60
Psychiatric disturbances, 427, 428
Pterygopalatine ganglion, 157
Pulmocutaneous artery, 25
Pulmonary alveolar macrophages (PAMs), 220–21,
    227
Pulmonary arterial blood pressure
    altitude and, 265, 283–95, 296
    in aminorex hypertension, 403, 404, 405, 406
    and atherogenesis, 247, 252
    brain influences on, 142, 143, 144
    and capillary pressure, 99, 100
    central nervous system and, 132, 135, 136–45
    in collagen vascular disease, 355, 358
    endotoxin infusion and, 100
    exercise and, 287–88, *illus.* 290, 310–11
    fetal, 162, 164, 315, 316, 319
    hematocrit and, 323
    in hepatic cirrhosis, 367–68
    heritable influences on, 301, 309–11
    hyperoxia and, 273
    increases in, sources of, 57
    mediators of, 96
    neonatal, 379
    in primary pulmonary hypertension, 455, 474,
        479, 502–3
    prostacyclin and, 517–18
    and pulmonary vascular resistance, 41–42, 51,
        54, 57, 92
    in pulmonary veno-occlusive disease, 349
    surgery and, 429
    in toxic oil syndrome, *illus.* 391, 393
    vascular transmural pressure (VTP), 28–29
    in vasodilator therapy, 480–81, 486–87, 488,
        493–94, 496
Pulmonary arterial hypertension, 54
Pulmonary arterial lesions, *illus.* 306, 307–9, 361
Pulmonary arterial vasomotor segment (PAVS), 23
Pulmonary arteries. *See also* Capillaries; Endothe-

lial cells; Small pulmonary arteries; Smooth
    muscle cells
    agenesis of, 425
    atherosclerosis, 245–54
    calf, *illus.* 317
    in chronic pulmonary hypertension, *illus.* 330
    elastic
        damage to, 329, *illus.* 330, 331
        fibrosis in, 460
        obstruction of, 333
    fetal, 264
    hypoxia and, 113
    intra-acinar, *illus.* 278
    muscular
        hyperreactive, 507, 508
        intimal fibrosis in, *illus.* 347, 462, 467
        medial hypertrophy in, *illus.* 328, 329, 337, 349
        in primary pulmonary hypertension, 460
        thromboemboli in, 333
    muscularization of
        in persistent pulmonary hypertension of the
            newborn, 373–74, 379
    normal circulation, 261–64, *illus.* 330
    in primary pulmonary hypertension, 453
    in pulmonary venous hypertension, 338, *illus.* 340
    in surgery, 427
    in thromboembolic pulmonary hypertension,
        illus. 419, *illus.* 422, *illus.* 423
    in veno-occlusive disease, 345, 349
Pulmonary arterioles
    adrenergic nerves in, 321
    constriction of, leukotrienes and, 226
    fetal, 319
    muscular, intimal fibrosis in, 467
    muscularization of
        in chronic pulmonary hypertension, 329,
            illus. 330
        hypoxia and, 176
        in plexogenic pulmonary arteriopathy, 335, 337
        in primary pulmonary hypertension, *illus.* 460,
            480
    and pulmonary vascular resistance, 134, 162
Pulmonary arteritis, 469
Pulmonary baroreceptors, 136
Pulmonary circulation, fetal, 161–68, 373–78
Pulmonary disease, fibrosing, 245–46
Pulmonary disease, obstructive, 245–46
Pulmonary edema
    altitude and, 310
    endothelial injury and, 178
    endotoxin infusion and, 99–100
    neutrophil and, 176
    platelet-activating factor and, 180–81
    reperfusion, 427–28
    in toxic oil syndrome, *illus.* 386
Pulmonary embolectomy, 426
Pulmonary embolism
    in thromboembolic pulmonary hypertension, 418,
        421, 425

in toxic oil syndrome, 390–91
and systemic venous thrombosis, 414–15
Pulmonary fibrosis, 356, 357, 389, 479
Pulmonary function testing, 355–57
Pulmonary hypertension, 95, 179. *See also* Primary
    pulmonary hypertension
  aminorex, 397–409
  and atherosclerosis, 253
  electrical stimulation and, 133
  endotoxemia and, 274–75
  growth factors and, 201, 205–8, 212–13
  heparin and, 199–200
  hyperoxia and, 58, 272
  hypoxia and, 124–25, 265
  nervous system and, 131, 145
  in newborn animals, 142
  obliterative, 311, 506
  reflex, 146
  toxic oil syndrome, 388–94
  and vascular remodeling, 259–60, 265–79
  venous, 54, 338
Pulmonary parenchymal disease, 353, 357, 399–400
Pulmonary phlebitis, 345
Pulmonary stenosis, peripheral, 398
Pulmonary vascular innervation, 134
Pulmonary vascular obstructive disease, 276–78
Pulmonary vascular reactivity (responsiveness),
    98, *illus.* 99, 110–12, 296. *See also* Vaso-
    constriction
  hypoxia and, 60, 291–95
  and pulmonary vascular resistance, 91
  vascular wall remodeling and, 60, 124
Pulmonary vascular resistance, 41–42, 91–96. *See*
    also Vasoconstrictors; Vasodilators
  acetylcholine and, 318
  in aminorex hypertension, 400, 403, 404, 405, 406
  anticoagulation and, 505
  arterioles and, 134
  brain and, 142, 145
  bronchial, 153, *fig.* 154, 157
  central nervous system and, 138, 141–42
  in cirrhosis and pulmonary hypertension, 362,
    367–68
  emboli and, 333
  fetal, 162–64, 371, 373–74, 376
  hypoxia and, 289–91
  in intermittent air breathers, 22–23, 25, 28
  irradiation and, *illus.* 99
  lesions and, 333, 393
  localization of, 163–64
  and mechanical energy balance, 45–47
  meclofenamate and, *illus.* 97
  neonatal, 315, 316, 379, 380, 381
  perinatal, 374–75, 376–78
  precapillary, 398
  pressure-flow relations, 47–54
  in primary pulmonary hypertension, 454,
    502–3
  pulmonary arterial, 248, 249

  and pulmonary arterial pressure, 41–42, 51, 54,
    57, 92
  surgery and, 421, 429
  in toxic oil syndrome, 391–93
  in vasodilator therapy, 479–80, 485, 486, 489,
    490, 492–93, 496
  veins and, 134
  wedge pressure, 42–45
Pulmonary vascular tone
  arachidonic acid metabolites and, 60, 67
  brain and, 131, 139–40, 142
  carotid baroreceptors and, 136
  changes in, mechanisms of, *illus.* 117, *illus.* 119,
    123, 393
  electrical stimulation and, 134–35
  fetal, neural control of, 164–65, 168
  initial, and hypoxia, 111–12, 125
  Raynaud's phenomenon and, 392
  smooth muscle, 57, 123
  vagus nerve and, 135
  in vasodilator therapy, 486
Pulmonary vasomotor nerves, 132
Pulmonary veins, 5
  arterialization of, 345, *illus.* 347, 349, 465
  blood pressure, 43–44, 380
  congestion of, 399–400
  lesions of, 276, 465
  obstruction of, 43, *illus.* 340, 343, *illus.* 346,
    illus. 347
  and pulmonary vascular resistance, 134
  in veno-occlusive disease, *illus.* 339, 344–45,
    349
Pulmonary veno-occlusive disease, *illus.* 339,
    343–49, 454, 459, 485, 507
  chest radiographs, 453
  etiology, 311, 338, 349–51
  familial, 301
  histopathology, 338, 465–66, 467
  in primary pulmonary hypertension registry,
    469
  treatment, 344
Pulmonary venous disease, 507
Pulmonary venous hypertension, 54, 338
Pulmonary venous obstruction, 390
Purine receptors, 70
Purines, 70
P wave, 502
Pyrrolizidine alkaloids, 338, 350. *See also*
    Monocrotaline

Rabbit
  atherogenesis studies, 248
  lung, *illus.* 4, *illus.* 5, *illus.* 7, *illus.* 10,
    illus. 11, *illus.* 12
  smooth muscle cells, 31, *illus.* 35
Racial differences
  in high altitude hypoxia, 287–88, 297, 311
Radiation
  and neutropenia, 323

Radiation (*continued*)
  and oxygen radicals, 219, 223, 227–28
  release, inflammatory mediators and, 178n,
    179–80
Radionuclide perfusion scans, 445, 446, 448
Rapeseed oil, 337, 361, 385, 387–88
Rat
  acinus, 264
  arteries, *illus.* 270, *illus.* 272
  endothelial cells, 58
  lung, *illus.* 74
  polycythemia in, 323
  pulmonary hypertension, 319–23
  smooth muscle cells, 268
Raynaud's phenomenon
  in familial pulmonary hypertension, 303
  mortality, 474
  in primary pulmonary hypertension, 438, 454
  in pulmonary hypertension and cirrhosis, 365, 367
  in pulmonary hypertension and collagen vascular
    disease, 355
  pulmonary veno-occlusive disease and, 350
  in toxic oil syndrome, 392
Recanalization, arterial, 345
Receptors
  aortic, 140–41
  baroreceptors, 136
  carotid body, 140–42, 153–54, 156, 158
  C3, 176
  endothelial cell, 76–77
  IgG, 176
  laryngeal, 138–39
  purine, 70
  systemic arterial, 153–54, 157–158
Red blood cells. *See* Erythrocytes
Reflex pulmonary hypertension, 146
Reflex pulmonary vasoconstriction, 140
Reflexes, 27
Regurgitant murmurs, 453
Relative hypoxia, 272–73. *See also* Hyperoxia
Relaxation, smooth muscle, 58–60
Renal artery constriction, 319
Renal transplantation, 350
Renin, 104
Reperfusion lung edema, 427–28
Reptiles, 17, 18, *illus.* 19, 24, 25
Resistance arteries, 263–64, 479
Respirator, 14
Respiratory alkalosis, 454, 455
Rheumatic heart disease, 249
Rheumatic mitral valvulitis, *illus.* 250–51,
    illus. 252
Rheumatic valvular disease, 253–54
Rheumatic vascular disease, 245
Rheumatoid arthritis, 357
Royal College of Surgeons, 515

S. minnesota Re mutant, 79
Salamander, 24

Sarafotoxins, 112
Sarcoplasmic reticulum, 33–35, 119, 123
Scavenging agents, 218, 223
Scavenging systems, 227
Schistosomiasis, 398, 466–67
Scleroderma, 337, 353, 446–47
Sclerosis
  hepatic vein, 363
  systemic, 356, 357, 462
Secondary pulmonary hypertension, 301, 329–40
Sepsis, and vascular remodeling, 260, 274–75
Septa, fibrous, 464
Septal pleat, *illus.* 10, *illus.* 11
Septicemia, 496
Serotonin
  and capillary pressure, 99
  and cell replication, 268
  cigarette smoking and, 254
  endothelial extraction of, 104
  and pulmonary vascular resistance, 100
  toxicity, 362–63
  as vasoconstrictor, 95, 96–97
  and wedge pressure, 43, 44–45
Sheep
  acinus, 264
  bronchial circulation, 151
  hypoxia and, 133, 136
  pulmonary vascular resistance, 93–95
Sheet flow theory, 28
Shunting, intracardiac, 444
  in cirrhosis with pulmonary hypertension, 362
  congenital, 334–36, 341
  left-to-right, 399–400
    and pulmonary artery pressure, 245
    and pulmonary artery atherosclerosis, 252
    small artery obstruction and, 246
  right-to-left
    heart-lung transplantation and, 514
    and hypoxemia, 360, 455
  neonatal, 145, 316, 371, 372, 375, 379
Sleep
  apnea, 310
  and hypoxia, 297–98
  and oxygen saturation, 296
  and pulmonary vasoconstriction, 296
Small pulmonary arteries
  in familial pulmonary hypertension, 307
  fetal and neonatal, 373–74
  hyperoxia and, *illus.* 270, *illus.* 271
  obstructive disease of, 246
  in persistent pulmonary hypertension of the
    newborn, 379, 381
  in primary pulmonary hypertension, *illus.* 277,
    455, 460, 486, 491
  in thromboembolic pulmonary hypertension, 414,
    416
  thrombosis in, 506–8
Smoking
  and atherosclerosis, 245, 247, 253, 254

in cirrhosis and pulmonary hypertension, 367
and laryngeal irritation, 146
and obstructive airways disease, 419
and oxygen radicals, 219
Smooth muscle
calf, *illus.* 317
hypertrophy, 124
hypoxia and, 113, *illus.* 117, 118
medial, 373, 461
relaxation of, vagal neurons and, 155
tone, 123
in vasodilator therapy, 488–89
Smooth muscle cells. *See also* Pericytes
communication with endothelial cells, 176
contraction in, 31–37, 85–87
endothelial cells and, 57–67
endothelium-derived products and, 76
hyperoxia and 273–74
medial, 201, 247, 261, 262, 263, 318
and heparan sulfate, 194–95, 199
migration of, 190
neonatal, 381
proliferation
in atherogenesis, 246–47
growth factors and, 64–65, 203, 205, 206, 207, 209
heparan sulfate inhibition, 194–98
heparin inhibition, 189–94, 199–200, 210
hypoxia and, 267, 268, 269
in medial hypertrophy, 201
in secondary pulmonary hypertension, 329–30
and vessel healing, 240
in pulmonary hypertension, 264, 320
superoxide production, 222
systemic arterial, 190–91
Smooth muscle elastogenic factor (SMEF), 318
Snakes, 25, 27
venom, 112
Sodium nitroprusside, 59
Species differences, 264, 403
central nervous system, 133, 134
Spinal cord, 143–44
Spirometry, 419
Starling resistance, 47, 49, 51
Starling resistors, 164
Stastny, Peter, 178n
Stellate ganglion stimulation
and autonomic nervous system, 154–55
effect on pulmonary circulation, *fig.* 132, 142
and pulmonary artery pressure, 135
Stenoses, *illus.* 424. *See also* Mitral stenosis
aortic, 427
branch, *illus.* 422, 425
peripheral pulmonary, 398
Strahler ordering system, 4
Streptococcal pneumonia, 372
Streptomyces protease (Pronase®), 195
Striated muscle, 37
Student's T-test, 355

Substance P, 111, 112, 226
antibodies, 157
N-sulfation, 188, 189
Superoxide ($O_2^-\cdot$)
biochemistry, 218, 219
production of, 220, 221, 222, 228
sites of damage, 223, 224, 226–27
Suppurative lung disease, 515
Surface vesicle, *illus.* 36
Surgery
cardiopulmonary bypass, 413, 421, 514, 519
thoracic, 515
in thromboembolic hypertension, 417, 421–33
Survival. *See* Mortality
Sustenacular cells, 116
Swimbladder. *See* Air-breathing organ
Syncope, 344, 362, 400, 453, 502, 516
Systemic circulation
arterial pressure
arachidonic acid and, 165
neural regulation of, 137, 140
in pulmonary hypertension with cirrhosis, 367–68
in vasodilator therapy, 493, 497
arterial smooth muscle cells, 190–91
blood pressure
aminorex and, 402
pulmonary circulation and, 104
in vasodilator therapy, 480
capillaries, 6–7
chemoreceptors, 140, 153–54, 157–58
hypertension in, 245, 252, 479
hypotension in, 494
hypoxemia in, 124, 155, 158
hypoxia in, 115–16, 140
in intermittent air breathers, 18, *illus.* 19, 22–23, 26
lung and, 69
perinatal, 374–75
sclerosis in, 356, 367, 462
vascular resistance
in lungfish, 22–23
neonatal, 377
nervous system and, 140, 146
in pulmonary hypertension with cirrhosis, 367–68
in vasodilator therapy, 479, 493
vasodilation, 122, 493
veins, 345

Tachycardia, 18–20, 22, 402
Tachyphylaxis, 482, 496
Tachypnea, 371
Testosterone, 294
Tetracaine, 138
Thoracic irradiation, 99
Thoracic surgery, 515
Thoracic vagosympathetic nerves, 132

Thrombi
in familial pulmonary hypertension, 307–9
in primary pulmonary hypertension, 466
in pulmonary veno-occlusive disease, *illus.* 339,
345, 349
surgical removal of, 427
in thromboembolic pulmonary hypertension,
illus. 332, *illus.* 423, *illus.* 424, 425, 430
Thrombin
antithrombin, 191
antithrombin III
deficiency, 311, 414–15
heparin mediation, 188, 189, 199, 232
and cell proliferation, 206, 209, 211
effects on endothelial cells, 78, 177, 178, 179, 180,
231, 238, 240
and prostacyclin production, 75, 175, 180
and vascular relaxation, 226
Thrombin-thrombomodulin-protein C system, 233,
237, 238–39
Thromboemboli
organized, 462, 464
and pulmonary hypertension, 361
recanalized, *illus.* 463
recurrent, 333
Thromboembolic disease, 446–47
recurrent, 479, 480, 502
Thromboembolic lesions, 467
Thromboembolic pulmonary arteriopathy, 465–66
Thromboembolic pulmonary hypertension, 307, 309,
400, 413–21, 469
anticoagulant therapy, 505
surgical correction, 421–33
Thromboembolism, 394, 398
atherosclerosis and, 249, 254
in high flow injury, 276–78
in primary pulmonary hypertension, 275, 344, 459
pulmonary, 311, 445
and pulmonary vascular resistance, 485
Thromboendarterectomy, 413, 416, 421, 426–27
Thromboplastin, 505
Thrombosis
atherosclerosis and, 249
in congenital heart disease, 508–9
endothelial cells and, 212, 213
infection and, 238
platelet-derived growth factor and, 206
in primary pulmonary hypertension, 469, 505–6
in pulmonary veno-occlusive disease, 348–49
in situ, 311, 337, 485, 508
in small pulmonary arteries, 506–8
thrombotic lesions, 212, 466, 468, 469
in toxic oil syndrome, 390–91
venous, 418, 421, 427, 465
prevention of, 428–29
Thrombotic arteriopathy, 507
Thrombotic pulmonary venopathy, 338
Thromboxane A$_2$ (TXA$_2$), 61, 62, 63, 95, 162, 167,
168, 376, 486
Thromboxane B$_2$ (TXB$_2$), 63, 95, 167, 410

Thromboxanes
effect on pulmonary circulation, 166–67
endothelial damage and, 60
metabolites of, 94
production of, 95–96, 102, 103, 162, 225
inhibition of, 323, 495
and pulmonary vascular tone, 67
Thromboxane synthetase, 168
inhibitor, 496
Tissue factor, 231, 238
Toad, 20, *illus.* 21
Tolazoline, 289, 392, 489
Tone. *See* Pulmonary vascular tone
Toronto Transplantation Group, 512
Toxic oil syndrome, 337, 385–94
Toxins, 350, 388
Trachea, 136, 512
Trachealis, smooth muscle in, 31
Tracheal mucosa, 158
Transduction mechanisms
endothelial, 75–80
in hypoxia, 119, 123
of oxygen, 85–86
Transforming growth factor alpha (TGF-α), 202,
203, 207
Transforming growth factor beta (TGF-β), 202,
203, 207–8, 210, 274
Transposition of the great vessels, 146
Trichloroacetic acid, 195
Tricuspid insufficiency, 427
Tricuspid regurgitation, *illus.* 331, 333, 418, 453
Tricuspid valve, 379
annulus, *illus.* 331, 333
Trypsin, 194
Tumor necrosis factor (TNF)
effects on endothelium, 80, 238, 240
endothelial cell activation, 104, 212
growth inhibition, 208, 210
and lung injury, 183
and transforming growth factor production, 274
as vasoconstrictor, 95
Tumor-promoting phorbol esters, 205
Turtle
apnea, 17, 29
cardiovascular changes, *illus.* 21, 22
pulmonary control mechanisms, 27
resistance sites, 25
tachycardia, 18–20
Tyrosine kinase, 204–5

Umbilical cord constriction, 319
Umbilical venous cells, 175
Unilateral pulmonary veno-occlusive disease, 350
Upper airway, 136–40
Urokinase, 234–36
United States Food and Drug Administration, 397n

Vagal stimulation, 135
Vagosympathetic nerves, thoracic, 132
Vagotomy, 138, 142, 154, 155

Vagus nerve
  and autonomic nervous system, 154
  and bronchial circulation, 155
  control of heart rate, 22, 27
  control of pulmonary circulation, 135, 164–65
Vascular disease, obliterative, 356
Vascular remodeling, 259–60, 265–79, 378–79
Vascular resistance. *See* Pulmonary vascular
    resistance
Vascular transmural pressure (VTP), 28–29
Vasculopathy
  congestive, 338–39
  dietary pulmonary, 337–38
  fibrosing pulmonary, 337
  hypoxic pulmonary, 335–36
Vasoactive intestinal peptide (VIP), 111, 112, 155, 226
  antibodies, 157
Vasoconstriction. *See also* Hypoxic pressor response
  arachidonic acid and, 168
  bronchial, 155, 157–58, 226
  central nervous system and, 132, 134, 135, 142
  chemoreceptors and, 141–42
  cholinergic, 24, 28
  chronic, *illus.* 334–35
  fetal, 164
  heritable influences on, 309–11
  hyperoxia and, 271, 272–73
  hypoxia and, 283, 289–91, 296, 297, 480
  mechanisms of, 85–87, 95, 96–98
  menstruation and, 507
  neonatal, 315–16, 377, 378
  and pulmonary hypertension, 259
  and pulmonary vascular resistance, 485
  reflex, 140
  in toxic oil syndrome, 391–93, 394
  vasodilator therapy and, 486, 487, 497
Vasoconstrictors
  endothelium and, 122
  fetal, 376
  systemic, 478
Vasodilation (dilatation)
  acetylcholine and, 318
  aneurysmal, *illus.* 424
  arterial, *illus.* 328, 329, 330
  bronchial, 155, 156–57, 158
  central nervous system and, 135
  fetal, 163
  neonatal, 377–78, 381
  and pulmonary hypertension, 493
Vasodilators, 114, 259
  calcium channel blockers, 448
  chronic use of, 495–97
  endothelial production of, 92, 122
  mediators of, 156–57
  nitrovasodilators, 26
  and pulmonary vascular resistance, 376
  in toxic oil syndrome, 392
Vasodilator therapy, xiii, 437, 449, 461
  primary pulmonary hypertension, 479–82
    acute, 485–95

  anticoagulant, 505
  chronic, 495–97
  prostacyclin, 517–18
  pulmonary arterial pressure in, 480–81, 486–87,
      488, 493–94, 496
  pulmonary vascular resistance in, 479–80, 485,
      486, 489, 490, 492–93, 496
Vasoreactivity. *See* Pulmonary vasoreactivity
Veins. *See also* Pulmonary veins
  arterialization of, 345, *illus.* 347, 349, 465
  bronchial, 337, 345
  femoral, 426
  iliac, 426
  oxygen pressure, 455
  oxygen saturation, 516, 517–18
  resistance in, 113
  systemic, 345
  thrombosis in, 418, 421, 427
    prevention of, 428–29
Venae cavae, 333, 426
Verapamil, 492, 493, 495
Verhoeff-van Gieson stain, 471
Vessel wall metabolism, 60–64
Vimentin, 66
Viral infections, 349–50
Viremia, 247
Voltage-dependent mechanisms, 118
Voltage-gated channels, 32
Von Willebrand factor, 275–76
  abnormalities in, 361, 508
  endothelial cell synthesis of, 80, 231

Warfarin, 311
Water, 218, 219, 220
Weaning, from hyperoxia, 260, 271, 272–73
Wedge pressure
  in diagnosis, 344
  endotoxin and, 100
  in primary pulmonary hypertension registry
      patients, 455
  and pulmonary vascular resistance, 42–45, 51
  surgery and, 429
Weibel, E. R., 6, 8
White blood cells. *See* Leukocytes
Wilcoxon Rank Sum test, 355
Women, 507
  Raynaud's phenomenon in, 454
World Health Organization
  disease classifications, 404, 459, 465–67, 507
  disease descriptions, 307, 344
  primary pulmonary hypertension meeting, 442

Xanthine oxidase (XO), 73, 220
Xenobiotic substances, metabolism by endothelial
    cells, 73–75
Xylose-serine linkages, 189, 197

Zonal perfusion, 12–14
Zone 1 conditions, 12, 13–14
Zone 2 conditions, 8, 11–14, 42, 47
Zone 3 conditions, 13–14, 49

LIBRARY-LRC
TEXAS HEART INSTITUTE